Ovarian Cancer

Ovarian Cancer

Edited by **Lester Price**

hayle
medical

New York

Published by Hayle Medical,
30 West, 37th Street, Suite 612,
New York, NY 10018, USA
www.haylemedical.com

Ovarian Cancer
Edited by Lester Price

International Standard Book Number: 978-1-63241-312-3 (Hardback)

Printed in China.

Contents

Preface

This book has been a concerted effort by a group of academicians, researchers and scientists, who have contributed their research works for the realization of the book. This book has materialized in the wake of emerging advancements and innovations in this field. Therefore, the need of the hour was to compile all the required researches and disseminate the knowledge to a broad spectrum of people comprising of students, researchers and specialists of the field.

An introductory account based on ovarian cancer is provided in this book along with descriptive information. Ovarian cancer causes more deaths across the planet than all the other gynecologic diseases together. Crucial general and biologic science issues relevant to this disease have been discussed in this book by several international leaders. The book elucidates the molecular biological characteristics of the disease and highlights molecular biology methodologies for the purpose of comprehending this cancer. These techniques are formulated to demonstrate tumor genetics, protein function, and expression, and to describe the genetic mechanisms by which immunotherapies and gene may be developed. It describes an overview of present research into aspects of malignant transformation, metastasis, and growth control. A wide range of topics have been encompassed providing updated information on management considerations and scientific discoveries.

At the end of the preface, I would like to thank the authors for their brilliant chapters and the publisher for guiding us all-through the making of the book till its final stage. Also, I would like to thank my family for providing the support and encouragement throughout my academic career and research projects.

Editor

1

Inflammation and Ovarian Cancer

Antonio Macciò[1] and Clelia Madeddu[2]
[1]*Department of Obstetrics and Gynecology, Sirai Hospital, Carbonia,*
[2]*Department of Medical Oncology, University of Cagliari, Cagliari*
Italy

1. Introduction

Epithelial ovarian cancer (EOC) is a highly lethal gynaecological cancer for which overall prognosis has remained poor over the past few decades. A number of theories have been postulated in an effort to explain the aetiology of EOC. Noteworthy, these theories likely are not mutually exclusive, as they all converge more or less on the role of inflammation in promoting ovarian tumorigenesis and cancer progression. The tumour milieu in which ovarian carcinoma develops has been described as one enriched with a broad spectrum of pro-inflammatory cytokines and chemokines. In particular, several of these cytokines (such as tumour necrosis factor-α (TNF-α), interleukin (IL)-1β, and IL-6) produced by tumour itself or/and activated immune cells, besides stimulating cancer cell growth, have been shown to influence clinical disease status and prognosis, by reducing responsiveness to chemotherapy and inducing symptoms such as anorexia, altered energy metabolism, anaemia, weight loss, depression and fatigue. Recent data show that cytokine antagonists may have a role to play in the treatment of ovarian cancer. Their action by inhibiting both production and activity of inflammatory cytokines seems to obtain the control of angiogenetic and apoptotic events, the reversal of chemoresistance, the improvement of systemic symptoms and prognosis. In the light of our scientific research and the most recent experimental and clinical advances our chapter will review the most relevant and recent findings on the role of proinflammatory cytokines in the pathogenesis and prognosis of ovarian cancer and the possible therapeutic implications.

2. Role of inflammation in the etiopathogenesis of ovarian cancer

A number of studies suggest that factors related to inflammation of the ovarian surface epithelium (OSE), such as ovulation, endometriosis and pelvic inflammatory diseases, are associated with an increased risk for EOC. In particular, inflammatory mediators and several cytokines produced by activated innate immune cells, such as TNF-α, IL-1β and IL-6 and IL-6, have been shown to promote EOC genesis, growth and progression (Nowak et al., 2010a, Clendenen et al., 2011).

The most important hypothesis to arise about EOC carcinogenesis was the ovulation theory, which relates ovarian cancer risk to incessant ovulation. To support this hypothesis, there is growing interest in the etiologic role of inflammation that accompanies each ovulation

(Landen et al., 2008). Ovarian surface epithelium adjacent to the site of ovulation may be exposed to inflammatory and oxidative status with consequent risk of malignant transformation. Intriguingly, the same ovulatory process together with the repair steps immediately after liberation of the ovum, are characterized by the generation of an enormous amount of cytokines/chemokines and matrix-remodeling enzymes, including prostaglandins, bioactive eicosanoids, plasminogen activators, collagenases, interleukins (ILs), TNF-α and various growth factors (Macciò et al., 1994) as well as by the recruitment of activated immune cells to the wounded epithelial surface, entailing the global activation of the pro-inflammatory network. Recently, it has been hypothesized that high grade serous ovarian cancer, endometrioid and clear cell cancers arise from fallopian tube epithelium and share a common pathogenic mechanism, i.e. iron-induced oxidative stress derived from retrograde menstruation. Fimbriae floating in bloody peritoneal fluid are exposed to the action of catalytic iron and to the genotoxic effect of reactive oxygen species, generated from haemolysis of erythrocytes by pelvic activated macrophages and by the cytokines secreted from themselves. In summary, both incessant ovulation and oxido-reductive fallopian tube epithelial damage hypotheses have provided evidence that inflammatory responses induced under physiological conditions may foster the development of EOC.

A growing body of evidence suggests that, although genetic events in the tumour cells themselves are definitely crucial, host and stromal factors in the tumour microenvironment are equally important. A clinically overt tumour includes not only cancer cells but also matrix components, stromal cells and inflammatory cells. In particular, in EOC peritoneal and stromal alterations alongside with their lymphomocytes components and associated cytokines may be permissive for cancer growth and spread. Likewise, cytokine production also by tumour cells themselves can both promote their growth and inhibits apoptosis in an autocrine manner. Therefore, inflammation seems to contribute to every step of carcinogenesis, including tumour initiation, promotion, and progression. On the other hand, tumour cells can produce immunogenic proteins that are recognized as foreign, potentially thus inducing an antineoplastic immune response. Actually, the tumour uses these immunological interactions to evade recognition and destruction by immune cells, i.e. Fas ligand production to induce lymphocyte apoptosis (Mantovani et al., 1999a) and HLA-G secretion to inhibit natural-killer cell activity. Then, although the importance of the host antitumor immune response, as demonstrated by the finding that increased T-cell infiltration into the tumour is associated with improved survival (Zhang et al., 2003), the real role of immune system in containing tumour growth remains to be fully defined (Landen, 2008).

3. Proinflammatory cytokines in the progression of EOC

Components of the inflammatory pathway, including free radicals, cytokines, NF-κB, signal transducer and activator of transcription-3 (STAT-3), inducible nitric oxide synthase (iNOS), cyclooxygenase-2 (COX-2), prostaglandins, and vascular endothelial growth factor (VEGF) have been shown to contribute to the development of various malignancies, including EOC. In particular, COX-2 was found to be highly expressed in non-mucinous ovarian cancers, and its expression was correlated with poor prognostic factors, such as stage, residual disease status and presence of ascites (Ferrandina et al. 2002a). Consistently with this hypothesis, patients with chronic aspirin, nonsteroidal anti-inflammatory drug, or acetaminophen use have a reduced risk of EOC (Altinoz & Korkmaz, 2004).

3.1 Cytokines as cancer growth factors

Multiple genetic alterations are implicated in ovarian carcinogenesis, but clinical and genetic evidence support two wide categories of EOC carcinogenesis: those of low-grade and high-grade pathways. Gene and protein analyses of tumours of these two different subtypes also suggest different pathogenesis: K-Ras, BRAF, and PTEN mutations are more frequently observed in low-grade tumours, whereas P53 mutation is predominantly present in high-grade tumours, but rarely in other subtypes or low malignant potential (LMP) tumors. Moreover, HER2 and AKT are overexpressed in high-grade carcinomas but rarely in low-grade and LMP tumours. Overexpression of human leukocyte antigen-G (HLA-G), which may provide a mechanism of immune escape for the tumour, has been noted in a high percentage of high-grade carcinomas but is absent in low-grade or LMP neoplasma (Landen, 2008). Moreover, the new proposed histological classification of EOC in type I slow growing tumours and type II rapidly growing and highly aggressive tumours is accompanied by a specific expression of the inflammatory markers: glucose transporter protein-1 (Glut-1), inducible nitric oxide synthase (iNOS), COX-1, COX-2) and nuclear factor kappa B. In detail, overexpression of COX-1, COX-2, iNOS, and Glut-1 was significantly higher in type II tumours and was associated with a poorer median survival as compared with those with type I tumours. Therefore, the distinct expression of these markers may explain the different biologic behaviour of these 2 tumour types and provide targets for therapy (Ali-Fehmi et al., 2011).

Although EOC can be subdivided by grade, their histological subtypes also differ. Serous, endometrioid, and mucinous adenocarcinomas have difference in clinical outcomes even if not as dramatic as those between high- and low-grade cancers. However, genomic studies have demonstrated that mucinous adenocarcinomas often harbour mutations and have peculiar gene expression similar to LMP tumours and to benign cystadenomas. Specifically, mutations in K-RAS have been described in borderline, low-grade tumours and mucinous adenocarcinomas, but are very rare in high-grade serous carcinomas. Moreover, endometrioid adenocarcinomas harbour PTEN mutations (similar to endometrioid tumours of the uterine endometrium) more frequently than do serous or mucinous subtype. The discovery of these genetic mutations allowed hypothesizing a model of multistep carcinogenesis of ovarian cancer (Landen, 2008). To become a clinically evident tumour ovarian cancer cells must overcome many protective mechanisms: these include unchecked proliferation, evading apoptosis, angiogenesis, stromal invasion, separation and survival away from the primary tumour, and implantation and growth within new tissues. Within the dual pathway model, it is clear that the tumour cell and its environment must acquire the above characteristics. Although the order in which these occur is likely variable, early alterations in dominant genes may dictate the specific path that is followed, such as K-RAS leading to an LMP tumour and early occurrence of a p53 alteration leading to genetic instability and rapid progression to a high-grade phenotype. Many researchers show a role for inflammation in tumour initiation, promotion, progression and metastatisation. In particular most studies focused their attention to IL-6 signalling which seems to play the main role (Lane et al., 2011). IL-6 is one of the major immunoregulatory cytokines present in the EOC microenvironment. Both ovarian cancer cells and tumor-associated macrophages produce IL-6, and it is to date known that high serum levels of IL-6 are related with specific immune and metabolic alterations which finally lead to cancer cachexia, the main cause of death of EOC patients. IL-6 has also been demonstrated to be involved in autocrine growth of ovarian cancer cells [19-21] as well as in tumorigenesis and progression of ovarian cancer cells particularly by increasing their capacity to secrete matrix metalloproteinase (MMP)-9 (Rabinovich et al., 2007). Then, IL-6 could stimulate the proliferation of tumour cells either directly and/or by promoting angiogenesis. In fact, IL-6 has an important role, precisely through tumour angiogenesis, in promoting the development of ascites as well as the spread of ovarian cancer thus leading to fast progression and short survival. (Lane, 2011; Lo, 2011). The high levels of IL-6 enhance the immune suppressive status of the tumour microenvironment by inhibiting IL-2 synthesis, T cell activation and proliferation, and promoting lymphocytes apoptosis (Macciò, 1998; Mantovani, 1999a). Furthermore, IL-6 may divert the immune response from Th1 towards a suppressive Th2 response although controversial data have been reported. Another inflammatory cytokine TNF-α that is constitutively expressed in the malignant ovarian surface epithelium generates and sustains a network of other mediators that promote tumour growth and peritoneal spread. Constitutive production of TNF-a is associated with greater release of IL-6 itself as well as other chemokines as: CCL2 and CXCL12, macrophage migration-inhibitory factor (MIF) and VEGF. In turn, these factors may act in an autocrine/paracrine manner to promote colonization of the peritoneum and neovascularization of developing tumour deposits. Moreover, also estrogens by the modulation of proinflammatory cytokines, and in particular IL-6, are involved in regulating the growth and progression of EOC. Estrogens not only enhance cytokines production but also modulate the expression of their receptors. In turn, IL-6 and IL-8 also promote ovarian cancer cells growth through an oestrogen receptor pathway. Therefore, these findings provide a novel mechanism that oestrogens, IL-6 and IL-8 may form a common amplifying signalling cascade to modulate ovarian cancer cells growth and progression (Yang et al., 2009).

From what has been written it can be deduced that IL-6 is the cytokine mainly involved in EOC carcinogenesis and progression. IL-6 is a 26-kDa glycopeptide whose gene is found on chromosome 7, produced by antigen presenting cells (APCs) such as dendritic cells, macrophages and B cells among other cells of the haematopoietic system. It is also produced by a variety of non-haematopoietic cells including keratinocytes, fibroblasts, epithelial cells, and neoplastic cells. IL-6 gene transcription is induced in many different normal tissues in response to stimuli, such as RNA and DNA virus infection, bacterial endotoxin, lipopolysaccharide and other inflammatory cytokines as TNF-α, IL-1, and platelet-derived growth factor (PDGF) and the interferons (IFNs). It has been previously named hepatocyte-stimulating factor, cytotoxic T-cell differentiation factor, B-cell differentiation factor, B-cell stimulatory factor 2, hybridoma/plasmacytoma growth factor, monocyte granulocyte inducer type 2 and thrombopoietin. The many names reflect the pleiotropism of IL-6. IL-6 affects virtually every organ, most notably the immune system and in particular, it is an essential factor for the normal development and function of both T and B lymphocytes and has broad actions on cells of the haematopoietic system. Efficient induction of the IL-6 promoter requires the interaction of several transcription factors, including the CAAT enhancer-binding protein (C/EBP) family members and nuclear factor kB (NF-kB). Nuclear factor for IL-6 (NF-IL6, C/EBP-b) and NF-kB interact with each other to synergistically up-regulate the IL-6 promoter, just like NF-IL6 (C/EBP-b) and NF-IL6b (C/EBP-d). The IL-6 promoter is inhibited by p53 and the retinoblastoma (Rb) gene product. The overexpression of IL-6 in many malignancies may occur as a result of the loss of one of these negative regulators of transcription.

The physiological activity of IL-6 is complex, including both pro-inflammatory and anti-inflammatory effects in the immune system. In fact, relative to its specific immunomodulating capacity, IL-6 is an activator or an inhibitor of T-cell responses, depending to the length of time of its activities. This combination of pro-inflammatory and anti-inflammatory effects suggests that IL-6 may play a role in regulating the control of immune system activation during the different phases of EOC evolution. IL-6 modulates the transcription of several liver-specific genes during acute inflammatory states, particularly C-reactive protein (CRP) and hepcidin. IL-6 can also up-regulates the multidrug resistance 1 (MDR-1) gene through activation of NF-IL6, which, in turn, transactivates the MDR-1 gene through a Y-box motif. IL-6 blood levels are high in numerous infectious, inflammatory, and autoimmune diseases and in cancer in association with increased synthesis of other cytokines and specific immunological challenge. Human diseases that involve prolonged inflammation and in particularly advanced EOC frequently exhibit cachexia with loss of muscle mass and IL-6 seems to be the key mediator of these processes as well. It is noteworthy that high circulating levels of IL-6 have also been linked to insulin resistance, high body mass index and obesity. IL-6 also exerts its effects on the central nervous system, where it regulates glial cell activation and modulate mood as well as induce severe depressive symptoms.

IL-6 signals primarily by its binding to a specific receptor (IL-6R) which is a member of the Class I cytokine receptor family. Functional Class I receptors contain high-affinity ligand-binding components and signal-transducing components, and are thus multichain receptor complexes that often share the signal-transducing element. Then, IL-6 signals through a protein complex including the membrane-bound non-signalling α-receptor subunit (IL-6R a-chain gp80 or CD126) and two signal-transducing gp130 subunits (IL6-Rβ-chain gp130 or CD130), this second chain of the receptor resulting in the formation of high-avidity IL-6 binding receptors (Lo, 2011). More precisely: the ligand-binding portion of the IL-6R is an 80-kDa molecule associates directly with IL-6 that exists both in a membrane-bound and a soluble form; the signal transducing component of the IL-6R complex is glycoprotein 130 (gp130), sometimes called IL-6Rb-chain. The gp130 functions as an affinity converter because the resulting affinity of IL-6 for the ternary complex is approximately 10^{-11} M instead of 10^{-9} M for IL-6R. While gp130 is expressed ubiquitously, gp80 is physiologically mainly expressed on hepatocytes and specialized subsets of leukocytes, including neutrophils, monocytes/macrophages, and T and B lymphocytes. However, IL-6 can also signal via a soluble receptor (sIL-6R or gp55 chain) that lacks the transmembrane and cytoplasmatic components. Soluble IL-6R (sIL-6R) can be generated by two mechanisms: 1) Metalloproteinase mediated cleavage ("shedding") of the membrane bound form of the IL-6R and 2) expression of an alternatively spliced IL-6R variant that lacks the transmembrane domain. Neutrophils and macrophages in addition to some cell lines have been shown to produce sIL-6R. Activated sIL-6R binds to membrane-bound gp130 subunits in a process known as trans-signalling. Therefore, unlike other soluble cytokine receptors, which are generally antagonists, sIL-6R is an agonist molecule, promoting IL-6 activity. This ability may explain a possible activation of gp130 despite the lack of gp80, if sIL-6R molecules circulate in great quantity, as demonstrated in certain pathological states. Accordingly, it was observed that cells lacking IL-6R expression are responsive to IL-6 stimulation especially during inflammatory conditions. As demonstrated in EOC, this alternate pathway serves as the major signalling in inducing endothelial hyperpermeability and increasing transendothelial migration of cancer cells, thus contributing to cancer progression. Moreover, elevated levels of sIL-6R in malignant ascites from ovarian cancer patients are associated with poor prognosis (Lo, Cancer Res 2011; 7: 424-34). The increase of IL6R expression as well as of the soluble spliced variant of IL6R in malignant ovarian tumours are regulated by cancer-associated inflammation (Rath et al., 2010). Therefore, in advanced EOC IL6R is overexpressed mainly because of increases in a sIL6R variant, which can influence its evolution and prognosis. In addition to sIL-6R, soluble gp130 (sgp130) also exists in human serum and acts as an antagonist of the IL-6/sIL-6R complex.

Once IL-6 binds its receptor and gp130 homodimerization occurs, a signalling cascade is triggered. X-Ray crystallography has shown that two heterotrimers of IL-6, IL-6R and gp130 associate to form a hexameric complex. Through formation of this complex, members of the cytoplasmic Janus kinase (Jak) family of tyrosine kinases bind to gp130 inducing phosphorylation of downstream targets. The Janus kinases activation is followed by the recruitment of signal transducers and activators of transcriptions (STATs). One phosphorylated, STATs translocate to the nucleus where they promote gene transcription. IL-6R stimulation also recruits other signal transduction molecules, including SH2 domain-containing tyrosine phosphatase (SHP2) and suppressor of cytokine signalling (SOCS). Both SHP2 and SOCS may subsequently down-regulate IL-6 signalling. Jak1 is thought to be the most relevant for IL-6 signalling although Jak2 and Tyk2 also transduce some of the IL-6 signals. In some instances, IL-6 acts with other factors, such as heparin-binding epithelial growth factor and hepatocyte growth factor in controlling proliferation and function of various cell types. Blocking IL-6 by specific anti-receptor drugs may thus be of benefit in many pathological situations.

The best-described substrate for Jaks in IL-6 signaling is the STAT 3, a transcription factor that in its inactive form remains in the cytoplasm but after phosphorylation forms homodimers that are actively being transported to the nucleus to induce gene transcription. Increasing evidence indicates that tumour cells express constitutively activated Stat proteins, particularly STAT3, independent of dysregulation of upstream molecules, disabled inhibitory mechanisms or identifiable ligand stimulation. Stat3 overexpression also may promote cell proliferation and transformation into a tumour phenotype. Overexpression and overactivation of Stat3 is found in EOC tissue and the constitutive activation of Stat3 signalling pathway may play an important role in the invasion and prognosis. The expressions of Stat3 and phosphorylated (p)-Stat3 in EOC are significantly higher than in normal ovarian epithelial tissues or benign ovarian tumour and the expression of Stat3 protein is highly correlated with the expression of p-Stat3 protein. The nuclear localization of p-Stat3 predicts a poor prognosis: in fact, pSTAT3 expression is significantly correlated with disease stage, degree of differentiation and lymph node metastasis (Min & Wei-hong, 2009). Recent studies suggest that STAT3 is a key factor for EOC chemoresistance, showing that STAT3 decoy oligodeoxynucleotides (ODN), its specific antagonist, inhibited cancer cell invasive power and enhanced sensitivity to paclitaxel. The mechanism involves the inhibition of EMMPRIN, P-gp, and pAkt by STAT3 decoy ODN. These three proteins are probably the target proteins of STAT3 (Zhang, 2010). Increased levels of pSTAT3 are correlated with increased expression of HER-2/neu, EGFR and proliferation but not apoptosis markers. Unlike other molecules involved in oncogenesis, no genetic mutations or amplifications have been identified for STAT3, suggesting that persistent STAT3 activity is caused mostly by the dysregulation of upstream molecules, such as receptors with intrinsic tyrosine kinase activity (e.g., EGFR or HER-2/neu) and, in particular, endogenous or exogenous IL-6. Moreover, the regulation and functions of Stat proteins are highly dependent on the cell type, the activating stimulus and the cellular context, especially the activity of other signalling pathways and transcription factors that interact with the Stat proteins. Consequently, depending on the cellular context, STAT3 may mediate conflicting responses in terms of cell proliferation, differentiation or apoptosis. For example, the concurrent coexpression of dominant-negative STAT3 and the oncoprotein Ras does not arrest Ras-induced transformation, suggesting that STAT3 signalling is only one of several pathways required for cell transformation induced by this oncogenic tyrosine kinase. In addition, STAT3 demonstrates a histotype-specific pattern of expression. High levels of expression were observed more commonly in those histotypes with aggressive biologic behaviour (undifferentiated, clear cell, and serous carcinomas) than in those histotypes with less aggressive behaviour (mucinous and endometrioid carcinomas).

Results from a recent study (Saydmohammed et al., 2010) confirm that IL-6 secretion increases during malignant progression of ovarian epithelial cells and found that IL-6 expression levels are not always correlated with the expression or subcellular location of pSTAT3 in ovarian carcinoma, supporting the finding that IL-6 is involved in other signalling pathways, independent of STAT3. Moreover, given the observations that cancer cells can constitutively express STAT3 in the absence of stimulation by any known ligand and that expression of STAT3 is higher in ovarian carcinoma than in normal ovarian tissue, it is possible to speculate that the constitutive activation of STAT3 in ovarian cancer cells could be because of aberrant EGFR signalling. In agreement with this possibility, it has been observed a significant correlation between high levels of pSTAT3 expression and the overexpression of EGFR and HER-2/neu in EOC (Bast et al., 1993). Alternatively, the constitutive activation of STAT3 in EOC may be caused by the elevation of Src and focal adhesion kinase levels (Rosen et al., 2006) More recently, a significant activation of both STAT-3 and its upstream activator JAK-2, has been demonstrate in high-grade ovarian carcinomas compared with normal ovaries and benign tumours. The association between STAT3 activation and migratory phenotype of ovarian cancer cells was investigated by EGF-induced epithelial-mesenchymal transition (EMT) in ovarian cancer cell lines. Ligand activation of EGFR induced a fibroblast-like morphology and migratory phenotype, consistent with the upregulation of mesenchyme-associated N-cadherin, vimentin and nuclear translocation of beta-catenin. This occurred concomitantly with activation of the downstream JAK2/STAT3 pathway. The cell lines expressed the IL-6R and treatment with EGF resulted in enhanced IL-6 expression and release in the serum-free medium. Exogenous addition of IL-6 stimulated STAT3 activation and enhanced migration. Blocking antibodies against IL-6R inhibited both IL-6 production and EGF- and IL-6-induced migration. Specific inhibition of STAT3 activation by a JAK2-specific inhibitor blocked STAT3 phosphorylation, cell motility, induction of N-cadherin and vimentin expression and IL6 production. These data suggest that the activated status of STAT3 in high-grade EOC may occur directly through activation of

EGFR or IL-6R or indirectly through induction of IL-6R signalling. Such activation of STAT3 suggests a rationale for a combination of anti-STAT3 and EGFR/IL-6R therapy to suppress the peritoneal spread of ovarian cancer (Colomiere et al., 2009).

In addition to STAT3 also the Ras protein can be activated in response to IL-6. After Ras activation, hyperphosphorylation of mitogen-activated protein kinase (MAPK) occurs as well as an increase in its serine/threonine kinase activity. MAPK then phosphorylates the NF-IL6 transcription factor on serine 231 and threonine 235, a process that is essential for DNA binding. NF-IL6 has a basic leucine zipper motif and is a member of the C/EBP family of transcription factors. NF-IL6 activates the promoter regions of various acute-phase protein genes in the liver. Thus, when IL-6 binds to a cell through IL-6Ra/gp130 complexes, a series of events takes place that leads to the activation of STATs and NF-IL6, switching on target genes. OSE cells immortalized with mutant H-Ras or K-Ras lead to cells that grow slowly but progressively with serous papillary histology in the peritoneal cavity. Gene expression profile analysis of these transformed cells showed an increased expression of several cytokines, mainly IL-6, which are up regulated by the NF-kB pathway. Each of these cytokines might provide targets for therapeutic intervention in EOC with RAS mutation.

3.2 Cytokines and modulation of immune system

The host immune response comprises a multitude of highly developed interconnected biological processes involving both cellular and humoral responses that cooperate to eliminate foreign bodies and repair the site of injury. The innate arm of the immune activity provides rapid reactions prior to the development of highly specific adaptive responses. In the context of a malignant tumour, many of the suppressive and stimulatory properties of innate immunity may influence tumour progression in both positive and negative ways. The activation of the cell-mediated immunity by macrophages, T lymphocytes, and natural killer cells has been suggested as a specific mechanism performed by the body to counteract oncogenesis and tumour growth. During their activation processes these cells release several soluble factors (cytokines) that send stimulatory or inhibitory signals to the different immune cell types. Interleukin-1, IL-2 and TNF-α are the main mediators of cell-mediated immune response. Interleukin-1 and TNF-α are potent inductors of IL-6 that, in turn, regulates their production, acts as a second signal for the production of IL-2 and induces on cytotoxic T lymphocytes the expression of IL-2 receptor (RIL-2). IL-2 is the key cytokine in the regulation of the antineoplastic immunity. The activity of IL-2 is strictly dependent on its binding to specific membrane receptor (IL-2R). Lymphocyte activation is followed by an increased expression of IL-2R and release of its α subunit from the membrane receptor in a soluble form (sIL-2R). Hence, sIL-2R serum levels provide direct evidence of immune system activation. Then, the synergistic effect of IL-2 and other cytokines deriving from the activated immune system may play an active role in the cytotoxic attack against tumour by counteracting neoplastic cells growth. However, some cytokines, such as IL-1, IL-6 and TNF-α may favour tumour progression. Indeed, several studies of our research group have shown in vitro that the immune system of EOC patients is inefficient to various mitogen stimuli in terms of lymphocyte proliferative response and that the severity of the immune deficit is proportionate to the stage of disease and to the performance status (PS) of patients (Mantovani et al., 2000, 2003). The reduced lymphocytes proliferative response to mitogens, such as phytohaemagglutinin (PHA) and anti-CD3 monoclonal antibody (mAb), must be considered as an index of more complex functional alterations. In fact, these mitogens induce in vitro a number of phenomena similar to those that follow antigenic activity in vivo. The secretion of macrophagic cytokines, the production of IL-2 by CD4+ lymphocytes and the RIL-2 expression on lymphocyte membrane are the defining moments of these events. For these reasons, the entity of the lymphocyte blastic response depends on the quantity of cytokines produced, the number of RIL-2 expressed and the physiologic interaction of IL-2 with its receptor. Lymphocytes inability both to produce adequate quantities of IL-2 and to express physiological amount of RIL-2 seems to be the crucial feature of this specific lymphocyte functional deficit in EOC patients. In our studies, patients peripheral blood mononuclear cells (PBMC) proliferative response to PHA, anti-CD3 mAb and human recombinant IL-2 (HurIL-2) alone was significantly lower in comparison to controls and it was not modified by the addition of human recombinant IL-2 (HurIL-2) to the culture media. Furthermore, also the expression of CD25 and CD122 subunits of membrane-bound IL-2R on patients' PBMC after stimulation with PHA or CD3mAb was lower than that seen in controls (Macciò et al., 1998). A very important finding of our researches highlights that this impairment of T cells response was associated with increased circulating levels of proinflammatory cytokines (IL-1α, IL-1β, IL-6, TNF-α) and other mediators of inflammation such as fibrinogen, CRP and sIL-2R (Figure 1).

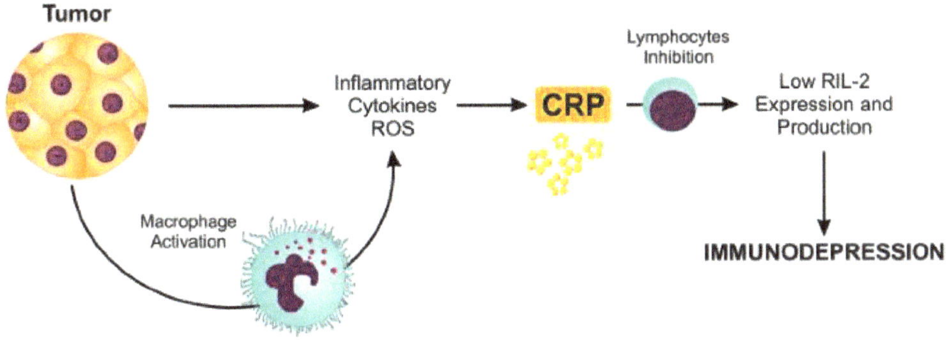

Fig. 1. Aspecific activation of immune system during the evolution of the ovarian cancer leads to immunodepression associated to high serum levels of inflammatory cytokines and acute phase proteins. Abbreviations: ROS, Reactive Oxygen Species, RIL-2, IL-2 receptor, CRP, C-reactive protein.

In particular, it is extremely interesting that IL-6 and CRP have been shown to be able to suppress T cell responses and several studies suggested that they might interfere with the immunological mechanisms underlying the antitumor activity of IL-2. Moreover, it is known that CRP, typically induced by IL-6, is involved in the binding of complement to cytotoxic CD3+ cells and plays a key role in the inhibition of cytotoxic activity of NK cells. Then, IL-6 can be an activator or an inhibitor of T-cell responses, depending its effects by the time and duration of its activity. This interaction of pro-inflammatory and anti-inflammatory activities suggests that IL-6 may play a role in regulating the control of immune system activation during the different phases of in EOC progression. A widely accepted model of tumour and immune cell interaction, termed immunoediting, describes an initial restriction of tumour cell growth, but maintains that the immune system ultimately selects for tumour cells with reduced immunogenicity that subsequently prevail over the host immune system. Therefore, whereas the immune system may initially be protective against tumour development, its efficacy may diminish over time and it may ultimately facilitate tumour progression. Indeed, the mechanisms by which the tumour can evade immune system control are manifold. Despite immune-cells have for long been known for their roles primarily in immune cancer surveillance, many tumour cell types secrete immunosuppressive cytokines such as transforming growth factor-beta, IL-6, IL-10 and IL-13, and chemokines that can also recruit cells that negatively regulate immunity such as T-regulatory cells, myeloid suppressor cells, NK cells and macrophage subsets (Robinson-Smith et al., 2007). Jeannin P et al. in a very recent work (Jeannin et al., 2011) reported that ovarian cancer ascites switched monocyte differentiation into tumour-associated macrophages (TAM)-like cells, that exhibit most phenotypic and functional characteristics of TAMs, suggesting that soluble mediators are involved in the differentiation of monocytes into TAM-like cells. TAMs, the most abundant immunosuppressive myeloid cells in the tumour microenvironment, exhibit an IL-10 (high) and IL-12 (low) profile called M2, opposite to the immunostimulatory M1. The same authors observed that the leukaemia-inhibitory factor and IL-6, present at high concentrations in ovarian cancer ascites, skew monocyte differentiation into TAM-like cells by increasing macrophage colony-stimulating factor consumption. These data reveal a new tumour-escape mechanism associated with TAMs generation through an IL-6 mediated effect. An interesting published study by Nowak et al. confirmed that in the presence of autologous ovarian cancer cells, peripheral blood mononuclear cells from patients with advanced EOC produced higher amount of immunosuppressive (Il-10, TGF-beta) and proinflammatory (IL-6) cytokines with downregulation of T cells response (Nowak et al., 2010b). In the context of EOC, two specific leukocyte subsets have been demonstrated to significantly promote tumour growth: regulatory T cells (Tregs) and pro-angiogenic/immunosuppressive myeloid cells, the latter exhibiting the phenotypic attributed of macrophages (Cubillos-Ruiz et al., 2010). Globally, all ovarian cancer-associated myeloid cell subsets impair the function of anti-tumour T cells, (Scarlett et al., 2009) the only element in the ovarian cancer microenvironment known to exert clinically relevant spontaneous immune pressure against tumour progression. The accumulation of tumour Tregs predicts poor survival in EOC patients. Curiel and colleagues (Curiel et al., 2004) first demonstrated a crucial role for Tregs in ovarian cancer-mediated immunosuppression. They showed that solid tumour masses and malignant ascites of human ovarian cancer accumulate variable levels of Tregs (CD3+CD4+CD25+ GITR+CTLA-4+CCR7+FoxP3hi), while non-malignant ascites or normal ovaries did not contain a significant proportion of these cells. Interestingly, Tregs were found to be specifically recruited to tumour locations via CCL22, a cytokine expressed by tumour cells and microenvironmental myeloid cells. Ovarian tumours and tumour microenvironment macrophages are major sources of CCL22. Tregs isolated from ovarian cancer ascites were functionally active, as they inhibited the proliferation of autologous T cells stimulated in vitro with DCs pulsed with tumour antigens, and also prevented the anti-tumour activity of adoptively transferred T cells. Giuntoli et al. reported that a high CD4+/CD8+ ratio in ascites, which may indicate the presence of Tregs, is associated with poor outcome (Giuntoli et al., 2009). Other studies investigating the significance of the role of intratumoral infiltrates (TIL) or tumour associated lymphocytes (TAL) in these events have been reported. By contrast, there is accumulating evidence that the presence both of TIL or TAL, such as those found in neoplastic effusions, is quantitatively related with improved clinical outcome in ovarian cancer (Kim et al., 2009). In fact, recent studies report on the infiltration of ovarian cancer by both CD4+ and CD8+ TILs and show a positive correlation between T-cell infiltration and prognosis (Yigit et al. 2010). Napoletano et al. demonstrated that primary debulking in ovarian cancer is associated with a reduction of circulating Tregs and an increase in CD8+ T-cell function (Napoletano et al., 2010). Leffers at al. reported that a high TIL/Treg ratio independently predicts increased survival and suggest that it is not so much the presence of Treg as the presence of TIL in general to be responsible for the observed survival effect (Leffers et al. 2009).

A central mechanism whereby both TIL and/or TAL contribute to invasive proliferation of tumour cells is through the production of the cytokines and chemokines that increase both the migration and survival of tumour cells. These cytokines present in the blood and in large quantities in neoplastic effusions can also be produced by cancer cells and have been associated with prognosis in EOC (Gavalas et al., 2010).

In conclusion the development of EOC is associated with changes in the peritoneal cavity microenvironment. Immune cells in the ovarian stromal microenvironment play an important role in ovarian tumorigenesis and progression (Wertel et al., 2011). In turn, tumour cells develop several mechanisms to evade anti-tumour immunity by developing an immunosuppressive microenvironment by the production of different factors (cytokines), which impairs differentiation, maturation, and function of antigen-presenting cells. Once transformed ovarian epithelial cells develop an immunoediting process occurs in which immune cells and their mediators dictate the growth and progression of EOC (Thompson & Mok, 2009). Then, as described above chronic inflammation is associated with initiation and/or progression of the most common EOC types and the balance between pro- and anti-inflammatory cytokines is critical for host immune response to tumours.

4. Proinflammatory cytokines and prognosis

Several studies, including some from our group (Macciò et al., 1998, 2009), demonstrated the correlation existing between the severity of chronic inflammation, advanced stage and poor outcome in patients with epithelial ovarian cancer. Epithelial ovarian cancer is an immunogenic tumour and exploits many suppressive ways to escape immune eradication. High circulating levels of proinflammatory cytokines, such as IL-1, Il-6, and TNF-α have been found in EOC patients with advanced stage of disease and an unfavourable prognosis. The prognostic role of various cytokines has been studied, but no absolutely firm conclusions can be drawn so far. It is likely that cytokines involved in Th1 response predict for better prognosis, while the opposite is expected in those associated with Th2 response. Moreover, proinflammatory cytokines play an important role in the mechanisms inducing the complex clinical condition known as cancer-related anorexia/cachexia (CACS). One of the metabolic changes present in this syndrome is the hepatic synthesis of C-reactive protein (CRP). High serum levels of CRP are associated with a poor prognosis in EOC patients and can negatively influence the therapeutic response to HurIL-2. This is extremely important since IL-2 initiates the activation of T and NK cells and it is also essential for the maintenance of self-tolerance through generation and maintenance of Tregs or by activation-induced cell death to eliminate self reactive T cells. Interestingly, IL-6 is a potent inducer of CRP exerting its regulatory effect on CRP synthesis at the pretranslational level. IL-6 levels have been shown to be increased in advanced ovarian cancer patients' serum and to correlate with poor prognosis and reduced overall survival (Scambia et al., 1995). Elevated levels are also present in malignant ascites from EOC patients (Plante et al., 1994) and a positive correlation has been found between IL-6 concentration in ascites and residual disease after debulking. Additionally, IL-6 levels are remarkably higher at recurrence compared to primary advanced disease, thus opening an opportunity for inhibition of IL-6 expression in the prevention of recurrence. EOC is known to spread primarily by tumour cell implantations in peritoneal cavity. Therefore, ascites may be an ideal fluid compartment to unravel the immune status of the peritoneal cavity (Mantovani et al, 1999, 1997). Recently, Yigit R et al. (Yigit et al., 2011) observed high expression of pro-inflammatory cytokines IL-6, IL-8 and immune suppressive cytokines IL-10, CCL22 and TGF-β in most samples of ovarian cancer ascites whereas Th1 (IL-12p70, IFN-γ) and Th2 (IL-4, IL-5) cytokines were only detectable in few samples. TGF-β was only detected in latent form, questioning its immune suppressive role. At advanced stage, they also observed a negative correlation with CCL22 levels and Th1/2 cytokine expression. A cytokine that seems to be heavily involved in tumour immunosuppression is the transforming growth factor beta (TGF-β), a protein that affects proliferation, activation, and differentiation of immune cells and inhibits antitumor immune response. In cancer cells, the production of TGF-β is increased and, in turn, raises their proteolytic activity and binding to cell adhesion molecules in the extracellular matrix. TGF-β can also convert effector T cells into Tregs. It has been reported that it can also promote angiogenesis and that this process can be blocked by anti-TGF-β antibodies. TGF-β blockade almost completely eradicate ascites formation and significantly inhibit the expression of VEGF, which is the major contributor to ascites formation. At the same time, TGF-β blockade prevent 'abnormalization' of diaphragm lymphatic vessels and improve ascites drainage (Liao et al., 2011). Also TNF-α is produced by tumour cells and can induce autocrine proliferation and disease progression in ovarian cancer. The autocrine action of TNFα may have direct effects on tumour cell spread via acting on the chemokine receptor CXCR4 and stimulating new blood vessel formation in the peritoneum by inducing expression of VEGF and CXCL12. In contrast, TNF-α levels have also been inversely correlated with the presence of CD4+ CD25+ cells, and have been shown to directly downregulate Tregs. This might indicate a favourable effect of this cytokine on prognosis and underlines the complexity of the functions that each of these factors may possess. Then, reports on whether TNF-α is a signature of poor or better prognosis vary. Another cytokine that was shown to be associated with the growth of cancer cells and tumour proliferation is IL-1. A family of proteins called chemokines (CC) may also be influencing cellular composition in biological fluids. Recent studies have demonstrated the presence of mRNA for CCL2, CCL3, CCL4, and CCL5 in EOC by in situ hybridization. Moreover, CCL5 has been shown to be secreted by CD4+ T cells, recruits CCR5+ dendritic cells to the tumour location, and activates them through CD40-CD40L interactions. The newly matured dendritic cells prime tumour-specific CD8+ cells thus providing with long-term protection. Also in the protein-rich ascitic fluid, different chemokine molecules are expressed, with CCL2 being the predominant one. In addition, chemokine stromal-derived factor-1 (CXCL-1) induced the migration of plasmacytoid dendritic cells (PDC) into the tumour microenvironment in cases of ovarian cancer and induced delivery of survival signals to PDC. In turn, the tumour microenvironmental PDC induced IL-10 expressing Tregs, which are correlated to poor prognosis and shorter progression-free survival. In the case of Tregs it has been exhibited that CCL22 plays a central role in inducing influx of these cells into tumour sites by binding to CCR4 that is expressed on Treg surface. Interferon gamma (IFN-γ) plays a stimulatory role for macrophages turning them from immunosuppressive to immunostimulatory cells. It also skewed monocyte differentiation from associated-associated macrophages (TAM) like cells to M1-polarized immunostimulatory macrophages. Taken together these data show that IFN-γ overcomes TAM-induced immunosuppression by preventing TAM generation and functions. Furthermore, cytokines such as IL-18 and stroma derived factor 1 (SDF-1) have been shown to be correlated with poor prognosis in ovarian cancer patients, but further studies are required to fully evaluate them in the tumour microenvironment and the periphery.

4.1 Inflammation and metabolic changes

In the course of its evolution cancer induces in the host changes of the immune system and energy metabolism that affect its clinical conditions so deeply that in some cases they are responsible for patient's death. Several symptoms are associated to these events and involve various organs and systems:

- Anorexia
- Nausea
- Weight loss (with reduction of lean mass and adipose tissue)
- increase of resting energy expenditure (with changes of the glucose, lipid and protein metabolism)
- Immunodepression
- Anaemia
- Fatigue

It is difficult to establish the exact moment when such changes actually start, but it could be hypothesized that they are the consequence of the interactions between the tumour and the host. The hypothesis that the presence of the tumour and its continuous growth are responsible for the increased energy expenditure and for the progressive weight loss has been considered the most reliable so far. Indeed, the presence in the host of continuously growing neoplastic tissue justifies by itself the increased energy needs; moreover, it is accompanied by enhanced energy expenditure associated with the chronic activation of the immune system, trying to counteract the tumour, which is energetically very costly (25-30% of the basal metabolic rate, i.e. 1750-2080 kJ/day) (Straub et al., 2010). The resulting metabolic scenario is that of two systems that require a continuous supply of energy substrates, particularly glucose. Glucose oxidation to CO_2 and H_2O is the main energy source produced as ATP, NADH and FADH. A further glucose amount is also involved for the synthesis, through the phosphate pentose pathway, of compounds with high reducing power as NADPH and reduced glutathione (GSH), essential for the neutralisation of reactive oxygen species (ROS) produced during the various steps of the energy metabolism. ROS are intermediate compounds derived from the univalent reduction of molecular oxygen by electrons and protons, characterized by the presence of an unpaired electron in the farthest external orbital, which makes them particularly unstable (hydrogen peroxide:

H_2O_2, superoxide anione: O_2^-; hydroxyl radical: OH°). As they are partly useful, but potentially toxic, compounds the body has a number of control mechanisms that limit their activity once they have been used for the scheduled objective. In particular superoxide dismutase (SOD) metabolises O_2^- to H_2O_2, whereas catalase and various glutathione peroxidase (GPx) metabolise it to H_2O and alcohol. ROS which have not been eliminated for the lack of these antioxidants, have a negative oxidative action on polyunsaturated fatty acids circulating proteins, membrane rich of disulphur bridge, enzymes and DNA, determining irreversible damage both to cell architecture and function. Under such conditions, detoxification systems, sustained by reducing compounds, should be adequately present. These reducing compounds, which are called natural detoxificants, are thus essential for a normal cell activity.

The energy metabolism in cancer patients is affected by the presence, during the disease evolution, of symptoms such as anorexia, nausea and vomiting, which prevent a normal nutrition and thus a regular supply of glucose, lipids, proteins and vitamins. Antiblastic treatments and the same molecules (cytokines), which regulate both the tumour development and the immune system functions, are responsible for these symptoms (Bennani-Baiti & Davis, 2008). In this context, the finding that neoplastic patients in advanced stages show a severe impairment of immunologic functions characterized by impaired cell-mediated immunity and elevated serum levels of macrophage cytokines (IL-1, IL-6, TNF-a) and inflammation acute phase proteins (fibrinogen and CRP) is of great importance (Macciò et al., 1998). Evidence that high serum concentrations of cytokines and inflammatory proteins are associated with high levels of ROS and low levels of SOD and GPx is also of particular interest (Mantovani et al., 2002).

Thus, in neoplastic patients tumour growth and immune system activation determine an overall metabolic picture characterized by:

- Increased glucose, lipid and protein requirements;
- Difficulty to introduce these substances with food because of anorexia, nausea and vomiting;
- Resorting to glucogenesis with depletion of protein and lipid stores and thus loss of weight;
- Difficult to use the newly formed glucose because of hypoinsulinemia and/or peripheral resistance to insulin;
- Oxidative damage induced by ROS on DNA, membrane lipoprotein, and enzymes and coenzymes that play a major role in the regulation of the main cell anabolic and catabolic pathways.

Therefore, the metabolic changes described in the neoplastic patients are to be attributed to the chronic action of some cytokines (in particular IL-1, IL-6 and TNF-α) produced both by activated immune system and tumour cells (Argiles & Lopez-Soriano, 1999; Delano & Moldawer, 2006). It may be hypothesised that, during the initial phases of neoplastic disease, the synthesis of proinflammatory cytokines leads to an efficient antineoplastic effect. However, the inability of the immune system to definitively counteract tumour growth (Hagemann et al., 2006) determines the chronicisation of cytokine activity with deleterious effects on cell metabolism, body composition, nutritional status and immune system efficiency. Indeed, the chronic action of cytokines is the main cause of the metabolic abnormalities characterising advanced ovarian cancer patient (Figure 2).

In detail, IL-1 exerts a specific effect on reducing food intake and influences meal size and duration: IL-1 has an anorectic action by directly decreasing neuropeptide Y (NPY) neurotransmission and secondarily by increasing corticotrophin-releasing factor (CRF), which in turn acts on the satiety circuitry inhibiting food intake. IL-1 has also been demonstrated to inhibit serum levels of growth hormone (GH) by increasing CRF and somatostatin levels. The decreased synthesis of GH leads to reduced synthesis of the insulin-like growth factors (IGFs), which in turn influences the muscle protein turnover and the autocrine and paracrine regulation of muscle mass proliferation. TNF-α has been shown to promote lipolysis and inhibit lipogenesis and plays a key role in the depletion of adipose tissue mass seen in cachexia. It has been proposed that an elevation in plasma levels of TNF-α is responsible for the metabolic alterations in adipose tissue seen in advanced cancer patients. Lipid metabolism is a complex sequence of events that determine whether the triglyceride pool within the adipocyte increases, due to the processes of free fatty acid (FFA) uptake and lipogenesis, or decreases, due to the process of lipolysis. Circulating lipoproteins and triglycerides are first converted into FFA by the action of lipoprotein lipase (LPL), which is secreted by the adipocyte. FFA can then enter the adipocyte via a fatty acid transporter and, once inside the adipocyte, they are converted into the triglyceride by a multi-step-regulated enzymatic reaction, which involves acyl-CoA synthetase. In addition, triglyceride can be formed from the uptake of glucose, via glucose transporters (GLUT) 1 and 4, into the adipocyte. The glucose can then be converted into triglyceride by the actions of a series of enzymes, which include acetyl-CoA carboxylase and fatty acid synthase. A large body of evidence now supports a role for TNF-α in modulating these processes. TNF-α inhibits LPL activity by down-regulating its protein expression. In addition, TNF-α has been shown to reduce the expression of FFA transporters in adipose tissue. TNF-α could thus hinder the synthesis and entry of FFA into the adipocyte, curtailing an increase in the intracellular triglyceride pool size. Studies have also suggested that TNF-α may decrease the expression of enzymes involved in lipogenesis. Specifically, it has been suggested that acetyl-CoA carboxylase and fatty acid synthase are down regulated. Acyl-CoA synthase expression and activity have also been suggested to be down regulated by TNF-α. TNF-α has been found to promote lipolysis. TNF-α has been implicated as a factor associated with the development of insulin resistance. A positive association between plasma insulin levels and TNF-α mRNA from subcutaneous adipose tissue has been found in women, finding which is supported by a further study showing increased adipose TNF-α secretion in obese patients with insulin resistance. Extensive research has highlighted several potential mechanisms by which TNF-α induces insulin resistance. These include: accelerated lipolysis and a concomitant increase in circulating FFA concentrations, down regulation of GLUT4 synthesis, down-regulation of insulin receptor, insulin receptor substrate-1 (IRS-1) synthesis and increased Ser/Thr phosphorylation of IRS-1. Interleukin-6 is another proinflammatory cytokine with cachectic effects. The presence of tumour in mouse models was associated with early CACS and production of IL-6, whom serum levels correlated with the severity of CACS. Vice versa, the administration of anti-IL-6 antibody inhibits the comparison of CACS symptoms thus demonstrating the central pathogenetic role of this cytokine in cachectic syndrome. In vitro studies have demonstrated that IL-6 induces, similarly to IL-1, the hypothalamic release of CRF. Moreover, IL-6 acts on β pancreatic cells similarly to IL-1 (Mantovani et al., 2001).

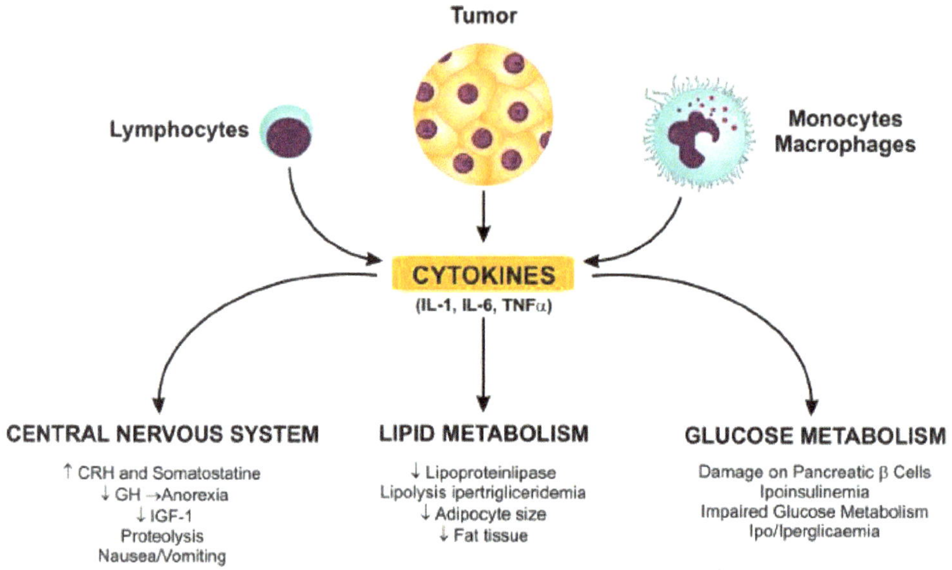

Fig. 2. Role of proinflammatory cytokines in inducing metabolic changes of advanced epithelial ovarian cancer patients. Abbreviations: IL, Interelukin; TNF, Tumour Necrosis Factor, CRH, corticotrophin releasing hormone; GH, growth hormone; IGF, Insulin growth factor.

Findings from our group demonstrated a relationship between serum levels of IL-6 and leptin, one of the most important parameters of the body energy metabolism (Macciò et al., 2008) in advanced EOC patients leptin levels were significantly lower in comparison to controls and were inversely correlated with weight, BMI, stage, PS, circulating cytokines, CRP and fibrinogen. Furthermore, multivariate regression analysis demonstrated that IL-6, besides stage of disease, was an independent predictive factor of leptin levels. These results are in accordance with those of other important studies performed on a wide population of newly diagnosed EOC patients (Mor et al., 2005; Visintin et al., 2008). Leptin, released from adipocytes into the systemic circulation proportionally to fat mass, acts as a master hormone controlling energy metabolism and weight balance. Additionally, this adipokine controls several other critical systems, including endocrine axis, bone metabolism, as well as the immune/inflammatory response. Noteworthy, our study showed that serum leptin levels evaluated in 104 ovarian cancer patients at different stage of disease (stage I-IV) were dependent both from stage of disease and serum IL-6 levels, independently of patient BMI. This finding was in contrast to the great majority of studies in cancer patients that have concluded that BMI and weight are the most important determinants of circulating leptin levels; however, it is to be noted that in the majority of these papers the impact of weight loss and the pattern of serum leptin concentration before diagnosis or study enrolment are unknown. Indeed, experimental and clinical studies have clarified that leptin production is not only strictly related to body weight and fat but it is also influenced by glucose utilization ability (Havel, 2004). Acute caloric deprivation and increased energy expenditure result in a large decrease of leptin synthesis, before major changes in body weight or fat mass have actually occurred (Chan et al., 2003). Consistently with this evidence and the findings obtained by some authors in tuberculosis patients (van Crevel et al., 2002), it can be suggested that the prolonged severe inflammatory response associated to the most advanced stages of EOC is responsible for the energy metabolism impairment thus down-regulating and exhausting leptin production. Indeed, the stimulation of leptin synthesis by aerobic glucose metabolism is mediated through the production of ATP and through the effect of glucose oxidation on cellular redox status and pyruvate cycling. Therefore, oxidative stress, in advanced cancer patients, consequent to the low energy reserves and the inability to utilize efficiently the energy substrates, particularly glucose, may be considered the direct evidence of the metabolic impairment of which leptin is the most important parameter. Accordingly, our results demonstrated that in advanced EOC patients the lowest leptin levels and the highest IL-6 levels correlated with the highest levels of ROS and the lowest levels of GPx, the most sensitive among antioxidants to nutritional status being a selenium-dependent enzyme. In keeping with these hypotheses, our prospective study, which analyzed the changes of the above reported parameters during the course of disease in advanced EOC patients, showed that in patients who achieved objective complete response after the primary antineoplastic treatment, IL-6 levels fell to normal values and leptin increased significantly. Then, patients who achieved progression of disease (PD) showed a significant increase of IL-6 accompanied by a significant decrease of leptin. The patients with further PD had a progressive increase of IL-6, which reached the highest concentrations in the terminal phases of disease, associated with a significant increase of CRP and fibrinogen and a further decrease of leptin. Importantly, when PD occurred leptin did not decreased proportionally to body weight that fell significantly only in the terminal phases of disease. Leptin changes strictly reflected changes of IL-6 in accordance to tumour response or disease progression (Maccio et al., 2009). It may be suggested that leptin variation reflected the changes of energy metabolism, induced by cytokines released from the tumour itself or by the aspecific activation of the immune system, even before they caused a significant body weight loss due to anorexia and muscle and fat wasting. In light of these results we can hypothesize that in EOC patients the reduced leptin production functions as a signal of increased energy expenditure and low energy reserves during the progression of the neoplastic disease. Leptin decrease in advanced EOC patients should induce an adaptative reduction of energy expenditure and an increase of appetite and food intake in response to the metabolic impairment induced by tumour growth and cancer-related inflammation. The signal activated by the drop of leptin levels might therefore constitute the evidence of the metabolic hyperactivity of the tumour and the host immune system and the subsequent defence attempt of the host to reduce energy expenditure when energy is scarce. Leptin levels fell together with a significant weight loss, probably induced by the prolonged action of inflammatory mediators, only in the last phases of the neoplastic disease. Indeed, chronic inflammation results in severe alterations of cell metabolism, with deleterious effects on body composition, nutritional status and immune system efficiency. Therefore, IL-6 and leptin play a central role as early markers of the main metabolic alterations associated to the progression of advanced EOC, and therefore their assessment should be included in monitoring the disease outcome, especially when cancer is no longer curable with standard antineoplastic treatments and quality of life becomes the primary endpoint.

4.2 Inflammation-related symptoms

As widely written on, several studies have shown that inflammatory cytokines, and in particular IL-6, play a central role in the evolution of EOC and the mechanisms by which IL-

6 may influence disease progression and outcome are extremely complex and multifactorial. In fact IL-6, as well as IL-1 and TNF-α, is responsible for symptoms such as anorexia, nausea and vomiting, weight loss and altered energy metabolism. Furthermore, high IL-6 levels are associated with an impaired efficiency of immune cells both in terms of PBMC reduced blastic response and membrane-bound IL-2 receptor expression (Macciò et al., 1998). In the same way, recent data shown that IL-6 exerts a central role in the pathogenesis of cancer-related anaemia. Additionally, elevated serum IL-6 levels account for its endocrine activity leading to severe impairment of physical, functional and psychosocial well-being (depression, anxiety, reduced social interaction) and fatigue.

4.2.1 Cancer-related anaemia

Anaemia is present in more than 30% of patients with EOC at the time of initial presentation. The severity of this particular form of anaemia called cancer-related anaemia (CRA) has been associated with more aggressive tumour hystotypes and is able to influence the response to treatment and the patients' performance status (PS). The biologic and hematologic characteristics of CRA are similar to those observed in anaemia occurring in chronic inflammatory diseases. Several *in vitro* and *in vivo* studies demonstrated that high levels of proinflammatory cytokines and increased oxidative stress contribute both to the development of anaemia and to the resistance to human recombinant erythropoietin (HurEPO) (Figure 3).

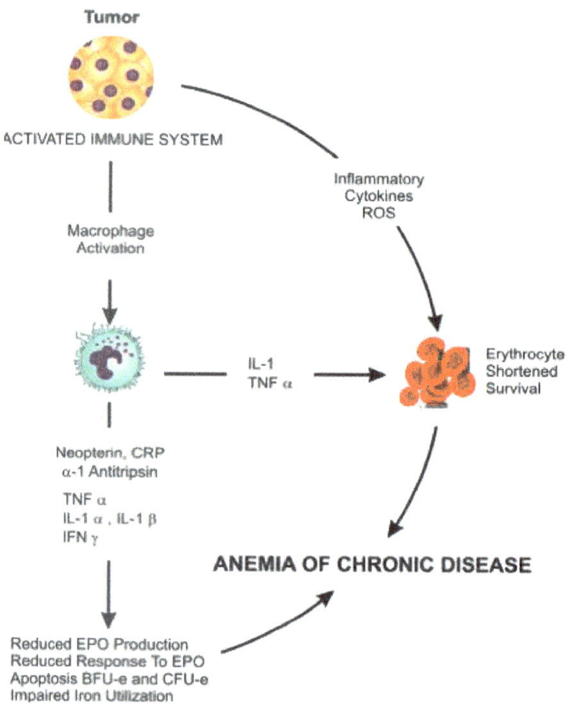

Fig. 3. Pathogenetic mechanisms of cancer-related anaemia. Abbreviations: ROS, Reactive Oxygen Species; IL, Interleukin; TNF, Tumor Necrosis Factor; IFN, Interferon; CRP, C-reactive protein; EPO, erythropoietin.

CRA is typically normochromic, normocytic with a low reticulocyte count. Bone marrow iron stores are adequate or increased, but iron reutilization is impaired, as shown by normal or increased ferritin levels and low serum iron levels and iron-binding capacity. In CRA, erythroid progenitor cells respond normally to erythropoietin (EPO), but EPO production is often not optimal for the level of anaemia. EOC patients and in particulary those in advanced stages of disease, suffer of anaemia similar to anaemia of inflammation. In these patients the lowest hemoglobin (Hb) levels are linked with the highest concentrations of markers of inflammation, such as proinflammatory cytokines (IL-6, IL-1, TNF-a), CRP, and Fibrinogen, and with the lowest leptin levels. Statistical analysis confirmed that Hb inversely correlates with stage and ECOG PS, proinflammatory cytokines, CRP, Fibrinogen, and ROS but positively correlated with leptin and GPx. By multivariate regression analysis, only stage of disease and IL-6 levels are independent factors in determining Hb levels. In accordance with these data, Van der Zee et al (van der Zee et al., 1995) demonstrated that higher levels of IL-6 in cystic fluids from patients with malignant versus benign ovarian tumors correlate with decreased Hb levels and increased platelet counts as marker of inflammatory status. Several researchers have also demonstrated that IL-6 is both necessary and sufficient for the induction of hepcidin, an iron regulatory hormone responsible for inflammation-induced iron disutilization resulting in the anaemia associated with acute and chronic infections, chronic kidney disease, and neoplastic disease. Of note, in an our study (Macciò et al., 2005) we demonstrated a significant positive correlation between IL-6 and other markers of inflammation and oxidative stress. Thus, high serum level of IL-6 may be considered an indicator of the inflammatory and pro-oxidative status of patients with EOC and they could be linked also with a specific production of IL-6 by ovarian cancer cells. Although, it is not completely clear the mechanism through which the high levels of inflammatory mediators could induce CRA, several studies showed that proinflammatory cytokines blunt HUrEPO response to anaemia and impair erythroid colony formation in response to HUrEPO. Additionally, proinflammatory cytokines and the acute-phase proteins impair iron metabolism, inhibiting the reticuloendothelial iron stores with low iron circulating levels. Furthermore, the presence of proinflammatory cytokines in patients with EOC is associated with increased production of ROS either as a reflection of inflammation or as a consequence of their metabolic effects. Several studies demonstrated that ROSs are capable of inhibiting the production of EPO from kidney tissue. Takeda et al. (Takeda et al., 2002) hypothesized that also nutritional status, probably through leptin action, may affect erythropoiesis and demonstrated that BMI and leptin were inversely correlated with rHuEPO dose required in patients receiving hemodialysis. Indeed, *in vitro* studies have suggested that leptin plays a role in enhancing erythropoiesis but, certainly, this hypothesis needs more definitive analysis. Therefore, the results we have reported suggest that anaemia in patients with EOC is, at least in part, the consequence of cancer-related chronic inflammation. Cancer-related anaemia must be recognized as a constitutional feature of patients with advanced neoplasms and not necessarily as just a consequence of antineoplastic treatments. Indeed, it has been widely demonstrated that CRA is associated with poor response to treatment and decreased survival, and with a decline in energy and activity levels, quality of life, and cognitive functions. An increased understanding of the pathogenesis of CRA may help identify the most appropriate treatment strategies.

4.2.2 Inflammation and depression

EOC patients, who have the poorest survival rate among gynaecologic cancer patients show high rates of depression. Depression among cancer patients has frequently been attributed to the stress of a potentially life-threatening diagnosis and the difficulties of cancer treatment. However, several recent studies among cancer patients have found associations between depression, elevated levels of the proinflammatory cytokine and/or dysregulation of the neuroendocrine hormone cortisol (Costanzo et al., 2005). Inflammation has been implicated in the pathogenesis of depression and it has been proposed that inflammatory cytokines such as IL-6 may contribute to depression in cancer patients. Also in healthy adults, elevated IL-6 has been associated with depressive symptoms and clinical depression. In particularly IL-6 has profound effects on the CNS, inducing a syndrome of "sickness behaviors" characterized by anhaedonia and vegetative symptoms including fatigue, malaise, anorexia, difficulty concentrating, reduced activity, sleep impairments, and disinterest in activities. Proinflammatory cytokines exert differential effects on affective and vegetative depression, with more prominent effects on vegetative symptoms. Affective and vegetative depressive symptoms are thought to occur via distinct mechanisms, with vegetative symptoms occurring significantly earlier than mood disturbance. Depressive symptoms are also associated with hypercortisolemia, downregulated glucocorticoid receptors, and general dysregulation of the hypothalamic pituitary adrenocortical (HPA) axis. With chronic stress and depression, the negative feedback system regulating cortisol may become impaired and diurnal cortisol rhythms altered, particularly with respect to evening cortisol. There is a well-characterized feedback loop whereby IL-6 stimulates HPA secretion of cortisol which, in turn, exerts negative feedback on IL-6 for inflammatory control. Persistent inflammation is associated with HPA abnormalities and may contribute to the hypercortisolemia seen in depression. In particular, in advanced-stage EOC patients, assessed prior to surgery, elevations of IL-6 associated with both affective and vegetative depressive symptoms have been documented (Lutgendorf et al., 2008). Early-stage patients had levels of IL-6 and depressive symptoms that were greater than those observed in LMP patients but lower than those in patients with advanced disease. Elevated IL-6 was also related to greater disturbances in the diurnal cortisol rhythm among advanced patients, with the elevated plasma and ascites levels of IL-6 related to higher evening cortisol as well as higher afternoon cortisol and cortisol AUC. These results are consistent with the "proinflammatory cytokine theory of depression" in suggesting that pathophysiologic elevations in circulating inflammatory mediators may lead to the appearance of depressive symptomatology via cytokine regulation of CNS function.

Proinflammatory cytokines influence the CNS via several direct pathways, including passage through permeability area of the blood-brain barrier and stimulation of afferent fibers in the vagus nerve. These fibers transmit information to specific brain nuclei with subsequent downstream effects on multiple central processes including induction of cytokines, neurotransmitters, stimulation of the HPA axis and development of sickness behaviors. Relationships between IL-6 and vegetative depression without any associations between affective depression and IL-6 are consistent with the possibility that inflammatory mechanisms may contribute specifically to vegetative symptoms, whereas other mechanisms may underlie affective symptoms of depression. Chronic inflammation can induce glucocorticoid resistance and lead to a hyperactive HPA axis. The resultant HPA dysregulation and high levels of cortisol may contribute to depression, providing an indirect pathway linking IL-6 and depression. Then, the excessive production of IL-6 by ovarian carcinomas may set up a chronic proinflammatory state, eliciting sickness behaviors in the CNS and hypersecretion and dysregulation of the HPA axis, both contributing to depressive symptomatology. Because of extremely high levels of tumor-secreted IL-6, particularly in ascites, secreted cortisol may be inadequate to suppress IL-6. In turn, depression may contribute to enhanced IL-6 secretion. In fact, depression has been associated with systemic elevations in norepinephrine which is known to enhance IL-6 secretion by ovarian tumor cells in vitro, potentially setting up a positive feedback loop for IL-6 in the tumor microenvironment. It is also possible that all of these pathways may operate simultaneously (Weinrib et al., 2010).

4.2.3 Inflammation and fatigue

Fatigue is one of the most common and distressing side effects of cancer and its treatment and may persist long after successful treatment completion. Subjective and objective evidence suggest that a third to half of patients developing EOC report symptoms at 3 or more months prior to diagnosis (Lurie et al., 2009; Arriba et al., 2010). Fatigue may be part of these symptom complex (Smith, 2006). Cancer-related fatigue (CRF) has been defined by National Comprehensive Cancer Network as "a distressing persistent subjective sense of tiredness or exhaustion related to cancer or cancer treatment that is not proportional to recent activity and interferes with usual functioning". It can adversely affect emotional, physical and mental well-being. CRF can also affect patients' abilities to function in terms of their usual social activities, and their ability to carry on with their normal working lives. The two most plausible mechanism include an abnormal or prolonged inflammatory response and/or disruption to the HPA axis. Emerging evidence suggests that inflammatory processes may be involved in cancer-related fatigue both during and after treatment. Indeed, a wide range of different changes of the immune system has been shown in patients suffering from fatigue. The most common are deficit of cell-mediated immunity associated with high serum levels of the proinflammatory cytokines. Each of these cytokines can determine by themselves the symptomatology typical of patient suffering from fatigue. Indeed, it is well known that these cytokines play important actions both on the central nervous system and the endocrine system and at various sites involved in the regulation of energy metabolism. The same proinflammatory cytokines involved in cachexia and associated with chronic inflammation are potent stimulators of the HPA axis. Moreover, changes in the HPA axis may be caused by a number of different factors relevant to neoplastic disease: cancer itself and/or cancer treatment can alter the function of the HPA axis resulting in endocrine changes that cause or contribute to fatigue. All these findings highlight multiple and complex mechanisms through which the immune system function disorders may lead to fatigue. Moreover, the close link between fatigue and depression in cancer patients suggests that a common mechanism could underlie the development of both. Since serotonin is a principal (but not a sole) contributor to depression, the model would predict that serotonin-influencing interventions effective against clinical depression might also prove beneficial for fatigue. Furthermore, it has been proposed that patients with cancer, particularly those with anorexia–cachexia, have altered muscle protein metabolism, which may also contribute to cancer-related fatigue.

Since the causes of fatigue are not fully understood, it is very difficult to treat it appropriately. The National Comprehensive Cancer Network's clinical guidelines also provide further options for cancer-related fatigue management. These suggest initially treating any underlying reversible causes of fatigue (e.g. anaemia, poor nutrition or depression) and attending to general supportive measures and psychosocial support. A recent review (Minton et al., 2010) has examined drug treatment for fatigue as it represents one of the ways this problem can be tackled. The review authors looked at trials in all types of cancer and at all stages of treatment. Fifty studies met the inclusion criteria but only 31 (7104 participants) were deemed suitable for detailed analysis as they explored fatigue in sufficient detail. They found mixed results with some drugs showing an effect on fatigue. In particular the authors concluded that Methylphenidate, a stimulant drug that improves concentration, is effective for the management of cancer-related fatigue but the small samples used in the available studies mean more research is needed to confirm its role. Erythropoietin and darbopoetin, drugs that improve anaemia, are effective in the management of cancer-related fatigue. Research on inflammation and cancer-related fatigue helps to elucidate the biological basis for this common and troublesome symptom and may also promote the development of targeted therapies. In particular, use of cytokine antagonists may be a promising direction for intervention efforts. There is preliminary evidence that TNF-α blockade with etanercept is safe and effective in reducing fatigue among patients with advanced cancer (Monk et al., 2006), but effects among patients with early stage cancer and cancer survivors have not been determined. Behavioural and mind–body interventions also show considerable promise for treating fatigue and other cancer-related symptoms, and there is preliminary evidence for their effects on immune function (Carlson et al., 2003; Fairey et al., 2005; Stevinson et al., 2009). These treatments may be more palatable to EOC patients than pharmacologic therapies and are another important avenue for research efforts.

4.3 Chemoresistance

It has been shown that increased IL-6 concentration in serum and ascites of EOC patients correlates with chemoresistance. In particular, the IL-6 signalling cascade in ovarian cancer cells has been associated with the development of cisplatin and paclitaxel resistance (Wang et al, 2010). The underlining mechanisms of IL-6-mediated chemoresistance in ovarian cancer cells are not so clear. However, some studies showed that IL-6 is associated with increased expression of multidrug resistance-related genes, apoptosis inhibitory proteins (Bcl-2, Bcl-xL and XIAP) as well as activation of Ras/MEK/Erk and PI3K/Akt signalling. Moreover, IL-6 signalling prevents chemotherapy-induced endothelial cells apoptosis (Lo et al., 2011). Thus, interference with IL-6 pathway may offer opportunities for new strategies in ovarian cancer therapy. Using a monoclonal antibody that specifically blocks IL-6 signalling (siltuximab), Guo et al. demonstrated *in vitro* that the combination of siltuximab with paclitaxel increased the sensitivity of ovarian tumour cells to paclitaxel (Guo et al., 2010).
In vitro studies with ovarian cancer cell lines confirm that generation of paclitaxel-resistant sublines is often associated with increased IL-6 mRNA expression and protein secretion. As well known, IL-6 acts through a hexametric receptor, which contains the ligand-binding IL-6a chain and the common cytokine receptor signal-transducing subunit gp130. The binding of IL-6 to gp130 activates multiple signal transduction pathways such as signal transducers and activators of transcription (JAK/STATs) pathway, Ras/MEK (mitogen-activated protein or extracellular signal-regulated kinase kinase)/ERK (extracellular signal-regulated kinase) pathway, and PI3K (phosphotidylinositol 3 kinase)/Akt pathway. Recently, evidence suggests that activation of Ras/MEK/ERK and PI3K/Akt signalling pathways play an important role in chemoresistance of EOC. A research by Wang et al (Wang et al., 2010) firstly demonstrated that autocrine production of IL-6 by ovarian cancer cell lines is

inversely associated with their response to cisplatin and paclitaxel. Moreover, both exogenous and endogenous IL-6 induce cisplatin and paclitaxel resistance in non-IL-6-producing cells, whereas deleting of endogenous IL-6 expression in IL-6-overexpressing cells promotes the sensitivity of these cells to these anticancer drugs. Meanwhile, IL-6-mediated resistance of EOC cells exhibits decreased proteolytic activation of caspase-3 and a number of studies have shown that the anti-apoptotic ability of IL-6 was associated with expression of the Bcl-2 family proteins that are typically associated with resistance to chemotherapy. Then, the main mechanism of drug resistance induced by IL-6 is exerted in a dose dependent manner by the increased expression of Bcl-2 family proteins. Other lines of evidence suggest that also the activation of Ras/MEK/ERK and PI3K/Akt, the most important cell survival signalling, protects EOC cells from chemotherapy. It has been shown that cisplatin treatment modulates ERK and that activation of ERK protects ovarian cancer cells from cisplatin-induced death. The inhibition *in vitro* of ERK signalling by a MEK1/2 inhibitor blocked ERK activation and increased cisplatin sensitivity in specific EOC cell lines. Also, the inactivation of Akt and its downstream targets sensitizes human ovarian cancer cells to cisplatin and paclitaxel. Worthy of note, it is specifically IL-6 to be able to induce activation of ERK and Akt in ovarian cancer cells and that the use of specific inhibitors of these two signal transducers, inhibits IL-6-induced cisplatin and paclitaxel resistance. Taken together, these data suggest that IL-6 promotes chemoresistance of ovarian cancer cells via activation of multiple signal transduction pathways including ERK cascade and PI3K/Akt pathway. These results provide support for these signal transduction pathways as a strategy for reversing drug resistance.

Another major downstream component of the IL-6 signalling pathway is STAT3. Duan et al. (Duan et al., 2006) has reported that inhibition of STAT3 expression increases the sensitivity of ovarian cancer cell lines to paclitaxel treatment *in vitro*, suggesting that the STAT3 pathway may also be involved in chemoresistance of ovarian cancer cells. They found that IL-6 induced phosphorylation of STAT3 in several, but not all, of the examined ovarian cancer cell lines. However, it is possible that STAT3 could be activated also through IL-6-independent mechanisms such as Src, epidermal growth factor receptor, or other cytokines like oncostatin in different cancer cells.

In conclusion, IL-6 secreted by ovarian cancer and/or immune cells may contribute to the refractoriness of these cells to conventional chemotherapy through down-regulation of various signalling step. IL-6-induced chemoresistance may be associated with increase of both multidrug resistance-related genes (MDR1 and GSTpi) and apoptosis inhibitory proteins (Bcl-2, BclxL and XIAP), as well as activation of Ras/MEK/ERK and PI3K/Akt. Then, modulation of IL-6 expression or its related signalling pathways may be a promising strategy of treatment for drug-resistant EOC.

Also COX-2 could represent a possible new marker of sensitivity to platinum-based chemotherapy in ovarian cancer. In a study by Ferrandina et al in a population of advanced ovarian cancer patients, COX-2 positivity was found in a statistically significant higher percentage of unresponsive cases than in patients responding to chemotherapy (Ferrandina et al., 2002b). The association between COX-2 positivity and poor chance of response to treatment was retained in multivariate analysis. The ability of COX-2 to predict tumour sensitivity to chemotherapy is not dependent on EGFR or Her-2/neu status and could be independently associated with prognosis. Therefore, in this context, the availability of agents able to specifically interfere with COX-2 is of potential interest.

5. Inflammation and possible therapeutic implications

Our knowledge on ovarian cancer-related inflammation offers innovative therapeutic strategies. For many years, all efforts to treat cancer have concentrated on the destruction/inhibition of tumour cells. Strategies to modulate the host microenvironment offer a complementary perspective. Primary proinflammatory cytokines represent the main targets and ongoing results in this direction justify continuing efforts (Colotta et al., 2009).

In particular, IL-6, as described above, plays a central role in EOC in promoting tumour growth and progression and influencing its prognosis and related symptoms. Collectively, all data available in the literature and reported in the previous sections of this chapter lead to hypothesize that IL-6 antagonists may have therapeutic activity in patients with ovarian cancer via inhibition of a tumour-promoting cytokine network. Accordingly to this evidence, Coward et al. (Coward et al., 2011) carried out an experimental study to assess the activity of the anti-human-IL-6 antibody siltuximab (CNTO328) in tissue culture of EOC and human ovarian cancer xenografts. The authors demonstrated that IL-6 is expressed both in malignant cells and infiltrating leukocytes, endothelial cells and stromal fibroblast. In addition, they found that high IL-6 expression in EOC cells was associated with poor prognosis. Vice versa, IL-6 inhibition prevents the constitutive production of IL-6 and other inflammatory and angiogenic mediators by EOC cells. Additionally, siltuximab had also a significant inhibitory effect on tumour cell proliferation, macrophage infiltration and angiogenesis. In the same paper Coward et al presented the results of a single arm phase II clinical trial of the anti-human IL-6 monoclonal antibody siltuximab in women with recurrent ovarian cancer. Interestingly, they showed that siltuximab, given as a single agent, has some clinical activity in recurrent, platinum-resistant ovarian cancer. A total of eight patients achieved radiological disease stabilisation, which lasted six months or more in four cases. One of these eight also had normalisation of CA125 that lasted for 12 weeks, giving an overall partial response by combined RECIST/CA125 criteria. Noteworthy, partial response was accompanied by a reduction in ^{18}F FDG uptake as detected by PET/TC imaging. Moreover, siltuximab treatment induced a decline in plasma levels of CRP, CCL2, CXCL12, VEGF and IL-8. Also a significant increase in Hb levels occurred in the majority of patients. The study by Coward et al is the first clinical study of anti-IL-6 therapy carried out in a population of EOC patients. Several experimental studies support the rationale for using this anti-IL-6 mAb in EOC. In fact, it has been demonstrated that siltuximab specifically suppress IL-6-induced STAT3 phosphorylation and STAT3 nuclear translocation, as well as the levels of Stat3 downstream proteins such as MCL-1, Bcl-X (L), and surviving, thus targeting the main intracellular mediator of the effects of cytokines on EOC cells growth (Guo et al., 2010).

Indeed, as well described above, STAT3 is constitutively active in EOC and leads to increased expression of genes regulating survival and proliferation, and drives the malignant behaviour of these cells. Therefore, the identification of novel compounds that selectively inhibit STAT3 activity may lead to additional useful tools to reduce cancer-associated cell proliferation, inflammation, and chemotherapeutic resistance. A potent and selective STAT3 inhibitor has been identified through the use of high throughput screening, synthetic medicinal chemistry, and molecular assays. Due to the central role of aberrant STAT3 signalling in ovarian cancer pathogenesis, this compound may provide a useful starting point for the development of chemical scaffolds to block STAT3 signalling for cancer therapy (Madoux et al., 2010). In particular, STAT3 dimerization inhibitors could play a significant role in the future of cancer and adjuvant cancer therapies (Lavecchia et al., 2011).

STAT3 activation is also induced by hypoxia that is commonly observed in many solid tumours and represents a major obstacle to chemo- or radiation therapy. In an experimental animal model it has been shown that exposure of mice containing human ovarian cancer xenograft tumour to hyperbaric oxygen (HBO) obtained a significant reduction in tumour volume, associated with a significant decrease of STAT3 (Tyr 705) activation and cyclin-D1 protein/mRNA levels. Interestingly, HBO exposure, in combination with weekly administration of cisplatin, also significantly reduced the tumour volume. Therefore, therapeutic strategies able to increase tumour oxygenation may be able to inhibit key steps, such as STAT3 activation, involved in the ovarian tumour progression. (Selvendiran et al., 2010). Moreover, the reduced effectiveness of conventional chemotherapeutic drugs cisplatin and taxol in eliminating the hypoxic ovarian cancer cells suggests a role for pSTAT3 in cellular resistance to chemotherapy. It has been shown that inhibition of STAT3 followed by treatment with cisplatin or taxol resulted in a significant increase in apoptosis supporting the hypothesis that hypoxia-induced STAT3 activation is responsible for chemoresistance (Selvendiran et al., 2009). According to this evidence the correction of anaemia and the maintenance of adequate Hb levels during cancer chemotherapy should be addressed as a fundamental outcome in the therapeutic strategies of EOC.

Disruption of STAT3 could also be therefore an effective approach to control EOC tumorigenesis. Among the several compounds tested for chemoprevention of EOC curcumin is one of the most interesting and studied. Curcumin is a dihydroxyphenolic compound, whose anti-tumour mechanisms involve regulation of STAT-3 and the negative regulators of STAT-3, including suppressors of cytokine signalling proteins (SOCS-1 and SOCS-3), protein inhibitors of activated STAT (PIAS-1 and PIAS-3), and SH2 domain-containing phosphatases (SHP-1 and SHP-2). Treatment of ovarian cancer cells with curcumin induced a dose- and time-dependent decrease of constitutive IL-6 expression and IL-6-induced STAT-3 phosphorylation, which is associated with decreased cell viability and increased cleavage of caspase-3. Moreover, curcumin suppresses JAK-STAT signalling also via activation of PIAS-3, thus attenuating STAT-3 phosphorylation and tumour cell growth (Saydmohammed et al., 2010). The activity of curcumin on STAT3 is also mediated by its ability to inhibit lysophosphatidic acid (LPA) which is a biolipid that stimulates tumour cell invasion and metastasis by inducing phosphorylation of STAT3 as well as IL-6 and IL-8 secretion, which in turn results in STAT3 phosphorylation. Treatment of the cells with curcumin inhibited LPA-induced IL-6 and IL-8 secretion and STAT3 phosphorylation, leading to blocked ovarian cancer cell motility (Seo et al., 2010).

Since the same inflammatory mediators that promote tumour growth also are responsible for cancer-related symptoms, i.e., cachexia/anorexia, anaemia, fatigue, pain, debilitation and shortened survival, a concerted effort should be made to attack inflammation alongside with other anticancer measures at initial diagnosis with the consequent probability of improving both patient quality of life and survival (MacDonald, 2007). Therefore, counteracting cancer-related inflammation is certainly a key target in the therapeutic approach of symptoms associated to advanced cancer, especially in EOC patients who are diagnosed at advanced stage and suffer of severe distressing symptoms. A suggestive example of how the modulation of inflammation may be useful in the care of EOC patients is represented by the efficacy of lactoferrin in association to rHuEPO in the treatment of chemotherapy-induced anaemia. In fact, lactoferrin is a specific protein involved in iron transport mechanisms, which has also an important role in host defence against infection and excessive inflammation. Results from a recent open label randomised phase III study of our group (Macciò et al., 2010), including EOC patients (20% in each arm), demonstrated that lactoferrin plus rHuEPO was able to increase Hb levels with a efficacy similar to iron i.v. in term of haematopoietic response but with a better capacity to modulate iron homeostasis and inflammation (as demonstrated by decrease of ferritin and CRP levels in patients treated with lactoferrin).

Specific inhibition of proinflammatory cytokines, and particularly IL-6, has also been tested in the therapeutic approach of cancer-related cachexia. Preliminary results form a phase I study showed that i.v. infusion of a specific anti-IL-6 MoAb was able to reverse fatigue, increase haemoglobin and albumin, and improve muscle strength (Clarke et al., 2009). However, according to the most recent findings, the best management of cancer-related symptoms, such as weight loss, muscle wasting, anorexia, anaemia, fatigue, which globally define the clinical picture of cachexia, requires a multimodal approach by a multi-disciplinary team and is best commenced earlier rather than later (Bosaeus, 2008). Intervention should include dietary counselling, nutritional and vitamin supplementation, exercise concordant with the patient's physical condition, anti-inflammatory agents, anabolic drugs and the most adequate symptom managements.

In the context of such combined approaches, one of the most intriguing ones was an open phase II trial published by our group (Mantovani et al., 2006) which aimed to test the safety and efficacy of an integrated treatment based on diet, pharmaconutritional support administered orally, and drugs in a population of cachectic patients with advanced cancer at different sites, including also a significant percentage of EOC patients. The treatment consisted of diet with high polyphenols content (400 mg), antioxidant treatment (300 mg/day alpha lipoic acid+2.7 g/day carbocysteine lysine salt+400 mg/day vitamin E+30,000 IU/day vitamin A+500 mg/day vitamin C), and pharmaconutritional support enriched with two cans per day (n−3)-PUFA (eicosapentaenoic acid and docosahexaenoic acid), 500 mg/day MPA and 200 mg/day selective cyclooxygenase-2 inhibitor celecoxib. The treatment duration was 4 months. Body weight increased significantly from baseline, as did LBM and appetite. There was an important decrease of proinflammatory cytokines IL-6 and TNF-α, and a negative relationship worthy of note was found between LBM and IL-6 changes. As for quality of life, there was a significant improvement in the European Organization for Research and Treatment of Cancer (EORTC) QLQ-C30, Euro QL-5D and fatigue assessed by Multidimensional Fatigue Symptom Inventory-Short Form (MFSI-SF) scores. The results overall showed the treatment to be both safe (without significant adverse events) and effective as for increase of body weight, increase of LMB, decrease of proinflammatory cytokines, improvement of quality of life parameters, amelioration of fatigue symptom. On the basis of these results, we started a phase III randomized clinical trial (Mantovani et al., 2010) to establish which was the most effective and safest treatment of CACS and oxidative stress in improving selected key variables as primary endpoints: increase of LBM, decrease of REE, increase of total daily physical activity, decrease of IL-6 and TNF-α, and improvement of fatigue. Three hundred thirty-two assessable patients with cancer-related anorexia/cachexia syndrome, including a significant proportion of advanced EOC patients, were enrolled. All patients were given as basic treatment polyphenols plus antioxidant agents alpha-lipoic acid, carbocysteine, and vitamins A, C, and E, all orally administered. Then patients were randomly assigned to one of five treatment arms: arm 1, MPA (500 mg/day) or MA (320 mg/day); arm 2, oral supplementation with EPA; arm 3, L-carnitine (4 g/day); arm 4, thalidomide (200 mg/day); and arm 5, a combination of the above (Figure 4).

Treatment duration was 4 months. Analysis of variance showed a significant difference between treatment arms. A post hoc analysis showed the superiority of arm 5 over the others for all primary endpoints. An analysis of changes from baseline showed that LBM (by dual-energy X-ray absorptiometry and by L3 computed tomography) significantly increased in arm 5. REE decreased significantly and fatigue improved significantly in arm 5. Appetite increased significantly in arm 5; IL-6 decreased significantly in arm 5 and arm 4; Glasgow Prognostic Score (GPS) and Eastern Cooperative Oncology Group (ECOG) performance status (PS) score decreased significantly in arm 5, arm 4, and arm 3. Toxicity was quite negligible, and was comparable between arms. In conclusion, the most effective treatment in terms of all three primary efficacy endpoints and the secondary endpoints appetite, IL-6, GPS, and ECOG PS score was the combination regimen that included all selected agents.

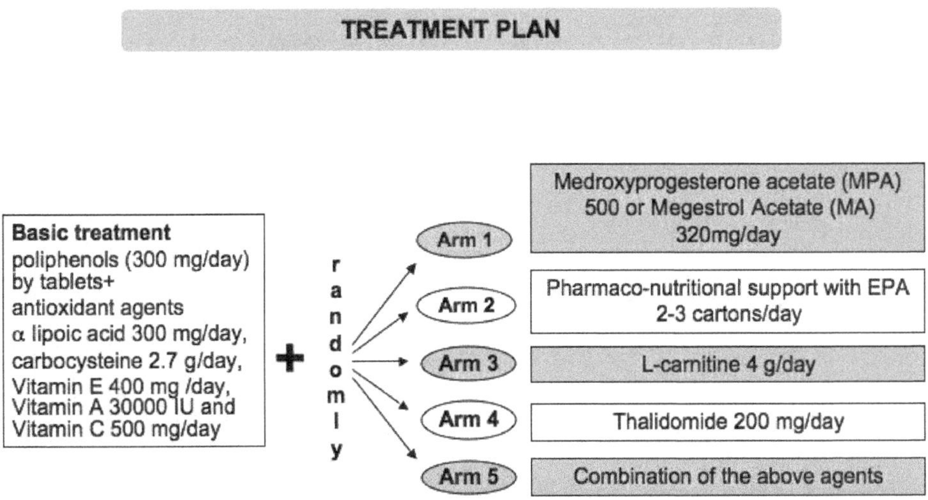

Fig. 4. Phase III randomised clinical trial of five different arms of treatment for cancer cachexia: treatment plan.

6. Conclusion

Proinflammatory cytokines, and in particular IL-6, as demonstrated in the present chapter, are involved in the development and progression of EOC. They are also associated with fatigue, depression, anaemia, pain and cachexia that impact significantly quality of life. Strategies to inhibit the effect of inflammation and such cytokines might therefore have a profound effect on quality of life and survival. In particular, IL-6 antagonism seems to have the most promising therapeutic activity in EOC patients but further clinical trials testing it both alone and in a multimodal approach are warranted. Certainly, from the body of evidence described in this chapter, it is clear that the assessment of inflammation markers, and especially IL-6, should be included in monitoring EOC during its course, from diagnosis to terminal stages, in order to develop the most appropriate care of EOC patients and allow the best supportive therapy considered as the irreplaceable therapeutic approach concurring to patients global well-being.

7. References

Ali-Fehmi, R., Semaan, A., Sethi, S., Arabi, H., Bandyopadhyay, S., Hussein, Y.R., Diamond, M.P., Saed, G., Morris, R.T., & Munkarah, A.R. (2011). Molecular typing of epithelial ovarian carcinomas using inflammatory markers. *Cancer* Vol. 117, No. 2 (January 2011), pp. 301-309

Altinoz MA, & Korkmaz R. (2004). NF-kappaB, macrophage migration inhibitory factor and cyclooxygenase-inhibitions as likely mechanisms behind the acetaminophen- and NSAID-prevention of the ovarian cancer. *Neoplasma* Vol. 51, No. 4, pp. 239-247

Argilés, J.M., & López-Soriano, F.J. The role of cytokines in cancer cachexia. *Medicinal Research Reviews* Vol. 19, No. 3 (May 1999), pp. 223-248

Arriba, L.N., Fader, A.N., Frasure, H.E., & von Gruenigen, V.E. (2010). A review of issues surrounding quality of life among women with ovarian cancer. *Gynecologic Oncology* Vol. 119, No. 2 (November 2010), pp. 390-396

Bast, R.C. Jr, Boyer, C.M., Jacobs, I., Xu, F.J., Wu, S., Wiener, J., Kohler, M., & Berchuck, A. (1993). Cell growth regulation in epithelial ovarian cancer. *Cancer* Vol. 71, no. 4 Suppl (February 1993), pp. 1597-1601

Bennani-Baiti, N., & Davis MP. (2008). Cytokines and cancer anorexia cachexia syndrome. *The American Journal of Hospice & Palliative Care* Vol. 25, No. 5 (October-November 2008), pp. 407-411

Bosaeus, I. (2008). Nutritional support in multimodal therapy for cancer cachexia. *Support Care Cancer* Vol. 16, No. 5 (May 2008), pp. 447-451

Carlson, L.E., Speca, M., Patel, K.D., & Goodey, E. (2003). Mindfulness-based stress reduction in relation to quality of life, mood, symptoms of stress, and immune parameters in breast and prostate cancer outpatients. *Psychosomatic Medicine* Vol. 65, No. 4 (July-August 2003), pp. 571-581

Chan, J.L., Heist, K., DePaoli, A.M., Veldhuis, J.D., & Mantzoros, C.S. (2003). The role of falling leptin levels in the neuroendocrine and metabolic adaptation to short-term starvation in healthy men. *Journal of Clinical Investigation* Vol. 111, No. 9 (May 2003), pp. 1409-1421

Clarke SJ, Smith JT, Gebbie C, Sweeney, C., & Olszewski, N. (2009). A phase I, pharmacokinetic (PK), and preliminary efficacy assessment of ALD518, a humanized anti-IL-6 antibody, in patients with advanced cancer humanized anti-IL-6 antibody, in patients with advanced cancer. J Clin Oncol, Vol. 27, No. 15s (suppl), abstr 3025.

Clendenen, T.V., Lundin, E., Zeleniuch-Jacquotte, A., Koenig, K.L., Berrino, F., Lukanova, A., Lokshin, A.E., Idahl, A., Ohlson, N., Hallmans, G., Krogh, V., Sieri, S., Muti, P., Marrangoni, A., Nolen, B.M., Liu, M., Shore, R.E., & Arslan, A.A. (2011). Circulating inflammation markers and risk of epithelial ovarian cancer. *Cancer epidemiology, biomarkers & prevention* 2011 Vol. 20, No. 5 (May 2011), pp. 799-810

Colomiere, M., Ward, A.C., Riley, C., Trenerry, M.K., Cameron-Smith, D., Findlay, J., Ackland, L., & Ahmed, N. (2009). Cross talk of signals between EGFR and IL-6R through JAK2/STAT3 mediate epithelial-mesenchymal transition in ovarian carcinomas. *British Journal of Cancer* Vol. 100, No. 1 (January 2009), pp. 134-144

Colotta, F., Allavena, P., Sica, A., Garlanda, C., & Mantovani, A. (2009). Cancer-related inflammation, the seventh hallmark of cancer: links to genetic instability. *Carcinogenesis* Vol. 30, No. 7 (July 2009), pp. 1073-1081

Costanzo, E.S., Lutgendorf, S.K., Sood, A.K., Anderson, B., Sorosky, J., & Lubaroff, D.M. (2005). Psychosocial factors and interleukin-6 among women with advanced ovarian cancer. *Cancer* Vol. 104, No. 2 (July 2005), pp. 305-313

Coward, J., Kulbe, H., Chakravarty, P., Leader, D.A., Vassileva, V., Leinster, D.A., Thompson, R., Schioppa, T., Nemeth, J.A., Vermeulin, J., Singh, N., Avril, N.E., Cummings, J., Rexhepaj, E., Jirstrom, K., Gallagher, W.M., Brennan, D.J., McNeish, I.A., & Balkwill, F.R. (2011). Interleukin-6 as a therapeutic target in human ovarian cancer. *Clin Cancer Res*. 2011 Jul 27.

Cubillos-Ruiz, J.R., Rutkowski, M., & Conejo-Garcia, J.R. (2010). Blocking ovarian cancer progression by targeting tumor microenvironmental leukocytes. *Cell Cycle* Vol. 9, No. 2 (January 2010), pp. 260-268

Curiel., T.J., Coukos, G., Zou, L., Alvarez, X., Cheng, P., Mottram, P., Evdemon-Hogan, M., Conejo-Garcia, J.R., Zhang, L., Burow, M., Zhu, Y., Wei, S., Kryczek, I., Daniel, B., Gordon, A., Myers, L., Lackner, A., Disis, M.L., Knutson, K.L., Chen, L., & Zou, W. (2004). Specific recruitment of regulatory T cells in ovarian carcinoma fosters immune privilege and predicts reduced survival. *Nature Medicine* Vol 10, No. 9 (September 2004), pp. 942-949

Delano, M.J., & Moldawer, L,L. (2006). The origins of cachexia in acute and chronic inflammatory diseases. *Nutr Clin Pract* Vol. 21, No. 1 (February 2006), pp. 68-81

Duan, Z., Foster, R., Bell, D.A., Mahoney, J., Wolak, K., Vaidya, A., Hampel, C., Lee, H., & Seiden, M,V. (2006). Signal transducers and activators of transcription 3 pathway activation in drug-resistant ovarian cancer. *Clin Cancer Res* Vol. 12, No. 17 (September 2006), pp. 5055-5063

Fairey, A.S., Courneya, K.S., Field, C.J., Bell, G.J., Jones, L.W., & Mackey, J.R. (2005). Randomized controlled trial of exercise and blood immune function in postmenopausal breast cancer survivors. *J Appl Physiol* Vol. 98, No. 4 (April 2005), pp. 1534-1540

Ferrandina, G., Ranelletti, F.O., Lauriola, L., Fanfani, F., Legge, F., Mottolese, M., Nicotra, M.R., Natali, P.G., Zakut, V.H., & Scambia, G. (2002). Cyclooxygenase-2 (COX-2), epidermal growth factor receptor (EGFR), and Her-2/neu expression in ovarian cancer. *Gynecologic Oncology* Vol. 85, No. 2 (May 2002), pp. 305-310

Ferrandina, G., Lauriola, L., Zannoni, G.F., Fagotti, A., Fanfani, F., Legge, F., Maggiano, N., Gessi, M., Mancuso, S., Ranelletti, F.O., & Scambia, G. (2002). Increased cyclooxygenase-2 (COX-2) expression is associated with chemotherapy resistance and outcome in ovarian cancer patients. *Annals of Oncology* Vol 13, No. 8 (August 2002), pp. 1205-1211

Gavalas, N.G., Karadimou, A., Dimopoulos, M.A., & Bamias, A. (2010). Immune response in ovarian cancer: how is the immune system involved in prognosis and therapy: potential for treatment utilization. *Clinical & Developmental Immunology* Vol. 2010 (January 2011), pp. 791603.

Giuntoli, R.L. 2nd, Webb, T.J., Zoso, A., Rogers, O., Diaz-Montes, T.P., Bristow, R.E., & Oelke, M. (2009). Ovarian cancer-associated ascites demonstrates altered immune environment: implications for antitumor immunity. *Anticancer Research* Vol. 29, No. 8 (August 2009), pp. 2875-2884

Hagemann, T., Wilson, J., Burke, F., Kulbe, H., Li, N.F., Plüddemann, A., Charles, K., Gordon, S., & Balkwill, F.R. (2006). Ovarian cancer cells polarize macrophages toward a tumor-associated phenotype. *J Immunol* Vol. 176, No. 8 (April 2006), pp. 5023-5032

Havel, P.J. (2004). Update on adipocyte hormones: regulation of energy balance and carbohydrate/lipid metabolism. *Diabetes* Vol. 53, Suppl. 1 (February 2004), pp. S143-S151

Jeannin, P., Duluc, D., & Delneste, Y. (2011). IL-6 and leukemia-inhibitory factor are involved in the generation of tumor-associated macrophage: regulation by IFN-γ. *Immunotherapy* Vol. 3, No. 4 Suppl (April 2011), pp. 23-26

Kim, S., Hagemann, A., & DeMichele, A. (2009). Immuno-modulatory gene polymorphisms and outcome in breast and ovarian cancer. *Immunological Investigations* Vol. 38, No. 3-4, pp. 324-340

Landen, C.N. Jr., Birrer, M.J., & Sood, A.K. (2008). Early events in the pathogenesis of epithelial ovarian cancer. *Journal of Clinical Oncology* Vol. 26, No. 6 (February 2008), pp. 995-1005

Lane, D., Matte, I., Rancourt, C., & Piché, A. (2011). Prognostic significance of IL-6 and IL-8 ascites levels in ovarian cancer patients. *BMC Cancer* Vol. 11 (May 2011), pp. 210

Lavecchia, A., Di Giovanni, C., & Novellino, E. (2011). STAT-3 inhibitors: state of the art and new horizons for cancer treatment. *Current Medicinal Chemistry* Vol 18, No. 16, pp. 2359-2375

Leffers, N., Gooden, M.J., de Jong, R.A., Hoogeboom, B.N., ten Hoor, K.A., Hollema, H., Boezen, H.M., van der Zee, A.G., Daemen, T., & Nijman, H.W. (2009). Prognostic significance of tumor-infiltrating T-lymphocytes in primary and metastatic lesions of advanced stage ovarian cancer. *Cancer Immunol Immunother* Vol. 58, No. 3 (March 2009), pp. 449-459

Liao, S., Liu, J., Lin, P., Shi, T., Jain, R.K., & Xu, L. (2011). TGF-beta blockade controls ascites by preventing abnormalization of lymphatic vessels in orthotopic human ovarian carcinoma models. *Clin Cancer Res* Vol. 17, No. 6 (March 2011), pp. 1415-1424

Lo, C.W., Chen, M.W., Hsiao, M., Wang, S., Chen, C.A., Hsiao, S.M., Chang, J.S., Lai, T.C., Rose-John, S., Kuo, M.L., & Wei, L.H. (2011). IL-6 trans-signaling in formation and progression of malignant ascites in ovarian cancer. *Cancer Research* Vol. 71, No. 2 (Jan 2011), pp. 424-434

Lurie, G., Thompson, P.J., McDuffie, K.E., Carney, M.E., & Goodman MT. (2009). Prediagnostic symptoms of ovarian carcinoma: a case-control study. *Gynecologic Oncology* Vol. 114, No. 2 (August 2009), pp. 231-236

Lutgendorf, S.K., Weinrib, A.Z., Penedo, F., Russell, D., DeGeest, K., Costanzo, E.S., Henderson, P.J., Sephton, S.E., Rohleder, N., Lucci, J.A. 3rd, Cole, S., Sood, A.K., & Lubaroff, D.M. (2008). Interleukin-6, cortisol, and depressive symptoms in ovarian cancer patients. *J Clin Oncol* Vol. 26, No. 29 (October 2008), pp. 4820-4827

Macciò, A., Mantovani, G., Turnu, E., Artini, P., Contu, G., & Volpe, A. (1994). Preovulatory human follicular fluid in vitro inhibits interleukin (IL)-1 alpha, IL-2, and production and expression of p55 chain IL-2 receptor of lymphomonocytes. *Fertility and Sterility* Vol. 62, No. 2 (August 1994), pp. 327-332

Macciò, A., Lai, P., Santona, M.C., Pagliara, L., Melis, G.B., & Mantovani, G. (1998). High serum levels of soluble IL-2 receptor, cytokines, and C reactive protein correlate with impairment of T cell response in patients with advanced epithelial ovarian cancer. *Gynecology Oncology* Vol 69, No. 3 (June 1998), pp. 248-252

Macciò, A., Madeddu, C., Massa, D., Mudu, M.C., Lusso, M.R., Gramignano, G., Serpe, R., Melis, G.B., & Mantovani G. (2005). Hemoglobin levels correlate with interleukin-6 levels in patients with advanced untreated epithelial ovarian cancer: role of inflammation in cancer-related anemia. *Blood* Vol. 106, No. 1 (July 2005), pp. 362-367

Macciò, A., Madeddu, C., Massa, D., Astara, G., Farci, D., Melis, G.B., & Mantovani, G. (2009). Interleukin-6 and leptin as markers of energy metabolic changes in advanced ovarian cancer patients. *Journal of Cellular and Molecular Medicine* Vol. 13, No. 9B (September 2009), pp. 3951-3959

Macciò, A., Madeddu, C., Gramignano, G., Mulas, C., Sanna, E., & Mantovani, G. (2010). Efficacy and safety of oral lactoferrin supplementation in combination with rHuEPO-beta for the treatment of anemia in advanced cancer patients undergoing chemotherapy: open-label, randomized controlled study. *Oncologist* Vol. 15, No. 8 (July 2010), pp. 894-902

MacDonald, N. (2007). Cancer cachexia and targeting chronic inflammation: a unified approach to cancer treatment and palliative/supportive care. The Journal of Supportive Oncology Vol. 5, No. 4 (April 2007), pp. 157-162

Madoux, F., Koenig, M., Sessions, H., Nelson, E., Mercer, B.A., Cameron, M., Roush, W., Frank, D., & Hodder, P. (2010). Modulators of STAT Transcription Factors for the Targeted Therapy of Cancer (STAT3 Inhibitors). Probe Reports from the NIH Molecular Libraries Program [Internet]. Bethesda (MD): National Center for Biotechnology Information (US) (August 2009) updated 2011 Mar 25

Mantovani, G., Macciò, A., Pisano, M., Versace, R., Lai, P., Esu, S., Massa, E., Ghiani, M., Dessì, D., Melis, G.B., & Del Giacco, G.S. (1997). Tumor-associated lympho-monocytes from neoplastic effusions are immunologically defective in comparison with patient autologous PBMCs but are capable of releasing high amounts of various cytokines. International Journal of Cancer Vol. 71, No. 5 (May 1997), pp. 724-731

Mantovani, G., Macciò, A., Massa, E., Lai, P., Manca, G., Mudu, C., Versace, R., & Pusceddu G. (1999). Relationships betxween Fas expression, activation molecule CD25, and functional activity of tumor-associated lymphomonocytes from neoplastic effusions. *Oncology Reports* Vol. 6, No. 1 (January-February 1999), pp. 235-239

Mantovani, G., Macciò, A., Melis, G., Mura, L., Massa, E., & Mudu, M.C. (2000). Restoration of functional defects in peripheral blood mononuclear cells isolated from cancer patients by thiol antioxidants alpha-lipoic acid and N-acetyl cysteine. *Int J Cancer* Vol 86, No. 6 (June 2000), pp. 842-847

Mantovani, G., Macciò, A., Massa, E., & Madeddu C. (2001). Managing cancer-related anorexia/cachexia. *Drugs* Vol. 61, No. 4, pp. 499-514

Mantovani, G., Macciò, A., Madeddu, C., Mura, L., Gramignano, G., Lusso, M.R., Mulas, C., Mudu, M.C., Murgia, V., Camboni, P., Massa, E., Ferreli, L., Contu, P., Rinaldi, A., Sanjust, E., Atzei, D., & Elsener, B. (2002). Quantitative evaluation of oxidative stress, chronic inflammatory indices and leptin in cancer patients: correlation with stage and performance status. *International Journal of Cancer* Vol. 98, No. 1 (March 2002), pp. 84-91

Mantovani, G., Macciò, A., Madeddu, C., Mura, L., Gramignano, G., Lusso, M.R., Massa, E., Mocci, M., & Serpe, R. (2003). Antioxidant agents are effective in inducing lymphocyte progression through cell cycle in advanced cancer patients: assessment of the most important laboratory indexes of cachexia and oxidative stress. *J Mol Med (Berl)* Vol. 81, No. 10 (October 2003), pp. 664-73

Mantovani, G., Macciò, A., Madeddu, C., Gramignano, G., Lusso, M.R., Serpe, R., Massa, E., Astara, G., & Deiana, L. (2006). A phase II study with antioxidants, both in the diet and supplemented, pharmaconutritional support, progestagen, and anti-cyclooxygenase-2 showing efficacy and safety in patients with cancer-related anorexia/cachexia and oxidative stress. Cancer Epidemiology Biomarkers & Prevention Vol. 15, No. 5 (May 2006), pp. 1030-1034

Mantovani, G., Macciò, A., Madeddu, C., Serpe, R., Massa, E., Dessì, M., Panzone, F., & Contu, P. (2010). Randomized phase III clinical trial of five different arms of treatment in 332 patients with cancer cachexia. *Oncologist* Vol. 15, No. 2 (February 2010), pp. 200-211.

Min, H., & Wei-hong, Z. (2009). Constitutive activation of signal transducer and activator of transcription 3 in epithelial ovarian carcinoma. *The journal of obstetrics and gynaecology research* Vol 35, No. 5 (October 2009), pp. 918-925

Minton, O., Richardson, A., Sharpe, M., Hotopf, M., & Stone, P. (2010). Drug therapy for the management of cancer-related fatigue. *Cochrane Database Syst Rev* 2010 Jul 7;(7):CD006704.

Monk, J.P., Phillips, G., Waite, R., Kuhn, J., Schaaf, L.J., Otterson, G.A., Guttridge, D., Rhoades, C., Shah, M., Criswell, T., Caligiuri, M.A., & Villalona-Calero, M.A. (2006). Assessment of tumor necrosis factor alpha blockade as an intervention to improve tolerability of dose-intensive chemotherapy in cancer patients. *J Clin Oncol* Vol. 24, No. 12 (April 2006), pp. 1852-1859

Mor, G., Visintin, I., Lai, Y., Zhao, H., Schwartz, P., Rutherford, T., Yue, L., Bray-Ward, P., Ward, D.C. (2005). Serum protein markers for early detection of ovarian cancer. *Proc Natl Acad Sci U S A* Vol. 102, No. 21 (May 2005), pp. 7677-7682

Napoletano C, Bellati F, Landi R, Pauselli S, Marchetti C, Visconti V, Sale P, Liberati M, Rughetti A, Frati L, Panici PB, Nuti M. Ovarian cancer cytoreduction induces changes in T cell population subsets reducing immunosuppression. J Cell Mol Med. 2010 Dec;14(12):2748-59. doi: 10.1111/j.1582-4934.2009.00911.x.

Nowak, M., Glowacka, E., Szpakowski, M., Szyllo, K., Malinowski, A., Kulig, A., Tchorzewski, H., & Wilczynski, J. (2010). Proinflammatory and immunosuppressive serum, ascites and cyst fluid cytokines in patients with early and advanced ovarian cancer and benign ovarian tumors. *Neuro Endocrinology Letters*, Vol. 31, No. 3, pp. 375-83

Nowak, M., Klink, M., Glowacka, E., Sulowska, Z., Kulig, A., Szpakowski, M., Szyllo, K., & Tchorzewski, H. (2010). Production of cytokines during interaction of peripheral blood mononuclear cells with autologous ovarian cancer cells or benign ovarian tumour cells. *Scand J Immunol* Vol 71, No. 2 (February 2010), pp. 91-98

Plante, M., Rubin, S.C., Wong, G.Y., Federici, M.G., Finstad, C.L., & Gastl, G.A. (1994). Interleukin-6 level in serum and ascites as a prognostic factor in patients with epithelial ovarian cancer. *Cancer* Vol. 73, No. 7 (April 1994), pp. 1882-1888

Rabinovich, A., Medina, L., Piura, B., Segal, S., & Huleihel, M. (2007). Regulation of ovarian carcinoma SKOV-3 cell proliferation and secretion of MMPs by autocrine IL-6. *Anticancer Research* Vol. 27, No. 1A (Jan-Feb 2007), pp. 267-272

Rath, K.S., Funk, H.M., Bowling, M.C., Richards, W.E., & Drew, A.F. (2010). Expression of soluble interleukin-6 receptor in malignant ovarian tissue. *American Journal of Obstetrics and Gynecology* Vol. 203, No. 3 (September 2010), pp. 230.e1-8

Robinson-Smith, T.M., Isaacsohn, I., Mercer, C.A., Zhou, M., Van Rooijen, N., Husseinzadeh, N., McFarland-Mancini, M.M., & Drew, A.F. (2007). Macrophages mediate inflammation-enhanced metastasis of ovarian tumors in mice. *Cancer Research* Vol 67, No. 12 (June 2007), pp. 5708-5716

Rosen, D.G., Mercado-Uribe, I., Yang, G., Bast, R.C. Jr, Amin, H.M., Lai, R., & Liu, J. (2006). The role of constitutively active signal transducer and activator of transcription 3 in ovarian tumorigenesis and prognosis. *Cancer* Vol. 107, No. 11 (December 2006), pp. 2730-2740

Saydmohammed, M., Joseph, D., & Syed V. (2010). Curcumin suppresses constitutive activation of STAT-3 by up-regulating protein inhibitor of activated STAT-3 (PIAS-3) in ovarian and endometrial cancer cells. *Journal of Cellular Biochemistry* Vol. 110, No. 2 (May 2010), pp. 447-456

Scambia, G., Testa, U., Benedetti Panici, P., Foti, E., Martucci, R., Gadducci, A., Perillo, A., Facchini, V., Peschle, C., & Mancuso, S. (1995). Prognostic significance of interleukin 6 serum levels in patients with ovarian cancer. *British Journal of Cancer* Vol. 71, No. 2 (February 1995), pp. 354-356

Scarlett, U.K., Cubillos-Ruiz, J.R., Nesbeth, Y.C., Martinez, D.G., Engle, X., Gewirtz, A.T., Ahonen, C.L., & Conejo-Garcia, J.R. (2009). In situ stimulation of CD40 and Toll-like receptor 3 transforms ovarian cancer-infiltrating dendritic cells from immunosuppressive to immunostimulatory cells. *Cancer Research* Vol. 69, No. 18 (September 2009), pp. 7329-7337

Selvendiran, K., Bratasz, A., Kuppusamy, M.L., Tazi, M.F., Rivera, B.K., & Kuppusamy, P. (2009). Hypoxia induces chemoresistance in ovarian cancer cells by activation of signal transducer and activator of transcription 3. *International Journal of Cancer* Vol. 125, No. 9 (November 2009), pp. 2198-2204

Selvendiran, K., Kuppusamy, M.L., Ahmed, S., Bratasz, A., Meenakshisundaram, G., Rivera, B.K., Khan, M., & Kuppusamy, P. (2010). Oxygenation inhibits ovarian tumor growth by downregulating STAT3 and cyclin-D1 expressions. *Cancer Biology & Therapy* Vol. 10, No. 4 (August 2010), pp. 386-390

Seo, J.H., Jeong, K.J., Oh, W.J., Sul, H.J., Sohn, J.S., Kim, Y.K., Cho do, Y., Kang, J.K., Park, C.G., & Lee, H,Y. (2010). Lysophosphatidic acid induces STAT3 phosphorylation and ovarian cancer cell motility: their inhibition by curcumin. *Cancer Letters* Vol. 288, No. 1 (February 2010), pp. 50-56

Smith, L.H. (2006). Early clinical detection of ovarian cancer: a review of the evidence. *Expert Rev Anticancer Ther* Vol. 6, No. 7 (July 2006), pp. 1045-1052

Stevinson, C., Steed, H., Faught, W., Tonkin, K., Vallance, J.K., Ladha, A.B., Schepansky, A., Capstick, V., & Courneya, K.S. (2009). Physical activity in ovarian cancer survivors: associations with fatigue, sleep, and psychosocial functioning. *Int J Gynecol Cancer* Vol. 19, No. 1 (January 2009), pp. 73-78

Straub, R.H., Cutolo, M., Buttgereit, F., & Pongratz, G. (2010). Energy regulation and neuroendocrine-immune control in chronic inflammatory diseases. Journal of Internal Medicine Vol. 267, No. 6 (June 2010), pp. 543-560

Takeda, A., Toda, T., Shinohara, S., Mogi, Y., & Matsui, N. Factors contributing to higher hematocrit levels in hemodialysis patients not receiving recombinant human erythropoietin. *Am J Kidney Dis* Vol. 40, No. 1 (July 2002), pp. 104-109

Thompson, M.S., & Mok, S.C. (2009). Immunopathogenesis of ovarian cancer. *Minerva Medica* Vol. 100, No. 5 (October 2009), pp. 357-370

van Crevel, R., Karyadi, E., Netea, M.G., Verhoef, H., Nelwan, R.H., West, C.E., & van der Meer, J.W. (2002) Decreased plasma leptin concentrations in tuberculosis patients are associated with wasting and inflammation. *Journal of Clinical Endocrinology and Metabolism* Vol 87, No. 2 (February 2002), pp. 758-763

van der Zee, A.G., de Cuyper, E.M., Limburg, P.C., de Bruijn, H.W., Hollema, H., Bijzet, J., Krans, M., & de Vries, E,G. (1995). Higher levels of interleukin-6 in cystic fluids from patients with malignant versus benign ovarian tumors correlate with decreased hemoglobin levels and increased platelet counts. *Cancer* Vol. 75, No. 4 (February 1995), pp. 1004-1009

Visintin, I., Feng, Z., Longton, G., Ward, D.C., Alvero, A.B., Lai, Y., Tenthorey, J., Leiser, A., Flores-Saaib, R., Yu, H., Azori, M., Rutherford, T., Schwartz, P.E., & Mor G. (2008). Diagnostic markers for early detection of ovarian cancer. *Clinical Cancer Research* Vol. 14, No. 4 (February 2008), pp. 1065-1072

Wang, Y., Niu, X.L., Qu, Y., Wu, J., Zhu, Y.Q., Sun, W.J., & Li, L.Z. (2010). Autocrine production of interleukin-6 confers cisplatin and paclitaxel resistance in ovarian cancer cells. *Cancer Letters* Vol. 295, No. 1 (September 2010), pp. 110-123

Weinrib, A.Z., Sephton, S.E., Degeest, K., Penedo, F., Bender, D., Zimmerman, B., Kirschbaum, C., Sood, A.K., Lubaroff, D.M., & Lutgendorf, S.K. (2010). Diurnal cortisol dysregulation, functional disability, and depression in women with ovarian cancer. *Cancer* Vol 116, No. 18 (September 2010), pp. 4410-4419

Wertel, I., Nowicka, A., Rogala, E., & Kotarski, J. (2011). Peritoneal immune system in patients with advance epithelial ovarian cancer. *International Reviews of Immunology* Vol. 30, No. 2-3 (Apr-Jun 2011), pp. 87-101

Yang, J., Wang, Y., Gao, Y., Shao, J., Zhang, X.J., & Yao, Z. (2009). Reciprocal regulation of 17beta-estradiol, interleukin-6 and interleukin-8 during growth and progression of epithelial ovarian cancer. *Cytokine* Vol. 46, No. 3 (June 2009), pp. 382-391

Yigit, R., Massuger, L.F., Figdor, C.G., & Torensma, R. (2010). Ovarian cancer creates a suppressive microenvironment to escape immune elimination. *Gynecologic Oncology* Vol. 117, No. 2 (May 2010), pp. 366-372

Yigit, R., Figdor, C.G., Zusterzeel, P.L., Pots, J.M., Torensma, R., & Massuger, L.F. (2011). Cytokine analysis as a tool to understand tumour-host interaction in ovarian cancer. *European Journal of Cancer* (April 2011)

Zhang, L., Conejo-Garcia, J.R., Katsaros, D., Gimotty, P.A., Massobrio, M., Regnani, G., Makrigiannakis, A., Gray, H., Schlienger, K., Liebman, M.N., Rubin, S.C., & Coukos, G. (2003). Intratumoral T cells, recurrence, and survival in epithelial ovarian cancer. *The New England Journal of Medicine* Vol. 348, No. 3 (January 2003), pp. 203-213

Zhang, X., Liu, P., Zhang, B., Wang, A., & Yang, M. (2010) Role of STAT3 decoy oligodeoxynucleotides on cell invasion and chemosensitivity in human epithelial ovarian cancer cells. *Cancer Genetic and Cytogenetics* Vol. 197, No. 1 (February 2010), pp. 46-53.

2

Epidemiology and Etiology of Ovarian Cancer

Ana Fernández Montes, Jesús García Gómez, Miguel Nuñez Viejo,
Miguel Alonso Bermejo, Susana Alonso Urrutia and Jesús García Mata
Complexo Hospitalario Universitario de Ourense
Spain

1. Introduction

Ovarian cancer is the second most common gynecological malignancy following uterine corpus cancer and it is the fifth leading cause of cancer death in women.

There are important differences in their incidence across the world. In Europe in 2008, estimated incidence was 66,734 cases with an estimated mortality of 41,929 women.

In United States, ovarian cancer was diagnosed in 21,880 with 13,850 cancer deaths last year. Both incidence and mortality are declining in USA and Europe.

Higher incidence rates are observed in North America and European countries exceeding 10 per 100.000 inhabitants. Lower rates are observed in South America (7,7 per 100.000) and Southern Asia (7,5 per 100.000). (Parkin et al, 2005)

Such geographical variations are due to differences in oral contraceptive use practices, pregnancy history, breast-feeding and other hormonal factors. (Permuth -Wey & Sellers, 2009)

The relative risk for developing ovarian cancer is 1.39% (lifetime risk). It affects 12.9 per 100,000 women per year. Incidence rate of ovarian cancer increases with aging, being more prevalent in the eighth decade of life.

At diagnosis, mean age is 63 years, and 62% of patients have advanced disease. Inherited ovarian cancer presents at younger age. (www.Seer.gov,Ferlay et al 2010)

Five year overall survival is 93.5% for localized disease, 73.4% for locoregional disease (regional lymph node involvement) and 27.6% for distant disease.

Genetic studies on ovarian cancer indicate that most of the cases are sporadic while 5 to 10 percent are inherited, generally due to germline mutations.

Three histological subgroups have been described: epithelial tumours, stromal tumours and germ-cell tumours. Ninety percent of cases are epithelial tumours arising from the ovarian surface epithelium or Mullerian derivatives. These tumours are typical in postmenopausal women. The World Health Organization classification defines six more histotypes: serous, mucinous, endometrioid, clear cell and squamous cell carcinomas.

According to their architectural features like glandular or papillary components, carcinomas have been classified into three histological grades, well differentiated, moderately differentiated, poorly or undifferentiated.

Malignant germ cell tumour affects younger women. (De Vita et al,2009)

Despite the high incidence, ovarian cancer etiology is still poorly understood.

The learning objective of this chapter is to review some hormonal, environmental, inherited risk and protective factors associated with ovarian cancer.

2. Risk and protective factors

2.1 Reproductive and hormonal factors

Hormones such as estrogen and progesterone are believed to be involved in promoting ovarian carcinogenesis. Several hypotheses have been postulated.

The "incessant ovulation theory" holds that the risk of ovarian cancer is increased through the repetitive ovulatory microtrauma to the ovarian epithelium. The number of ovulatory cycles increases the rate of cellular division associated with the repair of the surface epithelium after each ovulation, thereby increasing the likelihood of spontaneous mutations that might promote carcinogenesis.

Breast-feeding, pregnancy or oral anticonceptive that suppress ovulation would have a protective effect. (Casagrande et al,1979).

The "pituitary gonadotropin hypothesis" indicates that high levels of estrogens and gonadotropins such as luteinizing hormone and follicle-stimulating hormone would over estimulate ovarian epithelium causing increased proliferation and subsequent malignant transformation (Cramer et al,1983).

Another hypothesis has described that androgens may stimulate ovarian cancer formation whereas progestin are protective. (Risch et al,1998)

The "inflammation hypothesis" proposes that factors such as endometriosis, pelvic inflammatory disease and other inflammatory conditions may stimulate cancer formation. (Ness et al,2000)

The last hypothesis, also called "the ovarian stromal hypothesis" states that there may be a failure of the apoptosis of the granulose and theca cells after ovulation which continued producing steroid hormones, thereby stimulating the formation of cancer. (Vo et al,2007; Purdie et al,2003;Permuth-Wey & Sellers,2009)

2.1.1 Early menarche and late menopause

Due to support the incessant ovulation hypothesis early age at menarche (less than 12 years) and late age at menopause (more than 50 years) should increase the number of ovulatory cycles. Several epidemiological studies have examined this relationship showing a slight increase among women with early age at menarche, Odds Ratio (OR) ranging from 1,1-1,5 and women with late age at menopause with OR ranking from 1,4-4,6 (Permuth-Wey& Sellers,2009).

In contrast to these data another prospective study in healthy nurses found no association between age at menarche and menopause and ovarian cancer risk. (Hankinson et al,1995)

2.1.2 Pregnancy

Nulliparous women tend to have more ovulatory cycles than multiparous women. It has been shown that with each full ovulation year there is a 6 percent increase in risk of ovarian cancer. This finding is specially relevant in the 20 to 29 year age group in which the risk is highest with a 20 percent increase.(Purdie et al,2003) Pregnancy also causes anovulation and suppresses secretion of pituitary gonadotropins. Maternal age of last birth is also implicated in decreasing the risk of ovarian cancer if the last birth was at age of 35 or greater.

Several case-control studies have demonstrated that parous women are estimated to have a 30-60% lower risk for ovarian cancer. Increasing parity seems to reduce risk further. In a recent case-control study between parous and non parous women, higher parity, increased age at first or last birth, and time since last birth were associated with reduced risk of ovarian cancer. This was due to endometrioid and clear cell histology. This link was correlated with reduced risk of epithelial ovarian cancer in another studies. (Titus-Ernstoff et al,2001;Hinkula et al,2006;Whiteman et al,2000) In another prospective study which examined several hormonal factor in 121.700 healthy nurses between 35 to 55 years a statistically significant inverse association was observed between parity and ovarian cancer risk (relative risk [RR] = 0.84; 95% confidence interval [CI] = 0.77-0.91 per pregnancy) ; age at first birth was not associated independently with risk (Hankinson et al,1995). A history of incomplete pregnancy does not influence a woman's risk of epithelial ovarian cancer (Dick et al,2009). Age at last birth also has been strongly associated with a reduced risk of ovarian cancer. Women with a last birth after age 30 to 35 years have a 58% decreased risk for ovarian cancer compared with nulliparous women. One theory to explain this also called the exfoliate theory is based on the suspicion that older women are more likely than younger women to have accumulated transformed surface epithelial ovarian cells, and progestins as suggested before may induced apoptosis of this cells, reducing the account of cells susceptible of malignant transformation (Whiteman et al,2003).

2.1.3 Breastfeeding

Breastfeeding suppresses the secretion of pituitary gonadotropins leading to anovulation. Several studies have demonstrated an inverse association between ovarian cancer and lactation especially for non mucinous subtypes. An increasing period of breastfeeding has also been reported to decrease ovarian cancer risk. (Negri et al,2005;Chiafafrino et al,2005;Chiaffarino et al,2007;Jordan et al,2010) Danforth et al demonstrated that breastfeeding 18 or more months was associated with a significant decrease in ovarian cancer risk compared to never breastfeeding (RR=0.66, 95% CI 0.46-0.96). For each month of breastfeeding the relative risk decreased by 2 percent (RR=0.98 per month, 95% CI 0.97-1.00). (Danforth et al,2007)

2.1.4 Endometriosis

Endometriosis and its hormonally regulated lesions may trigger a local inflammatory reaction with activation of macrophages releasing cytokines and growth factors. Some clinical series have identified the coexistence of endometriosis and ovarian cancer particularly clear cell histology. (Ness et al,2000;Orezzoli et al,2008)

A Canadian cohort study also confirmed this association. They found an anticipation of 5, 5 years between people with endometriosis and ovarian cancer and also an increased risk of ovarian cancer. (Ariset al,2010)

2.1.5 Pelvic inflammatory disease and polycystic ovarian syndrome

Pelvic inflammatory disease has been linked to an increased risk of ovarian cancer, and more if it occurred at an early age, if the women were nulliparous, infertile or had experienced recurrent episodes.(Risch,1995)

Common clinical presentations of polycystic ovarian syndrome (PCOS) include obesity, hirsutism, infertility and menstrual abnormalities. Women with PCOS has an elevated luteinizing hormone to follicle stimulating hormone ratio, hyperandrogenism and abnormal estrogens secretion. Ovarian cancer risk seems higher among women who does not use oral contraceptives. However these data are controversial. Balen et al,2001)

2.1.6 Hormone replacement

The use of hormonal agents such as infertility treatment and their association with ovarian cancer has been subject of discussion for years. The Women's Health Initiative (WHI) study found an increased risk for ovarian cancer with a hazard ratio of 1,58.(Anderson et al,2003)

A metanalysis of eight cohort and 19 case-control studies found a summary relative risk (RR) of 1.24 (95% confidence interval [CI] 1.15-1.34) from cohort studies and a summary odds ratio [OR] of 1.19 (95%CI 1.02-1.40) from case-control studies for ever Hormone replacement therapy (HRT) use. Association was stronger among ERT (estrogen replacement treatment) user than EPRT (estrogen-progestin replacement treatment) user. Based on data abstracted from six case-control studies, duration of HRT use was not significant. The summary risk estimates for less than 5 years, 6-10, and more than 10 years use were 1.02, 1.13, and 1.21, respectively and 95%CI for each estimate crossed 1.0.(Zhou et al,2008) Another observational study from UK in postmenopausal women with no risk factor for ovarian cancer reported that current users of HRT were significantly more likely to develop and die from ovarian cancer than never users (relative risk 1.20 [95% CI 1.09-1.32; p=0.0002] for incident disease and 1.23 [1.09-1.38; p=0.0006] for death). Ovarian cancer increased with increasing duration of use, but did not differ significantly by type of preparation used, its constituents, or mode of administration. Serous carcinoma was more common associated than mucinous, endometrioid, or clear cell tumours. Past users of HRT were not at an increased risk of ovarian cancer. (Beral t al,2007)

The time association between the duration of use of HRT and the risk of development ovarian cancer seems to be between 5 and 10 years and may last up to 29 years after HRT use has stopped. (Danforth et al,2007) In contrast to these findings a recent Danish study found no overall increased risk of ovarian cancer was showed after any use of gonadotrophins, clomifene , human chorionic gonadotrophin , or gonadotrophin releasing hormone. Furthermore, no associations were found between all four groups of fertility drugs and number of cycles of use, length of follow-up, or parity.(Jense et al,2009)

2.1.7 Oral contraception

Several studies have demonstrated that oral contraception decreases the risk of ovarian cancer due to reduction in ovulatory cycles.

Women using oral contraceptives had a risk reduction of ovarian cancer of at least 30 to 40 percent with Lower risk with longer time of use. Use oral contraceptive for more than five years was found to have a stronger reduction than use for less than five years.

In a large review of twelve case-controlled studies in the United States , use of oral contraceptives and reduction ovarian cancer risk had an overall odds ratio of 0,67(95%CI 0,37-1,2) in white women.(Whittemore et al, 1992).

This protective effect continued 15 to 20 years after ceased and was independent of any specific type of oral contraceptive formulation. (Bosetti et al,2002;La Vecchia et al,2006).

In another reanalisis of data of 45 epidemiological studies use of oral contraceptives confers long-term protection against ovarian cancer suggesting that oral contraceptives have

already prevented some 200,000 ovarian cancers and 100,000 ovarian cancer related deaths.(Beral et al,2008)
This was also reported in both carriers and non-carriers of BRCA1 mutation. Reduced risk of ovarian cancer was associated with the use of oral contraceptives, odds ratio of 0.54 (95% confidence interval (CI): 0.26, 1.13) for carriers and 0.55 (95% CI: 0.41, 0.73) for non-carriers. Tubal ligation and increasing parity were also associated with reduced risk. (McGuire et al,2004)
Use for more than five years confers a protective factor for up to 10 years after discontinuation.

2.1.8 Tubal ligation and hysterectomy

Tubal ligation has been documented to decrease the risk of development epithelial ovarian cancer, especially endometrioid tumours. This has been postulated as a result of the reducing utero-ovarian flow and altering local hormonal and growth factor levels. This was also demonstrated for hysterectomy. (Parazzini et al,1993;Tung et al,2003)

3. Environmental factors

Obesity and increasing body mass index (BMI) have been associated with ovarian cancer risk. In a combined study of cohorts BMI was not associated with ovarian cancer risk in postmenopausal women but was positively associated with risk in premenopausal women (Schoute et al,2008). A metanalysis also concluded that being obese (defined as a body mass index over 30) or overweight in the premenopausal years is associated with an increased risk of ovarian cancer, suggesting a possible influence of menopausal status on the endogenous hormonal environment.(Olsen et al,2007)
The risk of ovarian cancer may result from changes in synthesis and bioavailability of endogenous sex esteroids seen in obese women. (Vo et al,2007)
Exposure to talc was associated with ovarian cancer risk due to perineal migration in the past. Noneless a metanalysis did not find any association.(Harlow et al,1992;Huncharek et al,2007)
Cigarette smoking increases risk of mucinous and borderline ovarian tumours but not other histological subtypes. (Zhang et al,2004;Rossing et al,2008).
Hankinson et al studied the relationship between ovarian cancer and several environmental factors. They found in a prospective study which examined 110,454 women that compared with never-smokers, neither current nor past smoking was associated with ovarian cancer risk overall; however, both situations were associated with mucinous tumors (n = 69; rate ratio [RR], past = 2.02 [95% confidence interval (CI), 1.15-3.55]; RR, current = 2.22 [95% CI, 1.16-4.24]). A modest inverse association between caffeine intake and ovarian cancer risk was observed (RR, top vs bottom quintile = 0.80; 95% CI, 0.60-1.07 [P = .03]), which was strongest for women who had never used either oral contraceptives (RR = 0.65; 95% CI, 0.46-0.92 [P for heterogeneity = .02]) or postmenopausal hormones (RR = 0.57; 95% CI, 0.36-0.91 [P for heterogeneity = .13]). Alcohol was not associated with ovarian cancer risk (Hankinson et al,2008).
Another data from alcohol and caffeine intake and ovarian cancer risk are inconclusive.
The impact of diet and physical activity is unknown.
La Vecchia et al found in a case- control study between italian women that meat consumption over 7 portions versus less than 4 portions of meat per week (RR:1,6;95%CI:1,21-2,12)

increased ovarian cancer risk and also the consumption of butter versus fat consumption (RR:1,9;95% CI:1,20-3,11). However some confounding factors were present in the study like body weight, parity, socioeconomic status and contraceptive use. The Women's Health Initiative Dietary Modification Randomized Controlled Trial demonstrated decreased ovarian cancer risk in postmenopausal women after four years of a low-fat diet, although this was not statistically significative. Increased daily fiber intake; the use of carotene, vitamin C, vitamin E, and unsaturated fatty acids; and increased physical activity were moderately associated with a decreased risk of ovarian cancer. However, several confounding factors may coexist, and there is limited evidence to support recommending specific lifestyle modifications to reduce ovarian cancer risk. (Prentice et al,2007)

Another prospective study did not find some relation between consumption of antioxidant vitamins from foods or supplements, or intake of fruits and vegetables, and the incidence of ovarian carcinoma (Fairfield et al,2001).

Milk, calcium and lactose intake were associated with reduced risk in another case-control study. The odds ratio for ovarian cancer was 0.46 (95% confidence interval: 0.27, 0.76) among women in the highest quartile of dietary calcium intake versus the lowest (p for trend = 0.0006). The significant dietary association was limited to dairy sources of calcium (p for trend = 0.003), although a nonsignificant inverse gradient in risk was also found in relation to calcium supplement intake (Goodman et al,2002).

Non steroidal anti-inflammatory drugs have been described as a protective factor of ovarian cancer.

Several hypotheses have been postulated like interruption prostaglandin synthesis, apoptosis induction and reduction local inflammatory processes.

Two case-control studies have found a relationship between acetaminophen use and reduction in ovarian cancer risk. (Rosenberg et al, 2000; Cramer et al,1998)

Despite this, the influence of environmental factors in the etiology of ovarian cancer is controversial.

4. Genetic factors

One of the most significant risk factors of ovarian cancer is a familial history of the disease. Mutations in genes involved in DNA repair (BRCA, MSH-2, MLH-1, PMS 1 and 2) increases risk of cancer in some individuals.

It is estimated that approximately 7 percent of women with ovarian cancer have a positive family history of the disease. (Nguyen et al, 1994)

Genetic factors account for 10 to 15 percent of ovarian cancer cases.

Population-based studies have identified a personal history of breast cancer (particularly at young age) or a family history of either breast or ovarian cancer as one of the strongest risk factors, increasing woman's risk two to six fold. Hereditary ovarian cancer generally occurs in women about 10 years earlier than sporadic disease (Negri et al,2003;Nguyen et al,1994; Parazzini et al 1992; Stratton et al 1998;Sutcliffe et al 2000; Ziogas et al 2000).

We should differentiate genetic factors into two different subtypes as are familiar ovarian cancer and hereditary ovarian cancer.

4.1 Familiar aggregation

Women with a single family member affected by epithelial ovarian cancer have a 4 to 5 percent risk, while those with two affected relatives have a 7 percent risk for developing the disease in absolute numbers (Carlson et al,1994). In relative numbers familiar ovarian cancer confers a 4,6 percent relative risk (95% CI =2,1-8,7) of this disease in the proband's mother and 1,66 relative risk (95% CI=0,2-5,9) in the proband's sister.(Ziogas et al,2000)

4.2 Hereditary factors

At least 10 percent of ovarian tumours are hereditary and associated with highly penetrant, autosomal dominant genetic predisposition.

The two most common hereditary cancer syndromes associated with ovarian cancer include Hereditary Breast Ovarian Cancer that accounts for approximately 90 percent of the cases and Ovarian Cancer and Hereditary Nonpoliposis Colorectal Cancer (Lynch Syndrome) that accounts for the 10 percent of the cases.(Russo et al,2009)

Hereditary ovarian cancer syndromes appears to be genotypically and phenotypically an heterogeneous disease characterized by variable clinical courses.

4.2.1 Hereditary Breast - Ovarian Cancer (HBOC) syndrome

Women who carry disease specific alleles for BRCA1 and BRCA2 are at significantly higher risk of epithelial ovarian cancer than general population. The BRCA1 is an oncosuppresor gene located on chromosome 17q21. It was first identified in 1994 and contains small delections or insertions that result in premature stop codons that shorten (truncate) its protein product. This gene participates in chromatin remodelling processes and when mutation occurs cellular controls are unchecked resulting in cellular overgrowing. Alterations in this gene are found in 75 percent of families with hereditary breast and ovarian cancer. On the other hand BRCA2 is a suppressor gene located on chromosome 13q. Its alterations are found in 10 to 20 percent of families with hereditary breast and ovarian cancer.

More tan 2600 mutations have been found in those chromosomes. They have been described in 1/800 people in the general (White) and 1/40-50 in ashkenazi Jewish. Mutations in these genes lead to inability to regulate cell death and uncontrolled cell growth leading to cancer. (Carroll et al,2008)

The average cumulative risks in BRCA1-mutation carriers by age 70 years were 39 percent (18%-54%) for ovarian cancer. The corresponding estimates for BRCA2 were 11 percent (2.4%-19%). (Antoniou et al,2003)

Type of Cancer	BRCA Mutation Carriers (%)	General Population (%)
Breast (women)	50-85	11
Breast (men)	≤6	Rare
Ovarian (BRCA1)	40-60	1,5
Ovarian (BRCA2)	10-20	1,5

Table 1. Estimated risk of developing cancer by age 70 in BRCA mutation carriers with the general population.

In contrast to Lynch syndrome there are no defined criteria for this hereditary syndrome. Some criteria have been described and these include several cases of breast cancer diagnosed before the age of 50, one or more relatives with both breast and ovarian cancer, the presence of BRCA1 or BRCA 2 germline mutation. These criteria vary between the different Cooperative Groups.

Independent of Family History • Patient with synchronous or metacronous breast and ovarian cancer • Breast cáncer before 30 years • Bilateral breast cancer before 40 years
Families with two affected breast or ovarian cancer an one of the next characteristics: • Male breast cancer • Ovarian, primary peritoneal or Fallopian tube cancer • Both two cases before 50 years • One bilateral case and the other before 50 years
Families with 3 or more affected members with breast or ovarian cancer

Table 2. Criteria for Mutation in BRCA1-BRCA 2 genes study.

Special mention deserves triple negative breast cancer associated with familiar history of breast or ovarian cancer and younger age at diagnosis. It confers a special risk for BRCA1 mutation although criteria have not yet been defined (Young et al, 2009;Haffty et al, 2006)

Some statistical models have been investigated to estimate the risk of having a germline mutation in BRCA1 and BRCA 2 genes like Boadicea, BRCAPRO, Manchester, IBIS, Myriad II, U Penn.

Ovarian cancers associated with BRCA1-2 mutation are typically high grade serous bilateral carcinomas.

There exist some controversies about the prognosis of these neoplasms. The information derives from retrospective studies, with intrinsic bias due to inadequate sample size and also the lack of adequate controls.

Some case-control and population studies found no difference in survival between general population and mutations carriers (Brunet et al,1997;Johannsson et al,1998) Another studies show a more favourable outcome in mutation carriers.(Rubin et al,1996)

Tan et al. described in a small case-control study that BRCA-positive patients had higher overall (95.5% v 59.1%; P = .002) and complete response rates (81.8% v 43.2%; P = .004) to first line chemotherapy treatment, higher responses to second and third line platinum-based chemotherapy (second line, 91.7% v 40.9% [P = .004]; third line, 100% v 14.3% [P = .005]) and longer progression free interval. A significant improvement in median OS in BRCA-positive patients compared with controls was observed from both time of diagnosis (8.4 v 2.9 years; P < .002) and time of first relapse (5 v 1.6 years; P < .001). BRCA status, stage, and length of first response were independent prognostic factors from time of first relapse. (Tan et al,2008)

Some preventive strategies like bilateral salpingo-oophorectomy or mastectomy have been developed to prevent these neoplasms.

Salpingo-oophorectomy has demonstrated a risk reduction of ovarian cancer over 90 percent and a 50 percent for breast cancer with a mean follow up time of 5 years. (Agnantis et al,2004;Dowdy et al,2004)

Rebbeck et al report that bilateral salpingo-oophorectomy was associated with a statistically significant risk reduction of BRCA1/2-associated ovarian or fallopian tube cancer (HR = 0.21; 95% CI = 0.12 to 0.39), which confers an absolute risk reduction near 80 percent of ovarian and fallopian tube neoplasm.(Rebbeck et al,2009)

Another neoplasm has been associated with these mutations. In BRCA 1 carriers primary peritoneal cancer, fallopian tube cancer and prostate cancer have been described. In BRAC 2 carriers there are also an increased risk for melanoma, pancreatic cancer, gastric cancer and biliary tract cancer. (Llort et al,2010)

4.2.2 Hereditary nonpolyposis colorectal cancer (lynch syndrome)

Lynch and co-workers described in 1966 a syndrome that conferred a susceptibility to colorectal cancer with predilection to the right of the splenic flexure but with no excess of adenomatous polyps in younger than expected in adult patients (<45 years) (Lynch et al,1967)

This is an autosomal dominant syndrome which increases risk of colorectal endometrial, ovarian, gastric, pancreatic , renal and biliary tract cancer and it is a result of mutations in mismatch repair (MMR) genes including at least four chromosomes (2p,3p,7p,2q).These genes form heterodimers which recognize and repair deoxyribonucleic acid mistakes during transcription.

Watson et al determined a 6,7 percent lifetime risk for ovarian cancer in proven or probable MSH2 and MSH1 mutation carriers (Watson et al,2008).

Some clinical criteria have been described to identificate Lynch syndrome.

Amsterdam criteria were first described in 1990 called Amsterdam I. They were revised in 1999 (Vasen et al, 1999).

Amsterdam I
1. At least 3 relatives with histologically confirmed colorectal cancer, 1 of whom is a first degree relative of the other 2 2. At least 2 successive generations involved. 3. At least 1 of the cancers diagnosed before age 50. 4. Familial adenomatous polyposis should be excluded.
Amsterdam II
1. 3 or more relatives with an associated cancer (colorectal cancer, or cancer of the endometrium, small intestine, ureter or renal pelvis); 2. 2 or more successive generations affected; 3. 1 or more relatives diagnosed before the age of 50 years; 4. 1 should be a first-degree relative of the other two; 5. Familial adenomatous polyposis (FAP) should be excluded in cases of colorectal carcinoma; 6. Tumours should be verified by pathologic examination

Table 3. Amsterdam I and II.

Then in 1996 Bethesda criteria were redacted to encompass a greater number of patients who may be carriers of a mutation.
They have found to be more sensitive than Amsterdam criteria.
Bethesda Criteria:

1. Individuals with cancer in families meeting the Amsterdam criteria
2. Individuals with two HNPCC-related cancers, including synchronous and metachronous colorectal cancers or associated extracolonic cancers an individual and a first-degree relative with:

- either colorectal cancer
- and/or HNPCC-related extracolonic cancer
- and/or a colorectal adenoma
- One of the cancers diagnosed at age <45 years, and the adenoma diagnosed at age <40 years

3. Individuals with colorectal cancer or endometrial cancer diagnosed at age <45 years.
4. Individuals with right-sided colorectal cancer with an undifferentiated pattern (solid/cribiform) on histopathology diagnosed at age <45 years
5. Individuals with signet-ring-cell-type colorectal cancer diagnosed at age <45 years.
6. Individuals with adenomas diagnosed at age <40 years

Revised Bethesda criteria:

1. CRC diagnosed in individual under age 50 years.
2. Presence of synchronous, metachronous colorectal, or other HNPCC-associated tumours, regardless of age.
3. CRC with the MSI-H histology (presence of tumor-infiltrating lymphocytes, Crohn's-like lymphocytic reaction, mucinous/signet-ring differentiation, or medullary growth pattern), in patient 60 years of age.
4. CRC in 1 or more first-degree relatives with an HNPCC-related tumor, with 1 of the cancers being diagnosed under age 50 years.
5. CRC diagnosed in 2 or more first- or second-degree relatives with HNPCC- related tumors, regardless of age.

(Rodriguez-Bigas et al,1997;Umar et al,2004)
Ovarian cancer from this syndrome at diagnosis is ten years earlier than in general population and survival is similar as sporadic ovarian cancer. It represents all histopathologic subtypes.(Crijnen et al,2005)
There are no proven strategies that have demonstrated an impact on survival in this setting.

Increased Risk	**Decreased Risk**
Delayed childbearing	Breastfeeding for 18 months or more
Early menarche	Early menopause
Endometriosis	Multiparity (risk decreases with each additional pregnacy)
Estrogen replacement therapy for more than five years	Hysterctomy
Family History suggesting genetic predisposition	Late menarche
Genetic syndromes	Low fat diet
Hight fat diet	Tubal Ligation
Late menopause	
Low parity	

Table 4. Risk Factors Associated with Ovarian Cancer.

5. Conclusion

Ovarian cancer is the second most common gynecological malignancy and the fifth leading cause of cancer death. Some histological subgroups have been described. Etiology is still poorly understood. Hypotheses relating to incessant ovulation, excessive gonadotropin secretion have been involved as etiological explanations. Based upon epidemiological research there is evidence that certain reproductive factors are associated with ovarian cancer risk. There are some hormonal factors that have special importance. Each childbirth incurs a 15 to 20 percent reduction risk. Breastfeeding also represents a protective factor. Oral contraceptive use for 5 years or longer reduced about half the risk compared to never users. In contrast to these protective factors hormone replacement therapy compared with never users increases the risk and this is associated with longer use. Some inflammatory disorders like pelvic inflammatory disease and endometriosis are associated with an increased risk. The significance of environmental factors like obesity, cigarette smoking, vegetable consumption etc is not yet established .Finally some genetic disorders like BRCA 1 and 2 mutations and Lynch syndrome have been involved as risk factors for this disease. A deeper understanding of these risk factors is important in order to establish preventive strategies for this fatal disease

6. References

Agnantis NJ, Paraskevaidis E, Roukos D. Preventing breast, ovarian cancer in BRCA carriers: rational of prophylactic surgery and promises of surveillance.Ann Surg Oncol. 2004 Dec;11(12):1030-4.

Anderson GL, Judd HL, Kaunitz AM, Barad DH, Beresford SA, Pettinger M et al. Effects of estrogen plus progestin on gynecologic cancers and associated diagnostic procedures: the Women's Health Initiative randomized trial. *JAMA.* 2003;290(13):1739-48.

Antoniou A, Pharoah PD, Narod S, Risch HA, Eyfjord JE, Hopper JL et al. Average risks of breast and ovarian cancer associated with BRCA1 or BRCA2 mutations detected in case Series unselected for family history: a combined analysis of 22 studies.Am J Hum Genet. 2003;72(5):1117-30.

Aris A. Endometriosis-associated ovarian cancer: A ten-year cohort study of women living in the Estrie Region of Quebec, Canada.J Ovarian Res. 2010 19;3:2.

Balen A. Polycystic ovary syndrome and cancer.Hum Reprod Update. 2001 Nov-Dec;7(6):522-5.

Beral V, Doll R, Hermon C, Peto R, Reeves G.Lancet .Ovarian cancer and oral contraceptives: collaborative reanalysis of data from 45 epidemiological studies including 23,257 women with ovarian cancer and 87,303 controls. Collaborative Group on Epidemiological Studies of Ovarian Cancer. 2008 ;371:303-14.

Beral V, Bull D, Green J, Reeves G, et al, Million Women Study Collaborators. Ovarian cancer and hormone replacement therapy in the Million Women Study.Lancet. 2007 ;369(9574):1703-10.

Bosetti C, Negri E, Trichopoulos D, Franceschi S, Beral V, Tzonou A et al. Long-term effects of oral contraceptives on ovarian cancer risk.Int J Cancer. 2002 ;102(3):262-5.

Brunet JS, Narod SA, Tonin P, Foulkes WD. BRCA1 mutations and survival in women with ovarian cancer N Engl J Med. 1997 ;336(17):1256.

Carroll JC, Cremin C, Allanson J, Blaine SM, Dorman H, Gibbons CA et al. Hereditary breast and ovarian cancers.Can Fam Physician. 2008 Dec;54(12):1691-2.

Casagrande JT, Louie EW, Pike MC, Roy S, Ross RK, Henderson BE. "Incessant ovulation" and ovarian cancer. Lancet. 1979 ;2:170-3.

Carlson KJ, Skates SJ, Singer DE. Screening for ovarian cancer.Ann Intern Med. 1994 Jul 15;121(2):124-32.

Chiaffarino F, Pelucchi C, Negri E, Parazzini F, Franceschi S, Talamini R et al. Breastfeeding and the risk of epithelial ovarian cancer in an Italian population. Gynecol Oncol. 2005 ;98:304-8.

Chiaffarino F, Pelucchi C, Danforth KN, Tworoger SS, Hecht JL, Rosner BA, Colditz GA, Hankinson SE. .Breastfeeding and risk of ovarian cancer in two prospective cohorts.Cancer Causes Control. 2007 ;18(5):517-23.

Cramer DW, Welch WR. Determinants of ovarian cancer risk. II. Inferences regarding pathogenesis.J Natl Cancer Inst. 1983 Oct;71(4):717-21.

Cramer DW, Harlow BL, Titus-Ernstoff L, Bohlke K, Welch WR, Greenberg ER. Over-the-counter analgesics and risk of ovarian cancer.Lancet. 1998 Jan 10;351(9096):104-7.

Crijnen TE, Janssen-Heijnen ML, Gelderblom H, Morreau J, Nooij MA, Kenter GG et al. Survival of patients with ovarian cancer due to a mismatch repair defect.Fam Cancer. 2005;4(4):301-5

Danforth KN, Tworoger SS, Hecht JL, Rosner BA, Colditz GA, Hankinson SE. A prospective study of postmenopausal hormone use and ovarian cancer risk. Br J Cancer. 2007 ;96(1):151-6.

De Vita,Hellman & Rosenberg's. Cancer: Principles and Pactice of Oncology.2008. pg 1568-1594. ISBN-13:987-0-7817-7207-5.

Dick ML, Siskind V, Purdie DM, Green AC; Australian Cancer Study Group (Ovarian Cancer); Australian Ovarian Cancer Study Group.Incomplete pregnancy and risk of ovarian cancer: results from two Australian case-control studies and systematic review.Cancer Causes Control. 2009 ;20(9):1571-85.

Dowdy SC, Stefanek M, Hartmann LC. Surgical risk reduction: prophylactic salpingo-oophorectomy and prophylactic mastectomy.Am J Obstet Gynecol. 2004 Oct;191(4):1113-23.

Fairfield KM, Hankinson SE, Rosner BA, Hunter DJ, Colditz GA, Willett WC. Risk of ovarian carcinoma and consumption of vitamins A, C, and E and specific carotenoids: a prospective analysis.Cancer. 2001 Nov 1;92(9):2318-26.

Ferlay J, Parkin DM, Steliarova-Foucher E. Estimates of cancer incidence and mortality in Europe in 2008. Eur J Cancer. 2010 ;46:765-81.

Goodman MT, Wu AH, Tung KH, McDuffie K, Kolonel LN, Nomura AM et al. Association of dairy products, lactose, and calcium with the risk of ovarian cancer. Am J Epidemiol. 2002 Jul 15;156(2):148-57.

Haffty BG, Yang Q, Reiss M, Kearney T, Higgins SA, Weidhaas J et al. Locoregional relapse and distant metastasis in conservatively managed triplenegative early-stage breast cancer.J Clin Oncol. 2006 Dec 20;24(36):5652-7.

Hankinson SE, Colditz GA, Hunter DJ, Willett WC, Stampfer MJ, Rosner B, Hennekens CH, Speizer FE. A prospective study of reproductive factors and risk of epithelial ovarian cancer.Cancer. 1995 Jul 15;76(2):284-90.

Harlow BL, Cramer DW, Bell DA, Welch WR.Obstet Gynecol. Perineal exposure to talc and ovarian cancer risk. 1992 ;80:19-26.

Huncharek M, Muscat J, Onitilo A, Kupelnick B. Use of cosmetic talc on contraceptive diaphragms and risk of ovarian cancer: ameta-analysis of nine observational studies. Eur J Cancer Prev. 2007;16:422-9.

Hinkula M, Pukkala E, Kyyrönen P, Kauppila A. Incidence of ovarian cancer of grand multiparous women--a population-based study in Finland.Gynecol Oncol. 2006 ;103:207-11.

Jensen A, Sharif H, Frederiksen K, Kjaer SK. Use of fertility drugs and risk of ovarian cancer: Danish Population Based Cohort Study. BMJ. 2009

Jóhannsson OT, Ranstam J, Borg A, Olsson H. Survival of BRCA1 breast and ovarian cancer patients: a population-based study from southern Sweden.J Clin Oncol. 1998 Feb;16(2):397-404.

Jordan SJ, Siskind V, C Green A, Whiteman DC, Webb PM. Breastfeeding and risk of epithelial ovarian cancer.Cancer Causes Control. 2010 ;21:109-16.

Llort Pursals G.Síndrome de Cancer de mama ovario hereditarios.Aspectos clínicos. Ed. Instituto Roche.Módulo III.pp 419-477.

Lynch HT, Krush AJ. Heredity and adenocarcinoma of the colon.Gastroenterology. 1967 ;53(4):517-27.

La Vecchia C. Oral contraceptives and ovarian cancer: an update, 1998-2004.Eur J Cancer Prev. 2006 Apr;15(2):117-24.

McGuire V, Felberg A, Mills M, Ostrow KL, DiCioccio R, John EM et al. Relation of contraceptive and reproductive history to ovarian cancer risk in carriers and noncarriers of BRCA1 gene mutations. Am J Epidemiol. 2004;160(7):613-8.

McLemore MR, Miaskowski C, Aouizerat BE, Chen LM, Dodd MJ. Epidemiological and genetic factors associated with ovarian cancer.Cancer Nurs. 2009;32:281-8.

Negri E, Pelucchi C, Franceschi S, Montella M, Conti E, Dal Maso L, Parazzini F, Tavani A, Carbone A, La Vecchia C.Family history of cancer and risk of ovarian cancer. Eur J Cancer. 2003 Mar;39(4):505-10.

Negri E, Parazzini F, Franceschi S, Talamini R,Montella M, Ramazzotti V et al. Breastfeeding and the risk of epithelial ovarian cancer in an Italian population.Gynecol Oncol. 2005 ;98(2):304-8.

Ness RB, Grisso JA, Cottreau C, Klapper J, Vergona R, Wheeler JE et al. Factors related to inflammation of the ovarian epithelium and risk of ovarian cancer.Epidemiology. 2000;11(2):111-7.

Nguyen HN, Averette HE, Janicek M. Ovarian carcinoma. A review of the significance of familial risk factors and the role of prophylactic oophorectomy in cancer prevention.Cancer. 1994 Jul 15;74(2):545-55.

Olsen CM, Green AC, Whiteman DC, Sadeghi S, Kolahdooz F, Webb PM. Obesity and the risk of epithelial ovarian cancer: a systematic review and meta-analysis. Eur J Cancer. 2007;43:690-709.

Orezzoli JP, Russell AH, Oliva E, Del Carmen MG, Eichhorn J, Fuller AF. Prognostic implication of endometriosis in clear cell carcinoma of the ovary.Gynecol Oncol. 2008;110:336-44.

Parkin DM, Bray F, Ferlay J, Pisani P. Global cancer statistics, 2002. CA Cancer J Clin. 2005 Mar-Apr;55(2):74-108.

Parazzini F, Negri E, La Vecchia C, Restelli C, Franceschi S. Family history of reproductive cancers and ovarian cancer risk: an Italian case-control study. Am J Epidemiol. 1992 Jan 1;135(1):35-40.

Parazzini F, Negri E, La Vecchia C, Luchini L, Mezzopane R. Hysterectomy, oophorectomy, and subsequent ovarian cancer risk.Obstet Gynecol. 1993 ;81(3):363-6.

Permuth-Wey J, Sellers TA. Epidemiology of ovarian cancer. Methods MolBiol.2009;472:413-37.

Prentice RL, Thomson CA, Caan B, Hubbell FA, Anderson GL, Beresford SA et al. Low-fat dietary pattern and cancer incidence in the Women's Health Initiative Dietary Modification Randomized Controlled Trial. J Natl Cancer Inst. 2007 ;99:1534-43.

Purdie DM, Bain CJ, Siskind V, Webb PM, Green AC. Ovulation and risk of epithelial ovarian cancer.Int J Cancer. 2003;104(2):228-32.

Rebbeck TR, Kauff ND, Domchek SM. Meta-analysis of risk reduction estimates associated with risk-reducing salpingo-oophorectomy in BRCA1 or BRCA2 mutation carriers.J Natl Cancer Inst. 2009 ;101(2):80-7.

Risch HA, Howe GR. Pelvic inflammatory disease and the risk of epithelial ovarian cancer.Cancer Epidemiol Biomarkers Prev. 1995 ;4:447-51.

Risch HA. Hormonal etiology of epithelial ovarian cancer, with a hypothesis concerning the role of androgens and progesterone.J Natl Cancer Inst. 1998 ;90:1774-86.

Rodriguez-Bigas MA, Boland CR, Hamilton SR, Henson DE, Jass JR, Khan PM et al. A National Cancer Institute Workshop on Hereditary Nonpolyposis Colorectal Cancer

Syndrome: meeting highlights and Bethesda guidelines. J Natl Cancer Inst. 1997 Dec 3;89(23):1758-62.

Rosenberg L, Palmer JR, Rao RS, Coogan PF, Strom BL, Zauber AG et al. A case-control study of analgesic use and ovarian cancer.Cancer Epidemiol Biomarkers Prev. 2000 Sep;9(9):933-7.

Rossing MA, Cushing-Haugen KL, Wicklund KG, Weiss NS. Cigarette smoking and risk of epithelial ovarian cancer.Cancer Causes Control. 2008 ;19:413-20.

Russo A, Calò V, Bruno L, Rizzo S, Bazan V, Di Fede G et al.Hereditary ovarian cancer.Crit Rev Oncol Hematol. 2009 ;69:28-44.

Rubin SC, Benjamin I, Behbakht K, Takahashi H, Morgan MA, LiVolsi VA et al. Clinical and pathological features of ovarian cancer in women with germ-linemutations of BRCA1.N Engl J Med. 1996 7;335(19):1413-6.

Stratton JF, Pharoah P, Smith SK, Easton D, Ponder BA. A systematic review and meta-analysis of family history and risk of ovarian cancer.Br J Obstet Gynaecol. 1998 May;105(5):493-9.

Schoute LJ, Rivera C, Hunter DJ, Spiegelman D, Adami HO, Arslan A et al. Height, body mass index, and ovarian cancer: a pooled analysis of 12 cohort Studies. Cancer Epidemiol Biomarkers Prev. 2008 ;17:902-12.

Sutcliffe S, Pharoah PD, Easton DF, Ponder B Ovarian and breast cancer risks to women in families with two or more cases of ovarian cancer Int J Cancer. 2000 Jul 1;87(1):110-7.

Tan DS, Rothermundt C, Thomas K, Bancroft E, Eeles R, Shanley S et al. "BRCAness" syndrome in ovarian cancer: a case-control study describing theclinical features and outcome of patients with epithelial ovarian cancerassociated with BRCA1 and BRCA2 mutations.J Clin Oncol. 2008 ;26(34):5530-6.

Tworoger SS, Gertig DM, Gates MA, Hecht JL, Hankinson SE. Caffeine, alcohol, smoking, and the risk of incident epithelial ovarian cancer.Cancer. 2008 Mar 1;112(5):1169-77.

Tung KH, Goodman MT, Wu AH, McDuffie K, Wilkens LR, Kolonel LN et al. Reproductive factors and epithelial ovarian cancer risk by histologic type: amultiethnic case-control study.Am J Epidemiol. 2003 ;158(7):629-38.

Titus-Ernstoff L, Perez K, Cramer DW, Harlow BL, Baron JA, Greenberg ER. Menstrual and reproductive factors in relation to ovarian cancer risk.Br J Cancer. 2001;84:714-21.

Umar A, Boland CR, Terdiman JP, Syngal S, de la Chapelle A, Rüschoff J et al. Revised Bethesda Guidelines for hereditary nonpolyposis colorectal cancer (Lynch syndrome) and microsatellite instability.J Natl Cancer Inst. 2004 Feb 18;96(4):261-8.

Vasen HF, Watson P, Mecklin JP, Lynch HT. New clinical criteria for hereditary nonpolyposis colorectal cancer (HNPCC, Lynch syndrome) proposed by the International Collaborative group on HNPCC.Gastroenterology. 1999 Jun;116(6):1453-6.

Vo C, Carney ME. Ovarian cancer hormonal and environmental risk effect.Obstet Gynecol Clin North Am. 2007 ;34(4):687-700.

WWW.SEER.cancer.gov

Watson P, Vasen HF, Mecklin JP, Bernstein I, Aarnio M, Järvinen HJ et al. The risk of extra-colonic, extra-endometrial cancer in the Lynch syndrome. Int J Cancer. 2008;123(2):444-9.

Whiteman DC, Murphy MF, Cook LS, Cramer DW, Hartge P, Marchbanks PA et al. Multiple births and risk of epithelial ovarian cancer. J Natl Cancer Inst. 2000;92:1172-7.

Whiteman DC, Siskind V, Purdie DM, Green AC. Timing of pregnancy and the risk of epithelial ovarian cancer.Cancer Epidemiol Biomarkers Prev. 2003 ;12(1):42-6.

Whittemore AS, Harris R, Itnyre J. Characteristics relating to ovarian cancer risk: collaborative analysis of 12 US case-control studies. IV. The pathogenesis of epithelial ovarian cancer. Collaborative Ovarian Cancer Group.Am J Epidemiol. 1992 Nov 15;136(10):1212-20.

Young SR, Pilarski RT, Donenberg T, Shapiro C, Hammond LS, Miller J et al.The prevalence of BRCA1 mutations among young women with triple-negative breast cancer BMC Cancer. 2009 9;9:86.

Zhou B, Sun Q, Cong R, Gu H, Tang N, Yang L et al. Hormone replacement therapy and ovarian cancer risk: a meta-analysis.Gynecol Oncol. 2008 ;108(3):641-51.

Zhang Y, Coogan PF, Palmer JR, Strom BL, Rosenberg L. Cigarette smoking and increased risk of mucinous epithelial ovarian cancer.Am J Epidemiol. 2004 ;159:133-9.

Ziogas A, Gildea M, Cohen P, Bringman D, Taylor TH, Seminara D et al. Cancer risk estimates for family members of a population-based family registry for breast and ovarian cancer. Cancer Epidemiol Biomarkers Prev. 2000 ;9(1):103-11.

3

Photonic Sensor System for Screening Serum Biomarker Proteins in Ovarian Cancer

Debra Wawro[1], Shelby Zimmerman[1], Robert Magnusson[1,2] and Peter Koulen[3]
[1]*Resonant Sensors Incorporated (RSI), Arlington, TX*
[2]*University of Texas at Arlington, Department of Electrical Engineering, Arlington, TX*
[3]*University of Missouri – Kansas City, School of Medicine, Departments of Ophthalmology and Basic Medical Science, Vision Research Center, Kansas City, MO USA*

1. Introduction

Ovarian cancer is among the most deadly types of cancers among women, with about 21,990 new cases diagnosed every year in the United States (American Cancer Society, 2011). About 15,460 of these women will die from ovarian cancer. If diagnosed while the cancer is still localized, survival rates of at least 5 years are likely. Unfortunately, less than 20% of cases are found at an early stage due to the absence of reproducible and definitive diagnostic tools. Because ovarian cancers occur deep in the pelvis, there are often few symptoms until the cancer is at an advanced stage. Furthermore, many of the symptoms of ovarian cancer (such as back pain, fatigue, and abdominal bloat) are common and difficult to distinguish from those not caused by cancer. Because of this lack of symptom specificity, most ovarian cancers are substantially advanced at the time of diagnosis. Staging of the cancer is critically important in order to determine the most effective treatment modality. Currently there are no routine clinical diagnostic assays using urinalysis or seranalysis for early screening or staging of ovarian cancer. However, there are several research studies (Bignotti et al., 2007; and Liotta et al., 2005) that identify potential biomarker indicators that can be used for this purpose.

When a woman is suspected of having ovarian cancer, medical diagnostics typically include an ultrasound of the abdomen and pelvis as well as a blood test that includes measurement of the CA-125 protein levels (American Cancer Society, 2011). CA 125 is a protein biomarker found in greater concentration in tumor cells than in other cells of the body. However, since CA-125 levels can be elevated due to other benign causes, it is primarily used to monitor women with a known cancer of the ovary to determine treatment efficacy. Measurement of CA-125 levels is not accepted as a sufficient test for an early screening indicator in ovarian cancer. Thus, improved methods are needed to provide a specific and early screen for this deadly disease.

Based on "Optical nanotechnology enables rapid label-free diagnostics for cancer biomarker screening," by D. Wawro, S. Zimmerman, R. Magnusson and P. Koulen which appeared in Proceedings of SPIE 8090, 80900S (2011).

In this work, we describe a high-accuracy, label-free biosensor system that can provide effective detection of an array of biomarker proteins in serum to accurately diagnose and stage ovarian cancer. While there are currently no established clinical diagnostic assays using urinalysis or seranalysis, experimentally and clinically identified targets (Bignotti et al., 2007; and Liotta et al., 2005) can be categorized into two groups: group 1 consists of biomarker proteins that are up-regulated twofold or higher in metastatic over primary ovarian serous papillary carcinoma (such as Fibronectin), and group 2 consists of biomarker proteins that are up-regulated twofold or higher in primary over metastatic ovarian serous papillary carcinoma (such as Apolipoprotein A-1). This differentiation yields accurate diagnosis of the disease and staging information that can be used to monitor pre-symptomatic aspects of the disease, disease progression, and the efficacy of therapies.

Conventional blood diagnostic testing methods such as immunoassay approaches require time-intensive processing and washing steps, and they are not easily integrated in a clinical setting. To address these needs, we utilize a real-time photonic biosensor technology that provides rapid results with minimal processing steps and the capability to test for an array of biomarkers in a single sample.

2. Label-free diagnostic approach

The diagnostic screening system that is central to this work applies an optical approach based on the guided-mode resonance (GMR) effect that occurs in subwavelength dielectric waveguide gratings. As shown in Fig. 1, when these diffractive elements are illuminated with a broadband light source, a specific wavelength of light is reflected (or transmitted) at a specific angle. The binding interaction between an immobilized receptor and its analyte can be monitored in real time without the use of reporter labels (such as fluorescent or radioactive tags) by following the corresponding resonance wavelength shift with an optical

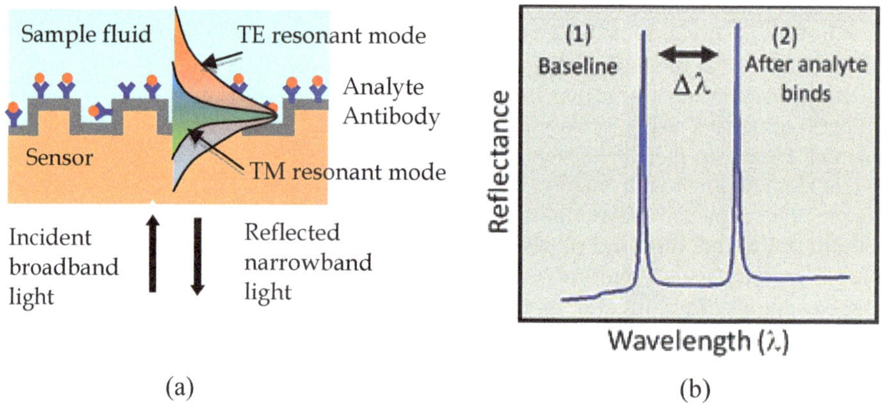

Fig. 1. (a) Schematic of a label-free GMR sensor system (single channel illustrated) operating in reflection mode. The collimated beam from a broadband source is incident on the sensor at normal incidence. The reflected spectral response is monitored in real time with an optical spectrum analyzer. (b) As binding events occur at the sensor surface, resonance peak changes (only one polarization depicted in plot) can be tracked as a function of the wavelength.

spectrum analyzer. Test time is limited solely by the chemical binding dynamics between the receptor and its target. Specificity is imparted on the sensor surface by covalently attaching a selective layer (such as antibodies). It is multifunctional as only the sensitizing surface layer needs to be chemically altered to detect different targets. Repeatable fabrication processes are in place to produce the resonant grating sensor element in low-cost polymer and other dielectric materials.

Since the resonance layer is polarization-sensitive, separate resonance peaks occur for incident TE (electric vector normal to the plane of incidence) and TM (magnetic vector normal to the plane of incidence) polarization states. This dual-peak feature provides cross-referenced data useful for increasing detection accuracy. These distinct resonant modes interact differently with the surrounding media, enabling the polarization-based differentiation. This sensor technology is broadly applicable to medical diagnostics, drug discovery and development, industrial process control, and environmental monitoring.

2.1 Guided-mode resonance technology overview

The coupling of a freely propagating electromagnetic wave to a state of confinement at a periodic surface is presently the subject of considerable research activity. Periodic structures with subwavelength features provide effective means of achieving such coupling. The resulting strong localization of energy at a dielectric (or metallic) layer is of interest for numerous photonic applications including biosensors, light sources, nonlinear frequency converters, and particle traps. Magnusson et al. disclosed GMR filters that were tunable on variation in resonance structure parameters (Magnusson & Wang, 1992). Wawro et al. presented GMR biosensor embodiments as well as system architectures (Wawro et al., 2000). Thus, spectral or angular variations induced via layer thickness change or on change in refractive index in surrounding media or in device layers can be used to sense these changes (Magnusson et al., 2011; Wawro et al., 2006; 2010). Additional aspects of GMR sensors in various applications have been discussed in the literature (Cunningham et al., 2002; Kikuta et al., 2001).

Thin-film structures containing waveguide layers and periodic elements, under the correct conditions, exhibit the GMR effect. Most commonly, GMR biosensors are designed to operate in reflection. In this configuration, an incident wave is phase-matched, by the periodic element, to a leaky waveguide mode. It is reradiated in the specular-reflection direction as it propagates along the waveguide and constructively interferes with the directly reflected wave. Conversely and equivalently, the phase of the reradiated leaky mode in the forward, directly transmitted wave direction is π radians out of phase with the direct unguided transmitted wave, thereby extinguishing the transmitted light (Rosenblatt, 1997). This picture of the resonance effect pertains to a reflection, or bandstop, filter. Other operation configurations are possible, such as in transmission mode, or as a bandpass filter.

Figure 2 shows the measured and calculated spectral reflectance of a dielectric GMR device (Priambodo et al., 2003). It acts as a bandstop filter with the spectrum of interest reflected in a narrow band with relatively low sidebands. Although the theoretical calculation predicts 100% peak efficiency for a plane wave incidence, it is diminished in practice by various factors such as material and scattering losses, incident beam divergence, and the lateral device size; here, the experimental peak is 90%.

These resonant structures, tunable on change of refractive index and/or thickness, have clear applications for biosensors. The buildup of the attaching biolayer can be monitored in real time, without use of chemical tags, by following the corresponding resonance shift.

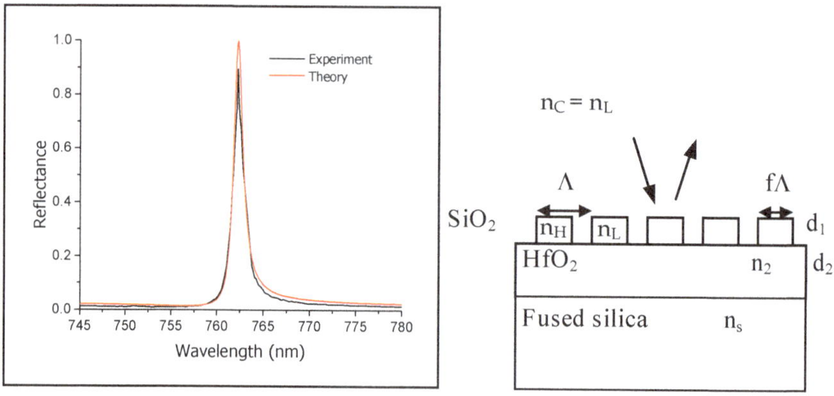

Fig. 2. Comparison between experiment and theory for a dielectric resonance element. The parameters used for the theoretical curve fit are close to the nominal values; they are n_C=1.0, nH=1.454 (SiO2), n2=1.975 (HfO2), ns=1.454, d1=135 nm, f=0.58, d2=208 nm, Λ=446 nm, normal incidence. Rigorous coupled-wave analysis (RCWA) is used for the computations (Gaylord & Moharam, 1985).

2.2 Biosensor operation

In addition to the reflection/transmission properties of propagating electromagnetic waves, the near-field properties of resonant periodic lattices, including localization and field-strength enhancement, are of interest in sensor applications. The near-field patterns associated with a typical filter, similar to that in Fig. 2 in structure, are shown in Figs. 3 and 4 with a normally incident TE-polarized wave. Numerical results are obtained with rigorous coupled-wave analysis (RCWA) (Gaylord & Moharam, 1985) to provide quantitative information on relative field strengths and spatial extents associated with the near fields. As shown in Fig. 3, the S_0 wave (S_0 denotes the electric field of the zero order) propagates with reflected-wave amplitude close to unity, producing the standing-wave pattern shown by interference with the unit-amplitude input wave used in our model. Thus, at resonance, most of the energy is reflected back. The evanescent, first-order diffracted waves S_1 and S_{-1} constitute the counter-propagating leaky modes. We see that the maximum field value is located in the HfO_2 layer with the evanescent tails gradually penetrating into the substrate and cover. Figure 4 shows the standing wave pattern formed by the counter-propagating S_{-1} and S_{+1} waves at a certain instant of time; the field scale is color coded as shown. Since the $S_{\pm 1}$ space harmonics correspond to localized waves, they can be very strong at resonance; here, the field enhancement is ~x10 as seen in Fig. 3. Depending on the level of grating modulation ($\Delta\varepsilon = n_H^2 - n_L^2$), the field amplitude can range from ~x10-x1000 in the layer relative to the input wave amplitude that represents a large increase in local intensity $I \sim S^2$. The maximum amplitude of S_1 is approximately inversely proportional to the modulation strength. In general, small modulation implies narrow linewidth $\Delta\lambda$ and a large resonator Q factor $Q=\lambda/\Delta\lambda$.

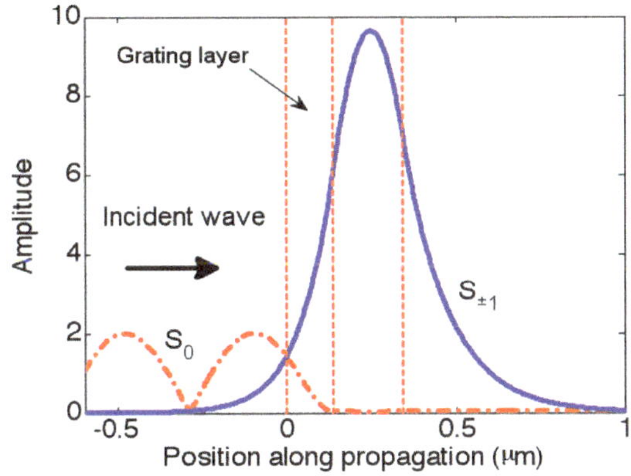

Fig. 3. Profile of the leaky mode at resonance for a typical GMR sensor device. The amplitude is normalized to the incident-wave amplitude.

The structure of the local fields associated with the resonant leaky modes is key to sensor applications. The leaky mode is a surface state that propagates along the surface, providing maximal interaction with any attached molecular or chemical layer. In the technology discussed herein, the sensing field (a resonant leaky mode) is maximized in the grating layer with an evanescent tail penetrating into the cover region (shown in Figs. 3 and 4).

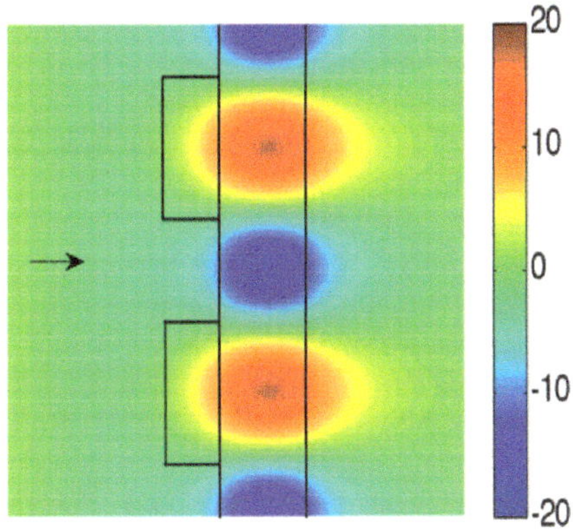

Fig. 4. Snapshot of the standing-wave pattern associated with the leaky mode in Fig. 3. The size of the region is $2\lambda \times 2\Lambda$. Results are obtained with rigorous coupled wave analysis.

2.3 Sensor element fabrication

The GMR biosensor devices used in this work are based upon a single-layer waveguide grating design. We fabricated these with low-cost submicron molding methods in our labs, and they can be purchased from numerous commercial sources. We utilize polymers that are imprinted with submicron grating patterns and coated with a high-index dielectric material (such as TiO_2 or HfO_2) to realize resonant sensors. Figure 5 shows an example of a GMR sensor.

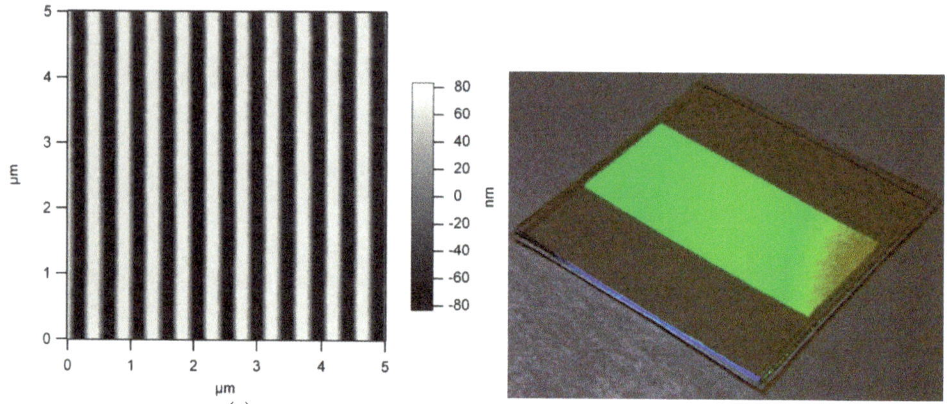

(a) (b)

Fig. 5. Submicron resonant grating. (a) Atomic force microscope (AFM) picture of a ~520-nm period grating contact printed in an optical polymer. (b) A picture of a submicron molded grating. The grating is coated with a thin high-index layer (TiO_2 or HfO_2) to realize a GMR sensor element.

2.4 Competing approaches

Numerous optical sensors for bio- and chemical detection have been developed commercially and in research literature. Key label-free technologies include the surface-plasmon resonance sensor (Homola, 2003; Raether, 1988), MEMS-based sensors, nano-sensors (rods and particles), resonant mirror, Bragg grating sensors, waveguide sensors, waveguide interferometric sensors, ellipsometry, and grating coupled sensors (Cunningham, 1998; Cooper, 2006). Other methods include immunomagnetic separation, polymerase chain reaction, and standard immunoassay approaches that incorporate fluorescent, absorptive, radioactive, and luminescence labels. The GMR sensor approach has advantages and distinctions relative to these technologies, including features such as polarization diversity and low-power, portable system formats.

In our opinion, although dramatically different in concept and function, the surface-plasmon resonance (SPR) sensor (Homola, 2003; Raether, 1988) comes closest in features and operation to the GMR sensor discussed here. The term surface plasmon (SP) refers to an electromagnetic field charge-density oscillation that can occur at the interface between a conductor and a dielectric (for example, gold/glass interface). An SP mode can be resonantly excited by parallel-polarized (TM, electric vector in the plane of the page) incident light but not with TE polarized light. Phase matching occurs by employing a metallized diffraction grating, or by using total internal reflection from a high-index material, such as in prism coupling or an evanescent field from a guided wave. When an SPR surface wave is excited, an absorption minimum occurs in a specific wavelength band. Since only a single polarization (TM) can physically be used for detection, refractive index and thickness attachments cannot simultaneously be resolved in one measurement. This is particularly important in chemical sensor applications where binding kinetics includes conformational and density changes at the sensor surface.

Standard label-based immunoassay tests involve extensive and complicated incubation and washing steps. In this approach, results are not obtained until 4-24 hours after starting the test. By using GMR sensor technology, real-time results can be obtained with no required washing steps. Results are limited only by the binding dynamics of the ligand-receptor interactions (typically less than 30 minutes). This greatly simplifies medical diagnostic testing approaches, and it will enable doctor offices and hospitals to perform routine screening on a much larger scale with dramatically less labor.

3. Experiments

Numerous characterization experiments have been performed for a variety of biological and chemical materials utilizing GMR sensors and the Vides bioassay spectroscopic reader system developed by Resonant Sensors Incorporated (shown in Fig. 6). In this work, we evaluate this label-free screening tool for the detection of biomarker proteins fibronectin and apolipoprotein A-1 (ApoA-1), which are relevant in ovarian cancer. The sensor plate (shown in Fig. 6(b)) is incorporated in the bottom of a bottomless microarray plate. Each well is sensitized to detect a target analyte by immobilizing a selective layer (such as highly specific antibodies). The spectroscopic sensor system approach (as shown in Fig. 1) tracks the GMR resonance peak wavelength changes as a function of time during a biochemical interaction. The relative peak shift is correlated to a concentration for a particular analyte in a serum or cell culture sample. We use an in vitro cell model for ovarian cancer to provide the relevant expressed biomarker proteins under test. Additionally, we investigate the impact of nonspecific binding and cross reactivity in complex samples such as human serum and cell media.

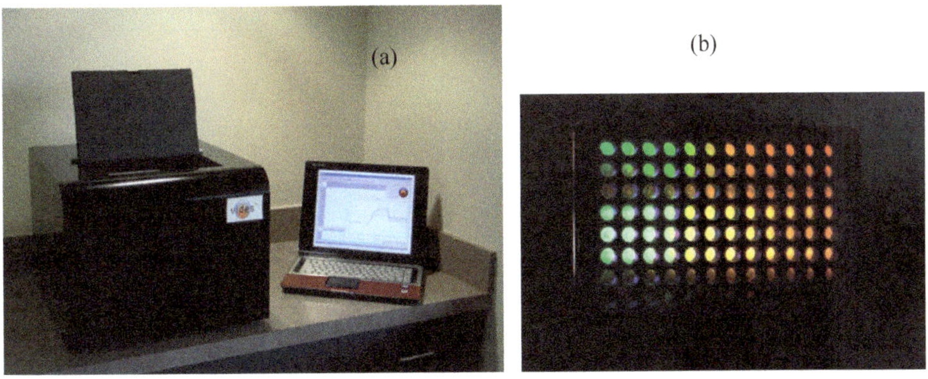

Fig. 6. (a) A benchtop spectroscopic detection system utilizing GMR biosensor technology developed by Resonant Sensors Incorporated (RSI). In this arrangement, the spectral reflectance is monitored with an optical spectrum analyzer, and the peak wavelength is tracked as a function of time during a biochemical event. (b) This bioassay reader utilizes 96-well (shown here) or 384-well (not shown) sensor array plates.

3.1 *In vitro* cell model

Human cell lines are used for the detection of relevant biomarker proteins and feasibility of sensor operation in complex samples. In order to combine the highest possible clinical relevance for the most financially viable research plan, the *in vitro* models for ovarian cancer are chosen based on human cell lines that had been derived directly from patients with ovarian cancer and are not from other types of cancer with ovarian side effects/metastases. Additionally, the *in vitro* models are established (used by ovarian cancer researchers in peer-reviewed publications) and reproducible (available through ATCC).

Two different cell lines are used to provide samples for the detection of ovarian cancer biomarker proteins as shown in Table 1. The cell culture supernatant, which contains the expressed biomarker proteins, is measured to determine the concentrations of fibronectin and apolipoprotein A-1 (detailed in next section). We culture both cell lines as follows:

3.1.1 Cell culture growth

Cells are thawed and transferred to a 15 ml conical tube. Cells are spun at 200 x g for 1 minute. The supernatant is removed and replaced with 1 ml of Complete Medium (MCDB 105 and Medium 199, with fetal bovine serum). A cell count is done on the Nexcelom T4 Cellometer (Nexcelom Bioscience LLC, Lawrence, MA). Cells are then seeded in two 75 cm^2 flasks per vial of cells.

Name	description	source	ATCC #	Ref.
Caov-3	Epithelial ovarian papillary adenocarcinoma	human	HTB-75	(Karlan & Lagasse, 1994)
TOV-21G	Epithelial ovarian poorly differentiated primary malignant adenocarcinoma; Stage IIIC	human	CRL-11730	(Provencher et al., 1993)

Table 1. Ovarian cancer cell lines used in this work.

3.1.2 Sub-culturing or passage

The media is removed and collected for supernatant. The media is replaced with 0.25% trypsin/EDTA, and the flask is placed in an incubator for approximately 3-5 minutes. Once cells are detached, the suspension is removed and placed in a 15 ml Falcon tube. The cell suspension is spun at 200 x g for 1 minute. The trypsin is removed, and the cell pellet is re-suspended in Complete Medium (amount varies depending on confluence). The suspension is seeded into a fresh flask.

3.1.3 Supernatant collection

To collect supernatant, the media is removed from the culture flask, placed in 50 ml Falcon tube, and spun at 300 x g for 1 minute. The supernatant is removed and placed in a fresh 50 ml falcon tube. The tubes are then frozen at -80°C.

3.2 Protein biomarker screening

Detection of the proteins fibronectin and ApoA-1 are performed in a variety of sample backgrounds, including a reagent diluent (containing bovine serum albumin, BSA), human serum, cell media, and cell culture supernatant. Figure 7 illustrates the spectral resonance peak shifts due to the binding of the ovarian cancer biomarker fibronectin in various concentrations. Fibronectin is a high-molecular weight (~440 kDa) extracellular matrix glycoprotein that is known to be produced by some ovarian cancer cell lines. To provide selectivity to fibronectin, anti-fibronectin monoclonal antibodies are immobilized on the sensor surface using commercial silane surface chemistries and cross-linking agents. Known standard concentrations of the target analyte fibronectin are diluted in a reagent diluent solution in phosphate buffered saline (PBS, pH 7.4). This reagent provides a BSA blocking agent to minimize nonspecific binding during the reaction. Both TE and TM polarization resonances are tracked for each concentration. Neat reagent diluent is used as a reference blank and subtracted from the data in Fig. 7. Binding is monitored for 1 hour at 37°C. At the end of the binding, any loose or unbound fibronectin is rinsed away in PBS, and a post-binding measurement is taken. Final data is shown using the relative peak shifts recorded pre- and post-binding in PBS. Both TE and TM resonances trend similarly, with the TM peak having slightly better detection sensitivity. The limit of detection for this assay is ~20 ng/ml.

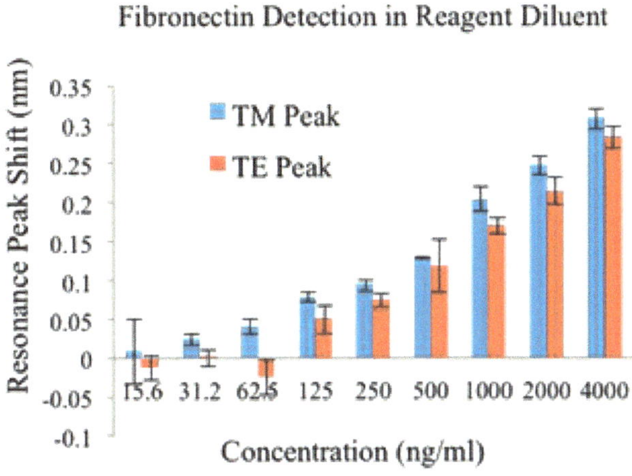

Fig. 7. Resonance peak shift as a function of concentration for fibronectin binding to its matched antibody on the sensor surface. Both TE and TM polarization resonances are tracked. Results are repeated in quadruplicate and averaged.

Figure 8 illustrates fibronectin detected in Caov-3 cell culture media and supernatant. The TM resonance peak shift for the test sample (unknown) is compared to the standard concentration (known) to obtain a measured concentration of 439.1 ng/ml for Caov-3 media and 996.7 ng/ml for Caov-3 supernatant. This indicates that the cell line is expressing fibronectin under culture conditions. Additional concentration measurements were performed for detection of fibronectin in TOV-21G media and cell culture supernatant. Summarized results comparing measured concentrations of both Caov-3 and TOV-21G are shown in Fig. 9. For TOV-21G (a stage IIIC ovarian cancer cell line), fibronectin levels are reduced during cell culture.

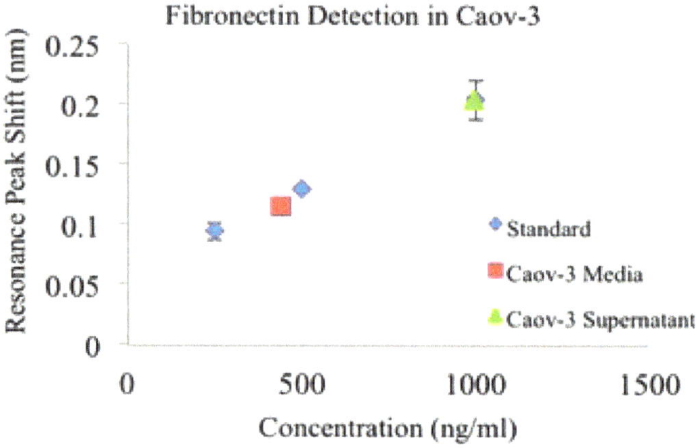

Fig. 8. Resonance peak shift as a function of concentration for detection of fibronectin. Standards are generated in a reagent diluent background. Caov-3 supernatant (green) and media (red) sample resonance shifts are compared to the known concentration resonance shifts (standard curve in blue) to obtain Fibronectin concentrations. All measurements are repeated in quadruplicate and averaged. Some standard deviations are too small to display on chart.

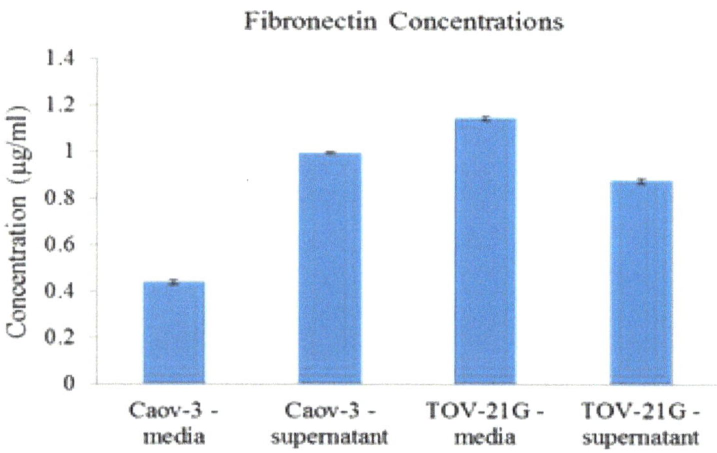

Fig. 9. Comparison of the measured fibronectin in cell culture media and expressed supernatant for two different ovarian cancer cell lines.

Detection of the expressed biomarker protein ApoA-1 in the ovarian cancer cell culture supernatant was also quantified for cell lines Caov-3 and TOV-21G. ApoA-1 is a protein component of high-density lipoprotein in plasma, and it has an approximate molecular weight of 28 kDa. In this experiment, anti-ApoA-1 antibodies are immobilized on the sensor surface to provide targeted selectivity for detection. Figure 10 illustrates measured TM-resonance shifts for standard known concentrations of ApoA-1 in reagent diluent (shown in blue). We also measure unknown amounts of ApoA-1 in fresh (unused) cell culture media and in ovarian cancer cell supernatant. The known standards are used to generate a linear calibration curve for the range from 32 ng/ml to 125 ng/ml (with an R_2 value of 0.989). Based on this linear fit, the fresh cell culture media is found to contain ~59 ng/ml ApoA-1 while the cell culture supernatant contains ~89 ng/ml. Binding is monitored for 1 hour at 37°C.

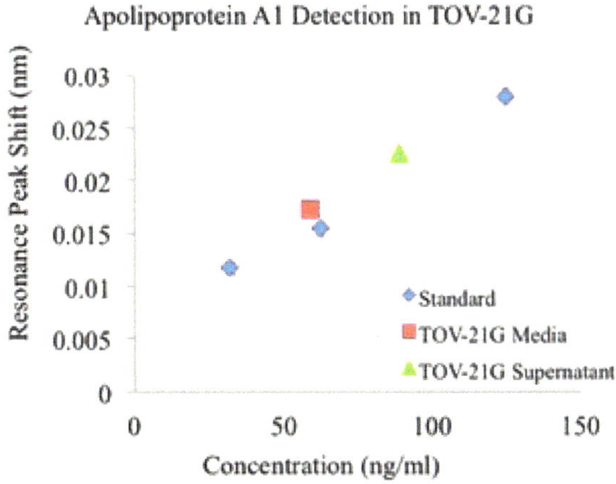

Fig. 10. Resonance peak shifts measured for detection of apolipoprotein A-1. Known standards are measured (shown in blue) to obtain a calibration curve that is used to quantify the unknown samples (shown in red and green). Samples are run in quadruplicate and averaged, with major outliers removed. Standard deviation is negligible (shown on plot).

Figure 11 illustrates detection of the biomarker ApoA-1 in culture media and supernatant for the Caov-3 and TOV-21G cell lines. The TM resonance peak shift for the test sample (unknown) is compared to the standard concentration (shown in Fig. 10) to obtain a measured concentration for each sample. Summarized results comparing measured concentrations of both cell media and culture supernatant are shown in Fig. 11. For the TOV-21G cell line, ApoA-1 is increased (or expressed) in the measured supernatant. In the Caov-3, the measured amount in the supernatant is reduced during culture. Tests are run in quadruplicate and averaged.

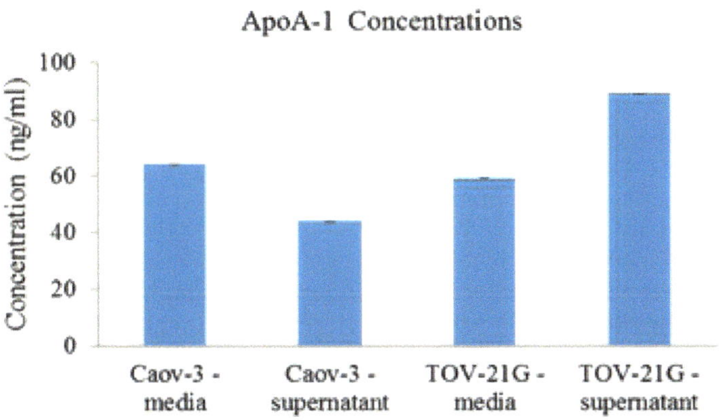

Fig. 11. Comparison of the measured ApoA-1 in cell culture media and expressed supernatant for two different ovarian cancer cell lines. Standard deviation is negligible (shown on plot).

3.3 Nonspecific binding

To investigate the amount of nonspecific binding that might occur during the media/supernatant and serum experiments, we prepare a negative reference well using a blocked silanized well (no antibodies attached); it is compared to wells containing specific antibodies for ApoA-1 and fibronectin. The capture antibodies for ApoA-1 and fibronectin are monoclonal mouse antibodies that are chemically attached to the sensor surface using a silane-based crosslinking agent. After antibody attachment, the unbound sites are blocked with a blocking buffer (BSA). In Figure 12, a cell culture media sample (having ApoA-1 naturally present) is incubated (1 hour) on sensor wells containing antibodies specific for ApoA-1 and wells that have no antibodies present. Figure 12 illustrates the minimal shift results from the negative reference well (no antibodies) as compared to the well containing the specific antibodies (large shift). We also investigate the use of human serum as a sample background in the detection of fibronectin. Figure 13 illustrates the resonance peak shift results from a serum sample (naturally containing fibronectin) after incubation (1 hour) on a negative reference well (no antibodies) compared to the specific antibody coated region. Both of these results are based on the difference of initial and final PBS baseline readings.

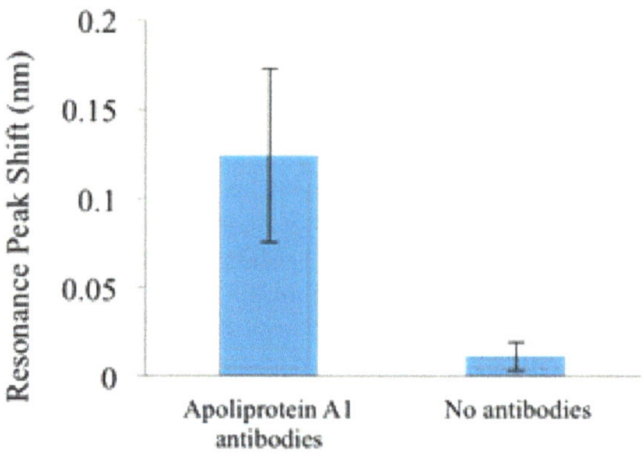

Fig. 12. Comparison of the TM resonant peak shift due to binding of the biomarker ApoA-1 (in a cell media background) to the ApoA-1 antibodies on the sensors surface versus nonspecific binding on the sensor elements not coated with antibodies.

Since the cell media and supernatant samples are made up of complex matrices, we used a spike and recovery method (Thermo, 2007) for each biomarker protein assay to determine whether the protein detection is affected by a difference between the diluent used to prepare the standard curve and the cell media sample matrix. In spike and recovery experiments, a known amount of protein standard is added to the sample matrix (corresponding growth media for each cell line) and compared to a standard curve measured in diluent. The two sets of total resonance peak shift measurements are compared. Table 2 shows results for spike and recovery experiments performed for fibronectin in both Caov-3 and TOV-21G cell culture media. Measurements are based on the difference of initial and final baseline readings with pure reagent diluent or pure media used as negative controls and subtracted from the data. In both cases, the detected amount was within ~10% of the target.

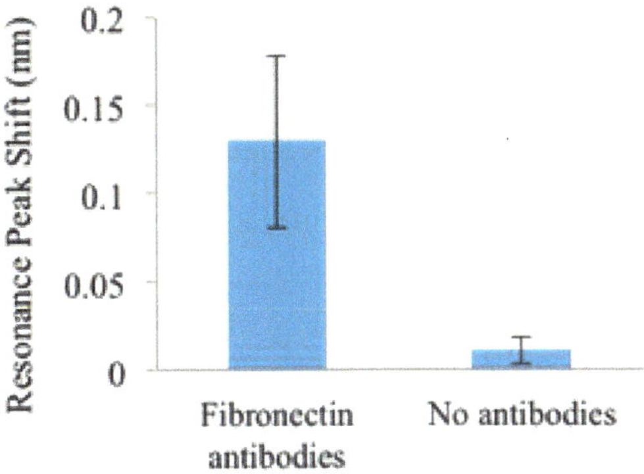

Fig. 13. Comparison of the TM resonant peak shift due to the binding of fibronectin (in human serum) to the fibronectin antibodies on the sensors surface versus the nonspecific binding on the sensor elements not coated with antibodies. Tests are run in quadruplicate and averaged.

Medium	Spike (ng/ml)	Standard Resonance Peak Shift (nm)	Spiked Resonance Peak Shift (nm)	Recovery %
Caov-3	500	0.129	0.135	104.7
TOV-21G	500	0.129	0.116	89.9

Table 2. Fibronectin Spike and Recovery.

4. Dual-peak analysis

As shown in Fig. 1, there are separate resonance peaks for each polarization (TE and TM) that shift in response to a given measurement. By backfitting this dual-peak response into our rigorous electromagnetic coupled wave analysis codes (Gaylord & Moharam, 1985), we can determine two unknowns: surface changes due to analyte binding and bulk refractive-index changes that occur due to sample background variations. First, we calculate and map the predicted TE and TM resonance peak shifts over a relevant range of added biolayer thicknesses (0 to 50 nm) and background index variations (n=1.33 to n=1.5). A simple matrix is applied to match the corresponding detection layer and background index when the two resonance peak shifts are known. This data is fitted assuming a known biolayer refractive index, with unknown values to be determined for the biolayer thicknesses and background index. To illustrate the utility of this approach, we use the ionic polymer poly (allylamine hydrochloride) to study binding interactions that involve biolayer adhesion and associated thickness change at the sensor surface (Magnusson et al., 2011). Two resonance peaks are tracked as the ionic polymer attaches a monolayer of material as shown in Fig. 14. After the polymer saturates, the measurement is paused and the sensor is washed to remove any unbound polymer. A post-binding measurement is made in DI water. The results in Fig. 15 show that the binding of the polymer layer to the sensor surface contributes most to the measured response. The fitted background drift is partially attributed to thermal changes in the sample during the measurement and imperfect model assumptions (such as polymer layer index). Improvements to the backfit model will further distinguish these contributions.

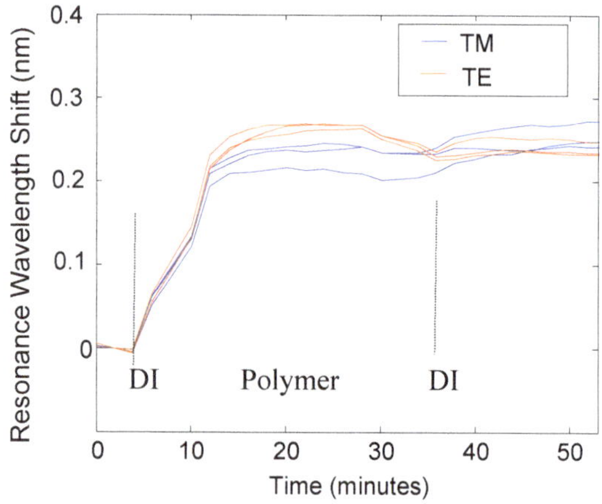

Fig. 14. Resonance peak shifts as a function of time for binding ionic polymer to the sensor surface. Both TE and TM resonances are monitored. This medium has a molecular weight of 56,000 kDa.

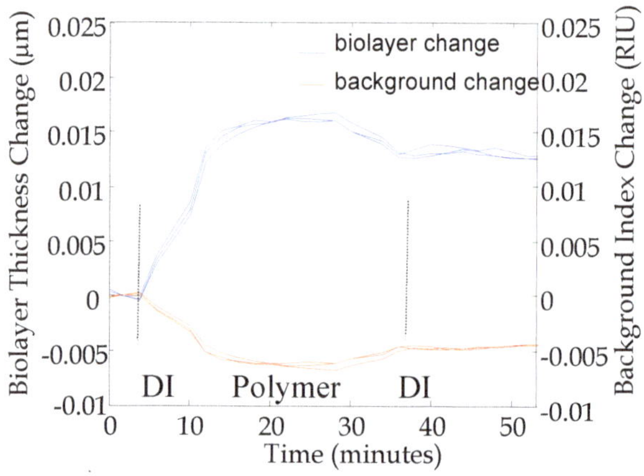

Fig. 15. Results of backfitting to a simple model, thereby differentiating contributions from biolayer adhesion and background changes.

5. Conclusions

A novel diagnostic system to detect biomarkers relevant for diagnosis of ovarian cancer has been developed. This label-free sensor system can accurately and rapidly detect an array of protein markers with minimal sample processing requirements. Sensor performance was characterized for the biomarker proteins fibronectin and apoliprotein A-1 with limits of detection measured to be ~20 ng/ml in backgrounds of cell culture media and human serum. An *in vitro* cell culture model was used with established ovarian cancer cell lines to provide relevant samples for this work. Nonspecific binding effects were investigated for operation in serum backgrounds with minimal impact. Additionally, due to inherent polarization diversity, these sensors employ multiple resonance peaks that are used to increase detection accuracy by providing multiple data points for each test. Work is ongoing to integrate this system into a portable detection unit that can be used in a point-of-care setting. Future work will include clinical sample validation and an expanded array of relevant biomarkers that can be tested in a single sample. This will provide a highly accurate rapid screening tool for early detection of ovarian cancer.

6. Acknowledgements

This work was supported in part by the National Science Foundation SBIR grant #0724407 (D.W), the National Cancer Institute SBIR grant #R43CA135960 (D.W. and P.K.) and the State of Texas Emerging Technology Fund (D.W.). Additional support was provided by the UT System Texas Nanoelectronics Research Superiority Award (R.M.), the Texas Instruments Distinguished University Chair in Nanoelectronics endowment (R.M.), the Vision Research Foundation of Kansas City (P.K.), and the Felix and Carmen Sabates Missouri Endowed Chair in Vision Research (P.K.). The content is solely the responsibility of the authors and does not necessarily represent the official views of the funding agencies.

7. References

American Cancer Society, (2011) *Ovarian Cancer Reference literature*, http://www.cancer.org.

Bignotti, E.; et al. (2007). Gene expression profile of ovarian serous papillary carcinomas: identification of metastasis-associated genes. *Am. J. Obstet. Gynecol.* 196:245.

Cooper, M. (2006). Current Biosensor Technologies in Drug Discovery. *Drug Discovery World*. 68-82.

Cunningham, A. (1998). Introduction to Bioanalytical Sensors. *John Wiley and Sons*, New York.

Cunningham, B.; Li, P.; Lin, B. & Pepper, J. (2002). Colorimetric resonant reflection as a direct biochemical assay technique. *Sens. Actuators* B. 81:316-328.

Gaylord, T. K. and Moharam, M. G. (1985). Analysis and applications of optical diffraction by gratings. *Proceedings of the IEEE*. 73:894-937.

Homola, J. (2003). Present and future of surface plasmon resonance biosensors. *Anal. Bioanal. Chem.* 377:528-539.

Karlan, B.Y. & Lagasse, L.D. (1994). Glucocorticoids stabilize HER-2/neu messenger RNA in human epithelial ovarian carcinoma cells. *Gynecologic Oncology* 53:70-77.

Kikuta, H.; Maegawa, N.; Mizutani, A.; Iwata, K.; & Toyota, H. (2001). Refractive index sensor with a guided-mode resonant grating filter. *Proceedings of the SPIE*. Yokohama, Japan. 4416:219-222.

Liotta, L.; Lowenthal, M.; & Mehta, A. (2005). Importance of communication between producers and consumers of publicly available experimental data. *J. Natl. Cancer Inst.* 97:310-314.

Magnusson, R. & S. S. Wang. (1992). New principle for optical filters. *Appl. Phys.* Lett. 61:1022-1024.

Magnusson, R.; Wawro, D.; Zimmerman, S.; & Ding, Y. (2011). Resonant Photonic Biosensors with Polarization-Based Multiparametric Discrimination in Each Channel, *Sensors*, 11, 1476-1488.

Priambodo, P.S.; Maldonado, T.A. & Magnusson, R. (2003). Fabrication and characterization of high-quality waveguide-mode resonant optical filters. *Appl. Phys. Lett.* 83, 3248-3250.

Provencher, D.M.; et al; (1993). Comparison of antigen expression on fresh and cultured ascites cells and on solid tumors of patients with epithelial ovarian cancer. *Gynecologic Oncology* 50:1,78-83.

Raether, H. (1988). Surface plasmons on smooth and rough surfaces and on gratings. *Springer Verlag*, Berlin.

Rosenblatt, D.; Sharon, A; & Friesem, A. (1997) Resonant Grating Waveguide Structures. *IEEE J. Quantum Electron.* 33, 2038.

Thermo Scientific Tech Tip #58. (2007) Spike-and-recovery and linearity-of-dilution assessment. www.thermo.com

Wawro, D.; Tibuleac, S.; Magnusson, R.; & Liu, H. (2000). Optical fiber endface biosensor based on resonances in dielectric waveguide gratings. *Proceedings of the SPIE*. San Jose, California. 3911:86-94.

Wawro, D.; Tibuleac, S.; & Magnusson, R. (2006). Optical waveguide-mode resonant biosensors. *Optical Imaging Sensors and Systems for Homeland Security Applications*. 367-384.

Wawro, D.; Koulen, P.; Ding, Y.; Zimmerman, S. & Magnusson, R. (2010). Guided-mode resonance sensor system for early detection of ovarian cancer. Optical Diagnostics and Sensing X: Toward Point-of-Care Diagnostics. *Proceedings of the SPIE*. San Francisco, California. 7572:75720D.

4

Apoptosis Pathways in Ovarian Cancer

Christine Sers[1], Reinhold Schafer[1] and Irina Nazarenko[2]
[1]*Institute of Pathology, University Medicine Charité, Berlin*
[2]*Institute of Toxicology and Genetics, Karlsruhe Institute of Technology, Karlsruhe*
Germany

1. Introduction

Tumour initiation and progression are driven by constitutively activated oncogenes mediating deregulation of the balance between cell death- and survival pathways. Among the most relevant signalling cascades activated in the majority of tumour types, the RAS/mitogen-activated protein kinase (Ras/MAPK), the phosphatidyl inositol-3-kinase/protein kinase B (PI3K/PKB) and the protein kinases C (PKC) signalling cascades were postulated (Weinstein, 1987; Nicosia et al., 2003; Roberts and Der, 2007; McCubrey et al., 2007; Breitkreutz et al., 2007). These cascades define individual characteristics of particular tumours and consequently their individual responsiveness to cancer therapy.

In this chapter, we will address the characteristics of the apoptotic signalling pathways in ovarian carcinomas. Particular attention will be given to the *HRS* family of tumour suppressor genes encoding proteins with phospholipase activity and suppressed in the majority of ovarian malignancies. We will describe signalling cascades down regulating two well-characterized members of this family H-REV107-1/HRLS3/PLA2G16 and TIG3/RARRES/RIG1 in tumour cells. Furthermore, potential therapeutic consequences of the re-expression of these genes defined as a class II tumour suppressors will be discussed.

2. The HRS class II tumour suppressors are important mediators of IFN-γ and retinoid-dependent growth suppression and cell death in ovarian cancer

The *H-REV107*-related genes (*TIG3, H-REV107-1, HRSL2*) are known as inhibitors of proliferation of tumour cells in vivo and in vitro. While being almost ubiquitously expressed in normal tissues, down-regulation or complete loss of these genes in tumours and tumour cell lines have been reported. Expression can be reconstituted by different anti-proliferative signals such as interferons and retinoids, as well as by the inhibition of oncogenic pathways and interference with DNA methylation (Alessi et al., 1994; Husmann et al., 1998; Akiyama et al., 1999; Siegrist et al., 2001; Ito et al., 2001; Roder et al., 2002; Huang et al., 2002; Higuchi et al., 2003; Duvic et al., 2003). Re-activation of the H-REV107-1-related proteins and over-expression of the genes induce apoptosis or differentiation of tumour cells.

2.1 HRS family members encode LRAT-related phospholipid-metabolizing enzymes

Two independent groups (Hughes and Stanway, 2000; Anantharaman and Aravind, 2003) have unfolded the phylogenetic relationship between *H-REV107-1*-related genes, LRAT (Lecithin retinol acyltransferase) and viral and bacterial peptidases in previous works.

Here we aimed to identify and describe H-REV107-1 homologs in different organisms in order to follow their origin and development during the evolution.

For that purpose, we performed an *in silico* analysis, using PSI-Blast and Blast-p screening in the NCBI non-redundant database. This analysis revealed 62 homologous proteins in eukaryotic and prokaryotic organisms. To identify phylogenetic relationships Tree Puzzle (Strimmer and von Haeseler, 1997) was applied (Fig. 1). The analysis revealed five closely related proteins, suggesting their origin from the same ancestor protein during the evolution. These proteins, including H-REV107-1 comprise a new protein family, which we designated here as the HRS (H-REV107-1-related proteins) protein family (Table 1).

The novel HRS family is composed of tumour suppressors, which negatively regulate cell survival, control signal transduction and induce differentiation.

Suggested nomenklature	*NCBI Synonyms*	*Chromosomal localization*	*Species*	*Publication - gene cloning*	*Acc. No gene*	*Acc. No protein*	*Function*
HRS1	HRASLS	3q29 (194440-1944470 K)	Human	Ito et al. Cytogenet. Cell Genet. 93:36-39 (2001)	NM_020386	NP_065119	Unknown
Hrs1	A-C1, Hrasls, 2810012B06Rik	16	Mouse	Akiyama et al. J. Biol. Chem. 274: 32192-32197 (1999)	NM_013751	NP_038779	Inhibits growth of HRAS-transformed cells
Hrs1	similar to Hrasls		Rat	Uyama et al., Biochim.Biophys.Acta (2009)	XM_213590	XP_213590	PE *N*-acyltransferase lysophospholipid *O*-acyltransferase
HRS2	**HRASLS2**	**11q12.3 (63076-63088 K)**	Human		NM_017878	NP_060348	
HRS3	**HRASLS3, H-REV107-1, H-REV107-3, hHrev-107, PLA2G16**	**11q12.3-q13.1 (63099-63138 K)**	Human	Husmann et al. Oncogene 17: 1305-1312 (1998)	NM_007069	NP_009000	Phospholipase 2A, Induces apoptosis in ovarian cancer cells
Hrs3	Hrasls3	19	Mouse	Roder et al. J: Biol. Chem. 277: 30543-30550 (2002); Jaworski et al., Nat Med. 2009	NM_139269	NP_644675	major adipocyte phosphoslipase
Hrs3	Hrasls3, H-Rev107	1q	Rat	Hajnal et al. Oncogene 9: 479-490 (1994)	NM_017060	NP_056756	Inhibits growth of Ras-transformed cells in vivo and in vitro
HRS4	**RARRES3, TIG3, RIG1, H-REV107-2**	**11q13.2 (63061-63070 K)**	Human	DiSepio et al. PNAS 95: 14811-14815 (1998)	NM_004585	NP_004576	phospholipid methabolizing enzyme, Induces apoptosis in ovarian cancer cells
HRS5	**HRLP5; iNAT**	**11q13.2 (62988-63015 K)**	Human	Jin et al., Biochim.Biophys.Acta (2009); Jin et al., J.Biol. Chem (2007)	NM_054108	NP_473449	Ca-independent phosphatidylethanolamine N-acyltransferase
Hrs5	Hrlp5		Mouse		NM_025731	NP_080007	
Hrs5	Hrlp5		Rat		XM219546	XP_219546	
Hrs	unnamed		Fish		CAG09755	CAAE01015008	
Hrs	MGC68773		Frog		BCO60489	AAH60489	
Hrs	unnamed		Amphioxus		AF391288	AAM18866	

Table 1. Members of the HRS family

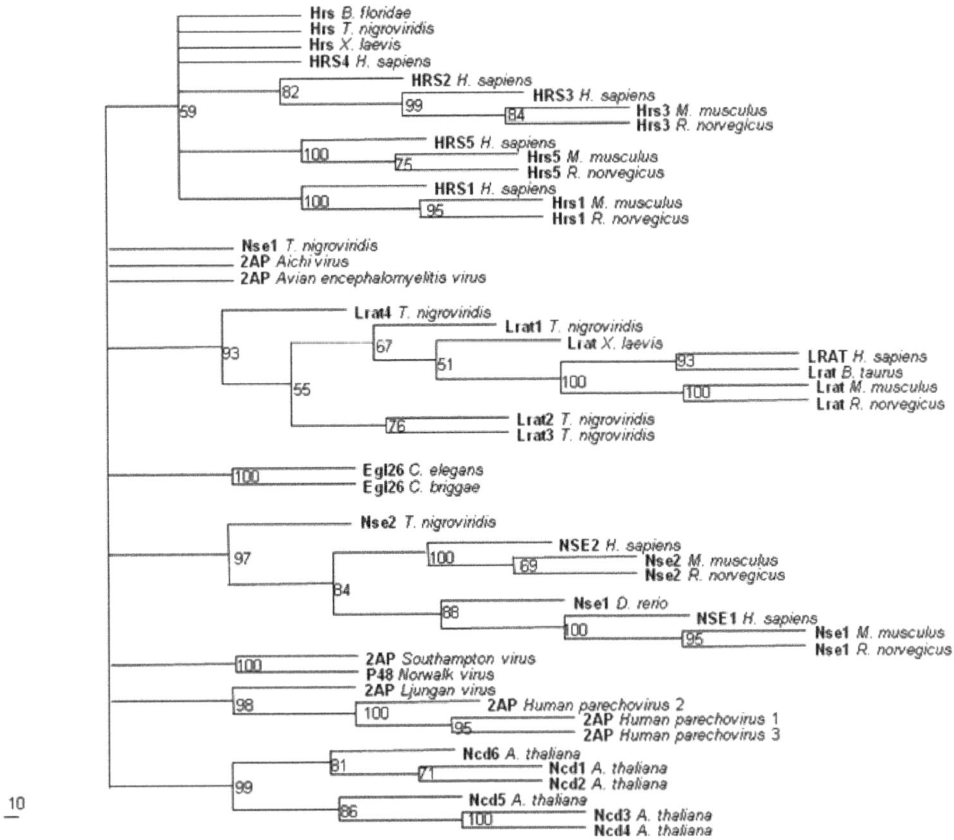

Fig. 1. Phylogeny of HRS and the related LRAT, NSE and NCD protein families
A maximum parsimony tree was generated with the help of Tree-Puzzle (Strimmer and von Haeseler 1997) and includes the eukaryotic members of the HRS, LRAT, NSE families, plant NC proteins, the *C.elegans* Egl26 proteins, and the viral 2A proteins.
First, only HRS proteins were aligned using the ClustlW algorithm (EMBL-EBI), then LRAT and NSE families. From the *C.elegans*, the viral and the plant proteins only regions with a high similarity to the HRS proteins were compared. Additional upstream and downstream motifs were cut out. As a result, all sequences had a comparable length of about 160 amino acid residues that corresponds the average length of the HRS proteins.
For the calculation of the phylogenetic relationships 1000 replicates were run. Branch support values are indicated at the nodes, distances are proportional to relative sequence divergence.

2.2 Clustered chromosomal localization of 4 human HRS genes on 11q13

Four of the five members of the human HRS family, *HRLS2, H-REV107-1, TIG3* and *HRLS5,* are localized in one cluster on chromosome 11q13, supporting the hypothesis of their origin from the same ancestor (Fig. 3). The *HRLS2* and *H-REV107-1* genes, encoding most closely related family members (Fig. 1A), are located next to each other. The *H-REV107-1* gene spans between 63099K and 63138K on the chromosome 11q, and directly downstream of it, from 63077K to 63088K, the *HRLS2* gene is located. The *TIG3* gene is positioned on the opposite DNA strand directly downstream of *HRLS2,* the gene has a small non-coding region and spans between 63070K and 63079K. The *HRLS5* gene 62897K and 63015K is also located on chromosome 11q13, but separated by two genes encoding the thymosin-like 5 (TMSL5) and the lectin, galactoside-binding, soluble, 12 (galectin 12/LGAL12) proteins, from the other HRS genes.

Earlier findings suggested that chromosomal alterations resulting in *HRS* gene down-regulation or loss are rather rare events in human carcinomas. Nevertheless, structural changes on 11q13 have been described in numerous cases and only recently methods such as array CGH and next generation sequencing (NGS) have improved the analysis such that the involvement of individual genes can now be analysed. Therefore, it cannot be excluded that future investigations might unravel smaller deletions influencing one of the clustered *HRS* genes on 11q13 in distinct tumour types.

2.3 Domain structure and enzymatic activity of the HRS family members

Phylogenetic analysis of HRS and HRS-related proteins revealed a high conservation within the so called NlpC/P60 domain (Anantharaman and Aravind, 2003). This sequence was indentified in LRAT proteins (lecithin retinol acyltransferase) as being essential for all-trans-retinol metabolism.

To analyse domain structure of other members of the HRS family, Clustl W alignment was performed. Using this program, 14 members of the HRS protein family found in the NCBI database, were analysed (Fig. 2).

The HRS proteins contain non-homologous proline-rich motifs on their N-termini (red line on the top of the alignment). The core parts of HRS proteins are highly conserved and contain the NlpC/P60 and NC domains (Fig. 2, blue and green boxes, respectively). We predicted three β-strands within the Nlpc/P60 domain (Fig. 2, blue arrows). The first and the second strand contain the conserved GDL and HWXXY motifs; the VXXLAP motif comprises the third strand. The region downstream the third β-strand with two conserved serine residues is likely to have the structure of α-helix (Fig. 2, green cylinder). The large NC domain depicted in Fig. 2 with a green box, contains a KALVK conserved motif of unknown function, two short stretches DXXG and NKXD, which are similar to conserved regions of GTPases (Akiyama et al., 1999; Bourne, Sanders, and McCormick 1990) and the NCEHFV conserved motif, characteristic for conventional NC domains. At the C-terminus, HRS proteins harbour a hydrophobic C-terminal α-helix,described as a membrane-binding domain.

Recently, a crystal structure of the NlpC/P60 domain of H-REV107-1 has being resolved (Ren et al., 2010b). Within this domain, a phospholipase active site consisting of a Cys-His-His triad was identified. The residues H23 and C113 play a pivotal role for the H-REV107-1 enzymatic activity (Ren et al., 2010a). Meantime, the enzymatic activity of the H-REV107-1, TIG3, HRASLS2 and HRLP5 proteins has been characterized as $PLA_{1/2}$- type hydrolysis, supporting a role of the HRS proteins in lipid metabolism.

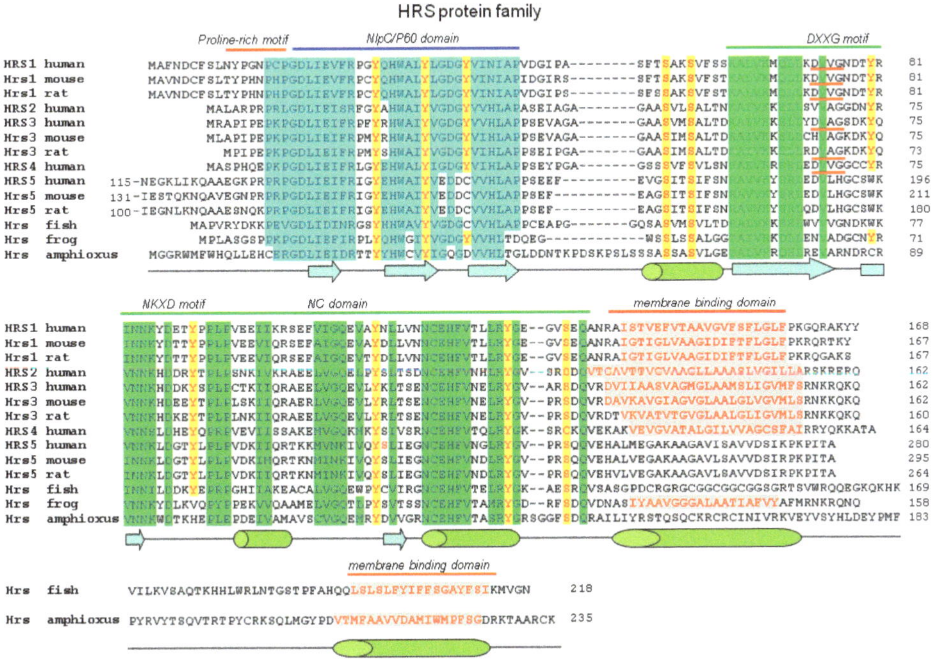

Fig. 2. HRS catalytic and protein-binding domains
Fourteen members of the HRS protein family found in the NCBI database were aligned using the Clustal W program as described in Figure 1B. Analysis, edition, and shading of conserved domains were performed with the help of the GenDoc freeware (http://www.psc.edu/biomed/genedoc/). The PSIPRED secondary structure prediction server was used to analyze potential secondary structures of the HRS protein sequences (http://bioinf.cs.ucl.ac.uk/psipred/) (McGuffin, Bryson, and Jones 2000).
The HRS proteins contain non-homologous proline-rich motifs on their N-termini (red line on the top of the alignment). The core parts of HRS proteins are highly conserved and contain the NlpC/P60 and NC domains (blue and green boxes, respectively). With a high prediction confidence of the PSIPRED standard analysis, three β-strands were defined within the Nlpc/P60 domain (blue arrows). The first and the second strand contain the conserved GDL and HWXXY motifs; the VXXLAP motif comprises the third strand. The region downstream the third β-strand with two conserved serine residues is likely to have a structure of α-helix (green cylinder). The large NC domain (green box) contains a KALVK conserved motif of unknown function, two short stretches DXXG and NKXD, which are similar to conserved regions of GTPases (Akiyama et al., 1999; Bourne, Sanders, and McCormick 1990) and the NCEHFV conserved motif, characteristic for conventional NC domains. At the C-terminus, HRS proteins harbour a hydrophobic C-terminal α-helix.

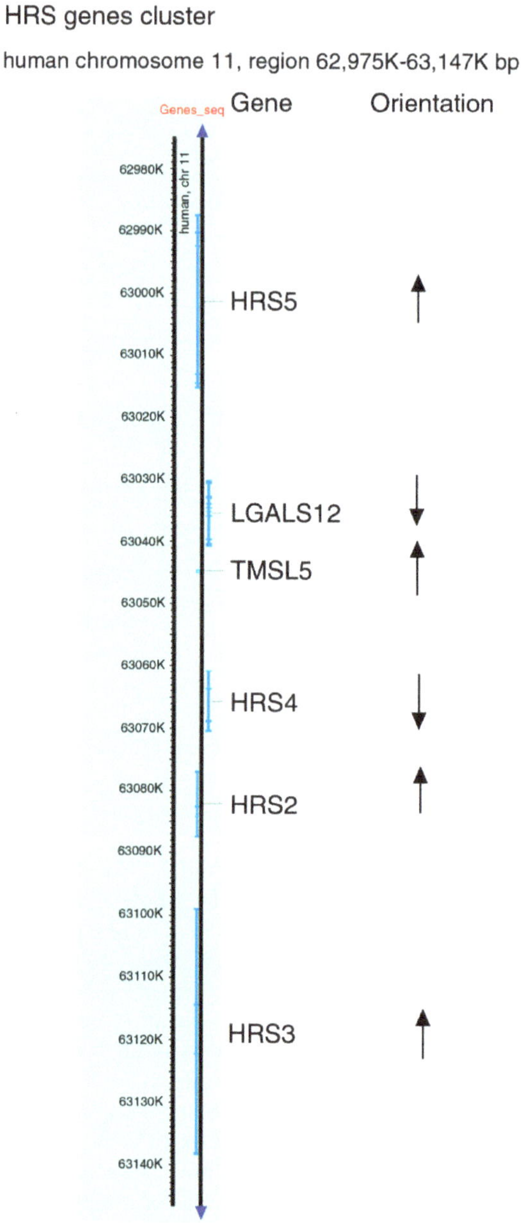

Fig. 3. *HRS2/HRLS2, HRS3/H-REV107-1/ HRS4/TIG3* and *HRS5/HRLS5* genes are localized on chromosome 11q13 in one cluster. Gene orientation, length and mapping of the chromosome regions are directly obtained from the NCBI Map View server.

Additionally to the NlpC/P60 domain, HRS proteins contain a proline-rich N-terminal domain, responsible for establishing protein-protein interactions and a variable hydrophobic C-terminal α-helix, which directs and transiently binds the protein to intracellular membranes (Husmann et al., 1998; Nazarenko et al., 2007). Furthermore, a DXXG domain, also termed G3 motif, characteristic for RAS small GTPases, and mediating the binding of magnesium and γ-phosphate of GTP via the aspartic acid and glycine residue, respectively was identified (Kjeldgaard et al., 1996). However, a functional role of these motifs in HRS proteins has not been defined yet.

2.4 Reversible Inhibition of the HRS genes H-REV107-1 and TIG3 by oncogenic signalling cascades in tumours

Members of the HRS gene family *H-REV107-1* and *TIG3* belong to the so called class II tumour suppressors. The major characteristic of this class, postulated in 1997 by Ruth Sager, is their down-regulation in tumours via reversible mechanisms, however not through mutations or deletions (Sager, 1997). Once re-expressed, these genes can exhibit their tumour-suppressive function and thereby contribute to the inhibition of tumour progression.

2.4.1 IFNγ-mediated re-expression of H-REV107-1 leads to the induction of apoptosis in ovarian cancer cells

Rat *H-Rev107-1*, the founder gene of the HRS family, was cloned from a subtractive cDNA library (Hajnal et al., 1994). The rat *H-Rev107-1* gene, expressed in immortalized rat fibroblasts, was identified as a gene suppressed in an HRAS-transformed derivative, but re-expressed in a revertant cell line. Further experiments suggested that repression of *H-Rev107-1* in HRAS-transformed cells was functionally involved in HRAS-dependent transformation (Hajnal et al., 1994; Sers et al., 1997).

Repression of *H-Rev107-1* was also detected in KRAS-transformed rat ovarian epithelial cells suggesting that in contrast to other HRS genes, *H-Rev107-1* suppression in response to RAS oncogenes is not associated with the RAS isoform. Most interestingly, *H-Rev107-1* down-regulation upon KRAS-transformation appeared to be reversible and identified the *H-Rev107-1* gene as a target negatively regulated by the MEK-ERK pathway. The same observation was also made in PA1 human teratocarcinoma cells, which harbour an activated NRAS oncogene (Alessi et al., 1994) and suggested that *H-REV107-1* might be negatively affected by RAS oncogene-dependent signalling in general.

The human *H-REV107-1*, first described in 1998, was found ubiquitously expressed in normal human epithelial tissues (;Husmann et al., 1998). When compared to differentiated cells in situ, *H-REV107-1* is down-regulated in human tumour cell lines and tumour samples at the mRNA and at the protein level. Loss of *H-REV107-1* mRNA until now was detected in tumours derived from breast, lung, ovary, kidney and testis (Sers et al., 1997;Siegrist et al., 2001). In human ovarian carcinomas, we also demonstrated strongly diminished levels or complete loss of the H-REV107-1 protein. In ovarian carcinomas sequencing of the *H-REV107-1* coding region revealed no alterations within this region suggesting that *H-REV107-1* acts as class II tumour suppressor gene in these tissues.

A functional involvement of H-REV107-1 inactivation in ovarian tumours was demonstrated by the finding that reactivation of endogenous H-REV107-1 in H-REV107-1-negative ovarian carcinoma cells induces apoptosis. In these cells, loss of *H-REV107-1* expression can be reconstituted upon administration of Interferon gamma (IFNγ), a finding reported earlier from rat astrocytoma cells (Bartel, 2004). Up-regulation of *H-REV107-1* in response to IFNγ works well at the mRNA level, yet only a small proportion of cells also express sufficient H-REV107-1 protein for detection. Most interestingly these cells undergo apoptosis (Sers et al., 2002). These observations made clear that H-REV107-1 is likely to interfere with the survival of ovarian cancer cells. Our work further supported this suggestion as we could show that H-REV107-1 is an inhibitor of PP2A whose function is required in ovarian carcinomas for cell survival (Nazarenko et al., 2007). This was the first hint indicating a role of the H-REV107-1 protein in the regulation of apoptotic intracellular signalling and will be discussed in part 3 of this chapter.

2.4.2 Mechanisms of H-REV107-1 suppression in ovarian carcinomas via anti-apoptotic pathways

The reversible down-regulation of *H-REV107-1* in ovarian cancer has prompted the investigation of the mechanisms responsible for suppression. The human *H-REV107-1* promoter is located directly upstream of a 408bp 5′UT sequence. The sequence harbours several potential transcription factor binding sites including an Interferon-responsive IRSE motif, a CREB site, potential AP-1 and c-REL binding sites (Fig. 4).

The IRSE site, a DNA-sequence bound by the Interferon regulatory factors IRF-1 and IRF-2, provides the structural basis for the observed induction of *H-REV107-1* upon administration of IFNγ and conditionally expressed IRF-1 (Alessi et al., 1994). Comparison of *IRF-1* and *H-REV107-1* levels between human ovarian carcinoma cells and immortalized human ovarian epithelial cells, revealed strongly diminished *IRF-1 and H-REV1017-1* levels in the tumour cell lines. This suggested that loss of *IRF-1* expression might be one of the mechanisms of *H-REV107-1* suppression in human ovarian carcinomas (Sers at al., 2002).

Surprisingly, there is no conservation between the human *H-REV107-1* and the mouse or rat *H-REV107-1* promoter region, suggesting a different regulation of human *H-REV107-1* and the rodent homologues. More importantly, it was shown that murine *H-REV107-1* can be regulated via DNA methylation. In view of human tumours, next steps will include addressing the question, whether this methylation-dependent suppression of *H-REV107-1* is a tumour-related process, or a developmental process during which tissue-specific expression profiles are established.

2.4.3 Physiological role of H-REV107-1 and its potential role in cancerogenesis

Meantime, the enzymatic function of H-REV107-1 has been defined (Ueda et al., 2009). The protein acts as a cytosolic Ca^{2+}-independent phospholipase Pla2G16, which catalyses esterolytic cleavage of glycerophospholipids to lysophospholipids. Supporting these data, a recent study in a knock-out model demonstrated that the H-rev107-1 physiological function is a major adipocyte phospholipase A_2 (AdPLA). The protein inhibited lipolysis in adipocytes, regulating adiposity on systemic level (Jaworski et al., 2009). Ablation of the H-rev107-1 led to a significantly higher rate of lipolysis, accompanied by an increase in cyclic AMP levels (Jaworski et al., 2009). The knock-out animals were resistant to high-fat feeding and leptin-deficiency mediated obesity. Albeit, a direct impact of the H-rev107-1 ablation on tumourigenesis in vivo has not been tested yet, the observed increase in lipolysis and elevated levels of cAMP, also common in tumour cells, suggest a potentially higher susceptibility of the H-rev107-1 knockout animals to tumour growth as compared to their wild type littermates.

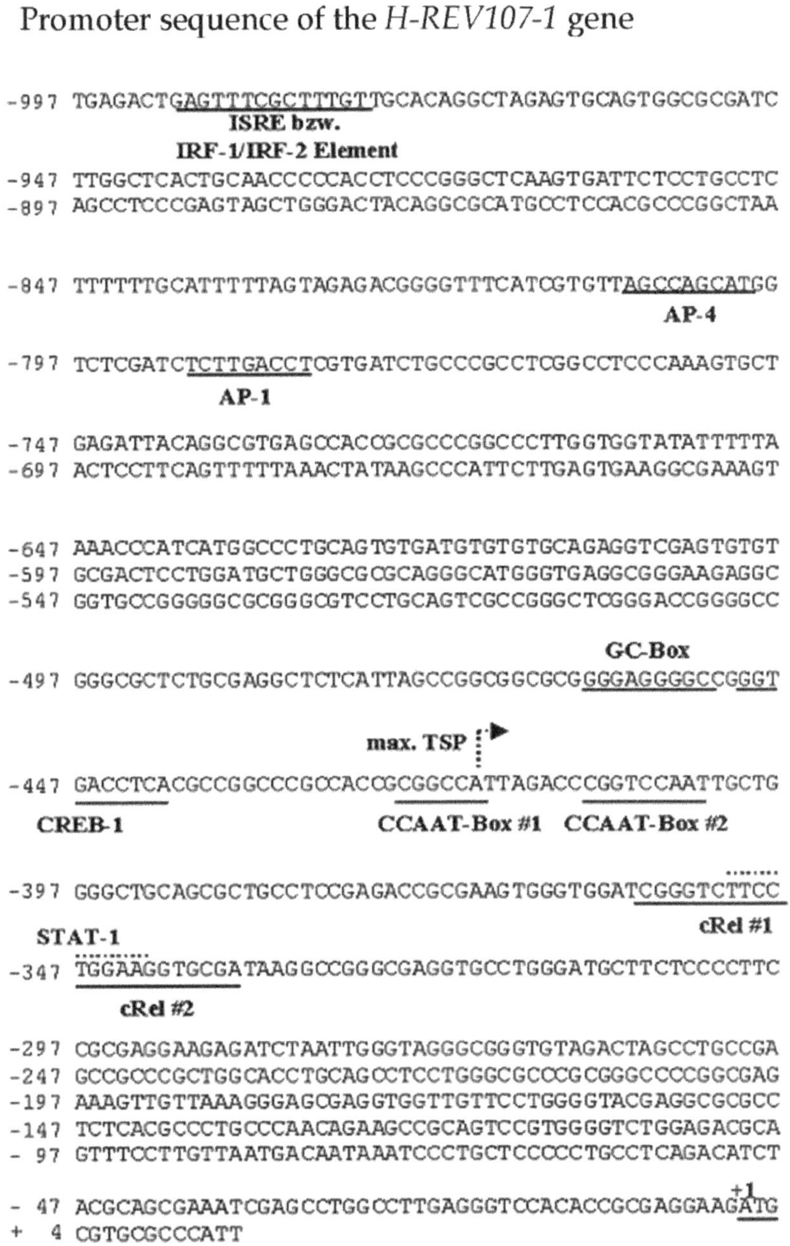

Fig. 4. Promoter sequence of the human *H-REV107-1* gene. The translatioal start site is indicated by +1, 997 base pairs of upstream sequence are shown. Individual sequence motifs as identified by MatInspector are indicated.

The H-rev107-1 knockout model provides a first link between lipid metabolism and a tumour suppressive effect of phospholipases. Alterations in lipid metabolism, especially in phospholipids-related pathways and fatty acid biosynthesis are known to occur in ovarian carcinomas (Tania et al., 2010). . Thus, FAS (fatty acid synthase) is up-regulated in cancer cells and mediates activity of HER-2 (Gansler at al., 1997; Menendez et al., 2004). It has been suggested that HER-2 functions as a cellular energy sensor in response to the metabolic stress, supporting therapeutic advantages of combinatorial inhibition of HER-2 and FAS in HER-2-positive tumours. However, phospholipases PLA2 were known to function as positive regulators of cell proliferation and migration (Song et al., 2007), playing rather a tumour-promoting role. In contrast to that, we and other uncovered a tumour-suppressive function of H-REV107-1 and its related proteins functioning as PLA2 enzymes.

It is likely that these observations provide a new link between malignant transformation, tumour progression and alteration in lipid metabolism, which needs further investigations. An important aspect needs to be refurbished according to the latest findings, is a change of lipid metabolic in tumour-surrounding stroma. Recent data clearly demonstrate a key role of adipocytes in the preferential metastasis of ovarian cancer to omentum, indicating their function as an energy source for homing tumour cells (Nieman et al, 2011). These and other data support a significant role of metabolism regulation in tumours and tumour stroma, and suggesting that inclusion of metabolism-regulating agents in cancer therapy should be re-examined with respect to a potential pronounced beneficial effect on the efficacy of the treatment on a system level.

2.5 TIG3, a target of the MAPK signalling pathway, acts as a tumour suppressor in ovarian cancer cells

The *TIG3* gene was described independently by two groups (Husmann et al., 1998; DiSepio et al., 1998). DiSepio et al. had identified a close homologue of the rat *H-rev107-1* gene, named *RARRES/TIG3*, which was isolated from a differential display approach using Tazarotene-treated human keratinocytes. Tazarotene is a synthetic retinoid, developed for the treatment of psoriasis (Weinstein et al., 1997). Husmann et al. also described a gene closely related to the human *H-rev107-1*, named *H-REV107-2*, isolated during a sequencing project by Merck and the University of Washington. The H-REV107-2 protein differed from RARRES/TIG3 in a longer C-terminal region however; this was recently identified as an artefact (Lotz et al., 2005). Re-sequencing of the *H-REV107-2* cDNA construct revealed that the cDNA is identical to the *RARRES/TIG3* gene, referred further as *TIG3*. In addition, a similar sequence cloned from human gastric carcinoma cells was described as RIG1 (Huang et al., 2000). According to sequence comparisons, all proteins are identical except a difference of two amino acids between the proteins deduced from the TIG3 and the RIG1 sequence.

Expression analysis for *TIG3* performed on Multiple Tissue Northern Blots and Cancer Profiling Arrays suggested expression of the gene in normal ovary and in many other tissues. Similar to *H-REV107-1*, *TIG3* expression was down-regulated in human ovarian carcinomas and tumour-derived cell lines (DiSepio et al., 1998;Duvic et al., 2000;Shyu et al., 2003;Higuchi et al., 2003;Sturniolo et al., 2003;Lotz et al., 2005) and can be re-expressed upon treatment with IFNγ or retinoid and its analogous (Weinstein et al., 1997).

Up-regulation of *TIG3* by IFNγ occurs in the same cells in which also *H-REV107-1* can be induced by this cytokine. Within the 5′ regulatory sequence of the *TIG3* gene an IRF-responsive element is present 84 base pairs upstream of the translational start site. However, compared to the related *H–REV107-1* gene, *TIG3* mRNA levels after IFNγ-administration follow a different kinetics suggesting that during the IFNγ-dependent apoptosis, these genes are involved at different stages of the process.

Deregulation of retinoic acid receptors has been involved in ovarian tumours, indicating an essential role of genes targeted by retinoic acid signalling in the prevention of transformation (Benoit et al., 2001;Sun and Lotan, 2002). Furthermore, retinoids represent a promising alternative chemotherapeutic approach for the treatment of late stage ovarian cancer (Zhang et al., 2000;Fields et al., 2007) Consequently, TIG3, involved into retinoic signalling, is likely to be one of the potential mediators for a successful anti-cancer therapy of ovarian carcinomas.

In addition to the retinoic acid responsiveness, we recently detected a negative regulation of *TIG3* via an activated MEK-ERK signalling pathway and a positive regulation via IFN-γ in ovarian carcinoma cells (Lotz et al., 2005). Thus, like the related *H-REV107-1* gene, *TIG3* is a target of the oncogenic MEK-ERK signalling pathway. TIG3 itself can dampen the activity of ERK, which suggests an involvement of TIG3 in a negative feedback loop for the control of ERK activity. Inducible and constitutive overexpression of *TIG3* cDNA, resulted in growth suppression of A27/80 ovarian carcinoma cells indicating a functional role of the protein in cell growth control (DiSepio et al., 1998; Lotz et al., 2005). However, the mechanisms of ovarian cancer-specific MEK-ERK-dependent TIG3-suppression are unknown.

An important finding was reported by Ou et al., showing that TIG3 mediates IFN-γ dependent down-regulation of HER-2 via regulation of the PI3-kinase pathway (Ou et al., 2008). Using human ovarian carcinoma cell lines OVCAR-3, SKOV-3, and TOV-21G, the group demonstrated an increase of the *TIG3* mRNA levels within 2 hours upon administration of IFN-γ to the cells. Up-regulation of *TIG3* correlated with the down-regulation of p185 protein, which could be restored by the application of siRNA against *TIG3*. A promoter activity assays allowed to demonstrate that TIG3 acts in a HER-2 dependent manner, by a diminishment of the HER-2 activity. Abrogation of HER-2 signalling resulted in a down-regulation of the p185 subunit of the PI3-Kinase. Additionally, VEGF (vascular endothelial growth factor) secretion was regulated in a TIG3-HER-2 dependent manner in a model system. The anti-proliferative, HER-2-inhibiting effect of TIG3 could be abrogated by overexpression of HGR, a member of the neuregulin family activating epidermal growth factor receptor family members and restoring p185 expression (Ou et al., 2008).

This work shows that TIG3 is an important regulator of survival signalling in ovarian carcinomas. Further experiments are necessary, verifying the in vitro observations in animal models of ovarian cancer. Additionally, examination of human ovarian carcinomas and a correlative analysis of TIG3, HER-2 and p185 expression will allow determining the general relevance the observed phenomenon.. Furthermore, due to the co-regulation of TIG3 and H-REV107-1 via IFN and MAPK signalling, a reactivation of both genes for therapeutic purposes might exhibit an enhanced anti-apoptotic effect.

3. H-REV107-1/HRLS3-driven interplay between PP2A and PKC signal transduction pathways in ovarian carcinomas

In our previous work, we demonstrated that the class II tumour suppressor H-REV107-1 defined as an enzyme with a phospholipase activity (Jaworski et al., 2009) induces apoptosis in ovarian cancer cells by inhibition of a specific pool of serine/threonine phosphatase PP2A followed by the activation of the atypical PKCζ (Nazarenko et al., 2007;Nazarenko et al., 2010).

The PKC family comprises 3 groups of kinases that display very distinct modes of activation and function. The classical PKCs (α,β,γ) are activated in a calcium-dependent manner through phosphatidylserine (PS) and diacylglycerol (DAG). The novel PKCs (δ, ε, η, θ), are also regulated through PS and DAG, but are calcium-independent. Finally, there are the atypical PKCs (ζ, ι/λ) that require neither calcium nor DAG, but in some cases PS, for activation (Parker and Murray-Rust, 2004;Mackay and Twelves, 2007;Breitkreutz et al., 2007). The different PKC isoenzymes are involved in the regulation of cell survival in normal organs and during tumourigenesis (Shayesteh et al., 1999;Leitges et al., 2001;Martin et al., 2002;Parker and Murray-Rust, 2004;Yin et al., 2005;Moscat et al., 2006). Among the classical PKCs, loss of PKCα in ovarian carcinoma was found to be correlated with increased malignancy (Weichert et al., 2003). While the classical PKCα is down-regulated in ovarian carcinomas, the novel PKCθ and PKCε were found up-regulated in this tumour, yet no functional consequence has been inferred from this deregulation. In addition to the novel PKCθ and PKCε, also the atypical PKCι is highly expressed in ovarian carcinomas and acts as a cooperating oncogene with mutant RAS (Zhang et al., 2006).

Recently, we demonstrated that forced expression of H-REV107-1 in ovarian carcinoma cell lines resulted in the inhibition of PP2A activity, re-activation of PP2A target proteins, among them PKCζ, and induction of apoptosis (Nazarenko et al., 2007). Importantly, not only tumour cell lines, but also primary tumour cells isolated from the ascites of patients with ovarian carcinomas were sensitive to the treatment with okadaic acid, an inhibitor of PP2A. Induction of apoptosis after okadaic acid treatment was accompanied by the phosphorylation of PKCζ, confirming a survival role of PP2A in ovarian cancer, and a potential pro-apoptotic function of PKCζ. Based on the in vitro cell culture work we analyzed how different members of the PKC family are regulated by H-REV107-1 or by the inhibition of PP2A activity with okadaic acid. Additionally, we verified an impact of the PI3-kinase pathway, a major survival kinase in ovarian carcinoma, in the regulation of PKC.

Analysis of novel PKCs revealed differences at the level of expression and phosphorylation. Thus, treatment with okadaic acid for 48 hours and overexpression of H-REV107-1 led to an increased expression of PKCε. Additionally, H-REV107-1 indirectly induced phosphorylation of the COOH-terminal residue Ser729, shown to enhance the enzymatic activity of PKCε (Parekh et al., 2000). This suggests that PKCε activity might be partially regulated in an H-REV107-1-dependent manner. Phosphorylation of Thr538 within the activation loop of PKCθ was elevated after 48 hours of treatment with okadaic acid and the AKT inhibitor LY294002, suggesting a negative but indirect regulation through PP2A and PI-3K. Additionally, Thr538 phosphorylation of PKCθ was increased in cells expressing H-REV107-1, suggesting a potential role of this kinase in H-REV107-1 signalling. The phosphorylation of Thr505 located within the activation loop of PKCδ increased already 15 minutes after the addition of okadaic acid or LY294002, indicating that PKCδ is directly inactivated by PP2A and PI3K. Although the levels of total PKCδ seemed to be slightly increased after long-term okadaic acid and LY294002 treatment, the phosphorylation was strongly diminished. H-REV107-1 negatively regulated the expression of PKCδ, supporting the finding that PKCδ is not involved in H-REV107-1-dependent cell death. Expression of atypical PKCι was increased following 48 hours of treatment with okadaic acid, but neither phosphorylation nor total levels were affected by H-REV107-1.

To correlate phosphorylation of kinases in the activation site and their intracellular kinase activity, we applied in vitro kinase assay described in detail elsewhere (Nazarenko et al., 2010) and measured direct changes in the activity of PKCs upon okadaic acid treatment. A significant elevation of the PKCθ and PKCε activity was detected 24 hours after okadaic acid incubation, confirming that these PKCs, although not known to be direct PP2A targets, are negatively regulated by PP2A signalling in OVCAR-3 cells.

As inhibition of PP2A is required for H-REV107 1 dependent apoptosis, we next asked if these kinases might be involved in H-REV107-1-induced cell death and tested if the abrogation of PKCθ and PKCε activity impairs the proapoptotic function of H-REV107-1. OVCAR-3 cells were transfected either with the H-REV107-1 expression vector or with a control plasmid. Twelve hours later, the PKCθ- and PKCε-specific peptides were added. Caspase-3 cleavage was tested after 48 hours using Western blot analysis. H-REV107-1 expression resulted in the induction of caspase-3 cleavage, which was however not altered after peptide applications. Additionally, PKCθ-specific peptide treatment of control cells revealed a weak toxic effect. This result suggests that although PKCε and PKCθ are clearly activated in a PP2A and H-REV107-1-dependent manner, they are not essential for the H-REV107-1 proapoptotic activity in OVCAR-3 cells.

An important finding was that the atypical PKCζ is uncoupled from the PI3K pathway in ovarian cancer cells and is more likely to be a PP2A target. This is in contrast to the situation in the majority of normal and malignant tissues, in which PKCζ functions as an insulin-dependent PI3K effector. Importantly, overexpression of wild type H-REV107-1, but not of its PP2A interaction-deficient mutant, led to PKC phosphorylation, suggesting a direct link between the ability of H-REV107-1 to inhibit PP2A and the activation of PKCζ.

Electroporation of the ovarian carcinoma cells with PKCζ-expression plasmid demonstrated that high levels of this kinase are sufficient to induce apoptosis. In our work we demonstrated an increase of the sub-G1 cell population and caspase-3 cleavage. Molecular mechanisms by mean of which PKCζ induces apoptosis remained elusive and need further investigations. A recent work of Peng et al. might provide an additional hint for the mechanisms of PKCζ-dependent apoptosis (Chen et al., 2008). Using a mouse model, the authors demonstrated that PKCζ directly interacts with ERK1/2 in Kupffer cells, mediating a translocation of NF-kB into the nucleus and inducing its activity. The novelty of this finding is a direct link between PKCζ, EKR1/2 and NF-kB. Consistently, a cross-talk between NF-kB and PKCζ is well- characterised for many systems (Moscat et al., 2001;Moscat and az-Meco, 2011). Next, a potential interaction between PKCζ, ERK1/2, and NF-kB in ovarian cancer cells should be verified. A hypothetical scheme of PKC apoptotic cascade and cross-talk with other pathways is represented on the Fig. 5.

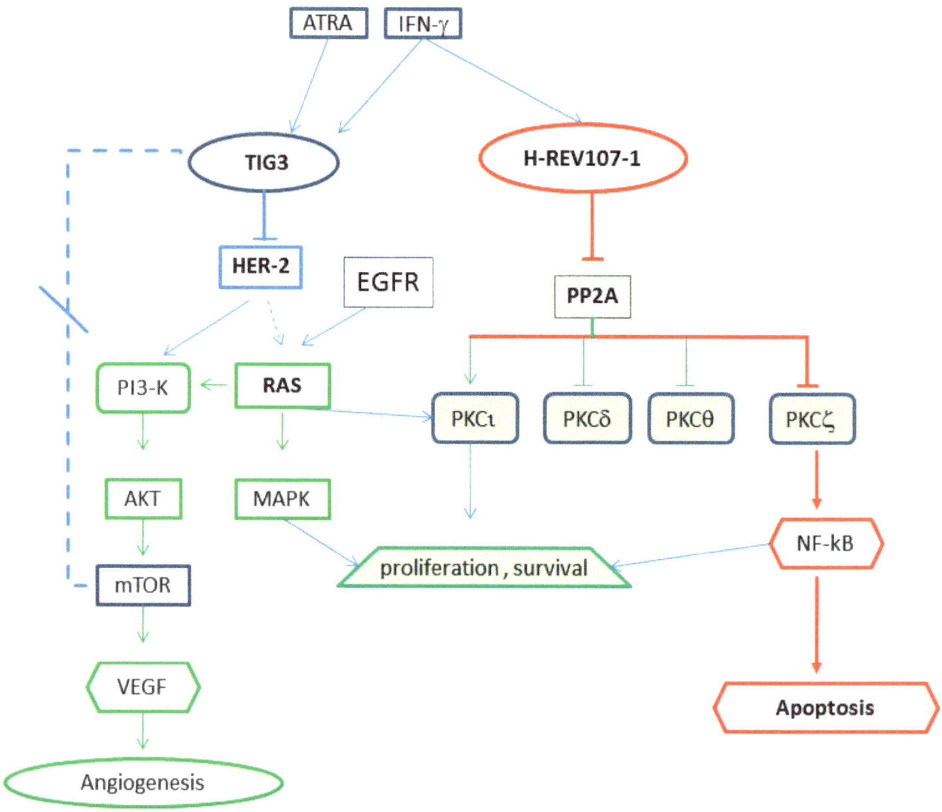

Fig. 5. Hypothetical scheme of the pro-apoptotic signal transduction network in ovarian cancer cells of two members of the HRS protein family, the H-REV107-1 (showed with red arrows) and TIG3 (showed with blue arrows). Both family members can be activated by IFNγ, whereas TIG3 can be additionally activated by ATRA. TIG3 mediates inhibition of HER-2, mediating herewith suppression of angiogenesis. H-REV107-1 inhibits PP2A, mediating activation of PKCζ. PKCζ functions as a major mediator of H-REV107-1-mediated cell death and is sufficient to induce apoptosis in a subset ovarian carcinoma cells, sensitive to the H-REV107-1--mediated apoptosis.

4. Receptor kinase pathway profiling in ovarian cancer cells

We applied the RPPA (reverse phase protein array) technique to define a potential regulation of PKCs by epidermal growth factor receptor inhibition. Earlier work on the H-REV107-1 tumour suppressor, an inhibitor of PP2A, has demonstrated that H-REV1071-1 is lost in a significant portion of ovarian tumours.

As a class II tumour suppressor gene, H-REV107-1 expression was reconstituted upon IFNγ treatment and MAPK inhibition and was able to induce specific phosphorylation of atypical PKC and the induction of apoptosis. These observations suggested to us that interference with oncogenic pathways might also have some impact on PKC isoform expression and/or activation. Therefore, we asked whether PKCζ phosphorylation, which is necessary for apoptosis induction in ovarian cancer cells, might also be regulated by inhibitors and therapeutic agents that target mitogenic and survival pathways. The most prominent candidates for such an approach appeared to be the family of epidermal growth factor receptors (EGFR), whose members are frequently mutated and activated in human malignancies, and specific inhibitors are used for the treatment of ovarian carcinomas (De Marinis et al., 2002;Blank et al., 2005).

We performed a reverse phase protein array analysis (RPPA) of OVCAR-3 cells treated with the EGFR inhibitors Cetuximab and Gefitinib/Iressa, and tested the expression and phosphorylation of PKCζ and the expression of PKCα and PKCδ with antibodies established for this approach. To test if other signalling cascades are similarly affected following inhibition of EGFR signalling, we applied antibodies against phosphorylated AKT and ERK proteins and against the Bad protein.

This analysis showed an increased protein level of PKCζ and of its phosphorylated form 24 hours after the treatment with EGFR inhibitors. The RPPA analysis of ERK, AKT and Bad proteins revealed a moderate effect of EGFR inhibition on the phosphorylation status of these proteins and their expression. While total levels of Akt/PKB and phosphorylation of Bad Ser112 were unchanged, Akt/PKC and ERK phosphorylation were moderately increased after application of inhibitors. In addition to PKCζ, RPPA analysis also revealed elevated levels of PKCα and PKCδ following incubation with the EGFR inhibitors, suggesting a role of these kinases in EGFR downstream signalling.

Our experimental data obtained through profiling with reverse phase protein arrays revealed that application of Cetuximab or Gefitinib to OVCAR-3 cells induced only a moderate effect on MAPK and PI3K signalling, and had no effect onto cell growth. This suggests that specific targeting of EGFR is not sufficient to switch the survival program to an apoptotic program in these cells. In addition, EGFR inhibition led to a transient activation of PKCζ and to an up-regulation of PKCα and PKCδ. Neither PKCα nor PKCδ seem to play a crucial role in apoptosis induction in the cell lines tested, while we provided clear evidence for an involvement of PKCζ in the induction of apoptosis. The transient activation of PKCζ following EGFR interference was not sufficient to induce apoptosis. Therefore, the inhibition of oncogenic tyrosine kinase receptors might be a prerequisite for full or partial reconstitution of the players involved in apoptosis, but an additional trigger such as chemotherapy might be necessary to actually execute the death program (Nazarenko et al., 2010).

5. Conclusion

This chapter describes the impact of a family of tumour suppressor proteins, and the specific PKCζ-mediated signalling on apoptosis induction in ovarian cancer. The genes encoding H-REV107-1/HRSL3 and TIG3 both act as tumour suppressor genes. While the functional impact of TIG3 is still somewhat elusive, H-REV107-1 governs the decision between survival and apoptosis. Of major importance for the future research is the newly described function of H-REV107-1 and its related proteins, being phospholipases. This function indicates a specific role of lipid metabolism in the control of transformation and potentially tumour progression.

Furthermore, high expression levels of PKCζ and a correlation with poor prognosis were observed in human ovarian carcinoma samples and only the activation of endogenous PKCζ by okadaic acid or by the HRSL3 tumour suppressor, correlated with the induction of apoptosis in primary and immortalized ovarian carcinoma cells. This suggests a potentially inaccessible pro-apoptotic action of this kinase, which might be negatively regulated by activated tyrosine kinase receptors in ovarian cancer. In future research, identification of yet unknown substrates of the members of the HRS family will support current knowledge on the mechanisms of their pro-apoptotic function. Possibly, new aspects of functions, opening novel horizons in the therapy of ovarian cancer therapy, will be developed.

6. Acknowledgment

We thank Andreas Weihe and Uwe Richter (Institute of Genetics, Humboldt University, Berlin, Germany) for their help in the phylogenetic analysis of the HRS and HRS-related families. Steffen Reich (Institute of Pathology, Charité, Berlin, Germany, for the analysis of H-REV107-1 human promoter.

7. References

Akiyama, H., Y. Hiraki, M. Noda, C. Shigeno, H. Ito, and T. Nakamura, 1999, Molecular cloning and biological activity of a novel Ha-Ras suppressor gene predominantly expressed in skeletal muscle, heart, brain, and bone marrow by differential display using clonal mouse EC cells, ATDC5: J.Biol.Chem., v. 274, no. 45, p. 32192-32197.

Alessi, D. R., Y. Saito, D. G. Campbell, P. Cohen, G. Sithanandam, U. Rapp, A. Ashworth, C. J. Marshall, and S. Cowley, 1994, Identification of the sites in MAP kinase kinase-1 phosphorylated by p74raf-1: EMBO J., v. 13, no. 7, p. 1610-1619.

Anantharaman, V., and L. Aravind, 2003, Evolutionary history, structural features and biochemical diversity of the NlpC/P60 superfamily of enzymes: Genome Biol., v. 4, no. 2.

Bartel, D. P., 2004, MicroRNAs: genomics, biogenesis, mechanism, and function: Cell, v. 116, no. 2, p. 281-297.

Benoit, G. R. et al., 2001, Autonomous rexinoid death signaling is suppressed by converging signaling pathways in immature leukemia cells: Mol.Endocrinol., v. 15, no. 7, p. 1154-1169.

Blank, S. V., R. Chang, and F. Muggia, 2005, Epidermal growth factor receptor inhibitors for the treatment of epithelial ovarian cancer: Oncology (Williston.Park), v. 19, no. 4, p. 553-559.

Breitkreutz, D., L. Braiman-Wiksman, N. Daum, M. F. Denning, and T. Tennenbaum, 2007, Protein kinase C family: on the crossroads of cell signaling in skin and tumor epithelium: J.Cancer Res.Clin.Oncol., v. 133, no. 11, p. 793-808.

Brown, L. A. et al., 2008, Amplification of 11q13 in ovarian carcinoma: Genes Chromosomes.Cancer, v. 47, no. 6, p. 481-489.

Chen, Y., Z. Liu, S. Liang, X. Luan, F. Long, J. Chen, Y. Peng, L. Yan, and J. Gong, 2008, Role of Kupffer cells in the induction of tolerance of orthotopic liver transplantation in rats: Liver Transpl., v. 14, no. 6, p. 823-836.

Choi, J. H., J. J. Sheu, B. Guan, N. Jinawath, P. Markowski, T. L. Wang, and I. Shih, 2009, Functional analysis of 11q13.5 amplicon identifies Rsf-1 (HBXAP) as a gene involved in paclitaxel resistance in ovarian cancer: Cancer Res., v. 69, no. 4, p. 1407-1415.

De Marinis, F., F. Nelli, and G. D'Auria, 2002, EGFR inhibitors: clinical results: Suppl Tumori, v. 1, no. 6, p. S5-S6.

DiSepio, D., C. Ghosn, R. L. Eckert, A. Deucher, N. Robinson, M. Duvic, R. A. S. Chandraratna, and S. Nagpal, 1998, Identification and characterization of a retinoid-induced class II tumor suppressor growth regulatory gene: Proc.Natl.Acad.Sci.U.S.A., v. 95, no. 25, p. 14811-14815.

Duvic, M. et al., 2000, Expression of a retinoid-inducible tumor suppressor, Tazarotene-inducible gene-3, is decreased in psoriasis and skin cancer: Clin.Cancer Res., v. 6, no. 8, p. 3249-3259.

Duvic, M., X. Ni, R. Talpur, K. Herne, C. Schulz, D. Sui, S. Ward, A. Joseph, and P. Hazarika, 2003, Tazarotene-induced gene 3 is suppressed in basal cell carcinomas and reversed in vivo by tazarotene application: J.Invest.Dermatol., v. 121, no. 4, p. 902-909.

Faratian, D., I. Um, D. S. Wilson, P. Mullen, S. P. Langdon, and D. J. Harrison, 2011, Phosphoprotein pathway profiling of ovarian carcinoma for the identification of potential new targets for therapy: Eur.J.Cancer, v. 47, no. 9, p. 1420-1431.

Fields, A. L., D. R. Soprano, and K. J. Soprano, 2007, Retinoids in biological control and cancer: J.Cell Biochem., v. 102, no. 4, p. 886-898.

Forbes, S. A. et al., 1997, Mapping of the gene encoding the B56 beta subunit of protein phosphatase 2A (PPP2R5B) to a 0.5-Mb region of chromosome 11q13 and its exclusion as a candidate gene for multiple endocrine neoplasia type 1 (MEN1): Hum.Genet., v. 100, no. 3-4, p. 481-485.

Gansler TS, Hardman W, Hunt DA, Schaffel S, Hennigar RA, 1997, Increased expression of fatty acid synthase (OA-519) in ovarian neoplasms predicts shorter survival: Hum Pathol., v. 28, p. 686–692

Hajnal, A., R. Klemenz, and R. Schafer, 1994, Subtraction Cloning of H-Rev107, A Gene Specifically Expressed in H-Ras Resistant Fibroblasts: Oncogene, v. 9, no. 2, p. 479-490.

Higuchi, E., R. A. Chandraratna, W. K. Hong, and R. Lotan, 2003, Induction of TIG3, a putative class II tumor suppressor gene, by retinoic acid in head and neck and lung carcinoma cells and its association with suppression of the transformed phenotype: Oncogene, v. 22, no. 30, p. 4627-4635.

Huang, S. L., R. Y. Shyu, M. Y. Yeh, and S. Y. Jiang, 2000, Cloning and characterization of a novel retinoid-inducible gene 1(RIG1) deriving from human gastric cancer cells: Mol.Cell.Endocrinol., v. 159, no. 1-2, p. 15-24.

Huang, S. L., R. Y. Shyu, M. Y. Yeh, and S. Y. Jiang, 2002, The retinoid-inducible gene I: Effect on apoptosis and mitogen-activated kinase signal pathways: Anticancer Res., v. 22, no. 2A, p. 799-804.

Hughes, P. J., and G. Stanway, 2000, The 2A proteins of three diverse picornaviruses are related to each other and to the H-rev107 family of proteins involved in the control of cell proliferation: J.Gen.Virol., v. 81, no. Pt 1, p. 201-207.

Husmann, K., C. Sers, E. Fietze, A. Mincheva, P. Lichter, and R. Schafer, 1998, Transcriptional and translational downregulation of H-REV107, a class II tumour suppressor gene located on human chromosome 11q11-12: Oncogene, v. 17, no. 10, p. 1305-1312.

Ito, H., H. Akiyama, C. Shigeno, and T. Nakamura, 2001, Isolation, characterization, and chromosome mapping of a human A-C1 Ha-Ras suppressor gene (HRASLS): Cytogenet.Cell Genet., v. 93, no. 1-2, p. 36-39.

Jaworski, K. et al., 2009, AdPLA ablation increases lipolysis and prevents obesity induced by high-fat feeding or leptin deficiency: Nat.Med., v. 15, no. 2, p. 159-168.

Kjeldgaard, M., J. Nyborg, and B. F. Clark, 1996, The GTP binding motif: variations on a theme: FASEB J., v. 10, no. 12, p. 1347-1368.

Leitges, M. et al., 2001, Targeted disruption of the zetaPKC gene results in the impairment of the NF-kappaB pathway: Mol.Cell, v. 8, no. 4, p. 771-780.

Lotz, K., T. Kellner, M. Heitmann, I. Nazarenko, A. Noske, A. Malek, A. Gontarewicz, R. Schafer, and C. Sers, 2005, Suppression of the TIG3 tumor suppressor gene in human ovarian carcinomas is mediated via mitogen-activated kinase-dependent and -independent mechanisms: Int.J.Cancer, v. 116, no. 6, p. 894-902.

Mackay, H. J., and C. J. Twelves, 2007, Targeting the protein kinase C family: are we there yet?: Nat.Rev.Cancer, v. 7, no. 7, p. 554-562.

Martin, P., A. Duran, S. Minguet, M. L. Gaspar, M. T. Diaz-Meco, P. Rennert, M. Leitges, and J. Moscat, 2002, Role of zeta PKC in B-cell signaling and function: EMBO J., v. 21, no. 15, p. 4049-4057.

McCubrey, J. A. et al., 2007, Targeting the RAF/MEK/ERK, PI3K/AKT and p53 pathways in hematopoietic drug resistance: Adv.Enzyme Regul., v. 47, p. 64-103.

Menendez JA, Vellon L, Mehmi I, et al., 2004, Inhibition of fatty acid synthase (f a s) suppresses h e r 2 / neu (ErbB-2) oncogene overexpression in cancer cells. Proc Natl Acad Sci U S A, v. 101, p 10715–10720.

Moscat, J., and M. T. az-Meco, 2011, Fine tuning NF-kappaB: new openings for PKC-zeta: Nat.Immunol., v. 12, no. 1, p. 12-14.

Moscat, J., L. Sanz, P. Sanchez, and M. T. az-Meco, 2001, Regulation and role of the atypical PKC isoforms in cell survival during tumor transformation: Adv.Enzyme Regul., v. 41, p. 99-120.

Moscat, J., P. Rennert, and M. T. Diaz-Meco, 2006, PKCzeta at the crossroad of NF-kappaB and Jak1/Stat6 signaling pathways: Cell Death.Differ., v. 13, no. 5, p. 702-711.

Nazarenko, I. et al., 2010, Atypical protein kinase C zeta exhibits a proapoptotic function in ovarian cancer: Mol.Cancer Res., v. 8, no. 6, p. 919-934.

Nazarenko, I., R. Schafer, and C. Sers, 2007, Mechanisms of the HRSL3 tumor suppressor function in ovarian carcinoma cells: J.Cell Sci., v. 120, no. Pt 8, p. 1393-1404.

Nicosia, S. V., W. Bai, J. Q. Cheng, D. Coppola, and P. A. Kruk, 2003, Oncogenic pathways implicated in ovarian epithelial cancer: Hematol.Oncol.Clin.North Am., v. 17, no. 4, p. 927-943.

Ou, C. C., S. C. Hsu, Y. H. Hsieh, W. L. Tsou, T. C. Chuang, J. Y. Liu, and M. C. Kao, 2008, Downregulation of HER2 by RIG1 involves the PI3K/Akt pathway in ovarian cancer cells: Carcinogenesis, v. 29, no. 2, p. 299-306.

Parekh, D. B., W. Ziegler, and P. J. Parker, 2000, Multiple pathways control protein kinase C phosphorylation: EMBO J., v. 19, no. 4, p. 496-503.

Parker, P. J., and J. Murray-Rust, 2004, PKC at a glance: J.Cell Sci., v. 117, no. Pt 2, p. 131-132.
Ren, X., J. Lin, C. Jin, and B. Xia, 2010a, 1H, 13C and 15N resonance assignments of human H-REV107 N-terminal domain: Biomol.NMR Assign., v. 4, no. 2, p. 175-178.
Ren, X., J. Lin, C. Jin, and B. Xia, 2010b, Solution structure of the N-terminal catalytic domain of human H-REV107--a novel circular permutated NlpC/P60 domain: FEBS Lett., v. 584, no. 19, p. 4222-4226.
Roberts, P. J., and C. J. Der, 2007, Targeting the Raf-MEK-ERK mitogen-activated protein kinase cascade for the treatment of cancer: Oncogene, v. 26, no. 22, p. 3291-3310.
Roder, K., M. J. Latasa, and H. S. Sul, 2002, Silencing of the mouse H-rev107 gene encoding a class II tumor suppressor by CpG methylation: J.Biol.Chem., v. 277, no. 34, p. 30543-30550.
Sager, R., 1997, Expression genetics in cancer: shifting the focus from DNA to RNA: Proc.Natl.Acad.Sci.U.S.A, v. 94, no. 3, p. 952-955.
Schafer, R., and C. Sers, 2010, RAS oncogene-mediated deregulation of the transcriptome: From molecular signature to function: Adv.Enzyme Regul..
Sers, C. et al., 2002, The class II tumour suppressor gene H-REV107-1 is a target of interferon-regulatory factor-1 and is involved in IFNgamma-induced cell death in human ovarian carcinoma cells: Oncogene, v. 21, no. 18, p. 2829-2839.
Sers, C., U. Emmenegger, K. Husmann, K. Bucher, A. C. Andres, and R. Schafer, 1997, Growth-inhibitory activity and downregulation of the class II tumor-suppressor gene H-rev107 in tumor cell lines and experimental tumors: J.Cell Biol., v. 136, no. 4, p. 935-944.
Shayesteh, L. et al., 1999, PIK3CA is implicated as an oncogene in ovarian cancer: Nat.Genet., v. 21, no. 1, p. 99-102.
Shyu, R. Y., S. Y. Jiang, J. M. Chou, Y. L. Shih, M. S. Lee, J. C. Yu, P. C. Chao, Y. J. Hsu, and S. W. Jao, 2003, RARRES3 expression positively correlated to tumour differentiation in tissues of colorectal adenocarcinoma: Br.J.Cancer, v. 89, no. 1, p. 146-151.
Siegrist, S., C. Feral, M. Chami, B. Solhonne, M. G. Mattei, E. Rajpert-De Meyts, G. Guellaen, and F. Bulle, 2001, hH-Rev107, a class II tumor suppressor gene, is expressed by post-meiotic testicular germ cells and CIS cells but not by human testicular germ cell tumors: Oncogene, v. 20, no. 37, p. 5155-5163.
Song Y., Wilkins P., Hu W., et al., 2007, Inhibition of calcium-independent phospholipase A2 suppresses proliferation and tumorigenicity of ovarian carcinoma cells: Biochem J, v 406, p.427–436.
Strimmer, K., and A. von Haeseler, 1997, Likelihood-mapping: a simple method to visualize phylogenetic content of a sequence alignment: Proc.Natl.Acad.Sci.U.S.A, v. 94, no. 13, p. 6815-6819.
Sturniolo, M. T., S. R. Dashti, A. Deucher, E. A. Rorke, A. M. Broome, R. A. S. Chandraratna, T. Keepers, and R. L. Eckert, 2003, A novel tumor suppressor protein promotes keratinocyte terminal differentiation via activation of type I transglutaminase: J.Biol.Chem., v. 278, no. 48, p. 48066-48073.
Sun, S. Y., and R. Lotan, 2002, Retinoids and their receptors in cancer development and chemoprevention: Crit Rev.Oncol.Hematol., v. 41, no. 1, p. 41-55.
Tanja, M.S., Khan, M.A., Song, Y. 2010, Association of lipid metabolism with ovarian cancer. Current Oncology., v. 17., no. 3, p. 6-11.

Weichert, W., V. Gekeler, C. Denkert, M. Dietel, and S. Hauptmann, 2003, Protein kinase C isoform expression in ovarian carcinoma correlates with indicators of poor prognosis: Int.J.Oncol., v. 23, no. 3, p. 633-639.

Weinstein, G. D. et al., 1997, Tazarotene gel, a new retinoid, for topical therapy of psoriasis: vehicle-controlled study of safety, efficacy, and duration of therapeutic effect: J.Am.Acad.Dermatol., v. 37, no. 1, p. 85-92.

Weinstein, I. B., 1987, Growth factors, oncogenes, and multistage carcinogenesis: J.Cell Biochem., v. 33, no. 3, p. 213-224.

Yin, L., N. Bennani-Baiti, and C. T. Powell, 2005, Phorbol ester-induced apoptosis of C4-2 cells requires both a unique and a redundant protein kinase C signaling pathway: J.Biol.Chem., v. 280, no. 7, p. 5533-5541.

Zhang, D., W. F. Holmes, S. Wu, D. R. Soprano, and K. J. Soprano, 2000, Retinoids and ovarian cancer: J.Cell Physiol, v. 185, no. 1, p. 1-20.

Zhang, L. et al., 2006, Integrative genomic analysis of protein kinase C (PKC) family identifies PKCiota as a biomarker and potential oncogene in ovarian carcinoma: Cancer Res., v. 66, no. 9, p. 4627-4635.

5

The Role of MUC16 Mucin (CA125) in the Pathogenesis of Ovarian Cancer

Claudine Rancourt, Isabelle Matte, Denis Lane and Alain Piché*
Département de Microbiologie et Infectiologie
Faculté de Médecine, Université de Sherbrooke
Canada

1. Introduction

The majority of epithelial ovarian carcinomas (EOCs) are derived from the ovarian surface epithelium (OSE). EOCs are the most lethal of all gynecological malignancies. Most patients present with advanced diseases in which tumor cells are disseminated throughout the peritoneal cavity. MUC16 serum level is a well-established marker for ovarian cancer (OC) progression and disease response to treatment. MUC16 is a high molecular weight, membrane associated-mucin, which is aberrantly expressed in advanced serous EOC. MUC16 is also expressed at the surface of corneal and respiratory epithelial cells, and the surface of female reproductive tract epithelium. It is however not expressed by the normal OSE. Like other membrane-bounded mucins, this glycosylated protein is primarily involved in the lubrification of epithelial luminal surfaces. MUC16 glycoprotein possesses unique structural motifs as compared with other membrane-bounded mucins. Its ectodomain is composed of a large heavily O-glycosylated N-terminus and a tandem repeat region with over 60 tandem repeats. MUC16 C-terminal domain (CTD) is composed of an extracellular unique region which contains a potential proteolytic cleavage site, a transmembrane domain and a short cytoplasmic tail with possible phosphorylation sites. MUC16 domains most likely have various functions resulting in activation of signalling pathways which regulate different tumor cell phenotypes. Indeed, recent functional studies have begun to uncover the unique role of MUC16 in the pathogenesis of OC. The present review will discuss the unique structure and functional roles of MUC16 in OC.

2. Ovarian cancer overview

OC is the fifth cause of cancer-related death in women in North America, the second most common gynecological cancer, and the leading cause of death from gynecological malignancies (Ozols *et al*, 2004). One in 78 women will develop OC during her lifetime (Jemal *et al.*, 2010). In 2010, nearly 22,000 new cases were estimated to occur in the United States and approximately 14,000 women are expected to die from this disease (Jemal *et al.*, 2010). Similar incidence and mortality has been observed in Canada, relative to the total population. Although survival rates approach 90% in OC patients diagnosed at early stage, most patients

* Corresponding Author

(~ 80%) are diagnosed with advanced diseases and metastases throughout the peritoneal cavity (Bast *et al.*, 2009). For these women, the 5-year survival rate is less than 30%.
Although OC may arise from all cell types composing the ovaries, EOC arising from the single-cell layer coelomic epithelium surrounding the ovaries, from postovulatory inclusion cysts or from the fimbriated end of the fallopian tube, are by far the most common (85-90% of all OC) (Ozols *et al*, 2004; Auersperg *et al.*, 2001; Landen *et al.*, 2008; Kindelberger *et al.*, 2007; Crum *et al.*, 2007 (2); Dubeau 2008; Kurman *et al.*, 2010). EOC presents substantial heterogeneity in terms of grade and histology. Most frequent EOCs divided into serous, mucinous, endometrioid and clear cell histotypes (Bast and al. 2009). Each histotype shows a distinctive gene expression and immunohistochemical profiling (Schwartz *et al.*, 2002; Ouellet *et al.*, 2005; Ouellet *et al.*, 2006; Ouellet *et al.*, 2008), and differs in the response to therapy (Bast *et al.*, 2009). Despite evidence of considerable heterogeneity in their histological phenotypes and molecular profiling (Bast *et al.*, 2009; Konstantinopoulos *et al.*, 2008; Soslow 2008), most cases of EOC are treated in a similar fashion.
Early detection of cancer patient remains an important objective in the field because over 70% of patients with EOC are diagnosed at late stage disease, with dissemination of tumor implants throughout the peritoneal cavity (Ozols *et al*, 2004; Aletti *et al.*, 2007; Goff *et al.*, 2000). Only 10-15% of these patients maintain a complete response after the initial therapy. The mean survival of patients that present with late stage disease, which is the case for most patients, is 39 months (Herzog 2004). Recurrence is associated with incurable diseases in most cases. The main obstacle to an effective treatment is the failure of the initial chemotherapy to eradicate a sufficient number of tumor cells to prevent disease recurrence. In this context, deficiency in the apoptotic cascade among tumor cells is a key hallmark of EOC.
The current standard treatment for advanced EOC consists of cytoreductive surgery and chemotherapy. Paclitaxel combined with platinum-based regimen is the standard first-line chemotherapy used for all patients with EOC (Colombo *et al.*, 2006). Serous EOC can be considered a chemosensitive neoplasm as most (80%) patients initially respond to the combination of paclitaxel and platinum-based drugs (McGuire *et al.*, 1996). However, 90% of the patients that initially responded will eventually develop chemotherapy-resistant diseases (Mano *et al.*, 2007). Although rarely curative, patients that do not respond to the first-line chemotherapy are given second-line and third-line regimens of chemotherapy in an attempt to prolong life and palliate symptoms.
Early on, MUC16 mucin has been recognized as a tumor-associated antigen because of its overexpression in EOC. Measurements of MUC16 serum level have been very useful over the years to monitor disease response or progression (Bast *et al.*, 2005). MUC16 is overexpressed in EOC, cleaved from the cell surface and detected into the peritoneal fluid and the blood. Since the characterization of the OC125 monoclonal antibody raised against the human ovarian cancer cell line OVCA433 in 1981 (Bast *et al.*, 1981; Bast *et al.*, 1983), a variety of MUC16-linked antibodies have been developed including VK8, M11 and 4H11 (Dharma Rao *et al.*, 2010; Nustad *et al.*, 2002). Except for 4H11 antibody, which recognizes an epitope in the noncleaved ectodomain of MUC16, other MUC16 antibodies bind to the glycosylated portion of the molecule. Measurement of serum MUC16 tumor antigen is an important part of the clinical management for EOC patients. Elevated levels of serum MUC16 are common in patients with advanced disease of serous histotype (~90%). It decreases to 50%-60% in patients with early stage OC. It was shown by several

groups that rising and falling levels of serum MUC16 correlate with progression and regression of the disease and this formed the basis for monitoring MUC16 serum levels for patient follow-up (Bast *et al.*, 1983; Canney *et al.*, 1984; Vergote *et al.*, 1987). However, up to 20% of patients with advanced EOC have normal serum level of MUC16. Furthermore, MUC16 levels can be elevated in various benign diseases including menstruation, first trimester pregnancy, endometriosis, adenomyosis, salpingitis, uterine fibroids, chronic renal failure or in inflammation of the pleura, peritoneum or pericardium (Bagdwell *et al.*, 2007; Xiaofang *et al.*, 2007). MUC16 is therefore not specific for EOC. MUC16, as a single modality, is not currently use for screening of EOC because of its lack of sensitivity and specificity.

Despite its recognized utility for the follow up of patients with EOC over the last three decades, the understanding of MUC16 structure became apparent only with the cloning of the gene in 2001. In addition, because of the lack of suitable cellular models, MUC16 functions have remained mostly unknown until very recently.

3. MUC16 structure

Although MUC16 was recognized as a high molecular weight glycoprotein a few years after the description of OC125 monoclonal antibody (Davis *et al.*, 1986), and its structure confirmed by subsequent studies (Lloyd *et al.*, 1997; Lloyd *et al.*, 2001), it took 20 years before the MUC16 gene could be cloned (Yin and Llyod, 2001; O'Brien *et al.*, 2001; Yin *et al.*, 2002). The gene is located on chromosome 19p13.2 (Yin and Lloyd, 2001). The deduced amino acid sequence of MUC16 demonstrated that it resembles other membrane-bounded mucins with high serine, threonine and proline content. With a molecular weight of > 2 MDa, MUC16 is the largest membrane-bounded mucin known to date (O'Brien *et al.*, 2001; O'Brien *et al.*, 2002). This glycoprotein is composed of three major domains: an N-terminal domain, a large multiple repeat domain (up to 60 tandem repeats of 156 amino acids each) and a C-terminal domain (O'Brien *et al.*, 2001) (Fig. 1). The N-terminal domain and the repeat domain are heavily glycosylated with both O- and N-linked oligosaccharides (Kui *et al.*, 2003). The C-terminal domain is composed of an extracellular domain with sea urchin sperm protein, enterokinase and agrin (SEA) domains, a transmembrane domain to anchor the protein to the cellular membrane and a short cytoplasmic tail (31 amino acids) with potential serine, threonine and tyrosine phosphorylation sites. The phosphorylation of MUC16 cytoplasmic tail has been associated with its secretion (Fendrick *et al.*, 1997). The secretion of MUC16 is stimulated by epidermal growth factor (EGF) or tyrosine phosphatases (Konishi *et al.*, 1994). Its shedding is decreased by glucocorticoids (Karlan *et al.*, 1988).

Human MUC16 differs from other mucins by having 16 SEA domains located near the membrane-spanning sequence. Other membrane-bounded mucins usually have a single SEA domain (Duraisamy *et al.*, 2006). SEA domains consist of about 120 amino acids. Sequence analysis of MUC16 SEA modules showed that they display some sequence variability. The second MUC16 SEA domain however is relatively conserved and most closely resembles the SEA domain found in other mucins. It may therefore provide the preferential cleavage site, like as in MUC1 and MUC3, which allows release of MUC16 from the cell surface. This, however, remains to be confirmed. Unlike MUC1 and MUC4, MUC16 lacks an EGF-like domain. Through their EGF-like motif located at C-terminal domain (extracellular portion), MUC1 and MUC4 bind to growth factor receptor tyrosine kinases (RTKs) such as erbB family and fibroblast growth factor receptor 3 (FGFR3) (Li *et al.*, 2001; Ren *et al.*, 2006; Schroeder *et al.*, 2001; Pochampalli *et al.*, 2007). The formation of heterodimer with RTKs causes cross-phosphorylation of their respective cytoplasmic domain leading to the activation of various signaling pathways (Bafna *et al.*, 2010). Because MUC16 lacks an RTK binding motif in its C-terminal domain, it is not clear whether MUC16-induced signaling is affected by RTKs although, as mentioned above, MUC16 release from the cell is stimulated by EGF. Consistent with the lack of an RTK binding motif, the intracellular interaction between MUC16 and β-catenin is not affected by EGF (Comamala *et al.*, 2011). MUC16 cytoplasmic tail contains a polybasic sequence of amino acids (RRRKK) which is predicted to bind to the ezrin/radixin/moesin (ERM) family of proteins (Fig. 2). This motif is not found in MUC1 and MUC4. The ERM proteins can interact with numerous membrane-associated proteins and the actin cytoskeleton. Consistently, MUC16 has recently been shown to interact with E-cadherin and β-catenin, and causes alteration in the actin cytoskeleton (Comamala *et al.*, 2011). However, it remains unclear whether MUC16/β-catenin and MUC16/E-cadherin interaction is mediated through the ERM motif of the MUC16 cytoplasmic tail. MUC1 cytoplasmic tail has been shown to bind to β-catenin and a serine-rich SXXXXXSSL motif in MUC1 is responsible for this interaction *in vitro* (Yamamoto *et al.*, 1997; Wen *et al.*, 2003; Huang *et al.*, 2005). This motif is notably absent in MUC16. Interestingly however, the binding of MUC1 to β-catenin in cells was independent of the serine-rich motif (Huang *et al.*, 2005). These observations suggest that MUC16 interaction with β-catenin is mediated by an indirect mechanism, probably through another protein. The positively charged R-K rich region of MUC16 cytoplasmic tail also constitutes a putative nuclear localization motif (Bafna *et al.*, 2010). Whether MUC16 cytoplasmic tail does indeed localize to the nucleus, as MUC1 cytoplasmic tail does (Wen *et al.*, 2003), remains to be determined. MUC1 nuclear localization suggests that it is cleaved and released from the membrane and traffic from the membrane to the cytoplasm and the nucleus.

Although MUC16 shares some structural similarities with other membrane-bounded mucins, it possesses many unique features suggesting that its signaling capabilities and functions may differ from other mucins.

4. Expression of MUC16 in normal tissues and ovarian tumors

Mucins are normally expressed by epithelial cells where they play a protective role. The extensive glycosylation of mucins provides a hydrophilic environment ideal for hydration and lubrication of epithelia. MUC16 is expressed at low levels in the normal airway epithelium but levels can increase in some chronic conditions such as cystic fibrosis (Hattrup *et al.*, 2008; Davies *et al.*, 2007; Gronowitz *et al.*, 2003). MUC16 is expressed at the apical surface of the ocular and conjonctival epithelium where it is part of the glycocalyx protecting corneal cells from bacterial infections and dryness (Argueso *et al.*, 2003; Blalock *et al.*, 2007). MUC16 is also found in lacrimal glands (Jäger *et al.*, 2007). Immunohistochemistry of human tissues using the OC125 antibody detected MUC16 expression in other epithelia such as the fetal coelomic epithelia and its derivatives such as Müllerian duct, fallopian tube, endometrium, and endocervix. MUC16 is also expressed by mesothelial cells of the peritoneum, pleura and pericardium (Kabawat *et al.*, 1983; Nap 1998). However, using OC125 or 4H11 antibodies, MUC16 expression is not found in normal adult colon, rectum, cervix, small intestine, liver, pancreatic ducts, spleen, kidney, skin and ovaries (Rao *et al.*, 2010).

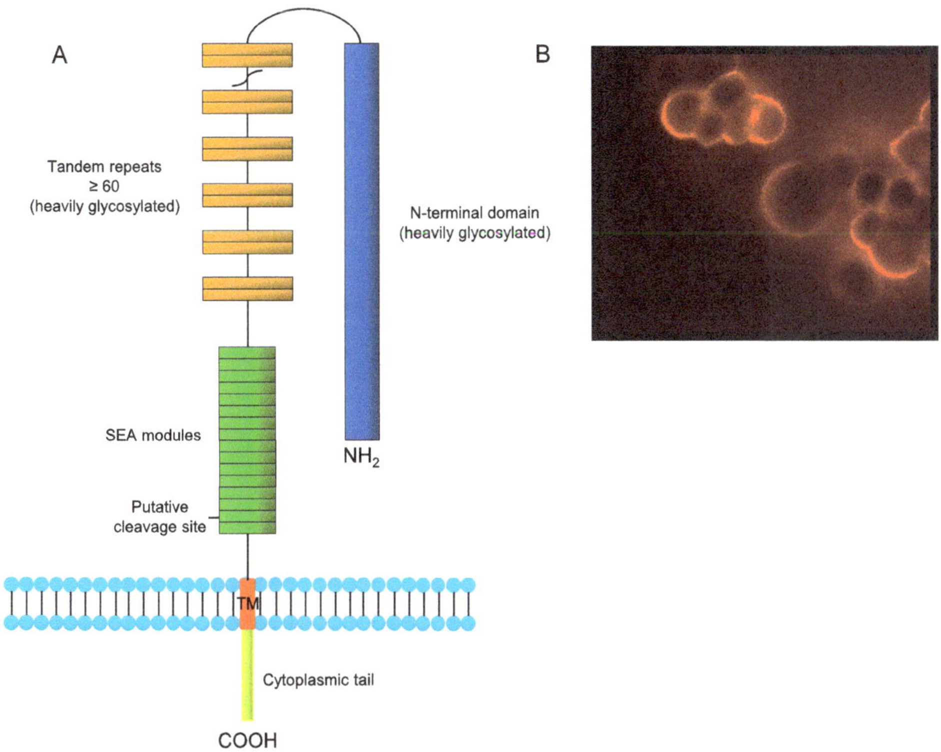

Fig. 1. Schematic structure of MUC16 mucin. A. The major domains of MUC16 include the N-terminal domain, the tandem repeat domain and the C-terminal domain. The SEA modules contain a putative proteolytic cleavage site which divides MUC16 in two subunits. The extracellular larger subunit consists of the N-terminal (> 12,000 a.a.) and tandem repeat domains (156 a.a. each), and are heavily glycosylated. The smaller subunit contains SEA domains, a transmembrane domain (TM) and the cytoplasmic tail (31 a.a.). B. MUC16 is usually expressed at the apical surface of normal epithelial cells. In EOC cells, this pattern of expression is lost and MUC16 is expressed through the entire surface of the tumor cells. The micrograph represents OVCAR3 cells probed with M11 antibody.

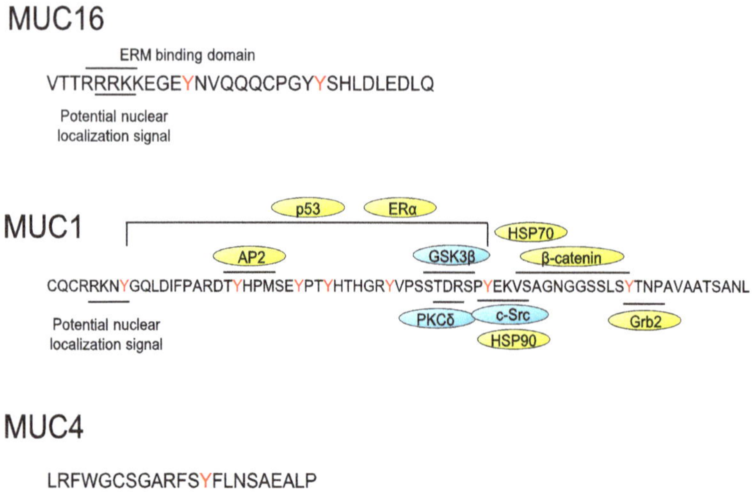

Fig. 2. Sequence of MUC1, MUC4 and MUC16 cytoplasmic tails. The intracellular sequence of the different mucins is shown along with protein interaction sites. MUC1 is the best characterized mucin. MUC1 cytoplasmic tail interacts with c-Src, GSK3β, PCKδ, β-catenin, p53, ERα, HSP70/90, Grb2, AP-2. Proteins with kinase activity are in blue whereas those without kinase activity are in yellow. HSP70 binds to MUC1 cytoplasmic tail in the same region as β-catenin. HSP90 binding to MUC1 depends on c-Src-induced Y-46 phosphorylation. MUC16 cytoplasmic tail has an ERM motif for potential interaction with the cytoskeleton. Both MUC1 and MUC16 contain a potential nuclear localization signal motif. MUC4 has no known interaction binding partners.

The expression of MUC16 in EOC tissues varies according to the histotype. Using tissues arrays, Hogdall *et al.*, reported that MUC16 was expressed by 85% of serous, 65% of endometrioid, 40% of clear cell and 36% of undifferentiated adenocarcinomas, but by only 12% of mucinous cancers (Hogdall *et al.*, 2007). Limited expression of MUC16 in mucinous EOC has also been reported by other groups (de la Cuesta *et al.*, 1999). These authors also showed that MUC16 tissues expression was significantly correlated with the FIGO stage but not with the histological grade (Hogdall *et al.*, 2007). In another study using tissues arrays, Rao *et al.*, found that 56%-66% of serous high grade EOC expressed MUC16 depending on the antibody used (OC125 vs 4H11) (Rao *et al.*, 2010). Other studies have also shown the lack MUC16 tissues expression in 15% to 25% of serous EOC (Lu *et al.*, 2004; Rosen *et al.*, 2005; Breitenecker *et al.*, 1989). MUC16 was also found to be expressed in a small percentage (3%-4%) of invasive breast carcinomas and 13% of lung carcinomas (Rao *et al.*, 2010).

Because MUC16 is expressed in a limited subset of early stage OC, in other types of cancers and in a number of benign conditions, its serum level is neither a sensitive nor a specific marker to detect early diseases. However, as mentioned previously, it is a useful marker to monitor response to treatment. In patients who reached complete response after standard primary treatment, MUC16 nadir serum values were associated with a significantly longer progression-free survival (PFS) and overall survival (Rustin *et al.*, 1996; Krivak *et al.*, 2009; van Altena *et al.*, 2010). Pretreatment MUC16 serum level is an independent predictor of PFS in patients with advanced EOC who received a standard chemotherapy regimen (Zorn *et al.*, 2009). In contrast, high MUC16 expression in EOC tissues has inconsistently been associated with overall survival. de la Cuesta *et al.*, found that, in a cohort of 50 EOC samples, patients with high tissue expression of MUC16 had a higher risk of death compared to patients with no expression (de la Cuesta *et al.*, 1999). However, in a much larger cohort of 778 EOC samples, Hogdall *et al.*, showed that late-stage patients that lacked MUC16 tissue expression had a significantly poorer survival (Hogdall *et al.*, 2007). In addition, MUC16 expression had no prognostic value in early stage EOC (Hogdall *et al.*, 2007). Because the immunohistochemical detection of tissues MUC16 was based on antibodies that recognize glycosylated epitopes in the tandem repeats in these studies, the expression of a cleaved MUC16 lacking the N-terminal and the tandem repeats domains could not have been detected. Furthermore, the fact that we recently shown that a MUC16 construct consisting of the last C-terminal 283 amino acid was sufficient to promote tumorigenicity (Thériault *et al.*, 2011), is not inconsistent with the observation that late-stage EOC lacking MUC16 (as assessed by immunohistochemistry) is associated with a worse prognosis.

5. MUC16 roles in the initiation and progression of ovarian cancer

Membrane-bounded mucins such as MUC1 and MUC4 are multifunctional molecules. Their large extracellular, heavily glycosylated domain promotes adequate hydration and lubrification of epithelia, and serve as a protective barrier with anti-adhesive properties. On the other hand, through their cytoplasmic tail, they activate various signaling pathways.

MUC16 is also seen as a multifunctional molecule with different domains involved in specific functions. Both secreted and membrane-bounded MUC16 have been shown to interact with galectin-1 (Seelenmeyer *et al.,*, 2002). The MUC16 C-terminal domain (last 1148 amino acids) appears to be sufficient for binding to galectin-1 but this interaction requires O-linked oligosaccharide chains which are found in the repeats of the MUC16. The biological significance of this interaction remains unclear but the cell surface recruitment of galectin-1 has been associated with processes such as regulation of cell adhesion (Perillo *et al.*, 1998). MUC16 facilitates cell-cell adhesion through its binding with mesothelin (Rump *et al.*, 2004; Gubbels *et al.*, 2006). The binding site for mesothelin on MUC16 is likely located in the 156 amino acid tandem repeats of the molecule (Gubbels *et al.*, 2006). MUC16 binds primarily to the N-terminus of the extracellular domain of mesothelin (residues 296-359) (Kaneko *et al.*, 2009). Mesothelin is a glycoprotein normally expressed on the mesothelial cells lining the peritoneal cavity (Chang *et al.*, 1996), and by ovarian tumor cells and mesotheliomas (Rump *et al.*, 2004). Mesothelin-MUC16 interaction could facilitate homotypic and heterotypic cell-cell adhesion and peritoneal metastasis of ovarian tumors through the adhesion with mesothelial cells. This is consistent with our recent observation that MUC16 knockdown abolished homotypic cell-cell adhesion (Comamala *et al.*, 2011). MUC16 knockdown also promotes EOC cell motility and invasiveness (Comamala *et al.*, 2011). By regulating cell adhesion, cell motility and invasiveness, the extracellular portion of MUC16, through its interaction with galectin-1 and mesothelin, may thus play an important role in metastasis.

MUC16 possesses immunosuppressive properties. Patankar *et al.*, reported that natural killer (NK) cells incubated with soluble MUC16 exhibited a 50–70% decrease in the lysis of tumor cells (Patankar *et al.*, 2005). MUC16-expressing EOC cells are also protected from lysis by primary NK cells (Gubbels *et al.*, 2010). Both soluble and membrane-bound MUC16 thus appear to be potent inhibitors of NK cells response *in vitro*. MUC16 downregulates CD16 expression in NK cells found in peritoneal fluids of patients with EOC (Patankar *et al.*, 2005; Belisle *et al.*, 2007). The secreted MUC16 binds to NK cells, B cells and monocytes via Siglec-9, a receptor found on immune cells that inhibits the NK cell response (Belisle *et al.*, 2010). The high levels of secreted MUC16 found in ascites may be one of the factors contributing to the immunosuppressive properties of ascites.

MUC1 and MUC4 mucins have been shown to promote the transformation of fibroblast cells. For example, when the C-terminal portion of MUC1 was stably transfected into 3Y1 fibroblast cells, soft agar colonies and subcutaneous tumors in nude mice were readily obtained (Li *et al.*, 2003). The transforming potential of MUC16 has not been reported yet but limited data from our laboratory showed that stable transfection of MUC16 C-terminal portion (extracellular unique region, transmembrane domain and full-length cytoplasmic tail) into normal ovarian cells failed to immortalized these cells as well as HFL-1 human fibroblast lung cells (Thériault, unpublished data). Recently, ectopic expression of MUC-16 C-terminal domain has been shown to increase tumorigenicity of SKOV3 ovarian cancer cell line in a xenograft mouse model (Thériault *et al.*, 2011). Deletion of the cytoplasmic tail completely abrogated this effect demonstrating that the enhanced tumorigenicity is mediated by interaction of the cytoplasmic tail with intracellular signaling molecules. Consistent with these results, single-chain antibody-mediated knockdown of cell surface MUC16 completely abrogated the formation of colonies in soft agar and subcutaneous tumors with OVCAR3 cells suggesting that MUC16 could be indeed an oncogene (Thériault *et al.*, 2011). Although MUC1 and MUC4 affect tumor progression through the interaction of their cytoplasmic tail with various intracellular signaling molecules (for review, see Bafna *et al.*, 2010), there is very limited data available on the signaling pathways activated by MUC16 cytoplasmic tail. Data from our laboratory suggest that the expression of anti-apoptotic proteins Bcl-2 and Bcl-XL and pro-apoptotic protein Bax is not affected by ectopic expression of MUC16 C-terminal domain (Matte *et al.*,, unpublished data). This observation contrasts with those of Raina *et al.*, which showed that stable transfection of MUC1 in rat 3Y1 fibroblast upregulates Bcl-XL but not Bcl-2 expression (Raina *et al.*, 2004). Growth factors induce tyrosine phosphorylation of MUC1 cytoplasmic tail (Ren *et al.*, 2006). This phosphorylation increases the binding of MUC1 to β-catenin and induces the translocation of MUC1 and β-catenin to the nucleus (Ren *et al.*, 2006). The dysregulation of β-catenin signaling contributes to the transformed phenotype of various cancers (Huang *et al.*, 2005). GSK3β phosphorylates β-catenin and targets it for ubiquitination and degradation (through β-Trcp, an E3 ubiquitin ligase) whereas the inhibition of GSK3β kinase activity results in the translocation of β-catenin from the cytosol to the nucleus where it acts as a transactivator of transcription. MUC1 increases the cytoplasmic and nuclear localization of β-catenin by inhibiting GSK3β-mediated phosphorylation and degradation of β-catenin (Huang *et al.*, 2005). Whether MUC16 could play a role similar to MUC1 is unknown. MUC16 cytoplasmic tail however lacks the β-catenin binding site. Nonetheless, MUC16 was shown to interact with β-catenin (Comamala *et al.*, 2011). In addition, MUC16 knockdown induces β-catenin relocalization from the cell membrane to the cytoplasm (Comamala *et al.,* 2011) and increases GKS3β activity (Comamala, unpublished data). It is thus possible that by regulating GKS3β activity, MUC16 regulates β-catenin subcellular localization/degradation. Importantly, β-catenin relocalization in MUC16 knockdown cells is associated with increase cell motility, migration and invasiveness *in vitro* (Comamala *et al.,* 2011). So far, there is no evidence that MUC16 cytoplasmic tail co-localizes with β-catenin in the cytoplasm or the nucleus. How does MUC16 regulates GKS3β activity is also not known. GKS3β has been shown to bind directly to MUC1 cytoplasmic tail and phosphorylates serine in a DRSP site adjacent to that for the β-catenin interaction (Li *et al.,* 1998). This GKS3β target motif is not present in MUC16 cytoplasmic tail and it has not been established yet whether MUC16 binds to GKS3β. The binding of GKS3β to MUC1 appears to be regulated by the phosphorylation of MUC1 by Src family members (Singh *et al.,* 2006). MUC16 cytoplasmic tail is phosphorylated by EGFR activation and its phosphorylation promotes the release of the extracellular domain. Other consequence of this phosphorylation event has not been yet reported.

MUC1 and MUC4 have been implicated in the regulation of cell growth through their interaction with tyrosine kinase growth factor although these mucins act through different mechanisms (Bafna *et al.,* 2010). MUC1 interacts with ErbB1 through its cytoplasmic tail and increases cell proliferation via the activation of ERK pathway (Jepson *et al.,* 2002). MUC4 probably interacts with ErbB2 through its extracellular domain which leads to the activation of ERK and Akt pathways to promote cell growth (Carraway *et al.,* 2007). MUC16 was also recently shown to affect the growth characteristics of ovarian cancer cells (Thériault *et al.,* 2011). Although the OVCAR3 cell growth rate was not affected by MUC16 knockdown, knockdown cells reached a stationary growth phase in a shorter time. There was no appreciable difference in spontaneous apoptosis between the MUC16 knockdown cells and control cells. Conversely, stable expression of the C-terminal domain into MUC16 negative SKOV3 cells prolonged anchorage dependent growth before they reached the stationary phase. Deletion of the cytoplasmic tail completely abrogated the effect of the MUC16 C-terminal domain on cell growth. It is not known how MUC16 affects tumor cell growth. Stable expression of the MUC16 C-terminal domain in SKOV3 cells did not alter the expression or phosphorylation of EGFR. Although these observations do not rule out the involvement of receptor tyrosine kinase, other partners are probably required to modulate cell growth.

A recent study showed that MUC16 confers protection against genotoxic agents such as cisplatin in p53 null ovarian cancer cells (Boivin *et al.,* 2009). Single-chain antibody-mediated downregulation of MUC16 sensitized the MUC16 overexpressing OVCAR3 cell line to cisplatin but not to taxol. Conversely, ectopic expression of MUC16 C-terminal domain increased SKOV3 cell line resistance to cisplatin. The downregulation of MUC16 in OVCAR3 cells activates the PI3K/Akt pathway (Comamala *et al.,* 2011). The authors also reported that MUC16 knockdown in these cells decreased FOXO3a nuclear localization. FOXO3a function is controlled in part by activation of the Akt pathway. Akt phosphorylates FOXO3a, resulting in binding of FOXO3a to 14-3-3 proteins and retention of FOXO3a in the cytoplasm. In contrast, dephosphorylation of FOXO3a induces its nuclear localization where it transactivates gene expression (Nemoto *et al.,* 2002). FOXO3a modulates the expression of several genes that regulate the cellular response to stress at the G2-M checkpoint. The growth arrest and DNA damage response gene Gadd54a is a target of FOXO3a that mediates part of FOXO3a's effects on DNA repair (Tran *et al.*, 2002). Thus, preventing the nuclear localization of FOXO3a contributes to the apoptotic response to genotoxic drugs. These data suggest that MUC16 knockdown sensitizes tumor cells to genotoxic drugs by activating Akt which in turn prevents FOXO3a nuclear localization. The knockdown of MUC1 has also been reported to sensitize carcinoma cells to apoptosis induced by genotoxic agents (Yin *et al.*, 2004; Ren *et al.*, 2004).

EOC is a highly metastatic disease which primarily metastasizes to the serosal cavities while dissemination through the vasculature is unusual (Naora *et al.*, 2005). During the progression to a metastatic phenotype, carcinoma cells undergo morphological changes, become motile and acquire the ability to migrate and invade to establish secondary tumors at distant sites. This epithelial to mesenchymal transition (EMT) is characterized by coordinated molecular and cellular changes including a reduction in cell-cell adhesion, the loss of apical-basolateral polarity, the loss of epithelial markers and the gain of mesenchymal markers (Vergara *et al*, 2010; Hugo *et al*, 2007). EMT is an important physiological process during embryogenesis and wound healing, but also a key step in cancer metastasis (Radisky, 2005). EMT is a necessary step towards metastatic tumor progression during detachment of tumor cells from the primary tumor site and attachment to metastatic sites. A key feature of EMT is the switch from E-cadherin expression at the cell surface to N-cadherin which promotes the interaction with stromal components (Cavallaro *et al.*, 2004). EMT results in enhanced cell motility and invasion. MUC16 was recently shown to be an important regulator of EMT in OC cells (Comamala *et al.*, 2011). Using a MUC16 knockdown OC cell model, the authors showed that downregulation of MUC16 cell surface expression prevents homotypic cell aggregation, enhances disruption of cell-cell junctions and increases cell motility and invasiveness. These effects were associated with the loss of epithelial markers such as E-cadherin and cytokeratin-18 and gain of mesenchymal markers such as N-cadherin and vimentin in knockdown cells. These data suggest that MUC16 is involved in the metastatic process. As mentioned previously, MUC16 knockdown induces an intracellular relocalization of E-cadherin. It is possible that the binding of MUC16 to E-cadherin complexes results in the surface localization of E-cadherin, which mediates cell contact and suppression of cell migration. Conversely, in the absence of MUC16, E-cadherin relocalizes in the cytoplasm, which abolishes its ability to promote cell contact formation. The cytoplasmic domain of E-cadherin binds to β-catenin, which forms complexes with α-catenin (Ozawa *et al*, 1990), actin (Adams *et al*, 1996), p120 (Staddon *et al*, 1995), EGFR (Hoschuetzky *et al*, 1994), and other proteins. It is possible that by forming a complex with E-cadherin and/or β-catenin, MUC16 re-distributes EGFR and consequently modulates its signaling pathway. Although expression of MUC16 C-terminal domain in SKOV3 cells does not affect EGFR phosphorylation, MUC16 knockdown activates EGFR resulting in increased activation of Akt, ERK1/2 and MMP-2 and MMP-9 (Comamala *et al.*, 2011). Activation of the MAPK-ERK pathway has been shown to upregulate MMP-9 and to enhance cell migration (Suyama *et al*, 2002). Akt activation has been associated with induction of EMT in carcinoma cells (Grille *et al*, 2003; Yan *et al*, 2009). In summary, the early steps in ovarian tumor metastasis involve shedding of the primary tumor through alterations of cell adhesive properties into ascites to form free floating cells or multicellular aggregates. Tumor cells from the primary site express MUC16, display a more epithelial phenotype and express E-cadherin. Shedding from the primary tumor site involves the loss of MUC16 and E-cadherin expression and the gain of mesenchymal markers leading to increased motility and loss of adhesive properties. Following this EMT, floating tumor cells revert to an epithelial phenotype and express MUC16 leading to adhesion to mesothelial cells via MUC16/mesothelin interaction and the formation of tumor implants in the peritoneal cavity.

MUC16 has been shown to alter tumorigenicity and metastasis of EOC cells (Thériault *et al.*, 2011). MUC16 knockdown inhibited cell growth in soft agar and abolished the formation of subcutaneous tumor nodule. Conversely, the MUC16 C-terminal domain appears to be sufficient to enhance *in vitro* and *in vivo* tumorigenicity, and promote dissemination of tumor cells throughout the peritoneal cavity of SCID mice. Importantly, deletion of MUC16 cytoplasmic tail completely abolished these effects. Although the mechanism by which MUC16 affects tumorigenicity and metastasis is unknown, this study suggests that MUC16 plays a critical role in the progression of EOC.

Although MUC16's functions are beginning to be elucidated in EOC cells, the normal function of MUC16 is for the most part unknown. As mentioned previously, it is expressed by various tissues, notably the conjonctiva and the lachrymal glands, were it can play a protective role against bacterial infection. Its expression in fallopian tube and endometrium suggests a role in reproduction. However, knockout mice have been shown to display a normal phenotype by 1 year of age demonstrating that MUC16 is not required for mouse development and reproduction (Cheon *et al.*, 2009). Consistent with these data, MUC1 null mice have normal fertility and development (Spicer *et al.*, 1995). One explanation that has been evoked for the lack of phenotype for MUC16 and MUC1 knockout mice is that functional redundancy can compensate for the loss of other mucins.

6. Conclusions and future directions

Since its discovery in the late 1970s, MUC16 glycoprotein has been recognized as a useful clinical biomarker in advance diseases. However, accumulating evidence suggests that MUC16 is more than a biomarker for disease progression; MUC16 contributes to the pathogenesis and progression of EOC. MUC16 appears to regulate cell survival, cell motility, invasiveness and tumorigenicity in EOC cells. These phenotypic effects are also shared by other membrane-bounded mucins such as MUC1 and MUC4. However, the underlying mechanisms responsible for the biological functions are likely to differ between mucins because of their structural differences, notably in their cytoplasmic tail. Although progress has been made regarding the role of MUC16 in tumor progression, the signaling pathways activated by its cytoplasmic tail are mostly unknown. The functional role of MUC16/β-catenin and MUC16/E-cadherin interactions is not known. Further studies are needed to understand the contribution of these interactions in tumor progression. Identifying the signaling molecules activated by MUC16 and elucidating their contribution to EOC progression will be critical in the near future as MUC16 may represent a target for EOC treatment.

7. References

Adams CL, Nelson WJ, Smith SJ. Quantitative analysis of cadherin-catenin-actin reorganization during development of cell-cell adhesion. J Cell Biol 1996;135:1899-1911.

Aletti GD, Dowdy SC, Podratz KC, Cliby WA. Relationship among surgical complexity, short-term morbidity, and overall survival in primary surgery for advanced ovarian cancer. Am J Obstet Gynecol. 2007;197:676 e1-7.

Argueso P, Spurr-Michaud S, Russo CL, Tisdale A, Gipson IK. MUC16 mucin is expressed by the human ocular surface epithelia and carries the H185 carbohydrate epitope. Invest Ophthalmol Vis Sci 2003;44:2487–2495.

Auersperg N, Wong AS, Choi KC, Kang SK, Leung PC. Ovarian surface epithelium: biology, endocrinology, and pathology. Endocr Rev 2001;22:255-288.

Badgwell D, Bast RC Jr. Early detection of ovarian cancer. Dis Markers 2007;23:397–410.

Bafna S, Kaur S, Batra SK. Membrane-bound mucins: the mechanistic basis for alterations in the growth and survival of cancer cells. Oncogene 2010;29:2893-2904.

Bast RC Jr, Badgwell D, Lu Z, Marquez R, Rosen D, Liu J, Baggerly KA, Atkinson EN, Skates S, Zhang Z, Lokshin A, Menon U, Jacobs I, Lu K. New tumor markers: CA125 and beyond. Int J Gynecol Cancer 2005;15(suppl 3):274-281.

Bast RC Jr, Feeney M, Lazarus H, Nadler LM, Colvin RB, Knapp RC. Reactivity of a monoclonal antibody with human ovarian carcinoma. J Clin Invest 1981;68:1331–1337.

Bast RC Jr, Hennessy B, Mills GB. The biology of ovarian cancer: new opportunities for translation. Nat Rev Cancer 2009;9:415-428.

Bast RC Jr, Klug TL, St John E, Jenison E, Niloff JM, Lazarus H, Berkowitz RS, Leavitt T, Griffiths CT, Parker L, Zurawski VR Jr, Knapp RC. A radioimmunoassay using a monoclonal antibody to monitor the course of epithelial ovarian cancer. N Eng J Med 1983;309:883-887.

Belisle JA, Gubbels JA, Raphael CA, Migneault M, Rancourt C, Connor JP, Patankar MS. Peritoneal natural killer cells from epithelial ovarian cancer patients show an altered phenotype and bind to the tumour marker MUC16 (CA125). Immunology 2007;122:418-429.

Belisle JA, Horibata S, Jennifer GA, Petrie S, Kapur A, André S, Gabius HJ, Rancourt C, Connor J, Paulson JC, Patankar MS. Identification of Siglec-9 as the receptor for MUC16 on human NK cells, B cells, and monocytes. Mol Cancer 2010;9:118.

Blalock TD, Spurr-Michaud SJ, Tisdale AS, Heimer SR, Gilmore MS, Ramesh V, Gipson IK. Functions of MUC16 in corneal epithelial cells. Invest Ophthalmol Vis Sci 2007;48:4509-18.

Boivin M, Lane D, Piché A, Rancourt C. CA125 (MUC16) tumor antigen selectively modulates the sensitivity of ovarian cancer cells to genotoxic drug-induced apoptosis. Gynecol Oncol 2009 115:407-413, .

Breitenecker G, Neunteufel W, Bieglmayer C, Kolbl H, Schieder K. Comparison between tissue and serum content of CA 125, CA 19-9, and carcinoembryonic antigen in ovarian tumors. Int J Gynecol Pathol 1989;8:97–102.

Canney PA, Moore M, Wilkinson PM, James RD. Ovarian cancer antigen CA125: a prospective clinical assessment of its role as a tumour marker. Br J Cancer 1984;50:765-769.

Carraway KL 3rd, Funes M, Workman HC, Sweeney C. Contribution of membrane mucins to tumor progression through modulation of cellular growth signaling pathways. Curr Top Dev Biol 2007;78:1-22.

Cavallaro U, Christofori G. Cell adhesion and signalling by cadherins and Ig-CAMs in cancer. Nat Rev Cancer 2004;4:118-132.

Chang K, Pastan I. Molecular cloning of mesothelin, a differentiation antigen present on mesothelium, mesotheliomas, and ovarian cancers. Proc Natl Acad Sci USA 1996;93:136-140.

Cheon DJ, Wang Y, Deng JM, Lu Z, Xiao L, Chen CM, Bast RC, Behringer RR. CA125/MUC16 is dispensable for mouse development and reproduction. PlosOne 2009;4:e4675.

Colombo N, Van Gorp T, Parma G, Amant F, Gatta G, Sessa C, Vergote I. Ovarian cancer. Crit Rev Oncol Hematol 2006;60:159-179.

Comamala M, Pinard M, Thériault C, Matte I, Albert A, Boivin M, Beaudin J, Piché A, Rancourt C. Downregulation of cell surface CA125/MUC16 induces epithelial-to-mesenchymal transition and restores EGFR signaling in NIH:OVCAR3 ovarian carcinoma cells. Br J Cancer 2011;104:989-999.

Crum CP, Drapkin R, Kindelberger D, Medeiros F, Miron A, Lee Y. Lessons from BRCA: the tubal fimbria emerges as an origin for pelvic serous cancer. Clin Med Res 2007;5:35-44.

Crum CP, Drapkin R, Miron A, Ince TA, Muto M, Kindelberger DW, Lee Y. The distal fallopian tube: a new model for pelvic serous carcinogenesis. Curr Opin Obstet Gynecol 2007;19:3-9.

Davies JR, Kirkham S, Svitacheva N, Thornton DJ, Carlstedt I. MUC16 is produced in tracheal surface epithelium and submucosal glands and is present in secretions from normal human airway and cultured bronchial epithelial cells. Int J Biochem Cell Biol 2007;39:1943-1954.

Davis HM, Zurawski VR Jr, Bast RC Jr, Klug TL. Characterization of the CA 125 antigen associated with human epithelial ovarian carcinomas. Cancer Res 1986;46:6143-6148.

de la Cuesta R, Maestro ML, Solana J, Vidart JA, Escudero M, Iglesias E, Valor R.. Tissue quantification of CA 125 in epithelial ovarian cancer. Int J Biol Markers 1999;14:106–114.

Dharma Rao T, Park KJ, Smith-Jones P, Iasonos A, Linkov I, Soslow RA, Spriggs DR. Novel Monoclonal Antibodies Against the Proximal (Carboxy-Terminal) Portions of MUC16. Appl Immunohistochem Mol Morphol 2010;18:462-472.

Dubeau L. The cell of origin of ovarian epithelial tumours. Lancet Oncol 2008;9:1191-1197.

Duraisamy S, Ramasamy S, Kharbanda S, Kufe D. Distinct evolution of the human carcinoma-associated transmembrane mucins, MUC1, MUC4 and MUC16. Gene 2006;373:28–34.

Fendrick JL, Konishi I, Geary SM, Parmley TH, Quirk JG Jr, O'Brien TJ. CA125 phosphorylation is associated with its secretion from the WISH human amnion cell line. Tumour Biol 1997;18:278-289.

Goff BA, Mandel L, Muntz HG, Melancon CH. Ovarian carcinoma diagnosis. Cancer 2000;89:2068-2075.

Grille SJ, Bellacosa A, Upson J, Klein-Szanto AJ, van Roy F, Lee-Kwon W, Donowitz M, Tsichlis PN, Larue L. The protein kinase Akt induces epithelial-mesenchymal transition and promotes enhanced motility and invasiveness of squamous cell carcinoma lines. Cancer Res 2003;63:2172-2178.

Gronowitz E, Pitkanen S, Kjellmer I, Heikinheimo M, Strandvik B. Association between serum oncofetal antigens CA 19-9 and CA 125 and clinical status in patients with cystic fibrosis. Acta Paediatr 2003;92:1267-1271.

Gubbels JA, Belisle J, Onda M, Rancourt C, Migneault M, Ho M, Bera TK, Connor J, Sathyanarayana BK, Lee B, Pastan I, Patankar MS. Mesothelin-MUC16 binding is a high affinity, N-glycan dependent interaction that facilitates peritoneal metastasis of ovarian tumors. Mol Cancer 2006;5:50.

Gubbels JA, Felder M, Horibata S, Belisle JA, Kapur A, Holden H, Petrie S, Migneault M, Rancourt C, Connor JP, Patankar MS. MUC16 provides immune protection by inhibiting synapse formation between NK and ovarian tumor cells. Mol Cancer 2010;9:11.

Hattrup CL, Gendler SJ. Structure and function of cell surface (tethered) mucins. Annu Rev Physiol 2008;70:431-457.

Herzog TJ. Recurrent ovarian cancer: how important is it to treat to disease progression? Clin Cancer Res 2004;10:7439-7449.

Hogdall EV, Christensen L, Kjaer SK, Blaakaer J, Kjaerbye-Thygesen A, Gayther S, Jacobs IJ, Hogdall CK. CA125 expression pattern, prognosis and correlation with serum CA125 in ovarian tumor patients from the danish "MALOVA" ovarian cancer study. Gynecol Oncol 2007;104:508-515.

Hoschuetzky H, Aberle H, Kemler R. β-catenin mediates the interaction of the cadherin-catenin complex with epidermal growth factor receptor. J Cell Biol 1994;127:1375-1380.

Huang L, Chen D, Liu D, Yin L, Kharbanda S, Kufe D. MUC1 oncoprotein blocks glycogen synthase kinase 3β—mediated phosphorylation and degradation of β-catenin. Cancer Res 2005;65:10413-10422.

Hugo H, Ackland ML, Blick T, Lawrence MG, Clements JA, Williams ED, Thompson EW. Epithelial-mesenchymal and mesenchymal-epithelial transitions in carcinoma progression. J Cell Physiol 2007;213:374-383.

Jäger K, Wu G, Sel S, Garreis F, Bräuer L, Paulsen FP. MUC16 in the lacrimal apparatus. Histochem Cell Biol 2007;127:433-438.

Jemal A, Siegel R, Xu J, Ward E. Cancer Statistics 2010. CA Cancer J Clin 2010;60:277-300.

Jepson S, Komatsu M, Haq B, Arango ME, Huang D, Carraway CA, Carraway KL. Muc4/sialomucin complex, the intramembrane erbB2 ligand, induces specific phosphorylation of ErbB2 and enhances expression of p27(kip), but does not activate mitogen-activated kinase or protein kinaseB/Akt pathways. Oncogene 2002;21:7524-7532.

Kabawat SE, Bast RC Jr, Bhan AK, Welch WR, Knapp RC, Colvin RB. Tissue distribution of a coelomic epithelium-related antigen recognized by the monoclonal antibody OC125. Int J Gynecol Pathol 1983;2:275-285.

Kaneko O, Gong L, Zhang J, Hansen JK, Hassan R, Lee B, Ho M. A binding domain on mesothelin for CA125/MUC16. J Biol Chem 2009;284:3739-3749.

Karlan B, Amin W, Casper SE, Littlefield BA. Hormonal regulation of CA125 tumor marker expression in human ovarian carcinoma cells: inhibition by glucocorticoids. Cancer Res 1988;48:3502-3506.

Kindelberger DW, Lee Y, Miron A, Hirsch MS, Feltmate C, Medeiros F, Callahan MJ, Garner EO, Gordon RW, Birch C, Berkowitz RS, Muto MG, Crum CP. Intraepithelial carcinoma of the fimbria and pelvic serous carcinoma: evidence for a causal relationship. Am J Surg Pathol 2007;31:161–9.

Konishi I, Fendrick JL, Parmley TH, Quirk JG Jr, O'Brien TJ. Epidermal growth factor enhances secretion of the ovarian tumor-associated cancer antigen CA125 from the human amnion WISH cell line. J Soc Gynecol Invest 1994;1:89-96.

Konstantinopoulos PA, Spentzos D, Cannistra SA. Gene-expression profiling in epithelial ovarian cancer. Nat Clin Pract Oncol 2008;5:577-587.

Krivak TC, Tian C, Rose GS, Armstrong DK, Maxwell GL. A Gynecologic Oncology Group Study of serum CA-125 levels in patients with stage III optimally debulked ovarian cancer treated with intraperitoneal compared to intravenous chemotherapy: an analysis of patients enrolled in GOG 172. Gynecol Oncol 2009;115:81–85.

Kui WN, Easton RL, Panico M, Sutton-Smith M, Morrison JC, Lattanzio FA, Morris HR, Clark GF, Dell A, Patankar MS. Characterization of the oligosaccharides associated with the human ovarian tumor marker CA125. J Biol Chem 2003;278:28619-28634.

Kurman RJ, Shih IM. The origin and pathogenesis of epithelial ovarian cancer: a proposed unifying theory. Am J Surg Pathol 2010;34:433-443.

Landen CN Jr, Birrer MJ, Sood AK. Early events in the pathogenesis of epithelial ovarian cancer. J Clin Oncol 2008;26:995–1005.

Li Y, Bharti A, Chen D, Gong J, Kufe D. Interaction of glycogen synthase kinase 3β with the DF3/MUC1 carcinoma-associated antigen and β-catenin. Mol Cell Biol 1998;18:7216-7224.

Li Y, Liu D, Chen D, Kharbanda S, Kufe D. Human DF3/MUC1 carcinoma-associated protein functions as an oncogene. Oncogene 2003;22:6107-6110.

Li Y, Ren J, Yu W, Li Q, Kuwahara H, Yin L Carraway KL 3rd, Kufe D. The epidermal growth factor receptor regulates interaction of the human DF3/MUC1 carcinoma antigen with c-Src and beta-catenin. J Biol Chem 2001;276:35239-35242.

Lloyd KO, Yin BW, Kudryashov V. Isolation and characterization of ovarian cancer antigen CA 125 using a new monoclonal antibody (VK-8): identification as a mucin-type molecule. Int J Cancer 1997;71:842-850.

Lloyd KO, Yin BW. Synthesis and secretion of the ovarian cancer antigen CA 125 by the human cancer cell line NIH:OVCAR-3. Tumour Biol 2001;22:77-82.

Lu KH, Patterson AP, Wang L, Marquez RT, Atkinson EN, Baggerly KA, Ramoth LR, Rosen DG, Liu J, Hellstrom I, Smith D, Hartmann L, Fishman D, Berchuck A, Schmandt R, Whitaker R, Gershenson DM, Mills GB, Bast RC Jr. Selection of potential markers for epithelial ovarian cancer with gene expression arrays and recursive descent partition analysis. Clin Cancer Res 2004;10:3291–3300.

Mano MS, Rosa DD, Azambuja E, Ismael G, Braga S, D'Hondt V, Piccart M, Awada A. Current management of ovarian carcinosarcoma. Int J Gynecol Cancer 2007;17:316-24.

McGuire WP, Hoskins WJ, Brady MF, Kucera PR, Partridge EE, Look KY, Clarke-Pearson DL, Davidson M. Cyclophosphamide and cisplatin versus paclitaxel and cisplatin: a phase III randomized trial in patients with suboptimal stage III/IV ovarian cancer (from the Gynecologic Oncology Group). Semin Oncol. 1996;5 (Suppl 12):40-7.

Naora H, Montell DJ. Ovarian cancer metastasis: integrating insights from disparate model organisms. Nat Rev Cancer 2005;5:355-366.

Nap M. Immunohistochemistry of CA125. Unusual expression in normal tissues, distribution in the human fetus and questions around its application in diagnostic pathology. Int J Biol Markers 1998;13:210–215.

Nemoto S, Finkel T. Redox Regulation of Forkhead Proteins Through a *p66shc*-Dependent Signaling Pathway. Science 2002;295:2450-2452.

Nustad K, Lebedin Y, Lloyd KO, Shigemasa K, de Bruijn HW, Jansson B, Nilsson O, Olsen KH, O'Brien TJ. Epitopes on CA125 from cervical mucus and ascites fluid and characterization of six new antibodies. Third report from the ISOBM TD-1 workshop. Tumour Biol 2002;23:303–314.

O'Brien TJ, Beard JB, Underwood LJ, Dennis RA, Santin AD, York L. The Ca125 gene: an extracellular superstructure dominated by repeat sequences. Tumour Biol 2001;22:348-466.

O'Brien TJ, Beard JB, Underwood LJ, Shigemasa K. The CA 125 gene: a new discovered extension of the glycosylated N-terminal domain doubles the size of this extracellular superstructure. Tumour Biol 2002;23:154-169.

Ouellet V, Guyot MC, Le Page C, Filali-Mouhim A, Lussier C, Tonin PN, Provencher DM, Mes-Masson AM. Tissue array analysis of expression microarray candidates identifies markers associated with tumor grade and outcome in serous epithelial ovarian cancer. Int J Cancer 2006;119:599-607.

Ouellet V, Ling TH, Normandin K, Madore J, Lussier C, Barrès V, Bachvarov D, Rancourt C, Tonin PN, Provencher DM, Mes-Masson AM. Immunohistochemical profiling of benign, low malignant potential and low grade serous epithelial ovarian tumors. BMC Cancer 2008;8:346.

Ouellet V, Provencher DM, Maugard CM, Le Page C, Ren F, Lussier C, Novak J, Ge B, Hudson TJ, Tonin PN, Mes-Masson AM. Discrimination between serous low malignant potential and invasive epithelial ovarian tumors using molecular profiling. Oncogene 2005;24:4672-4687.

Ozawa M, Ringwald M, Kemler R. Uvomorulin-catenin complex formation is regulated by a specific domain in the cytoplasmic region of the cell adhesion molecule. Proc Natl Acad Sci USA 1990;87:4246-4250.

Ozols RF, Bookman MA, Connolly DC, Daly MB, Godwin AK, Schilder RJ, Xu X, Hamilton TC. Focus on epithelial ovarian cancer. Cancer Cell 2004;5:19-24.

Patankar MS, Jing Y, Morrison JC, Belisle JA, Lattanzio FA, Deng Y, Wong NK, Morris HR, Dell A, Clark GF. Potent suppression of natural killer cell response mediated by the ovarian tumor marker CA125. Gynecol Oncol 2005;99:704-713.

Perillo NL, Marcus ME, Baum LG. Galectins : versatile modulators of cell adhesion, cell proliferation, and cell death. J Mol Med 1998;76:402-412.

Pochampalli MR, el Bejjani RM, Schroeder JA. MUC1 is novel regulator of ErbB1 receptor trafficking. Oncogene 2007;26:1693-1701.

Radisky DC. Epithelial-mesenchymal transition. J Cell Sci 2005;118:4325-4326.

Raina D, Kharbanda S, Kufe D. The MUC1 oncoprotein activates the anti-apoptotic phosphoinositide 3-kinase/Akt and Bcl-XL pathways in rat 3Y1 fibroblast. J Biol Chem 2004;279:20607-20612.

Ren J, Agata N, Chen D, Li Y, Yu WH, Huang L, Raina D, Chen W, Kharbanda S, Kufe D. Human MUC1 carcinoma-associated protein confers resistance to genotoxic anticancer agents. Cancer Cell 2004;5:163:175.

Ren J, Raina D, Chen W, Li G, Huang L, Kufe D. MUC1 oncoprotein functions in activation of fibroblast growth factor receptor signaling. Mol Cancer Res 2006;4:873-883.

Rosen DG, Wang L, Atkinson JN, Yu Y, Lu KH, Diamandis EP, Hellstrom I, Mok SC, Liu J, Bast RC Jr. Potential markers that complement expression of CA125 in epithelial ovarian cancer. Gynecol Oncol 2005;99:267–77.

Rump A, Morikawa Y, Tanaka M, Minami S, Umesaki N, Takeuchi M, Miyajima A. Binding of ovarian cancer antigen CA125/MUC16 to mesothelin mediates cell adhesion. J Biol Chem 2004;279:9190-9198.

Rustin GJ, Nelstrop AE, Tuxen MK, Lambert HE. Defining progression of ovarian carcinoma during follow-up according to CA 125: a North Thames Ovary Group Study. Ann Oncol 1996;7:361-364.

Schroeder JA, Thompson MC, Gardner MM, Gendler SJ. Transgenic MUC1 interacts with epidermal growth factor receptor and correlates with mitogen-activated protein kinase activation in the mouse mammary gland. J Biol Chem 2001;276:13057-13064.

Schwartz DR, Kardia SL, Shedden KA, Kuick R, Michailidis G, Taylor JM, Misek DE, Wu R, Zhai Y, Darrah DM, Reed H, Ellenson LH, Giordano TJ, Fearon ER, Hanash SM, Cho KR. Gene expression in ovarian cancer reflects both morphology and biological behavior, distinguishing clear cell from other poor-prognosis ovarian carcinomas. Cancer Res 2002;62:4722-4729.

Seelenmeyer C, Wegehingel S, Lechner J, Nickel W. The cancer antigen CA125 represents a novel counter receptor for galectin-1. J Cell Sci 2003;116:1305-1318.

Singh PK, Hollingsworth MA. Cell surface-associated mucins in signal transduction. Trends Cell Biol 2006;16:467-476.

Soslow RA. Histologic subtypes of ovarian carcinoma: an overview. Int J Gynecol Pathol 2008;27:161-174.

Spicer AP, Rowse GJ, Lidner TK, Gendler SJ. Delayed mammary tumor progression in Muc-1 null mice. J Biol Chem 1995;270:30093-30101.

Staddon JM, Smales C, Schulze C, Esch FS, Rubin LL. p120, a p120-related protein (p100), and the cadherin/catenin complex. J Cell Biol 1995;130:369-381.

Suyama K, Shapiro I, Guttman M, Hazan RB. A signaling pathway leading to metastasis is controlled by N-cadherin and the FGF receptor. Cancer Cell 2002;2:301-314.

Thériault C, Pinard M, Comamala M, Migneault M, Beaudin J, Matte I, Boivin M, Piché A, Rancourt C. MUC16 (CA125) regulates epithelial ovarian cancer cell growth, tumorigenesis and metastasis. Gynecol Oncol 2011;121:434-443.

Tran H, Brunet A, Grenier JM, Datta SR, Fornace AJ Jr, DiStefano PS, Chiang LW, Greenberg ME. DNA repair pathway stimulated by the forkhead transcription factor FOXO3a through the Gadd45 protein. Science 2002;296:530-534.

Van Altena AM, Kolwijck E, Spanjer MJ, Hendriks JC, Massuger LF, de Hullu JA. CA125 nadir concentration is an independent predictor of tumor recurrence in patients with ovarian cancer: a population-based study. Gynecol Oncol 2010;119:265-269.

Vergara D, Merlot B, Lucot JP, Collinet P, Vinatier D, Fournier I, Salzet M. Epithelial-mesenchymal transition in ovarian cancer. Cancer Lett 2010;291:59-66.

Vergote IB, Bormer OP, Abeler VM. Evaluation of serum CA 125 levels in the monitoring of ovarian cancer. Am J Obstet Gynecol 1987;157:88-92.

Wen Y, Caffrey T`C, Wheelock MJ, Johnson KR, Hollingsworth MA. Nuclear association of the cytoplasmic tail of MUC1 and β-catenin. J Biol Chem 2003;278:38029-38039.

Xiaofang Y, Yue Z, Xialian X, Zhibin Y. Serum tumour markers in patients with chronic kidney disease. Scand J Clin Lab Invest 2007;67:661-667.

Yamamoto M, Bharti A, Li Y, Kufe D. Interaction of the DF3/MUC1 breast carcinoma-associated antigen and β-catenin in cell adhesion. J Biol Chem 1997;272:12492-12494.

Yan W, Fu Y, Tian D, Liao J, Liu M, Wang B, Xia L, Zhu Q, Luo M. PI3 kinase/Akt signaling mediates epithelial-mesenchymal transition in hypoxic hepatocellular carcinoma cells. Biochem Biophys Res Commun 2009;382:631-636.

Yin BW, Dnistrian A, Lloyd KO, Ovarian cancer antigen CA125 is encoded by the MUC16 mucin gene. Int J Cancer 2002;98:737-740.

Yin BW, Lloyd KO. Molecular cloning of the CA125 ovarian cancer antigen: identification as a new mucin, MUC16. J Biol Chem 2001;276:27371-27375.

Yin L, Huang L, Kufe D. MUC1 oncoprotein activates the FOXO3a transcription factor in a survival response to oxidative stress. J Biol Chem 2004;279:45721-45727.

Zorn KK, Tian C, McGuire WP, Hoskins WJ, Markman M, Muggia FM, Rose PG, Ozols RF, Spriggs D, Armstrong DK. The prognostic value of pretreatment CA 125 in patients with advanced ovarian carcinoma: a Gynecologic Oncology Group Study. Cancer 2009;115:1028-1035.

6

Dysregulated TGFβ Signaling in Ovarian Cancer

Kyle Bauckman[2], Christie Campla[1] and Meera Nanjundan[1,2]
[1]*University of South Florida, Department of Cell Biology, Microbiology, and Molecular Biology,*
[2]*Moffitt Cancer Center, Cancer Biology Program, Tampa, Florida*
USA

1. Introduction

Ovarian cancer is one of the most lethal gynecological cancers in the United States. NCI estimates ~21,880 new cases with ~13,850 deaths in 2011 (http://www.cancer.gov/cancertopics/ types/ovariancancer). Unfortunately, the majority of these cases are only discovered at advanced stages (stage III or IV) due to the cancer's asymptomatic nature which has an overall survival rate between 5-25% (Bast et al., 2009; Hennessy et al., 2008). Hence, the inability to detect this disease during early stages has led to poor prognosis. Despite improvements in medicine and patient care, reasonable screening measures for detecting early stage ovarian cancers are presently lacking. Thus, a better understanding of the molecular events that underlie ovarian cancer development are needed.

The current strategy for treatment of ovarian cancer is surgical debulking followed by chemotherapy (Bast et al., 2009; Hennessy et al., 2008). Although ~70% of ovarian cancers respond to a combination of platinum and taxane-based chemotherapy administered after surgery, current treatments are of limited efficacy in preventing tumor recurrence and progression (Bast et al., 2009; Hennessy et al., 2008). Thus, new anti-neoplastic agents are urgently needed to increase the chemotherapeutic sensitivity of ovarian cancer cells.

Recently, evidence has emerged revealing the importance of genomic aberrations in the progression of ovarian cancer (Gorringe & Campbell, 2009; Gray et al., 2003). Through the use of high throughput technologies (i.e. array comparative genomic hybridization (aCGH), microarray, and SNP arrays), specific genomic regions have been identified to be either amplified or silenced in tumor progression (Gorringe & Campbell, 2009; Gray et al., 2003). One such region which we and others (Nanjundan et al., 2007; Osterberg et al., 2009) have previously identified to be frequently amplified early in serous epithelial ovarian cancer development is the 3q26.2 region which harbors Transforming Growth Factor β pathway (TGFβ) co-repressors, ecotropic viral integration site-1 (EVI1) (Nanjundan et al., 2007) and SnoN/SkiL (Nanjundan et al., 2008). A large amount of work has recently emerged involving the intricacies of TGFβ signaling and its role in cancer progression. Importantly, this signaling pathway is dysregulated in ovarian carcinomas.

2. Dual functionality of TGFβ signaling in cancer

There exist three isoforms of TGFβ, namely TGFβ1, TGFβ2, and TGFβ3, which are initially present in the inactive latent form (L-TGFβ) (Elliott & Blobe, 2005; Meulmeester & Ten Dijke,

2011). In its active dimeric form, the TGFβ ligand binds to the TGFβ receptor type II (TGFβRII) leading to heterotetrameric receptor complex formation with TGFβRI. In addition, the co-receptor, TGFβRIII or proteoglycan (a.k.a. endoglin), aids binding of the ligand to the TGFβRII (Elliott & Blobe, 2005; Meulmeester & Ten Dijke, 2011). The activated receptors then recruit receptor regulated SMADs (R-SMADs) such as SMAD2/3 which form a complex with a Co-SMAD, SMAD4, and then shuttles into the nucleus. These activated SMADs associate with DNA binding transcription factors to enhance DNA binding to regulate transcription of TGFβ target genes such as cyclin-dependent kinase inhibitors (i.e. p21, involved in regulating cell survival) (Elliott & Blobe, 2005) (Figure 1). The TGFβ pathway is regulated via several mechanisms including (1) phosphorylation, (2) ubiquitination, (3) inhibitory SMADs (i.e. SMAD6 and SMAD7), and (4) transcriptional co-repressors (i.e. SnoN/SkiL and EVI1) (Elliott & Blobe, 2005; Meulmeester & Ten Dijke, 2011). In addition to the canonical SMAD dependent pathway, there exists the non-canonical pathway involving (1) TRAF5/TAK1/p38-JNK, (2) RhoA/ROCK, and (3) ERK/MAPK (Elliott & Blobe, 2005; Meulmeester & Ten Dijke, 2011).

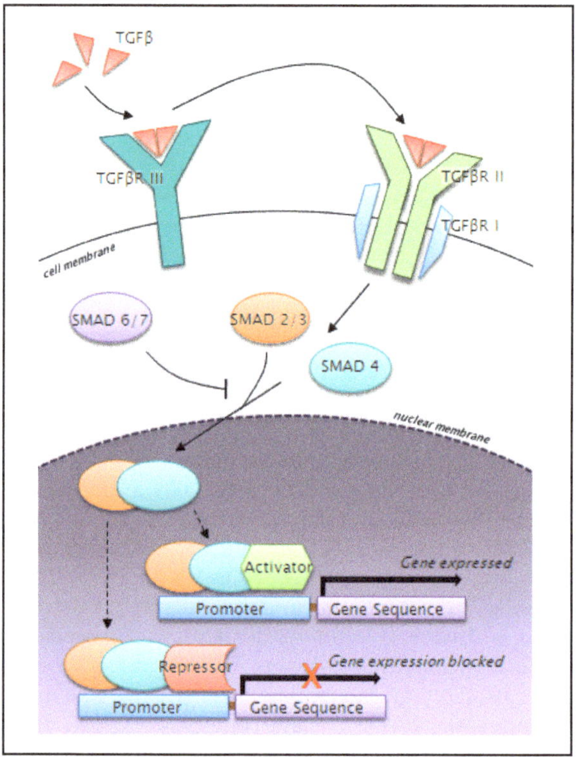

Fig. 1. The TGFβ signaling pathway. Active dimeric TGFβ ligand binds to TGFβRII on the cell surface leading to complex formation with TGFβRI. Endoglin (TGFβRIII) assists in recruitment of the active TGFβ ligand to bind to the cell surface receptors. Following receptor activation, receptor SMADs (SMAD2/3) become phosphorylated and form a complex with the Co-SMAD (SMAD4) which then translocate into the nuclear compartment to regulate transcription of various TGFβ target genes.

The TGFβ signaling pathway has the ability to transition from a tumor suppressor (in normal or early stage cancers) to a tumor promoter (late stages of cancer) (Elliott & Blobe, 2005; Meulmeester & Ten Dijke, 2011) (Figure 2). During the early stages of epithelial tumorigenesis, TGFβ inhibits tumor development and growth by inducing cell cycle arrest, senescence, and apoptosis; this aids in maintaining cellular homeostasis critical for prevention of continuous cell proliferation and thus tumor formation (Elliott & Blobe, 2005). This functionality is elicited via induction of cyclin-dependent kinase inhibitors (CDK), namely p15, p21, and p27. TGFβ also represses expression of the c-myc oncogene which leads to activation of these CDK inhibitors (Elliott & Blobe, 2005; Meulmeester & Ten Dijke, 2011). Additional molecules that are involved in the TGFβ apoptotic functional response include the death receptor FAS, GADD45b, BIM, and DAPK (Elliott & Blobe, 2005; Meulmeester & Ten Dijke, 2011).

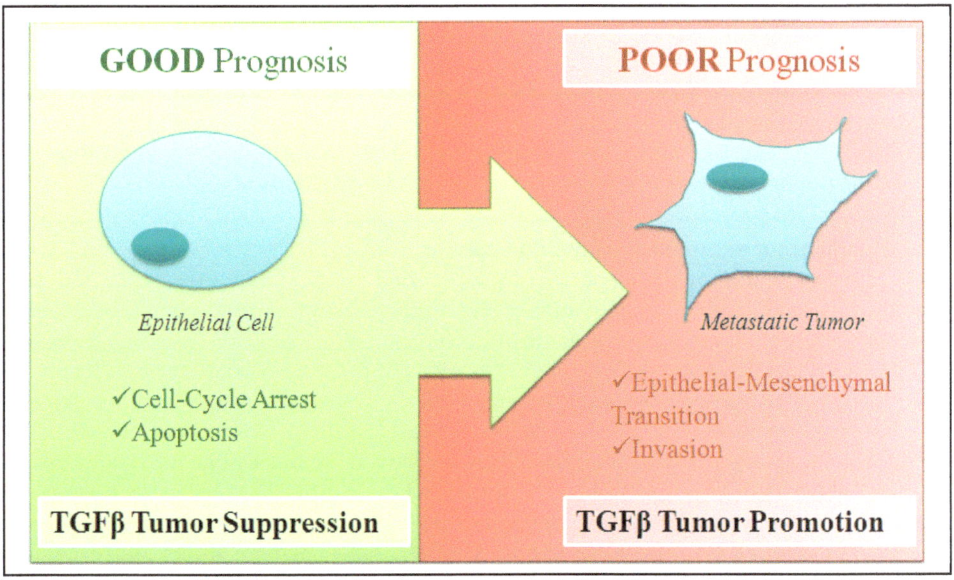

Fig. 2. The TGFβ signaling pathway elicits dual functionality. The pathway can transition from a tumor suppressive (normal or early stages of cancer) role to a tumor promoting role (late stages of cancer).

During the progression of cancer, mutations in these components may lead to disruption of TGFβ mediated control of cell proliferation. In late stages of tumor progression, tumor cells become resistant to growth inhibition due to inactivation of the TGFβ signaling pathway thus leading to altered cell cycle control (Elliott & Blobe, 2005). TGFβ becomes capable of inducing metastatic functions via increased cellular migration, invasiveness, loss of epithelial markers, and a corresponding acquisition of mesenchymal characteristics.

3. Dysregulated TGFβ signaling in ovarian cancer

Several components of the TGFβ signaling pathway have been reported to be dysregulated in ovarian cancers and are summarized in the subsections below.

3.1 TGFβ ligand expression in ovarian cancer

By immunohistochemical and in situ hybridization approaches, all of the three TGFβ ligands (TGFβ1, TGFβ2, and TGFβ3) are markedly elevated in ovarian cancer cells (Henriksen et al., 1995). Similar results were obtained via RNAse protection assay in primary ovarian cancer specimens (Bartlett et al., 1997). Northern blot analysis indicated that mRNA levels of both TGFβ1 and TGFβ3 are increased in recurrent ovarian cancers (Bristow et al., 1999). Using enzyme-linked immunosorbant assay (ELISA), TGFβ1 levels are increased in plasma and peritoneal fluid of advanced stage ovarian cancer patients (Santin et al., 2001). Increased expression of TGFβ appears to be correlated with a poor patient survival outcome which is associated with peritoneal metastasis, expression of vascular endothelial growth factor (VEGF), and microvessel density (markers of angiogenesis) (Nakanishi et al., 1997).

Mutational analysis of TGFβ1 assessed by PCR-SSCP (polymerase chain reaction single-strand conformational polymorphism) uncovered defects in the coding region of exons 5, 6, and 7 (Cardillo et al., 1997). However, these alterations were not associated with histological type of the tumor or its transcript/protein expression levels (Cardillo et al., 1997).

3.2 TGFβ receptor expression in ovarian cancer

There appears to be some discrepancy in the reported levels of TGFβ receptors in ovarian cancer which may be due to the nature of the cell lines and tumor specimens assessed. In one study, the proximal components of the TGFβ signaling pathway (receptor expression and its phosphorylation status) appeared to be intact in primary ovarian cancer cell cultures; this indicated that downstream mechanisms could be responsible for growth resistance to TGFβ such as increased matrix metalloproteinase-2 (MMP2) expression (Yamada et al., 1999). Yet in another report, TGFβRII transcripts were undetectable in TGFβ resistant ovarian cancer cell lines (AZ224 and AZ547) whereas SKOV3 cells were positive for TGFβRII expression (Zeinoun et al., 1999). TGFβRII was also detectable in an additional 14 ovarian cancer cell lines (Hu et al., 2000) (Xi et al., 2004). A more recent study reported reduced TGFβRII levels which was determined via microarray analysis and validated via real-time PCR (qPCR) (Sunde et al., 2006).

Via northern blot analysis, expression of TGFβRI and TGFβRIII was markedly reduced in recurrent ovarian tumors (Bristow et al., 1999). In an independent study, TGFβRIII was notably decreased or absent in ovarian cancers at the RNA and protein levels (Hempel et al., 2007).

Mutational analysis of TGFβRI and TGFβRII uncovered mutations in a minority of ovarian cancers (Ding et al., 2005). Specifically, a frameshift mutation has been identified in Exon 5 of TGFβRI in 31% of ovarian tumors (Wang et al., 2000b), in exons 2, 3, 4, and 6 of TGFβRI (catalytic domain of the kinase) in 33% primary ovarian cancers (Chen et al., 2001), and deletions in exon 1 of TGFβRI in <30% of ovarian tumors (Antony et al., 2010). Likewise, missense mutations have been identified in TGFβRII (Francis-Thickpenny et al., 2001) and deletions in exon 3 of TGFβRII in ovarian tumors (Antony et al., 2010).

3.3 SMAD expression in ovarian cancer

Decreased expression of SMAD4 has been described in several ovarian cancer cell lines (Hu et al., 2000) which appears to correlate with dysregulated expression of p21 and c-myc (Antony et al., 2010).

Unlike pancreatic cancer in which ~50% of SMAD4 is mutated (Elliott & Blobe, 2005), reports of the presence of SMAD4 variants in ovarian cancers are lacking (Wang et al., 2000b). However, mutational analysis of additional SMAD family members showed that 35% and 23%, respectively, of ovarian tumor specimens contained a polymorphism in intron 2 of SMAD6 and a polymorphism at codon 208 in SMAD7. Neither of these mutations were associated with amino acid changes and thus, are unlikely to be important in ovarian cancer development (Wang et al., 2000a). Similarly, 42% of ovarian tumor specimens had a polymorphism for SMAD2 which was not associated with an amino acid change; thus it is also unlikely that this mutation is significant in the development of ovarian cancer (Wang et al., 1999).

3.4 TGFβ transcriptional co-regulator/co-factor expression in ovarian cancer

Ecotropic viral integration site-1 (EVI1), a TGFβ corepressor, was elevated up to 40-fold in ovarian carcinoma cells via RNAse protection assay (Brooks et al., 1996). Similarly, via microarray analysis and qPCR validation, EVI1 was found to be upregulated in advanced stage ovarian cancers (Sunde et al., 2006). In our analysis, we identified that EVI1 and MDS1/EVI1 are amplified in advanced stage serous epithelial ovarian cancers at the DNA, RNA, and protein levels via aCGH, transcriptional profiling/qPCR analysis, and western blot analysis (Nanjundan et al., 2007). Further, SnoN/SkiL, another TGFβ corepressor, is likewise increased at the DNA and RNA levels (cCGH and qPCR) in advanced stage serous epithelial ovarian cancers (Nanjundan et al., 2008). In addition, c-myc, an oncogenic transcriptional regulator, is upregulated in ovarian cancers (Garte, 1993).

3.5 Other TGFβ mediator expression in ovarian cancer

Other TGFβ mediators whose expression is altered in ovarian cancers include DACH1 and BMP7 which are both upregulated and inhibit TGFβ signaling (Sunde et al., 2006). Mediators in ovarian cancers that are downregulated include PCAF and TFE3 (which enhance TGFβ signaling) (Sunde et al., 2006). Other molecules that could attenuate TGFβ proliferative control include FOXG1 which is overexpressed in high-grade ovarian cancers and suppresses p21 WAF1/CIP1 transcription (Chan et al., 2009). BAMBI (BMP and activin membrane-bound inhibitor) is overexpressed in ovarian cancers promoting resistance to TGFβ mediated apoptosis by shuttling into the nuclear compartment with SMAD2/3 in a TGFβ dependent manner (Pils et al., 2011). EZH2 is increased in ovarian cancers and appears to be involved in altering metastatic potential by upregulating TGFβ1 (Rao et al., 2010). A SMAD4 target gene, RunX1T1, is a tumor suppressor in ovarian cancers and is repressed by histone modifications (Yeh et al., 2011).

4. SnoN/SkiL, a TGFβ transcriptional modulator, in ovarian cancer

SnoN/SkiL belongs to the Ski family (i.e. Ski, SnoN, Fussel-15, and Fussel-18), a group of proto-oncogenes involved in early developmental processes sharing structural and functional features characteristic of winged-helix/forkhead class of DNA binding proteins (Deheuninck & Luo, 2009). However, these proteins do not directly bind to DNA but associate to DNA via interaction via nuclear proteins (i.e. SMADs) (Deheuninck & Luo, 2009). Thus, the mechanism of repression of TGFβ signaling occurs by transcriptional modulation by recruitment of nuclear corepressors (i.e. N-CoR), histone deacetylase complex (HDAC), and interference of SMAD-mediated binding to the transcriptional coactivator, p300/CBP (Deheuninck & Luo, 2009). Ski and SnoN genes have an overall homology of 50% and both are tightly regulated at multiple levels via: (1) transcriptional regulation, (2) protein degradation, (3) post-translational modifications, and (4) subcellular localization (Deheuninck & Luo, 2009; Luo, 2004; Pan et al., 2009). SnoN is not only phosphorylated by TGFβ activating kinase (TAK1) but can also physically associate with TAK1 leading to SnoN degradation (Kajino et al., 2007). SnoN is degraded rapidly via proteasome-mediated degradation upon TGFβ stimulation via SMURF2, APC, and Arkadia (RNF111) E3 ubiquitin ligases (Inoue & Imamura, 2008; Izzi & Attisano, 2004; Levy et al., 2007). SnoN can also interact with promyelocytic leukemia protein (PML) which promotes its association with PML nuclear bodies to stabilize p53 leading to induction of premature senescence (Lamouille & Derynck, 2009; Pan et al., 2009). SnoN can be sumoylated via SUMO E3 ligase PIAS independently of TGFβ signaling and its ubiquitination status (Hsu et al., 2006; Wrighton et al., 2007). Although sumoylation does not alter its stability or subcellular localization, it may augment SnoN-mediated repression of TGFβ signaling on specific promoters such as the myogenin promoter (Hsu et al., 2006). Although SnoN is predominantly nuclear localized, it can be cytoplasmically localized in normal cells under non-pathological conditions (Krakowski et al., 2005).

Both Ski and SnoN are expressed in all adult tissues at low levels and are involved in differentiation of neural and muscle cells (Deheuninck & Luo, 2009; Luo, 2004; Pan et al., 2009). Expression of Ski and SnoN are altered in numerous disease states including cancer (Deheuninck & Luo, 2009; Luo, 2004; Pan et al., 2009). Our research indicates that SnoN levels are upregulated in serous epithelial ovarian cancers via different mechanisms including gene amplification, altered protein stability, and transcriptional activation (Nanjundan et al., 2008). Further, siRNA targeting SnoN leads to reduction in ovarian cancer cell proliferation implicating a pro-oncogenic function (Nanjundan et al., 2008; Smith et al., 2010). In addition, attenuated SnoN protein via siRNA is detrimental to breast and lung cancer cellular transformation in both *in vitro* and *in vivo* mouse xenograft models (Zhu et al., 2007). Strikingly, SnoN has also been implicated in a tumor suppressive function. Deletion of one copy of SnoN leads to increased susceptibility to carcinogen-induced tumor development (Deheuninck & Luo, 2009; Luo, 2004; Pan et al., 2009). Furthermore, long-term stable expression of SnoN in an ovarian cell line leads to induction of senescence (i.e. oncogene-induced senescence similar to that described for Ras) (Nanjundan et al., 2008). In another study, SnoN induces premature senescence in a PML and p53-dependent fashion; it also inhibits epithelial-mesenchymal transition (EMT) and tumor metastasis in breast and lung cancer cells (Pan et al., 2009; Zhu et al., 2007). Collectively, these findings suggest that SnoN elicits multiple roles in cancer development.

5. EVI1, a TGFβ transcriptional modulator, in ovarian cancer

EVI1, ecotropic viral integration site-1 protein, now called MECOM (MDS1 and EVI1 complex) is located at the 3q26.2 locus. It was initially identified as a site for viral integration in mouse cancer models; it has been well studied as an oncogene in acute myeloid leukemia (AML) and in myelodysplastic syndrome (MDS) (Levy et al., 1994; Morishita et al., 1992b). Functions of EVI1 include (1) proliferation of leukemic cells (Tanaka et al., 1995), (2) cellular transformation (Kilbey & Bartholomew, 1998), (3) inhibition of growth factor mediated differentiation and survival (Morishita et al., 1992a), (4) induction of neural and megakaryocyte differentiation, and (5) inhibition of interferon (Buonamici et al., 2005) and TGFβ signaling (Izutsu et al., 2001; Soderholm et al., 1997; Sood et al., 1999; Vinatzer et al., 2003; Vinatzer et al., 2001). Notably, EVI1 represses transcription via binding to SMADs and recruiting CtBP1/HDAC (Izutsu et al., 2001; Palmer et al., 2001; Senyuk et al., 2002) to target promoter elements, increasing AP-1 activity (Tanaka et al., 1994), disrupting JNK induced apoptosis (Maki et al., 2008), inhibiting PML function (Buonamici et al., 2005), binding to BRG1 (Chi et al., 2003), and activating PI3K by reducing TGFβ and drug induced apoptosis (Liu et al., 2006; Yoshimi et al., 2011). Supporting its role as an inducer of cellular proliferation, EVI1 knockout mice are embryonically lethal due to hypocellularity across multiple organ sites (Hoyt et al., 1997). There exist multiple splice variants of EVI1 whose functions are presently unclear (Alzuherri et al., 2006; Jazaeri et al., 2010; Vinatzer et al., 2003). In particular, the MDS1/EVI1 is a read-through splice form which contains a novel PR (PRD1-BF1-RIZ homology) domain; its functionality is unclear and is suggested to be context or cell type dependent (either eliciting functionality similar or antagonistic to EVI1 (Vinatzer et al., 2003). Structurally, EVI1 contains 2 zinc finger domains, an intervening region required for transformation, and a repressor domain necessary for binding to CtBP1/HDAC (Nanjundan et al., 2007).

In ovarian cancer, the first report of altered EVI1 expression in ovarian carcinoma cells demonstrated up to a 40-fold increase in its mRNA levels via RNAse protection assay compared to the normal ovary; these initial findings implicate a novel role for EVI1 in solid tumor carcinogenesis (Brooks et al., 1996). A decade later, increased EVI1 levels in advanced stage ovarian cancers supported these initial findings via oligonucleotide arrays profiling and validation via qPCR analysis (Sunde et al., 2006). The same researchers also found that the EVI1 gene locus was amplified in 43% of the tumors with a significant correlation between gene copy and EVI1 gene expression levels (Sunde et al., 2006). They also reported that EVI1 inhibited TGFβ signaling in normal immortalized ovarian epithelial cells (Sunde et al., 2006). Our research has also uncovered increased copy number at the EVI1 locus in advanced stage serous epithelial ovarian carcinomas via aCGH analysis (Nanjundan et al., 2007). We found that EVI1 DNA copy number increases were associated with at least a 5-fold increase in RNA transcript levels in the majority of advanced ovarian cancers (Nanjundan et al., 2007). More recent whole genome aCGH analysis of stage III ovarian serous carcinomas also identified a gain at 3q26.2 with their gene expression analysis demonstrating elevated EVI1 expression (Osterberg et al., 2009). Protein level determination via western blotting analysis showed a corresponding increase in MDS1/EVI1 and EVI1 expression in ovarian cancers and multiple ovarian cancer cell lines (Nanjundan et al., 2007). Interestingly, functional studies by transient transfection into normal immortalized epithelial cells demonstrated that EVI1 and MDS1/EVI1 increased cell proliferation, migration, and decreased TGFβ-mediated plasminogen activator inhibitor-1 (PAI-1) promoter activity (Nanjundan et al., 2007). In yet another recent study, highest expression of EVI1 and a splice variant, Del324 (EVI1s), was observed in ovarian cancer specimens with a constant ratio between the two splice variants across all specimens assessed (Jazaeri et al., 2010). However, their analysis did not identify an altered expression protein pattern between serous ovarian cancers and fallopian tube fimbria or benign neoplasms (Jazaeri et al., 2010). In support of our functional studies in OVCAR8 cells (Nanjundan et al., 2007), when EVI1 was expressed exogenously in this ovarian carcinoma cell line (which harbors a deletion at the EVI1 locus), there was no altered proliferation (Jazaeri et al., 2010). Furthermore, with knockdown of specific EVI1 forms (via siRNA and shRNA) in ovarian cancer cells, there was no alteration in functionality (Jazaeri et al., 2010). Although their data do not support a role for EVI1 in ovarian cancer cell proliferation (Jazaeri et al., 2010), further investigations are warranted to determine the functional relevance of disrupted TGFβ signaling via EVI1 in ovarian cancer.

5.1 Epigenetic aberrations, EVI1, and ovarian cancer

Epigenetic modifications refers to changes in gene expression as a result of DNA methylation, histone modification, nucleosome repositioning, and post-transcriptional gene regulation by micro-RNAs (Balch et al., 2009). DNA methyltransferases are involved in adding methyl groups to the cytosine-5 position within CpG dinucleotides (Balch et al., 2009). CpG dense regions, however, are normally unmethylated in normal specimens (Balch et al., 2009). Histone modifications are extensive and can regulate transcription in an open or closed conformation on the chromatin structure (Balch et al., 2009). These regions can be extensively altered in disease states such as cancer with a general DNA hypomethylation status and localized hypermethylation of promoter associated CpG islands in cases of tumor suppressor genes (Balch et al., 2009). Further, dysregulation of miRNA expression has been also linked to cancer development (Balch et al., 2009). A number of epigenetic aberrations are well noted in ovarian cancer (Balch et al., 2009).

Based on homology to proteins with PR domains, MDS1/EVI1 (which contains such a domain) has the potential to elicit protein methyltransferase activity (Vinatzer et al., 2003; Vinatzer et al., 2001). However, we did not detect any such activity associated with MDS1/EVI1 via *in vitro* methyltransferase activity assays using free histones as substrate (Nanjundan et al., 2007). There was some weak associated activity which we suggested to be due to co-immunoprecipitating molecules, possibly SWI/SNF components or proteins associated with methyltransferase activity (Nanjundan et al., 2007). Indeed, EVI1 has recently been shown to physically interact with molecules which have such activities (Cattaneo & Nucifora, 2008; Lugthart et al., 2011; Pradhan et al., 2011; Senyuk et al., 2011; Spensberger & Delwel, 2008).

Indeed, links between DNA hypermethylation and EVI1 are observed in AML (Lugthart et al., 2011); further, EVI1 physically interacts with DNA methyltransferase 3A/3B (DNMT3A/3B) (Senyuk et al., 2011). Thus, EVI1 is likely involved in promoter DNA methylation in leukemia and possibly in other solid tumors such as ovarian cancers. EVI1 regulates the expression of microRNA-124 which is involved in regulation of differentiation and cycling of hematopoietic cells (De Weer et al., 2011; Dickstein et al., 2010). This was demonstrated to occur via methylation of CpG dinucleotides upstream of the miRNA leading to its repression and hence, increased expression of genes involved in cell division such as Bmi1 and cyclin D3 (De Weer et al., 2011; Dickstein et al., 2010). Through its interaction with DNMT3, the EVI1 complex binds to regulatory regions of the miRNA to regulate its expression (De Weer et al., 2011; Dickstein et al., 2010). Of further interest is the recent identification of the physical interaction between EVI1 and SIRT1, a histone deacetylase which is itself a direct target of EVI1. Interaction between SIRT1 and EVI1 leads to EVI1 degradation (Pradhan et al., 2011). SIRT1 is increased in AML patient samples where EVI1 is elevated (Pradhan et al., 2011). In addition, EVI1 interacts directly with SUV39H1 and G9a, both histone methyltransferases, which elicit methyltransferase activities and enhance the repressive activity of EVI1 (Cattaneo & Nucifora, 2008; Spensberger & Delwel, 2008). Thus, the oncogenic activity of EVI1 may be involved in deacetylation and methylation events which would lead to altered chromatin structure and, thus, transcriptional events.

6. Novel perspective into the functionality of TGFβ: Autophagy

More recently, TGFβ has been implicated in regulating autophagy (Gajewska et al., 2005; Kiyono et al., 2009), a self eating process whereby damaged cellular organelles and other cellular material are sequestered within autophagosomes. These double-membrane structures eventually fuse with single-membrane lysosomes leading to degradation of the inner contents (Huang & Klionsky, 2007; Yang & Klionsky, 2009) (Figure 3). Autophagy is activated in response to multiple stresses during cancer progression including nutrient starvation, the unfolded protein response (UPR), hypoxia, and cellular treatment with cytotoxic chemotherapeutic agents (Huang & Klionsky, 2007; Yang & Klionsky, 2009). It has been suggested that autophagy promotes tumorigenic development; thus, it would be an ideal target for tumor ablation. Indeed, increased levels of autophagy are observed in tumor cells following treatment of cells with chemotherapeutic agents (Kondo et al., 2005; Kondo & Kondo, 2006).

The isolation membrane of the autophagosome arises due to complex formation between beclin-1 and hVps34 (Geng & Klionsky, 2008; Klionsky, 2005; Wang & Klionsky, 2003; Yorimitsu & Klionsky, 2005). The membrane elongates via activation of ubiquitin-like conjugation system. ATG12 is activated by ATG7 which is then transferred to ATG10 and finally covalently attached to ATG5 (Geng & Klionsky, 2008). The ATG12-ATG5 conjugate localizes to autophagosome precursors and dissociates prior to or following completion of formation of the autophagic vacuole. Another ubiquitin-like modification system involving LC3 (microtubule associated protein 1 light chain 3) completes autophagosome formation (Geng & Klionsky, 2008). The cytosolic precursor of LC3 (LC3-I) becomes cleaved at its C-terminus by ATG4 and is conjugated to phosphatidylethanolamine (PE) to generate the membrane bound LC3-II form; this process requires ATG7 and ATG3 activities (Geng & Klionsky, 2008; Klionsky, 2005; Wang & Klionsky, 2003; Yorimitsu & Klionsky, 2005). LC3-II is specifically targeted to ATG12-ATG5 associated autophagosomal precursor membranes. Following fusion of autophagosomes with lysosomes, LC3-II becomes delipidated and returns to the cytosolic pool to be recycled (Geng & Klionsky, 2008; Klionsky, 2005; Wang & Klionsky, 2003; Yorimitsu & Klionsky, 2005).

The initial finding that TGFβ induces autophagy was observed in bovine mammary epithelial BME-UV1 cells; both LC3 and beclin-1 expression were induced following TGFβ1 treatment leading to cell death (Gajewska et al., 2005). Following reports support this finding in a number of cell lines including hepatocellular and breast carcinoma cell lines

(Kiyono et al., 2009). TGFβ was noted to induce autophagosome formation with a corresponding conversion of LC3-I to LC3-II and increased expression of autophagic markers including beclin-1, ATG5, ATG7, and DAPK (Kiyono et al., 2009). In addition, knockdown of SMADs and other targets in the non-canonical SMAD pathways decreased TGFβ mediated autophagy (Kiyono et al., 2009). Autophagy induction led to induction of BIM and BMF (proapoptotic markers) which occurred prior to initiation of apoptosis (Kiyono et al., 2009).

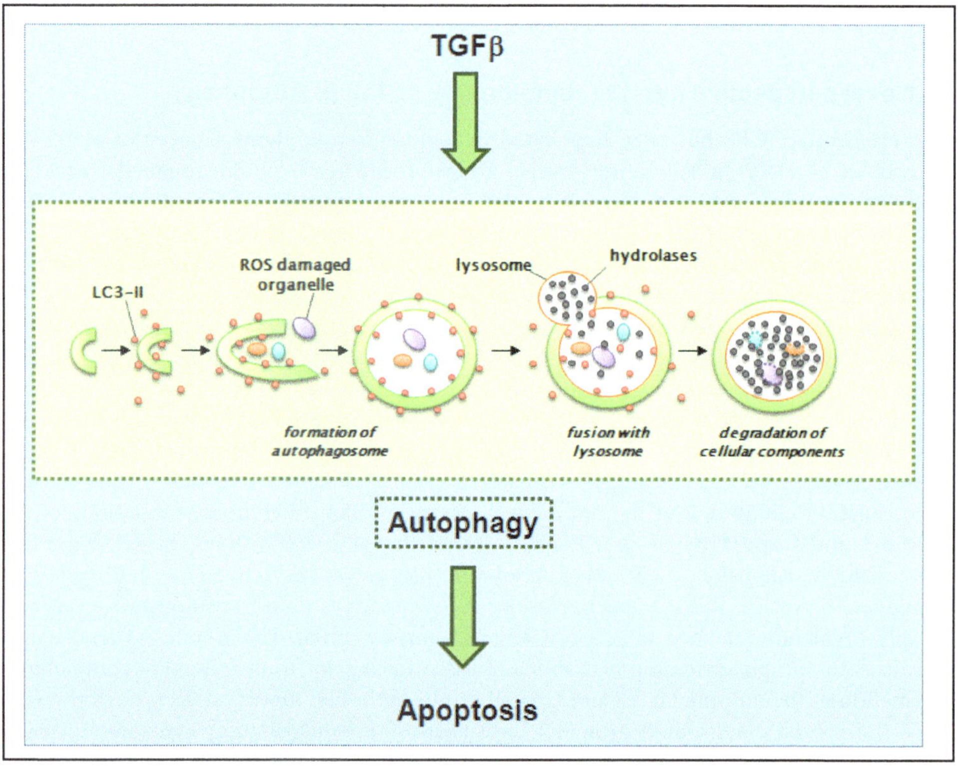

Fig. 3. Activation of the TGFβ signaling pathway induces autophagy. TGFβ can induce autophagosome formation in cancer cell lines via enhanced expression of autophagic markers (i.e. beclin-1, ATG5, and ATG7) and enhanced conversion of LC3-I to LC3-II. Induction of TGFβ -mediated autophagy occurs prior to apoptosis.

Supporting reports of TGFβ-induced autophagy arise from studies of renal epithelial cells which is involved in induction of peritubular fibrosis and degeneration of nephrons (Koesters et al., 2010). Opposing the concept that TGFβ leads to autophagic mediated cell death, TGFβ was reported to protect mesangial cells from apoptosis as a protective mechanism for survival during serum starvation via a TAK1 and AKT dependent pathway (Ding et al., 2010).

Our recent work has shown that upon exposure to reactive oxygen generating conditions (i.e. arsenic trioxide (As_2O_3) which is used to treat patients with acute promyelocytic leukemia (APL)), SnoN protein levels increase which coincides with induction of autophagy in a beclin-1 independent manner (Smith et al., 2010). Other TGFβ signaling mediators were examined and As_2O_3 was found to reduce the protein expression of EVI1, TAK1, SMAD2/3, and TGFβRII while increasing SnoN (Smith et al., 2010). Knockdown of SnoN via siRNA markedly reduced autophagy with a corresponding increase in apoptosis (Smith et al., 2010). Thus, disruption of induction of autophagy may be a novel therapeutic strategy to re-establish or increase sensitivity to therapeutic agents.

7. Targeting the TGFβ signaling pathway for therapy

Strategies need to be carefully designed for successful treatment of ovarian cancer patients via inhibition of TGFβ signaling pathway due to the apparent bifunctionality of TGFβ signaling. In particular, TGFβ levels, TGFβ receptor expression, and tumor stage/progression need to be assessed. There are in essence three major groups of TGFβ signaling therapeutics: (1) ligand traps including monoclonal TGFβ neutralizing antibodies and soluble TGFβRI/RII; (2) antisense molecule mediated silencing strategies for targeting TGFβ ligands; and (3) small molecule inhibitors targeting TGFβRI/RII and downstream mediators (Chou et al., 2010; Iyer et al., 2005; Korpal & Kang, 2010; Nagaraj & Datta, 2010).

Neutralizing antibodies are designed to disrupt the interactions between TGFβ ligands and their cell-surface receptors (Chou et al., 2010). Some of these include 2G7 and 1D11 monoclonal antibodies which hinder the activity of all three TGFβ ligands to reduce tumor growth and metastasis (Chou et al., 2010). GC1008 is yet another neutralizing antibody which entered a Phase I/II clinical trial for advanced malignant melanoma and renal cell carcinoma patients (Chou et al., 2010). Soluble ligand traps include soluble TGFβRII/III which hinder TGFβ interaction with its cognate cell surface receptors leading to inhibition of tumor growth and metastasis in athymic murine models (Chou et al., 2010). Antisense oligonucleotides are yet another route to block TGFβ signaling, specifically against TGFβ1 gene expression which reduced tumor survival and metastasis in mouse models (Chou et al., 2010). In particular, AP12008, an antisense molecule which targets TGFβ2, effectively targets pancreatic and melanoma cell lines; it entered a Phase IIb clinical trial for patients with high grade gliomas with successful outcomes (Chou et al., 2010). However, the effectiveness of these large molecule inhibitors has limitations including adequately targeting a solid tumor due to physical barriers (Chou et al., 2010). Thus, small molecule inhibitors may be more effective and have been developed to initially target TGFβRI kinase activity with specificity (i.e. SB0431542, SD-208, LY580276, etc.). These act as competitive inhibitors of the ATP binding site of TGFβRI kinase (Chou et al., 2010). In addition, there now exists a dual inhibitor of TGFβRI and TGFβRII (LY2109761) which hinders metastatic process effectively (Chou et al., 2010). Other strategies that are being developed include small molecule inhibitors to directly inhibit SMAD-specific pathways as opposed to the non-canonical pathways (Chou et al., 2010).

In addition to the above targeting strategies, epigenetic therapy may also be another valuable therapeutic strategy for ovarian cancers with respect to targeting TGFβ transcriptional co-regulators such as EVI1. This strategy could potentially alter the epigenetic status leading to restoration of the expression of tumor suppressor genes with a

corresponding reduction in the expression of genes involved in mestastasis. For example, ADAM19, FBXO32, and RunX1T1 (tumor suppressors) are reduced in ovarian cancers but are normally increased in response to TGFβ; these genes are epigenetically silenced by promoter hypermethylation or histone modification (Balch et al., 2009).
With respect to SnoN/SkiL (Figure 4), based on our results with As_2O_3 in ovarian carcinoma cells, targeting of this TGFβ transcriptional co-regulator in ovarian cancers may lead to increased sensitivity to various chemotherapeutic agents.

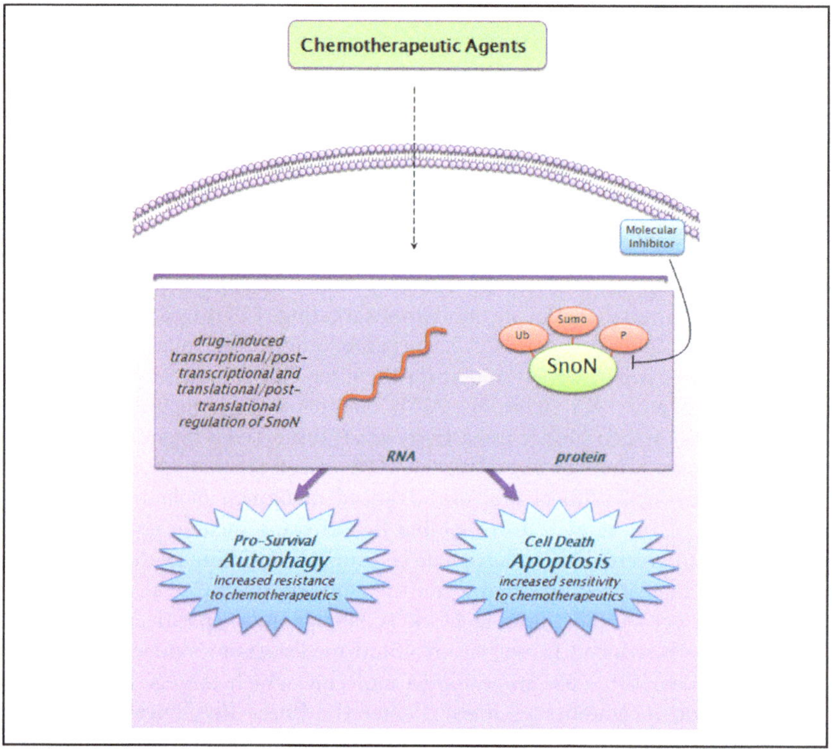

Fig. 4. Targeting of SnoN/SkiL to increase the sensitivity of ovarian cancer cells to chemotherapeutics. SnoN/SkiL levels increase following As_2O_3 treatment leading to induction of autophagy and increased resistance to the agent. Targeting of SnoN/SkiL with specific inhibitors may be a strategy to improve the sensitivity of the chemotherapeutic agents in ovarian cancer patients.

8. Conclusion

Although significant progress has been made in improving our understanding of the TGFβ signalling pathway, there remain numerous areas for further investigation to improve our understanding of the regulation of the TGFβ pathway. Thus, future research could possibly lead to development of novel and improved strategies for treatment of ovarian cancer patients.

9. Acknowledgements

We acknowledge RO1 CA123219 which supported our ovarian cancer studies we have reported in this review.

10. References

Alzuherri H., McGilvray R., Kilbey A. and Bartholomew C., 2006. Conservation and expression of a novel alternatively spliced Evi1 exon. Gene, 384, 154-162.

Antony M.L., Nair R., Sebastian P. and Karunagaran D., 2010. Changes in expression, and/or mutations in TGF-beta receptors (TGF-beta RI and TGF-beta RII) and Smad 4 in human ovarian tumors. J Cancer Res Clin Oncol, 136, 351-361.

Balch C., Fang F., Matei D.E., Huang T.H. and Nephew K.P., 2009. Minireview: epigenetic changes in ovarian cancer. Endocrinology, 150, 4003-4011.

Bartlett J.M., Langdon S.P., Scott W.N., Love S.B., Miller E.P., Katsaros D., Smyth J.F. and Miller W.R., 1997. Transforming growth factor-beta isoform expression in human ovarian tumours. Eur J Cancer, 33, 2397-2403.

Bast R.C., Jr., Hennessy B. and Mills G.B., 2009. The biology of ovarian cancer: new opportunities for translation. Nat Rev Cancer, 9, 415-428.

Bristow R.E., Baldwin R.L., Yamada S.D., Korc M. and Karlan B.Y., 1999. Altered expression of transforming growth factor-beta ligands and receptors in primary and recurrent ovarian carcinoma. Cancer, 85, 658-668.

Brooks D.J., Woodward S., Thompson F.H., Dos Santos B., Russell M., Yang J.M., Guan X.Y., Trent J., Alberts D.S. and Taetle R., 1996. Expression of the zinc finger gene EVI-1 in ovarian and other cancers. Br J Cancer, 74, 1518-1525.

Buonamici S., Li D., Mikhail F.M., Sassano A., Platanias L.C., Colamonici O., Anastasi J. and Nucifora G., 2005. EVI1 abrogates interferon-alpha response by selectively blocking PML induction. J Biol Chem, 280, 428-436.

Cardillo M.R., Yap E. and Castagna G., 1997. Molecular genetic analysis of TGF-beta1 in ovarian neoplasia. J Exp Clin Cancer Res, 16, 49-56.

Cattaneo F. and Nucifora G., 2008. EVI1 recruits the histone methyltransferase SUV39H1 for transcription repression. J Cell Biochem, 105, 344-352.

Chan D.W., Liu V.W., To R.M., Chiu P.M., Lee W.Y., Yao K.M., Cheung A.N. and Ngan H.Y., 2009. Overexpression of FOXG1 contributes to TGF-beta resistance through inhibition of p21WAF1/CIP1 expression in ovarian cancer. Br J Cancer, 101, 1433-1443.

Chen T., Triplett J., Dehner B., Hurst B., Colligan B., Pemberton J., Graff J.R. and Carter J.H., 2001. Transforming growth factor-beta receptor type I gene is frequently mutated in ovarian carcinomas. Cancer Res, 61, 4679-4682.

Chi Y., Senyuk V., Chakraborty S. and Nucifora G., 2003. EVI1 promotes cell proliferation by interacting with BRG1 and blocking the repression of BRG1 on E2F1 activity. J Biol Chem, 278, 49806-49811.

Chou J.L., Chen L.Y., Lai H.C. and Chan M.W., 2010. TGF-beta: friend or foe? The role of TGF-beta/SMAD signaling in epigenetic silencing of ovarian cancer and its implication in epigenetic therapy. Expert Opin Ther Targets, 14, 1213-1223.

De Weer A., Van der Meulen J., Rondou P., Taghon T., Konrad T.A., De Preter K., Mestdagh P., Van Maerken T., Van Roy N., Jeison M., et al., 2011. EVI1-mediated down regulation of MIR449A is essential for the survival of EVI1 positive leukaemic cells. Br J Haematol.

Deheuninck J. and Luo K., 2009. Ski and SnoN, potent negative regulators of TGF-beta signaling. Cell Res, 19, 47-57.

Dickstein J., Senyuk V., Premanand K., Laricchia-Robbio L., Xu P., Cattaneo F., Fazzina R. and Nucifora G., 2010. Methylation and silencing of miRNA-124 by EVI1 and self-renewal exhaustion of hematopoietic stem cells in murine myelodysplastic syndrome. Proc Natl Acad Sci U S A, 107, 9783-9788.

Ding W., Tang Q., Espina V., Liotta L.A., Mauger D.T. and Mulder K.M., 2005. A transforming growth factor-beta receptor-interacting protein frequently mutated in human ovarian cancer. Cancer Res, 65, 6526-6533.

Ding Y., Kim J.K., Kim S.I., Na H.J., Jun S.Y., Lee S.J. and Choi M.E., 2010. TGF-{beta}1 protects against mesangial cell apoptosis via induction of autophagy. J Biol Chem, 285, 37909-37919.

Elliott R.L. and Blobe G.C., 2005. Role of transforming growth factor Beta in human cancer. J Clin Oncol, 23, 2078-2093.

Francis-Thickpenny K.M., Richardson D.M., van Ee C.C., Love D.R., Winship I.M., Baguley B.C., Chenevix-Trench G. and Shelling A.N., 2001. Analysis of the TGF beta functional pathway in epithelial ovarian carcinoma. Br J Cancer, 85, 687-691.

Gajewska M., Gajkowska B. and Motyl T., 2005. Apoptosis and autophagy induced by TGF-B1 in bovine mammary epithelial BME-UV1 cells. J Physiol Pharmacol, 56 Suppl 3, 143-157.

Garte S.J., 1993. The c-myc oncogene in tumor progression. Crit Rev Oncog, 4, 435-449.

Geng J. and Klionsky D.J., 2008. The Atg8 and Atg12 ubiquitin-like conjugation systems in macroautophagy. 'Protein modifications: beyond the usual suspects' review series. EMBO Rep, 9, 859-864.

Gorringe K.L. and Campbell I.G., 2009. Large-scale genomic analysis of ovarian carcinomas. Mol Oncol, 3, 157-164.

Gray J.W., Suzuki S., Kuo W.L., Polikoff D., Deavers M., Smith-McCune K., Berchuck A., Pinkel D., Albertson D. and Mills G.B., 2003. Specific keynote: genome copy number abnormalities in ovarian cancer. Gynecol Oncol, 88, S16-21; discussion S22-14.

Hempel N., How T., Dong M., Murphy S.K., Fields T.A. and Blobe G.C., 2007. Loss of betaglycan expression in ovarian cancer: role in motility and invasion. Cancer Res, 67, 5231-5238.

Hennessy B.T., Murph M., Nanjundan M., Carey M., Auersperg N., Almeida J., Coombes K.R., Liu J., Lu Y., Gray J.W., et al., 2008. Ovarian cancer: linking genomics to new target discovery and molecular markers--the way ahead. Adv Exp Med Biol, 617, 23-40.

Henriksen R., Gobl A., Wilander E., Oberg K., Miyazono K. and Funa K., 1995. Expression and prognostic significance of TGF-beta isotypes, latent TGF-beta 1 binding protein, TGF-beta type I and type II receptors, and endoglin in normal ovary and ovarian neoplasms. Lab Invest, 73, 213-220.

Hoyt P.R., Bartholomew C., Davis A.J., Yutzey K., Gamer L.W., Potter S.S., Ihle J.N. and Mucenski M.L., 1997. The Evi1 proto-oncogene is required at midgestation for neural, heart, and paraxial mesenchyme development. Mech Dev, 65, 55-70.

Hsu Y.H., Sarker K.P., Pot I., Chan A., Netherton S.J. and Bonni S., 2006. Sumoylated SnoN represses transcription in a promoter-specific manner. J Biol Chem, 281, 33008-33018.

Hu W., Wu W., Nash M.A., Freedman R.S., Kavanagh J.J. and Verschraegen C.F., 2000. Anomalies of the TGF-beta postreceptor signaling pathway in ovarian cancer cell lines. Anticancer Res, 20, 729-733.

Huang J. and Klionsky D.J., 2007. Autophagy and human disease. Cell Cycle, 6, 1837-1849.

Inoue Y. and Imamura T., 2008. Regulation of TGF-beta family signaling by E3 ubiquitin ligases. Cancer Sci, 99, 2107-2112.

Iyer S., Wang Z.G., Akhtari M., Zhao W. and Seth P., 2005. Targeting TGFbeta signaling for cancer therapy. Cancer Biol Ther, 4, 261-266.

Izutsu K., Kurokawa M., Imai Y., Maki K., Mitani K. and Hirai H., 2001. The corepressor CtBP interacts with Evi-1 to repress transforming growth factor beta signaling. Blood, 97, 2815-2822.

Izzi L. and Attisano L., 2004. Regulation of the TGFbeta signalling pathway by ubiquitin-mediated degradation. Oncogene, 23, 2071-2078.

Jazaeri A.A., Ferriss J.S., Bryant J.L., Dalton M.S. and Dutta A., 2010. Evaluation of EVI1 and EVI1s (Delta324) as potential therapeutic targets in ovarian cancer. Gynecol Oncol, 118, 189-195.

Kajino T., Omori E., Ishii S., Matsumoto K. and Ninomiya-Tsuji J., 2007. TAK1 MAPK kinase kinase mediates transforming growth factor-beta signaling by targeting SnoN oncoprotein for degradation. J Biol Chem, 282, 9475-9481.

Kilbey A. and Bartholomew C., 1998. Evi-1 ZF1 DNA binding activity and a second distinct transcriptional repressor region are both required for optimal transformation of Rat1 fibroblasts. Oncogene, 16, 2287-2291.

Kiyono K., Suzuki H.I., Matsuyama H., Morishita Y., Komuro A., Kano M.R., Sugimoto K. and Miyazono K., 2009. Autophagy is activated by TGF-beta and potentiates TGF-beta-mediated growth inhibition in human hepatocellular carcinoma cells. Cancer Res, 69, 8844-8852.

Klionsky D.J., 2005. Autophagy. Curr Biol, 15, R282-283.

Koesters R., Kaissling B., Lehir M., Picard N., Theilig F., Gebhardt R., Glick A.B., Hahnel B., Hosser H., Grone H.J., et al., 2010. Tubular overexpression of transforming growth factor-beta1 induces autophagy and fibrosis but not mesenchymal transition of renal epithelial cells. Am J Pathol, 177, 632-643.

Kondo Y., Kanzawa T., Sawaya R. and Kondo S., 2005. The role of autophagy in cancer development and response to therapy. Nat Rev Cancer, 5, 726-734.

Kondo Y. and Kondo S., 2006. Autophagy and cancer therapy. Autophagy, 2, 85-90.

Korpal M. and Kang Y., 2010. Targeting the transforming growth factor-beta signalling pathway in metastatic cancer. Eur J Cancer, 46, 1232-1240.

Krakowski A.R., Laboureau J., Mauviel A., Bissell M.J. and Luo K., 2005. Cytoplasmic SnoN in normal tissues and nonmalignant cells antagonizes TGF-beta signaling by sequestration of the Smad proteins. Proc Natl Acad Sci U S A, 102, 12437-12442.

Lamouille S. and Derynck R., 2009. Oncogene and tumour suppressor: the two faces of SnoN. Embo J, 28, 3459-3460.

Levy E.R., Parganas E., Morishita K., Fichelson S., James L., Oscier D., Gisselbrecht S., Ihle J.N. and Buckle V.J., 1994. DNA rearrangements proximal to the EVI1 locus associated with the 3q21q26 syndrome. Blood, 83, 1348-1354.

Levy L., Howell M., Das D., Harkin S., Episkopou V. and Hill C.S., 2007. Arkadia activates Smad3/Smad4-dependent transcription by triggering signal-induced SnoN degradation. Mol Cell Biol, 27, 6068-6083.

Liu Y., Chen L., Ko T.C., Fields A.P. and Thompson E.A., 2006. Evi1 is a survival factor which conveys resistance to both TGFbeta- and taxol-mediated cell death via PI3K/AKT. Oncogene, 25, 3565-3575.

Lugthart S., Figueroa M.E., Bindels E., Skrabanek L., Valk P.J., Li Y., Meyer S., Erpelinck-Verschueren C., Greally J., Lowenberg B., et al., 2011. Aberrant DNA hypermethylation signature in acute myeloid leukemia directed by EVI1. Blood, 117, 234-241.

Luo K., 2004. Ski and SnoN: negative regulators of TGF-beta signaling. Curr Opin Genet Dev, 14, 65-70.

Maki K., Yamagata T. and Mitani K., 2008. Role of the RUNX1-EVI1 fusion gene in leukemogenesis. Cancer Sci, 99, 1878-1883.

Meulmeester E. and Ten Dijke P., 2011. The dynamic roles of TGF-beta in cancer. J Pathol, 223, 205-218.

Morishita K., Parganas E., Matsugi T. and Ihle J.N., 1992a. Expression of the Evi-1 zinc finger gene in 32Dc13 myeloid cells blocks granulocytic differentiation in response to granulocyte colony-stimulating factor. Mol Cell Biol, 12, 183-189.

Morishita K., Parganas E., William C.L., Whittaker M.H., Drabkin H., Oval J., Taetle R., Valentine M.B. and Ihle J.N., 1992b. Activation of EVI1 gene expression in human acute myelogenous leukemias by translocations spanning 300-400 kilobases on chromosome band 3q26. Proc Natl Acad Sci U S A, 89, 3937-3941.

Nagaraj N.S. and Datta P.K., 2010. Targeting the transforming growth factor-beta signaling pathway in human cancer. Expert Opin Investig Drugs, 19, 77-91.

Nakanishi Y., Kodama J., Yoshinouchi M., Tokumo K., Kamimura S., Okuda H. and Kudo T., 1997. The expression of vascular endothelial growth factor and transforming growth factor-beta associates with angiogenesis in epithelial ovarian cancer. Int J Gynecol Pathol, 16, 256-262.

Nanjundan M., Cheng K.W., Zhang F., Lahad J., Kuo W.L., Schmandt R., Smith-McCune K., Fishman D., Gray J.W. and Mills G.B., 2008. Overexpression of SnoN/SkiL, amplified at the 3q26.2 locus, in ovarian cancers: a role in ovarian pathogenesis. Mol Oncol, 2, 164-181.

Nanjundan M., Nakayama Y., Cheng K.W., Lahad J., Liu J., Lu K., Kuo W.L., Smith-McCune K., Fishman D., Gray J.W., et al., 2007. Amplification of MDS1/EVI1 and EVI1, located in the 3q26.2 amplicon, is associated with favorable patient prognosis in ovarian cancer. Cancer Res, 67, 3074-3084.

Osterberg L., Levan K., Partheen K., Delle U., Olsson B., Sundfeldt K. and Horvath G., 2009. Potential predictive markers of chemotherapy resistance in stage III ovarian serous carcinomas. BMC Cancer, 9, 368.

Palmer S., Brouillet J.P., Kilbey A., Fulton R., Walker M., Crossley M. and Bartholomew C., 2001. Evi-1 transforming and repressor activities are mediated by CtBP co-repressor proteins. J Biol Chem, 276, 25834-25840.

Pan D., Zhu Q. and Luo K., 2009. SnoN functions as a tumour suppressor by inducing premature senescence. Embo J, 28, 3500-3513.

Pils D., Wittinger M., Petz M., Gugerell A., Gregor W., Alfanz A., Horvat R., Braicu E.I., Sehouli J., Zeillinger R., et al., 2011. BAMBI is overexpressed in ovarian cancer and co-translocates with Smads into the nucleus upon TGF-beta treatment. Gynecol Oncol, 117, 189-197.

Pradhan A.K., Kuila N., Singh S. and Chakraborty S., 2011. EVI1 up-regulates the stress responsive gene SIRT1 which triggers deacetylation and degradation of EVI1. Biochim Biophys Acta, 1809, 269-275.

Rao Z.Y., Cai M.Y., Yang G.F., He L.R., Mai S.J., Hua W.F., Liao Y.J., Deng H.X., Chen Y.C., Guan X.Y., et al., 2010. EZH2 supports ovarian carcinoma cell invasion and/or metastasis via regulation of TGF-beta1 and is a predictor of outcome in ovarian carcinoma patients. Carcinogenesis, 31, 1576-1583.

Santin A.D., Bellone S., Ravaggi A., Roman J., Smith C.V., Pecorelli S., Cannon M.J. and Parham G.P., 2001. Increased levels of interleukin-10 and transforming growth factor-beta in the plasma and ascitic fluid of patients with advanced ovarian cancer. Bjog, 108, 804-808.

Senyuk V., Chakraborty S., Mikhail F.M., Zhao R., Chi Y. and Nucifora G., 2002. The leukemia-associated transcription repressor AML1/MDS1/EVI1 requires CtBP to induce abnormal growth and differentiation of murine hematopoietic cells. Oncogene, 21, 3232-3240.

Senyuk V., Premanand K., Xu P., Qian Z. and Nucifora G., 2011. The Oncoprotein EVI1 and the DNA Methyltransferase Dnmt3 Co-Operate in Binding and De Novo Methylation of Target DNA. PLoS One, 6, e20793.

Smith D.M., Patel S., Raffoul F., Haller E., Mills G.B. and Nanjundan M., 2010. Arsenic trioxide induces a beclin-1-independent autophagic pathway via modulation of SnoN/SkiL expression in ovarian carcinoma cells. Cell Death Differ, 17, 1867-1881.

Soderholm J., Kobayashi H., Mathieu C., Rowley J.D. and Nucifora G., 1997. The leukemia-associated gene MDS1/EVI1 is a new type of GATA-binding transactivator. Leukemia, 11, 352-358.

Sood R., Talwar-Trikha A., Chakrabarti S.R. and Nucifora G., 1999. MDS1/EVI1 enhances TGF-beta1 signaling and strengthens its growth-inhibitory effect but the leukemia-associated fusion protein AML1/MDS1/EVI1, product of the t(3;21), abrogates growth-inhibition in response to TGF-beta1. Leukemia, 13, 348-357.

Spensberger D. and Delwel R., 2008. A novel interaction between the proto-oncogene Evi1 and histone methyltransferases, SUV39H1 and G9a. FEBS Lett, 582, 2761-2767.

Sunde J.S., Donninger H., Wu K., Johnson M.E., Pestell R.G., Rose G.S., Mok S.C., Brady J., Bonome T. and Birrer M.J., 2006. Expression profiling identifies altered expression of genes that contribute to the inhibition of transforming growth factor-beta signaling in ovarian cancer. Cancer Res, 66, 8404-8412.

Tanaka T., Mitani K., Kurokawa M., Ogawa S., Tanaka K., Nishida J., Yazaki Y., Shibata Y. and Hirai H., 1995. Dual functions of the AML1/Evi-1 chimeric protein in the mechanism of leukemogenesis in t(3;21) leukemias. Mol Cell Biol, 15, 2383-2392.

Tanaka T., Nishida J., Mitani K., Ogawa S., Yazaki Y. and Hirai H., 1994. Evi-1 raises AP-1 activity and stimulates c-fos promoter transactivation with dependence on the second zinc finger domain. J Biol Chem, 269, 24020-24026.

Vinatzer U., Mannhalter C., Mitterbauer M., Gruener H., Greinix H., Schmidt H.H., Fonatsch C. and Wieser R., 2003. Quantitative comparison of the expression of EVI1 and its presumptive antagonist, MDS1/EVI1, in patients with myeloid leukemia. Genes Chromosomes Cancer, 36, 80-89.

Vinatzer U., Taplick J., Seiser C., Fonatsch C. and Wieser R., 2001. The leukaemia-associated transcription factors EVI-1 and MDS1/EVI1 repress transcription and interact with histone deacetylase. Br J Haematol, 114, 566-573.

Wang C.W. and Klionsky D.J., 2003. The molecular mechanism of autophagy. Mol Med, 9, 65-76.

Wang D., Kanuma T., Mizumuma H., Ibuki Y. and Takenoshita S., 2000a. Mutation analysis of the Smad6 and Smad7 gene in human ovarian cancers. Int J Oncol, 17, 1087-1091.

Wang D., Kanuma T., Mizunuma H., Takama F., Ibuki Y., Wake N., Mogi A., Shitara Y. and Takenoshita S., 2000b. Analysis of specific gene mutations in the transforming growth factor-beta signal transduction pathway in human ovarian cancer. Cancer Res, 60, 4507-4512.

Wang D., Kanuma T., Takama F., Mizumuma H., Ibuki Y., Wake N., Mogi A., Shitara Y., Hagiwara K. and Takenoshita S., 1999. Mutation analysis of the Smad3 gene in human ovarian cancers. Int J Oncol, 15, 949-953.

Wrighton K.H., Liang M., Bryan B., Luo K., Liu M., Feng X.H. and Lin X., 2007. Transforming growth factor-beta-independent regulation of myogenesis by SnoN sumoylation. J Biol Chem, 282, 6517-6524.

Xi L., Hu W., Meng L., Zhou J., Lu Y., Wang C. and Ma D., 2004. Dysregulation of the TGF-beta postreceptor signaling pathway in cell lines derived from primary or metastatic ovarian cancer. J Huazhong Univ Sci Technolog Med Sci, 24, 62-65.

Yamada S.D., Baldwin R.L. and Karlan B.Y., 1999. Ovarian carcinoma cell cultures are resistant to TGF-beta1-mediated growth inhibition despite expression of functional receptors. Gynecol Oncol, 75, 72-77.

Yang Z. and Klionsky D.J., 2009. An overview of the molecular mechanism of autophagy. Curr Top Microbiol Immunol, 335, 1-32.

Yeh K.T., Chen T.H., Yang H.W., Chou J.L., Chen L.Y., Yeh C.M., Chen Y.H., Lin R.I., Su H.Y., Chen G.C., et al., 2011. Aberrant TGFbeta/SMAD4 signaling contributes to epigenetic silencing of a putative tumor suppressor, RunX1T1 in ovarian cancer. Epigenetics, 6, 727-739.

Yorimitsu T. and Klionsky D.J., 2005. Autophagy: molecular machinery for self-eating. Cell Death Differ, 12 Suppl 2, 1542-1552.

Yoshimi A., Goyama S., Watanabe-Okochi N., Yoshiki Y., Nannya Y., Nitta E., Arai S., Sato T., Shimabe M., Nakagawa M., et al., 2011. Evi1 represses PTEN expression and activates PI3K/AKT/mTOR via interactions with polycomb proteins. Blood, 117, 3617-3628.

Zeinoun Z., Teugels E., De Bleser P.J., Neyns B., Geerts A. and De Greve J., 1999. Insufficient TGF-beta 1 production inactivates the autocrine growth suppressive circuit in human ovarian cancer cell lines. Anticancer Res, 19, 413-420.

Zhu Q., Krakowski A.R., Dunham E.E., Wang L., Bandyopadhyay A., Berdeaux R., Martin G.S., Sun L. and Luo K., 2007. Dual role of SnoN in mammalian tumorigenesis. Mol Cell Biol, 27, 324-339.

7

New Tumor Biomarkers in Ovarian Cancer and Its Prognostic and Clinical Relevance

Malgorzata Banys[1,2], Natalia Krawczyk[1] and Tanja Fehm[1]
[1]*Department of Obstetrics and Gynecology, University of Tuebingen, Tuebingen,*
[2]*Department of Obstetrics and Gynecology, Marienkrankenhaus Hamburg, Hamburg*
Germany

1. Introduction

In Europe and the United States, ovarian cancer is currently the major cause of death from gynecological malignancy. Up to 60% ovarian cancer patients die from locally advanced disease. Nonetheless, even patients treated with optimal cytoreduction may subsequently suffer from metastatic disease. Since treatment strategies are developed to control locoregional cancer growth, it may be anticipated that more patients will die of distant metastases. The lack of early disease signals further contributes to the fact that only one-fourth of ovarian cancers are identified at stage I. Ovarian cancer remains thus undetected due to late symptoms and the lack of reliable and clinically applicable screening tools. Further, the identification of new biomarkers could optimize prediction and monitoring of anticancer therapies and provide insights into ovarian cancer progression.

Presence of disseminated tumor cells (DTC) in bone marrow is a common phenomenon observed in solid epithelial tumors. As shown by a multi-center analysis of bone marrow (BM) specimens from more than 4,700 patients, DTC detection at the time of breast cancer diagnosis is strongly correlated with poor clinical outcome (level-I-evidence) [1]. There is growing evidence that hematogenous tumor cell dissemination may occur in other tumors, such as prostate, colon and gynecologic malignancies. DTC, as surrogate parameter for occult hematogenous spread, are routinely detected in 22-51% ovarian cancer patients. Interestingly, ovarian metastases to the bone are only rarely observed [2], [3], [4]. Whether bone marrow serves in these patients as a temporary compartment from where persistent DTC are able to migrate, remains unclear. It has been demonstrated that dissemination of isolated tumor cells to secondary sites occurs as early as in FIGO stage I disease [4]. Single tumor cells acquire thus the potential to disseminate to extraperitoneal compartments early in the process of the disease.

Of all prognostic factors, monitoring of minimal residual disease is the only one available after the tumor has been removed. Beside monitoring of tumor markers, there is currently a major effort to identify other biological markers which can be assessed with minimally invasive methods and persist beyond surgery. We previously reported on a significant correlation of positive bone marrow status with shortened relapse-free survival in ovarian cancer patients [5]. DTC persistence after completion of platinum-based chemotherapy was also found to be prognostically relevant [6]. Further, the identification of molecular biomarkers may represent excellent targets for new treatment strategies for chemoresistant

ovarian cancer patients. Recently, attempts have been made to target DTC by using antibody-based therapy with catumaxomab [7]. However, data on DTC detection in gynecological malignancies are so far limited [4], [8], [9], [10], [11].
In the following chapter, we discuss new biomarkers and circulating tumor cells. Data on prognostic and clinical relevance are presented.

2. Disseminated and circulating tumor cells in ovarian cancer

High mortality in patients with ovarian malignancies is mostly due to their locally advanced tumor rather than to distant metastatic disease. According to autopsy studies, however, occult metastatic tumors are encountered frequently at distant sites (e.g. liver, lung, bone, central nervous system) [3]. Up to 38% of patients with ovarian cancer developed metastases consistent with Stage IV disease at some time during the natural history of their disease. These results suggest that hematogenous dissemination of single tumor cells is a phenomenon much more common than would be expected from the clinical course of the disease.
Numerous techniques have been developed to isolate and quantify disseminated tumor cells in epithelial carcinomas. So far, no specific antigen or marker gene has been described for ovarian cancer. Therefore, the most widely used DTC detection assays rely on antibody-based capture of tumor cells, which express epithelial markers that are absent from normal leukocytes (Figure 1). Commonly targeted antigens are cytokeratin and EpCAM because their expression is relatively constant and universal in cells of epithelial origin [2, 6, 11].

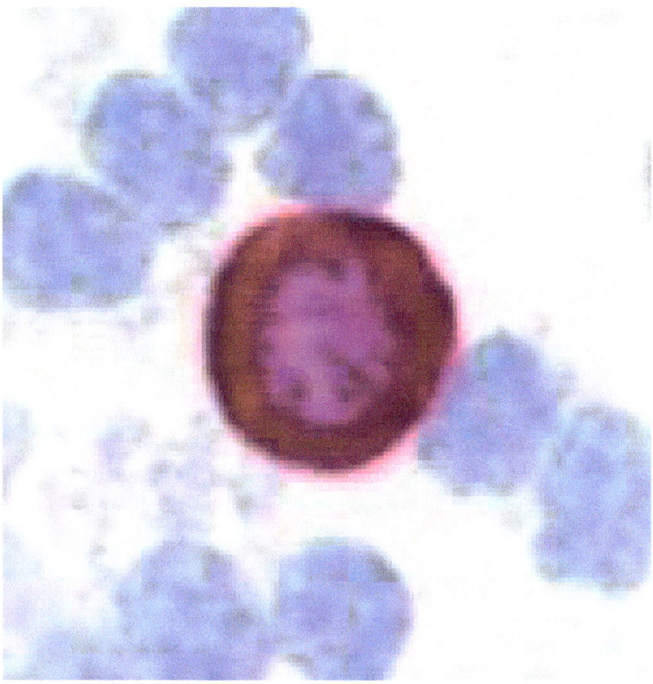

Fig. 1. Disseminated tumor cell from ovarian cancer patient with typical cytomorphology and immunophenotype (positive cytokeratin-staining, large nucleus, high nuclear to cytoplasmic ratio, nucleus partially covered by CK-staining, nucleus granular [12].

Disseminated tumor cells can be detected in 22-51% of ovarian cancer patients stage FIGO I-III [2, 4, 6, 11]. This relatively high incidence suggests that single tumor cells acquire the potential to disseminate to secondary sites outside the peritoneum early in the course of the disease, and that blood-borne dissemination in ovarian malignancy is a common rather than random occurrence. The number of detected cytokeratin-positive cells generally ranges in bone marrow from 1 to 30 per $2x10^6$ mononuclear cells [5, 6].
The influence of primary tumor's characteristics on DTC presence is unclear. Based on a group of 108 primary ovarian cancer patients, Braun et al. reported no correlation between classical prognostic factors, such as FIGO stage, tumor type, residual intraperitoneal tumor, the presence of ascites, peritoneal metastasis or lymph node involvement, and DTC status [4]. The only parameter associated with BM positivity was grading ($p = 0.02$). In a study collective of 112 patients, we could confirm this observation [5]. Similar results were reported by others [6, 10, 11, 13].

2.1 Prognostic relevance of DTC/CTC in ovarian cancer

For ovarian cancer, there is only limited data on prognostic value of DTC detection (Table 1). Braun et al. reported reduced distant disease-free survival in patients with detectable DTC at the time of diagnosis [4]. This correlation was confirmed in a subgroup of 64 optimally debulked patients, which indicated the importance of bone marrow status in patients who received successful surgical cytoreduction. We previously demonstrated that DTC positivity affects disease-free survival in a group of 112 ovarian cancer patients stage FIGO I-III [5]. Interestingly, positive DTC status was also an indicator for early local recurrence which is mostly due to suboptimal tumor debulking surgery and abdominal spread. Therefore, it might be speculated that DTC are indicators of a more aggressive phenotype of the primary disease that is likely to cause local recurrence. In contrast, other authors reported no

Author	N	Method	Median follow-up [months]	Prognostic significance
Banys [5]	112	DTC (ICC)	12	DFS
Braun [4]	108	DTC (ICC)	45	DFS
Aktas [13]	95	DTC (ICC)	28	n.s.
Fehm [2]	69	DTC (ICC)	5	n.s.
Schindlbeck [11]	90	DTC (ICC)	28	DDFS
Marth [10]	73	DTC (immunobeads)	25	n.s.
Wimberger [16]	62	DTC (ICC)	18	DFS [1]
Cain [14]	50	DTC (ICC)		n.s.
Wimberger et al. [6]	30	DTC (ICC)	18 [2]	PFS

Abbreviations: DFS - disease-free survival, DDFS - distant disease-free survival, DTC - disseminated tumor cells in bone marrow, ICC - immunocytochemistry, n.s. - not significant, PFS - progression-free survival

[1] DTC detected after chemotherapy

[2] Mean

Table 1. Prognostic relevance of disseminated tumor cells and other biomarkers in ovarian cancer.

significant correlation between bone marrow status and survival in ovarian cancer patients [10, 14]. One possible explanation for this discrepancy might be the time point of bone marrow aspiration. For instance, Marth et al. showed no association between the presence of tumor cells in BM and survival [10]. However, all samples were collected after surgery, whereas other authors aspirated BM immediately preoperatively [4, 5]. A transient dissemination of cancer cells from the primary tumor due to intraoperative manipulation could contribute to false-positive results and therefore affect further analysis [15].

2.2 Circulating tumor cells

One limitation of bone marrow sampling is its invasiveness. Since BM biopsy is not well tolerated by many patients, translational research have focused increasingly on circulating tumor cell (CTC) detection in the blood. In breast cancer, a significant impact of CTC detection on survival has already been established both in primary and metastatic situation [17, 18]. Currently, two commercially available kits for CTC detection in breast cancer are in use: antibody-based CellSearch and Multiplex-RT-PCR AdnaTest. Both tests were modified and validated in ovarian cancer patients (Table 2). The largest trial so far is the recently published study by Poveda et al. including 216 patients diagnosed with relapsed ovarian cancer [19]. Elevated numbers of CTC (> 1 cell / 7.5 ml blood) detected by the CellSearch assay before start of therapy predicted unfavorable prognosis. Aktas et al. used a modified AdnaTest assay to isolate cells expressing EpCAM, MUC-1, HER-2 or CA 125-transcripts [13]. Patients with detectable CTC has significantly shorter survival, irrespective of time point of blood sampling (before surgery or after chemotherapy). Further, Fan et al. examined 66 primary ovarian patients using a cell invasion assay and reported a significant decrease in disease-free survival in CTC-positive ovarian patients

Author	N	Method	Median follow-up [months]	Prognostic significance
Poveda [19]	216	CTC (ICC: CellSearch) [1]		PFS, OS
Sehouli [8]	167	CTC (ICC)	46	n.s.
Marth [10]	90	CTC (immunomagnetic beads)	25	n.s.
Aktas [13]	86	CTC (Multiplex-RT-PCR: AdnaTest)	28	OS [2]
Heubner [23]	68	Circulating 20S-proteasomes	19	OS
Fan [20]	66	CTC (immunofluorescence, cell invasion assay)	18	DFS
Wimberger [16]	62	Circulating nucleosomes, DNA, protease and caspase activity	18	DFS, OS
Judson [24]	53	CTC (ICC)	19 [3]	n.s.

Abbreviations: CTC – circulating tumor cells in peripheral blood, DFS – disease-free survival, ICC – immunocytochemistry, n.s. – not significant, PFS – progression-free survival

[1] Relapsed ovarian cancer

[2] Both before and after chemotherapy

[3] Mean

Table 2. Prognostic relevance of circulating tumor cells in ovarian cancer.

[20]. In contrast, Marth et al. reported a 12% incidence throughout all tumor stages but observed no correlation with clinical outcome [10]. Interestingly, positive finding in the blood was highly associated with DTC detection in bone marrow. Smaller studies showed varying CTC incidence, depending on methodology [21, 22].

2.3 Therapy monitoring

Beyond the prognostic value of DTC detection, monitoring of minimal residual disease following treatment represent a promising parameter for the assessment of residual risk of relapse. Tumor markers such as CA125 are clinically accepted tools for therapy monitoring in advanced ovarian cancer. Nevertheless, CA125 levels generally decline rapidly during chemotherapy and are mostly below cut-off level at the end of treatment even though a significant proportion of patients will face a relapse of the disease within five years. Moreover, the clinical utility of serial CA125 measurements for early therapy of a relapse is currently controversially debated [25]. In this context, the presence of isolated tumor cells in bone marrow and possibly in peripheral blood, might indicate occult tumor load after first line therapy and serve as a parameter for suboptimal response to therapy. For other tumor entities, such as breast cancer, DTC persistence after treatment is an independent indicator of reduced clinical outcome [26]. Whether therapy-resistant DTC also affect survival in ovarian cancer, is a subject of current studies. Wimberger et al. correlated changes in DTC counts before and after first-line chemotherapy to clinical course of disease in 30 ovarian cancer patients. DTC persistence was observed in half of the patients after chemotherapy. Patients with marked increase in DTC numbers had significantly shortened progression-free survival [6].

So far, assessment of therapy efficacy in asymptomatic ovarian cancer patients after completion of standard chemotherapy has not been possible until patient's eventual relapse. A reliable therapy monitoring tool could identify high-risk patients in need of additional therapy. Whether persistent DTC, as surrogate parameter of minimal residual disease, may be targeted by secondary adjuvant therapy is currently under investigation and should be further studied.

2.4 Stem cell hypothesis

As to progression of ovarian cancer, an interesting hypothesis has been introduced recently. According to 'classical' model of carcinogenesis, any cell may be source of malignant transformation and lead to tumor growth. However, emerging evidence has suggested that the capability of cancer to grow, proliferate and eventually relapse is dependent on a small subpopulation of tumor cells, called cancer stem cells (CSC). These cells are considered especially significant on the background of drug resistance, tumor dormancy, minimal residual disease, and disease recurrence. Several cancer entities, such as ovarian cancer, retinoblastoma, gastrointestinal and breast cancer might arise from a small population of cells with stem cell properties that sustain tumor formation and growth [27]. This 'stem cell hypothesis' assumes an important role of tumor-initiating progenitor cells in tumor progression. Accordingly, cancer stem cells, but not the remaining cells in the primary tumor, have the ability to self-renew, propagate tumorigenesis and are drug-resistant [28]. Ovarian cancer cell lines were demonstrated to feature "side population" cells with ability to differentiate into cancers with different histologies, similar to the assumed pluripotent character of stem cells [29]. Such cells has been detected in various solid tumors, such as colon [30], breast [31] and ovarian cancer [32-34]. Based on animal models and natural course of the disease (e.g. high recurrence rates, multidrug resistance), it has been postulated that cancer stem cells play a crucial role in ovarian cancer [32, 35]. Szotek et al. detected side population (SP) not only in human ovarian cancer cell lines, but also in primary ascites cancer cells [32]. Hosonuma et al. analyzed 28 samples obtained from ovarian cancer patients with respect to the expression of SP as a marker for the presence of cancer stem cells [29]. Side population was encountered more often in recurrent and metastatic patients and SP+ patients had significantly reduced survival. Further, although advanced ovarian cancer mostly initially responds to platinum-based combination treatment, it is usually followed by the chemotherapy-resistant phenotype. One possible explanation for this phenomenon is the CSC-induced drug-resistance: standard therapies fail to target tumor-initiating cells [32]. Recently, cisplatin chemotherapy has been shown to generate residual cells with mesenchymal stem cell-like characteristics *in vitro* [36]. Therefore, these cells need to be targeted with different approaches by identification of specific antigens. However, very few tumor antigens have been described to target the CSC subpopulation.

One currently debated hypothesis is the theory that disseminated and circulating tumor cells, the surrogate marker for minimal residual disease and possibly precursor of systemic metastasis, are cancer stem cells. In breast cancer, Balic et al. reported that early DTC express stem cell phenotype [37] and circulating tumor cells often exhibit epithelial-mesenchymal transition markers [31]. In addition, Abraham et al. has shown that a high percentage of CD44+/CD24- cells in the primary tumor correlate with a higher prevalence of distant metastasis [38]. Since the majority of CTC in breast cancer are triple-negative, irrespective of primary tumor's phenotype [39], we may assume that some of these cells reflect stem cell-like subpopulation. This issue, however, has not been studied in ovarian cancer. Whether isolated tumor cells in extraperitoneal sites, such as blood and bone marrow, are in fact ovarian cancer stem cells, remains yet to be cleared.

3. Novel biomarkers in ovarian cancer

To date, the only tumor marker that has proven to detect ovarian cancer prior to the onset of clinical symptoms and is commonly used in clinical practice is CA125 [40]. However, numerous other biomarkers have been developed over the years and are currently being tested for their usefulness as screening, prognostic or therapy monitoring tools.

3.1 Osteopontin

Osteopontin (OPN) is a cell surface and secretory glycoprotein containing an arginine-glycine-aspartate motif and is one of the candidate markers identified by high-throughput cDNA microarray techniques. Osteopontin plays a critical role in cellular proliferation, metastasis and apoptosis. Preoperative plasma levels are significantly higher in ovarian cancer patients than in women with benign tumors or in healthy women [41]. OPN levels also seem to correlate with stage of disease. It has been speculated that OPN may complement CA125 expression in a marker panel for recurrence monitoring [42, 43]. When combined with CA125, OPN reaches high sensitivity of 94%. Further, like other cell-surface proteins, OPN may serve as a potential target for the antibody-based therapies. *In vitro*, humanized anti-osteopontin antibody, hu1A12, was effective in inhibiting the cell adhesion, migration, invasion and colony formation and may be a promising therapeutic agent in breast cancer, and possibly other tumor entities, including ovarian cancer, as well [44].

3.2 Haptoglobin

In a manner similar to other acute phase proteins, increased levels of haptoglobin are observed in inflammatory processes, infections and various cancers, including breast, lung and bladder cancers [45]. Elevation of haptoglobin in blood of ovarian cancer patients has been reported in several studies [46-48]. Zhao et al. has shown that elevated haptoglobin at the time of diagnosis is associated with reduced overall survival in a multivariate analysis [45].

3.3 Human Epididymis Protein 4 (HE4)

Human Epididymis Protein 4 is a stable disulfide core protein associated with the *WFDC2* gene that is overexpressed in ovarian cancer, particularly serous and endometrioid histologies. Serum HE4 levels were found to be elevated in ovarian cancer patients in numerous studies [49]. Conclusive data on the feasibility as a screening assay is pending. Holcomb et al. reported a superior specificity of HE4 compared to CA125 for the identification of malignant adnexal masses [50]. An evaluation of a marker panel ROMA (Risk of Ovarian Malignancy Algorithm) utilizing CA125 and HE4 initially yielded promising results [51]. However, subsequent validation in clinical setting did not confirm any benefit compared to use of CA125 alone [52, 53]. As to prognostic relevance, Peak et al. have shown that an elevated serum HE4 level was associated with reduced progression-free survival [54].

3.4 Mesothelin

Mesothelin is a cell surface glycoprotein that is present on normal mesothelial cells and overexpressed in mesothelioma, ovarian cancer and other malignant tumors [55-57]. As a screening tool, mesothelin was shown to perform comparably to CA125 and might improve cancer detection as a combined marker panel [58].

3.5 B7-H4

B7-H4 is one of the B7 family members that serve as negative regulators of T cell function. Its overexpression promotes cellular transformation and has been shown in a variety of cancers. Elevated levels of B7-H4 are detected in early-stage ovarian cancer [59].

3.6 Additional markers

Numerous other biomarkers, such as prostasin, VEGF, macrophage colony stimulating factor, kallikrein 6 and 10, mucin 1, interleukins 6 and 8, apolipoprotein A1, OVX1 and many others, have been identified and yielded promising results [60, 61]. In 2009, the U.S. Food and Drug Administration approved the blood test panel OVA1 for the preoperative assessment of pelvic masses [62]. OVA1 incorporates five markers: CA125-II, transferrin, transthyretin, apolipoprotein AI, and beta 2 microglobulin. To date, none of the currently discussed novel markers has a real potential to replace CA125 in clinical routine.

Biomarker	Function	Useful as a screening tool	Useful for therapy monitoring	Clinical relevance
Osteopontin	Cell surface protein; plays a role in cellular proliferation, metastasis and apoptosis	Low specificity; possibly useful in combination with CA125 [41, 43]	Possibly yes; in combination with CA125 [42]	Limited data on prognostic relevance [63]; possible use in targeted therapy [44, 64]
Haptoglobin	Acute phase protein	Low specificity [46, 48]	Unclear; mostly decrease during chemotherapy [47]	Prognostic relevance - yes (data from small studies) [45]
Human epididymis protein 4	Secreted glycoprotein	Unclear due to partly contradictory results [50, 52, 65]	No conclusive data	Prognostic relevance - yes (data from small studies) [54]
Mesothelin	Surface antigen of mesothelial cells	Not superior to CA125, however use in combination with CA125 possible [58]	No conclusive data	Possible use in targeted therapy [66, 67]
B7-H4	Negative regulator of T cell function	Possibly yes in combination with CA125 [59]	No conclusive data	No prognostic value [59, 68]

Table 3. Novel biomarkers in ovarian cancer and their potential impact on diagnostics and therapy.

4. Conclusions

Despite advances in diagnostics and therapy, 60% of women diagnosed with ovarian cancer will eventually suffer from a relapse, resulting in a poor overall survival. Currently, efficacy of therapy is evaluated by physical examinations, radiographic imaging, and evaluation of CA125 levels. There continues to be a need to identify new biomarkers for better prediction and prognostication.

Early hematogenous tumor cell dissemination is a common phenomenon in solid epithelial cancers. There is growing evidence that detection of single tumor cells in blood or bone marrow of ovarian cancer patients is associated with reduced clinical outcome. Whether these patients benefit from a more aggressive or prolonged treatment remains to be evaluated.

5. References

[1] Braun S, Vogl FD, Naume B, Janni W, Osborne MP, Coombes RC, Schlimok G, Diel IJ, Gerber B, Gebauer G *et al*: A pooled analysis of bone marrow micrometastasis in breast cancer. *N Engl J Med* 2005, 353(8):793-802.

[2] Fehm T, Becker S, Bachmann C, Beck V, Gebauer G, Banys M, Wallwiener D, Solomayer EF: Detection of disseminated tumor cells in patients with gynecological cancers. *Gynecol Oncol* 2006, 103(3):942-947.

[3] Dauplat J, Hacker NF, Nieberg RK, Berek JS, Rose TP, Sagae S: Distant metastases in epithelial ovarian carcinoma. *Cancer* 1987, 60(7):1561-1566.

[4] Braun S, Schindlbeck C, Hepp F, Janni W, Kentenich C, Riethmuller G, Pantel K: Occult tumor cells in bone marrow of patients with locoregionally restricted ovarian cancer predict early distant metastatic relapse. *J Clin Oncol* 2001, 19(2):368-375.

[5] Banys M, Solomayer EF, Becker S, Krawczyk N, Gardanis K, Staebler A, Neubauer H, Wallwiener D, Fehm T: Disseminated tumor cells in bone marrow may affect prognosis of patients with gynecologic malignancies. *Int J Gynecol Cancer* 2009, 19(5):948-952.

[6] Wimberger P, Heubner M, Otterbach F, Fehm T, Kimmig R, Kasimir-Bauer S: Influence of platinum-based chemotherapy on disseminated tumor cells in blood and bone marrow of patients with ovarian cancer. *Gynecol Oncol* 2007, 107(2):331-338.

[7] Wimberger P, Heubner M, Lindhofer H, Jager M, Kimmig R, Kasimir-Bauer S: Influence of catumaxomab on tumor cells in bone marrow and blood in ovarian cancer. *Anticancer Res* 2009, 29(5):1787-1791.

[8] Sehouli J, Konsgen D, Nimpsch R, Stengel D, Oskay G, Mustea A, Oertel J, Lichtenegger W: Prognostic significance of epithelial cells in the blood of patients with gynaecological malignancies. *Anticancer Res* 2003, 23(5b):4133-4140.

[9] Janni W, Hepp F, Strobl B, Rack B, Rjosk D, Kentenich C, Schindlbeck C, Hantschmann P, Pantel K, Sommer H *et al*: Patterns of disease recurrence influenced by hematogenous tumor cell dissemination in patients with cervical carcinoma of the uterus. *Cancer* 2003, 97(2):405-411.

[10] Marth C, Kisic J, Kaern J, Trope C, Fodstad O: Circulating tumor cells in the peripheral blood and bone marrow of patients with ovarian carcinoma do not predict prognosis. *Cancer* 2002, 94(3):707-712.

[11] Schindlbeck C, Hantschmann P, Zerzer M, Jahns B, Rjosk D, Janni W, Rack B, Sommer H, Friese K: Prognostic impact of KI67, p53, human epithelial growth factor receptor 2, topoisomerase IIalpha, epidermal growth factor receptor, and nm23 expression of ovarian carcinomas and disseminated tumor cells in the bone marrow. *Int J Gynecol Cancer* 2007.

[12] Fehm T, Braun S, Muller V, Janni W, Gebauer G, Marth C, Schindlbeck C, Wallwiener D, Borgen E, Naume B *et al*: A concept for the standardized detection of disseminated tumor cells in bone marrow from patients with primary breast cancer and its clinical implementation. *Cancer* 2006, 107(5):885-892.

[13] Aktas B, Kasimir-Bauer S, Heubner M, Kimmig R, Wimberger P: Molecular profiling and prognostic relevance of circulating tumor cells in the blood of ovarian cancer patients at primary diagnosis and after platinum-based chemotherapy. *Int J Gynecol Cancer* 2011, 21(5):822-830.

[14] Cain JM, Ellis GK, Collins C, Greer BE, Tamimi HK, Figge DC, Gown AM, Livingston RB: Bone marrow involvement in epithelial ovarian cancer by immunocytochemical assessment. *Gynecol Oncol* 1990, 38(3):442-445.

[15] Camara O, Kavallaris A, Noschel H, Rengsberger M, Jorke C, Pachmann K: Seeding of epithelial cells into circulation during surgery for breast cancer: the fate of malignant and benign mobilized cells. *World J Surg Oncol* 2006, 4:67.

[16] Wimberger P, Roth C, Pantel K, Kasimir-Bauer S, Kimmig R, Schwarzenbach H: Impact of platinum-based chemotherapy on circulating nucleic acid levels, protease activities in blood and disseminated tumor cells in bone marrow of ovarian cancer patients. *Int J Cancer* 2010.

[17] Cristofanilli M, Budd GT, Ellis MJ, Stopeck A, Matera J, Miller MC, Reuben JM, Doyle GV, Allard WJ, Terstappen LW *et al*: Circulating tumor cells, disease progression, and survival in metastatic breast cancer. *N Engl J Med* 2004, 351(8):781-791.

[18] Rack BK, Schindlbeck C, Andergassen U, Schneeweiss A, Zwingers T, Lichtenegger W, Beckmann M, Sommer HL, Pantel K, Janni W: Use of circulating tumor cells (CTC) in peripheral blood of breast cancer patients before and after adjuvant chemotherapy to predict risk for relapse: The SUCCESS trial. ASCO Annual Meeting 2010. *J Clin Oncol* 2010, 28:15s (suppl; abstr 1003).

[19] Poveda A, Kaye SB, McCormack R, Wang S, Parekh T, Ricci D, Lebedinsky CA, Tercero JC, Zintl P, Monk BJ: Circulating tumor cells predict progression free survival and overall survival in patients with relapsed/recurrent advanced ovarian cancer. *Gynecol Oncol* 2011.

[20] Fan T, Zhao Q, Chen JJ, Chen WT, Pearl ML: Clinical significance of circulating tumor cells detected by an invasion assay in peripheral blood of patients with ovarian cancer. *Gynecol Oncol* 2009, 112(1):185-191.

[21] Ntouroupi TG, Ashraf SQ, McGregor SB, Turney BW, Seppo A, Kim Y, Wang X, Kilpatrick MW, Tsipouras P, Tafas T *et al*: Detection of circulating tumour cells in peripheral blood with an automated scanning fluorescence microscope. *Br J Cancer* 2008, 99(5):789-795.

[22] Engel H, Kleespies C, Friedrich J, Breidenbach M, Kallenborn A, Schondorf T, Kolhagen H, Mallmann P: Detection of circulating tumour cells in patients with breast or ovarian cancer by molecular cytogenetics. *Br J Cancer* 1999, 81(7):1165-1173.

[23] Heubner M, Wimberger P, Dahlmann B, Kasimir-Bauer S, Kimmig R, Peters J, Wohlschlaeger J, Sixt SU: The prognostic impact of circulating proteasome concentrations in patients with epithelial ovarian cancer. *Gynecol Oncol* 2011, 120(2):233-238.

[24] Judson PL, Geller MA, Bliss RL, Boente MP, Downs LS, Jr., Argenta PA, Carson LF: Preoperative detection of peripherally circulating cancer cells and its prognostic significance in ovarian cancer. *Gynecol Oncol* 2003, 91(2):389-394.

[25] Rustin GJ, van der Burg ME, Griffin CL, Guthrie D, Lamont A, Jayson GC, Kristensen G, Mediola C, Coens C, Qian W *et al*: Early versus delayed treatment of relapsed

ovarian cancer (MRC OV05/EORTC 55955): a randomised trial. *Lancet* 2010, 376(9747):1155-1163.

[26] Janni W, Rack B, Schindlbeck C, Strobl B, Rjosk D, Braun S, Sommer H, Pantel K, Gerber B, Friese K: The persistence of isolated tumor cells in bone marrow from patients with breast carcinoma predicts an increased risk for recurrence. *Cancer* 2005, 103(5):884-891.

[27] Setoguchi T, Taga T, Kondo T: Cancer stem cells persist in many cancer cell lines. *Cell Cycle* 2004, 3(4):414-415.

[28] Dyall S, Gayther SA, Dafou D: Cancer stem cells and epithelial ovarian cancer. *J Oncol* 2010, 2010:105269.

[29] Hosonuma S, Kobayashi Y, Kojo S, Wada H, Seino K, Kiguchi K, Ishizuka B: Clinical significance of side population in ovarian cancer cells. *Hum Cell* 2011, 24(1):9-12.

[30] Ricci-Vitiani L, Lombardi DG, Pilozzi E, Biffoni M, Todaro M, Peschle C, De Maria R: Identification and expansion of human colon-cancer-initiating cells. *Nature* 2007, 445(7123):111-115.

[31] Aktas B, Tewes M, Fehm T, Hauch S, Kimmig R, Kasimir-Bauer S: Stem cell and epithelial-mesenchymal transition markers are frequently overexpressed in circulating tumor cells of metastatic breast cancer patients. *Breast Cancer Res* 2009, 11(4):R46.

[32] Szotek PP, Pieretti-Vanmarcke R, Masiakos PT, Dinulescu DM, Connolly D, Foster R, Dombkowski D, Preffer F, Maclaughlin DT, Donahoe PK: Ovarian cancer side population defines cells with stem cell-like characteristics and Mullerian Inhibiting Substance responsiveness. *Proc Natl Acad Sci U S A* 2006, 103(30):11154-11159.

[33] Bapat SA, Mali AM, Koppikar CB, Kurrey NK: Stem and progenitor-like cells contribute to the aggressive behavior of human epithelial ovarian cancer. *Cancer Res* 2005, 65(8):3025-3029.

[34] Challen GA, Little MH: A side order of stem cells: the SP phenotype. *Stem Cells* 2006, 24(1):3-12.

[35] Ponnusamy MP, Batra SK: Ovarian cancer: emerging concept on cancer stem cells. *J Ovarian Res* 2008, 1(1):4.

[36] Latifi A, Abubaker K, Castrechini N, Ward AC, Liongue C, Dobill F, Kumar J, Thompson EW, Quinn MA, Findlay JK *et al*: Cisplatin treatment of primary and metastatic epithelial ovarian carcinomas generates residual cells with mesenchymal stem cell-like profile. *J Cell Biochem* 2011.

[37] Balic M, Lin H, Young L, Hawes D, Giuliano A, McNamara G, Datar RH, Cote RJ: Most early disseminated cancer cells detected in bone marrow of breast cancer patients have a putative breast cancer stem cell phenotype. *Clin Cancer Res* 2006, 12(19):5615-5621.

[38] Abraham BK, Fritz P, McClellan M, Hauptvogel P, Athelogou M, Brauch H: Prevalence of CD44+/CD24-/low cells in breast cancer may not be associated with clinical outcome but may favor distant metastasis. *Clin Cancer Res* 2005, 11(3):1154-1159.

[39] Fehm T, Hoffmann O, Aktas B, Becker S, Solomayer EF, Wallwiener D, Kimmig R, Kasimir-Bauer S: Detection and characterization of circulating tumor cells in blood of primary breast cancer patients by RT-PCR and comparison to status of bone marrow disseminated cells. *Breast Cancer Res* 2009, 11(4):R59.

[40] Moore RG, Maclaughlan S: Current clinical use of biomarkers for epithelial ovarian cancer. *Curr Opin Oncol* 2010, 22(5):492-497.
[41] Nakae M, Iwamoto I, Fujino T, Maehata Y, Togami S, Yoshinaga M, Douchi T: Preoperative plasma osteopontin level as a biomarker complementary to carbohydrate antigen 125 in predicting ovarian cancer. *J Obstet Gynaecol Res* 2006, 32(3):309-314.
[42] Schorge JO, Drake RD, Lee H, Skates SJ, Rajanbabu R, Miller DS, Kim JH, Cramer DW, Berkowitz RS, Mok SC: Osteopontin as an adjunct to CA125 in detecting recurrent ovarian cancer. *Clin Cancer Res* 2004, 10(10):3474-3478.
[43] Rosen DG, Wang L, Atkinson JN, Yu Y, Lu KH, Diamandis EP, Hellstrom I, Mok SC, Liu J, Bast RC, Jr.: Potential markers that complement expression of CA125 in epithelial ovarian cancer. *Gynecol Oncol* 2005, 99(2):267-277.
[44] Dai J, Li B, Shi J, Peng L, Zhang D, Qian W, Hou S, Zhao L, Gao J, Cao Z *et al*: A humanized anti-osteopontin antibody inhibits breast cancer growth and metastasis in vivo. *Cancer Immunol Immunother* 2010, 59(3):355-366.
[45] Zhao C, Annamalai L, Guo C, Kothandaraman N, Koh SC, Zhang H, Biswas A, Choolani M: Circulating haptoglobin is an independent prognostic factor in the sera of patients with epithelial ovarian cancer. *Neoplasia* 2007, 9(1):1-7.
[46] Ye B, Cramer DW, Skates SJ, Gygi SP, Pratomo V, Fu L, Horick NK, Licklider LJ, Schorge JO, Berkowitz RS *et al*: Haptoglobin-alpha subunit as potential serum biomarker in ovarian cancer: identification and characterization using proteomic profiling and mass spectrometry. *Clin Cancer Res* 2003, 9(8):2904-2911.
[47] Ahmed N, Barker G, Oliva KT, Hoffmann P, Riley C, Reeve S, Smith AI, Kemp BE, Quinn MA, Rice GE: Proteomic-based identification of haptoglobin-1 precursor as a novel circulating biomarker of ovarian cancer. *Br J Cancer* 2004, 91(1):129-140.
[48] Bertenshaw GP, Yip P, Seshaiah P, Zhao J, Chen TH, Wiggins WS, Mapes JP, Mansfield BC: Multianalyte profiling of serum antigens and autoimmune and infectious disease molecules to identify biomarkers dysregulated in epithelial ovarian cancer. *Cancer Epidemiol Biomarkers Prev* 2008, 17(10):2872-2881.
[49] Moore RG, Brown AK, Miller MC, Skates S, Allard WJ, Verch T, Steinhoff M, Messerlian G, DiSilvestro P, Granai CO *et al*: The use of multiple novel tumor biomarkers for the detection of ovarian carcinoma in patients with a pelvic mass. *Gynecol Oncol* 2008, 108(2):402-408.
[50] Holcomb K, Vucetic Z, Miller MC, Knapp RC: Human epididymis protein 4 offers superior specificity in the differentiation of benign and malignant adnexal masses in premenopausal women. *Am J Obstet Gynecol* 2011.
[51] Moore RG, Jabre-Raughley M, Brown AK, Robison KM, Miller MC, Allard WJ, Kurman RJ, Bast RC, Skates SJ: Comparison of a novel multiple marker assay vs the Risk of Malignancy Index for the prediction of epithelial ovarian cancer in patients with a pelvic mass. *Am J Obstet Gynecol* 2010, 203(3):228 e221-226.
[52] Van Gorp T, Cadron I, Despierre E, Daemen A, Leunen K, Amant F, Timmerman D, De Moor B, Vergote I: HE4 and CA125 as a diagnostic test in ovarian cancer: prospective validation of the Risk of Ovarian Malignancy Algorithm. *Br J Cancer* 2011, 104(5):863-870.

[53] Jacob F, Meier M, Caduff R, Goldstein D, Pochechueva T, Hacker N, Fink D, Heinzelmann-Schwarz V: No benefit from combining HE4 and CA125 as ovarian tumor markers in a clinical setting. *Gynecol Oncol* 2011, 121(3):487-491.
[54] Paek J, Lee SH, Yim GW, Lee M, Kim YJ, Nam EJ, Kim SW, Kim YT: Prognostic significance of human epididymis protein 4 in epithelial ovarian cancer. *Eur J Obstet Gynecol Reprod Biol* 2011.
[55] Rein BJ, Gupta S, Dada R, Safi J, Michener C, Agarwal A: Potential markers for detection and monitoring of ovarian cancer. *J Oncol* 2011, 2011:475983.
[56] Hassan R, Remaley AT, Sampson ML, Zhang J, Cox DD, Pingpank J, Alexander R, Willingham M, Pastan I, Onda M: Detection and quantitation of serum mesothelin, a tumor marker for patients with mesothelioma and ovarian cancer. *Clin Cancer Res* 2006, 12(2):447-453.
[57] Scholler N, Fu N, Yang Y, Ye Z, Goodman GE, Hellstrom KE, Hellstrom I: Soluble member(s) of the mesothelin/megakaryocyte potentiating factor family are detectable in sera from patients with ovarian carcinoma. *Proc Natl Acad Sci U S A* 1999, 96(20):11531-11536.
[58] McIntosh MW, Drescher C, Karlan B, Scholler N, Urban N, Hellstrom KE, Hellstrom I: Combining CA 125 and SMR serum markers for diagnosis and early detection of ovarian carcinoma. *Gynecol Oncol* 2004, 95(1):9-15.
[59] Simon I, Katsaros D, Rigault de la Longrais I, Massobrio M, Scorilas A, Kim NW, Sarno MJ, Wolfert RL, Diamandis EP: B7-H4 is over-expressed in early-stage ovarian cancer and is independent of CA125 expression. *Gynecol Oncol* 2007, 106(2):334-341.
[60] Lu KH, Patterson AP, Wang L, Marquez RT, Atkinson EN, Baggerly KA, Ramoth LR, Rosen DG, Liu J, Hellstrom I *et al*: Selection of potential markers for epithelial ovarian cancer with gene expression arrays and recursive descent partition analysis. *Clin Cancer Res* 2004, 10(10):3291-3300.
[61] Visintin I, Feng Z, Longton G, Ward DC, Alvero AB, Lai Y, Tenthorey J, Leiser A, Flores-Saaib R, Yu H *et al*: Diagnostic markers for early detection of ovarian cancer. *Clin Cancer Res* 2008, 14(4):1065-1072.
[62] Ueland FR, Desimone CP, Seamon LG, Miller RA, Goodrich S, Podzielinski I, Sokoll L, Smith A, van Nagell JR, Jr., Zhang Z: Effectiveness of a multivariate index assay in the preoperative assessment of ovarian tumors. *Obstet Gynecol* 2011, 117(6):1289-1297.
[63] Bao LH, Sakaguchi H, Fujimoto J, Tamaya T: Osteopontin in metastatic lesions as a prognostic marker in ovarian cancers. *J Biomed Sci* 2007, 14(3):373-381.
[64] Matsuura M, Suzuki T, Suzuki M, Tanaka R, Ito E, Saito T: Statin-mediated reduction of osteopontin expression induces apoptosis and cell growth arrest in ovarian clear cell carcinoma. *Oncol Rep* 2011, 25(1):41-47.
[65] Chang X, Ye X, Dong L, Cheng H, Cheng Y, Zhu L, Liao Q, Zhao Y, Tian L, Fu T *et al*: Human Epididymis Protein 4 (HE4) as a Serum Tumor Biomarker in Patients With Ovarian Carcinoma. *Int J Gynecol Cancer* 2011, 21(5):852-858.
[66] Hassan R, Cohen SJ, Phillips M, Pastan I, Sharon E, Kelly RJ, Schweizer C, Weil S, Laheru D: Phase I clinical trial of the chimeric anti-mesothelin monoclonal antibody MORAb-009 in patients with mesothelin-expressing cancers. *Clin Cancer Res* 2010, 16(24):6132-6138.

[67] Ho M, Feng M, Fisher RJ, Rader C, Pastan I: A novel high-affinity human monoclonal antibody to mesothelin. *Int J Cancer* 2011, 128(9):2020-2030.

[68] Kryczek I, Wei S, Zhu G, Myers L, Mottram P, Cheng P, Chen L, Coukos G, Zou W: Relationship between B7-H4, regulatory T cells, and patient outcome in human ovarian carcinoma. *Cancer Res* 2007, 67(18):8900-8905.

8

Oncogenic Pathway Signatures and Survival Outcome

Xuan Bich Trinh[1,2], Peter A. Van Dam[1], Luc Y. Dirix[1],
Steven J. van Laere[1] and Wiebren A. A. Tjalma[2]
[1]*Translational Cancer Research Unit, St Augustinus GZA Hospitals, Antwerp*
[2]*Department of Gynaecological Oncology, Antwerp University Hospital, Antwerp*
Belgium

1. Introduction

Recent microarray technology and bioinformatics have shown the ability of analysing oncogenic cellular signalling pathways based upon gene signatures in cancers. (Bild et al., 2006; Dressman et al., 2007; Gatza et al., 2010) Epithelial ovarian cancer (EOC) is the most important cause of mortality among gynaecological cancers. Patients with EOC often present in an advanced stage. Treatment modalities consist in general of the sequence of surgical cytoreduction and platinum-taxane based chemotherapy. (Cannistra, 2004) Although the disease is relatively sensitive to cytotoxics, relapses occur in a majority of patients with advanced stage. (Cannistra, 2004) The emergence of resistance to conventional chemotherapeutics is an often-deadly event in the management of ovarian cancer patients. There is an urgent need for additional therapies that increase survival and/or quality of life in these patients.

The objective of our study was to look for cellular pathways that have an effect on survival outcome by a bioinformatical approach. (Trinh et al., 2011) These pathways may guide us to find interesting targets in ovarian cancer. Survival can be used as a measure to quantify the biological relevance in this disease. Ideally, evaluation of survival outcome should be made in a homogenous population with a uniform treatment to avoid treatment-induced biases and uniform histology to find subtler differences independent from histology. Another methodology of estimating prognostic value may be the correlation with documented prognostic gene signatures that have shown to be of prognostic value in breast cancer and other types of cancer. The invasiveness gene signature (IGS) was generated using stem cell-like or tumorigenic breast cancer cells.(Liu et al., 2007) This signature has shown prognostic value in lung cancer, medulloblastoma and prostate cancer. The Wound healing response (WHR) signature, based upon genes induced by wound healing, also has shown its prognostic value in breast cancer, NSLC and bladder cancer. (Chang et al., 2005; Lauss, Ringnér, & Höglund, 2010; Mostertz et al., 2010) The genomic grade index (GGI) is a signature that divides low-grade versus high-grade breast carcinomas. (Sotiriou et al., 2006) Interestingly, using this signature, histological intermediate-grade tumours could be classified as low- or high-grade tumours with the preservation of the gene signatures' prognostic value.

2. Oncogenic pathways

The oncogenic gene signatures were derived from a recent paper by Gatza and colleagues and applied similarly. (Gatza et al., 2010) These pathway signatures were mainly generated by activating or silencing specific genes in cell lines experiments. The signatures were robustly validated afterwards. For each pathway, a pathway activation score was calculated based upon the gene signature to quantify the activation by a score.

Briefly, for each array-sample the pathway-specific informative genes were identified. Next a pathway score was calculated by adding up the products of the gene expression for each gene and its corresponding regression coefficient, which indicates the weight (amplitude of regression coefficient) and the effect (sign of regression coefficient) of the corresponding gene for activation of the corresponding pathway. Finally, the pathway scores were scaled using the intercept values provided in the original manuscript and standardized for comparability by median-centering and setting the standard deviation to 1. Pathways included in the analysis were AKT, β-Catenin, E2F1, EGFR, ER, HER2, INFα, INFγ, MYC, p53, p63, PI3K, PR, RAS, SRC, STAT3, TNFα, and TGFβ.

Since PARP inhibitors and VEGF-A inhibitors have shown promising results in ovarian cancer, the BRCA pathway and VEGF-A pathway was also studied. (Audeh et al., 2010; Burger et al., 2010; Fong et al., 2009; 2010) For the BRCA signature, we used one that was published by Konstantinopoulos and colleagues. (Konstantinopoulos et al., 2010) For a VEGF-A signature we have used and validated genes that were reported by Hu et al. (Hu et al., 2009) A BRCA activation score was applied using the same methodology with 60 genes, their weight and sign. (Konstantinopoulos et al., 2010) Prognostic gene signatures (IGS, GGI and WHR) were also applied by previously described methodology. (Chang et al., 2005; Liu et al., 2007; Sotiriou et al., 2006) All gene signature activation scores were handled as a continuous variable. The same standardisation (Median=0; SD=1) was applied for each gene signature.

For the VEGF-A activation signature we used the 13 genes reported by Hu and colleagues. (Hu et al., 2009) To validate and transform this gene signature into a VEGF-A activation probability score we performed subsequent analysis using publicly available gene expression data sets on naïve and VEGF-A treated HUVEC cell lines (GSE18913 (N=21), GSE10778 (N=9; only the HGU133A samples were used) and GSE15464 (N=4)). Each data set was normalised using the GC-RMA algorithm and informative genes (above log 2(100) in at least 25% of the genes) were filtered in. First, we applied a principal component analysis on the GSE18913 data set using the informative VEGF-A signatures genes only (N=10). Only 10 out of 13 genes (*FABP5, UCHL1, PLOD, DDIT4, VEGF, ADM, ANGPTL4, NDRG1, NP* and *SLC16A3*) were reliably measured (high signal-to-noise ratio). Using these 10 genes in a principal component analysis (PCA) we were able to demonstrate a significant segregation of VEGF-A treated and naïve HUVEC's along the first principal component. Class label permutation analysis revealed that the observed Euclidean distance between the centroids of the VEGF-A treated and naïve HUVEC's on the 2D scatterplot representation of the PCA was significantly different from the expected Euclidean distance (Figure 1A; Observed Euclidean distance=2.185, Expected Euclidean distance=0.682, $P<0.0001$).

Next, we transformed the VEGF-A signature into a VEGF-A activation probability score adopting the methodology described by Gatza and his colleagues. (Gatza et al., 2010). Therefore, we used the regression coefficients that define the first principal component and multiplied these with the gene expression values of their corresponding genes. The products were summed and the resulting score was compared between VEGF-A treated and naïve HUVEC's using a Mann-Whitney U-test (Median VEGF-A treated HUVEC's: 6.416, Median naïve HUVEC's: 4.276, P<0.0001). The boxplot representation is provided in Figure 1B. In addition, we observed a strong correlation between the VEGF-A activation probability scores and the time of VEGF-A incubation of HUVEC's (Correlation coefficient = 0.762; P=0.038). (Figure 1C). To validate our procedure, we applied our algorithm on the samples in gene expression data sets GSE10778 and GSE15464.

FIG I

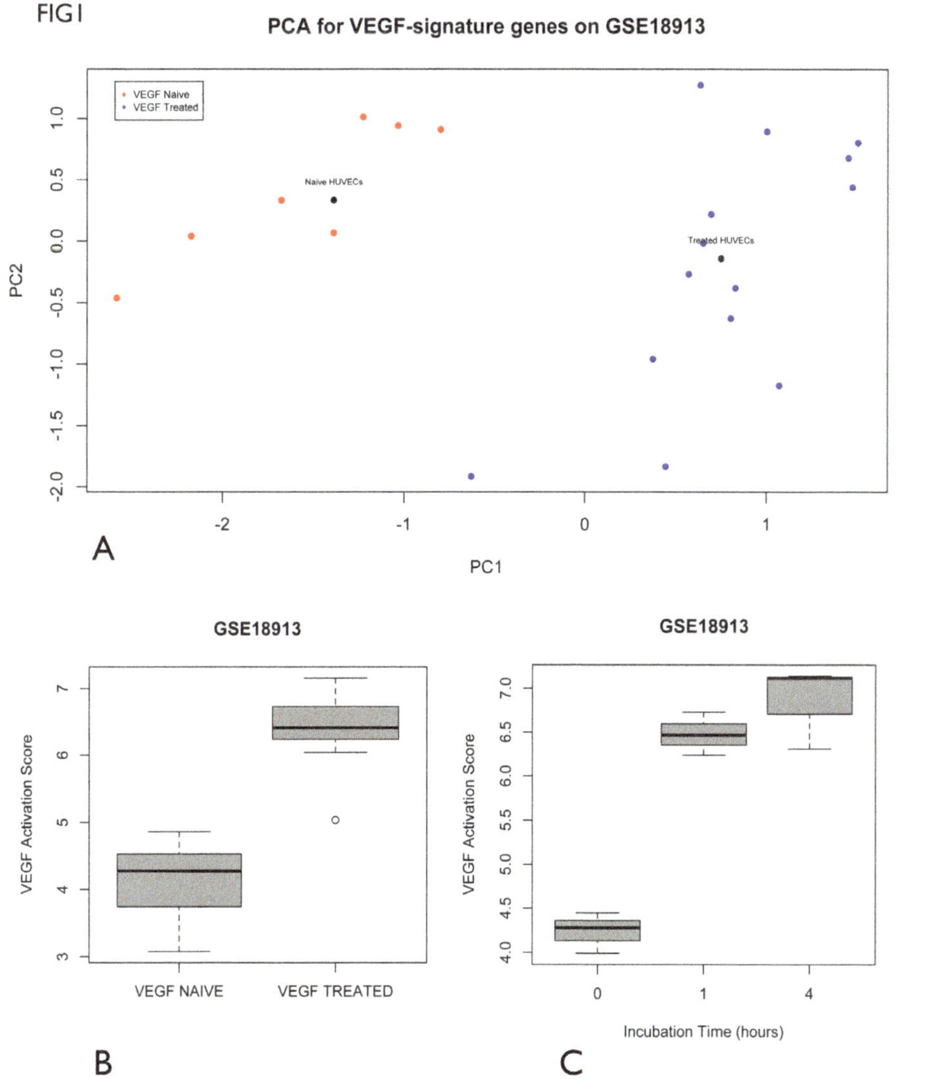

Fig. 1. Principal Component Analysis Plot (A) segregates VEGF-A treated cells versus untreated cells. The calculated activation scores were higher in treated cells versus untreated cells in an apparent time dependent way. (B+C)

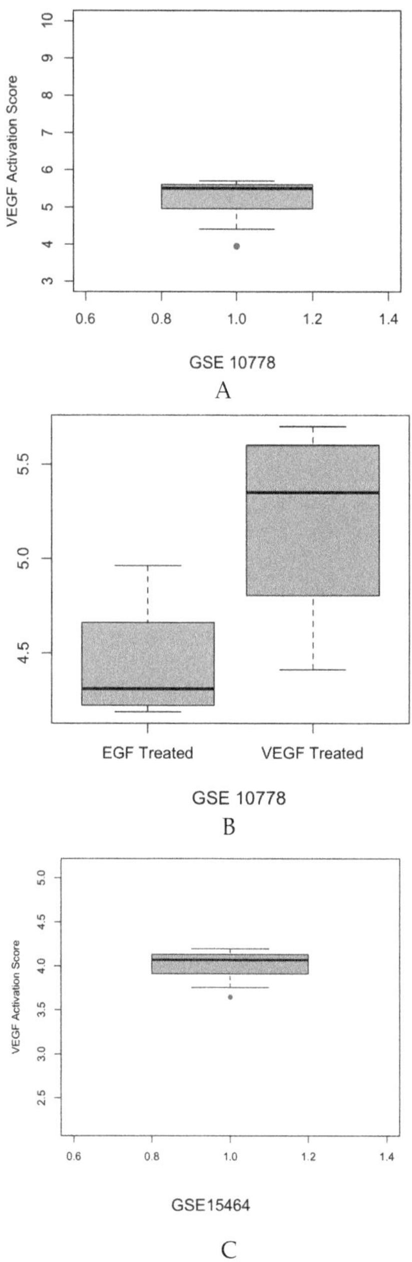

Fig. 2. Validation of the VEGF-A activation score methodology in data derived from two other experiments. The activation scores of VEGF-A treated cells were higher than the untreated condition (red dot). The higher activation scores were observed for VEGF-A treated cells but not for EGF treated cells, suggesting he specificity of the activation score for VEGF-A.

3. Patient datasets

A dataset of 285 patients (Melbourne dataset) was obtained though the Gene Expression Omnibus GEO database (GSE 9891) together with the clinical annotation data file. Only patients that had carcinomas of serous histology in advanced stages (III/IV) were included for analysis. Patients were selected that received platinum and taxane based chemotherapy. Other patients who did not receive chemotherapy or received only one agent, platinum or taxane, were also excluded. After this selection N=165 patients were eligible for further analysis. This dataset contained gene expression data derived from the Affymetrix U133_plus2 platform, which already underwent normalisation using the Robust Multiarray Averaging (RMA) method and subsequent filtering by excluding log expression values of <7 and a variance of <0.5. After filtering there were 8,732 probe sets left that are considered informative. Progression free survival was used in further analysis. (Tothill et al., 2008)

A second dataset GSE3149 N=153 (North Carolina dataset) with clinical data was also obtained from the GEO website. Here, the same criteria for patient selection were used. After selection N=107 were further analysed. The North Carolina dataset used the same Affymetrix U133_plus2 platform. The raw data were processed in Bioconductor in R software packages. Filtering was done by selecting expressions below a threshold (log 2 of 100) that are present in at least 25% of the arrayed samples. Normalisation was done using GC-Robust Multiarray Averaging. The number of probe sets that were informative was 7,741. Overall survival data was used, as there was no progression free survival data available. (Bild et al., 2006) A third dataset (Québec dataset) were patients (N=20) that were selected to be either chemoresistant versus chemosensitive. Here, raw microarray data based upon the Agilent platform Human 1A (v2) oligonucleotide microarray were normalised using the Lowess normalisation method. Hereafter, 16,096 genes were eligible for further analysis. Progression free survival data were used. RAW gene expression data is publicly available according to MIAME guidelines through the GEO database (Accession number: GSE 28739). (Bachvarov et al., 2006) A fourth dataset (Niigata Dataset-GSE 17260) contained samples that originated from patients who met the inclusion criteria from present study. Progression free survival data were available. The authors used the Agilent Whole Human Genome Oligo Microarray platform and normalised the data using upper quartile normalisation. 28,446 genes were found to be informative. (Yoshihara et al., 2010) A fifth and sixth dataset (Boston dataset A +B - GSE19829) were derived from a report studying BRCAness in ovarian cancer. (Konstantinopoulos et al., 2010) Progression free survival data was used. After selection, (N=26) and (N=36) patients were eligible. These datasets were RMA-normalised. 35252 and 5626 probe set ID's were informative after filtering. Gene expression data was derived from two platforms: the Affymetrix U133_plus2 platform and the Affymetrix 95UAv2.

4. Correlation of pathway activation scores with prognostic signatures

We applied the oncogenic pathways on the six datasets. These datasets together represent a total of N=464 advanced serous papillary carcinomas. A summary of these 6 datasets is listed in Table 1. Since these are selected oncogenic pathways, it is plausible that many significant correlations were found between pathway activations and the 3 prognostic

Dataset	N=464	Platform	Norma-lisation	Clinical outcome	Uniform treat-ment	Advanced stage/ serous papillary histology
Québec 2006	20	Agilent Human 1A (v2)	Lowess	PFS	yes	yes
North Carolina 2006	107	Affymetrix U133_plus2	GC-RMA	OS	yes	yes
Melbourne 2008	165	Affymetrix U133_plus2	RMA	PFS	yes	yes
Niigata 2010	110	Agilent Whole Human Genome Oligo Microarray	Upper quartile	PFS	yes	yes
Boston A 2010	26	Affymetrix U133_plus2	RMA	PFS	yes	yes
Boston B 2010	36	Affymetrix U95_A2	RMA	PFS	yes	yes

Table 1. A summary of datasets that were used in the meta-analysis.

Pearson Rho	WHR	IGS	GGI
Québec	0.65	0.62	0.67
	p=3.4 E-4	p=0.001	p=2.0 E-4
North Carol	0.81	0.89	0.6
	p=7.7 E-40	p=9.9 E-59	p=8.0 E-18
Melbourne	0.73	0.54	0.79
	p=2.8 E-22	p=6.9 E-11	p=5.6 E-28
Niigata	0.77	0.73	0.79
	p=2.4 E-19	1.0 E-22	p=4.5 E-25
Boston A	0.83	0.48	0.87
	p=1.2 E-7	p=0.013	p=5.5 E-9
Boston B	0.75	0.56	0.26
	p=1.8 E-7	p=3.7 E-4	p=0.13
Meta Analysis	0.73	0.62	0.79
	p<0.0001	p<0.0001	p<0.0001

Table 2. This shows the consistent correlations of the β-Catenin activation scores and WHR/IGS/GGI in each separate dataset (Québec, North Carolina, Melbourne, Niigata, Boston A and Boston B dataset). Overall Rho Coefficients were estimated by a meta-analysis approach using random models effects.

signatures (IGS, WHR and GGI). The β-Catenin pathway showed consistent and strong correlations. (Table 2) Since the six datasets were generated on different platforms with different methodologies, we estimated the overall effect of a pathway activation score by using a meta-analysis approach (Table 2). Similar meta-analysis of correlation coefficients showed that the BRCA, E2F1, EGFR, HER2, MYC, p53, p63 and PI3K showed steady correlations with the WHR, GGI and IGS. The RAS pathway and TGFβ pathway showed significant correlations with 2/3 prognostic signatures. Table 3 shows the overall correlation estimates, which were the most significant. While most pathway activation scores showed a positive correlation, the EGFR, HER2, p53 and TGFβ pathway showed a negative correlation.

Rho estimates	WHR	IGS	GGI
β-Catenin	0.73	0.62	0.79
	p<0.0001	p<0.0001	p<0.0001
BRCA	0.43	0.36	0.36
	p<0.0001	p<0.0001	p<0.0001
E2F1	0.51	0.42	0.54
	p<0.0001	p<0.0001	p<0.0001
EGFR	-0.52	-0.43	-0.42
	p<0.0001	p<0.0001	p<0.0001
HER2	-0.45	-0.5	-0.26
	p<0.0001	p<0.0001	p<0.0001
MYC	0.69	0.53	0.4
	p<0.0001	p<0.0001	p<0.0001
p53	-0.59	-0.42	-0.72
	p<0.0001	p<0.0001	p<0.0001
p63	0.46	0.29	0.36
	p<0.0001	p=0.001	p<0.0001
PI3K	0.43	0.33	0.29
	p<0.0001	p<0.0001	p=0.002
RAS	0.51	0.2	0.4
	p<0.0001	p=0.017	p<0.0001
TGFβ	-0.23	-0.3	-0.13
	p=0.0001	p<0.0001	p=0.004

Table 3. Estimates of Pearson rho correlation coefficients after meta-analysis of six datasets between pathway activation scores and prognostic gene signatures: wound healing response signature (WHR)/ Invasiveness gene signature IGS and Genomic grade Index (GGI). Most significant correlations are shown. (Threshold p-value adjusted for multiple testing=0.0025)

5. Association of pathway activation scores with survival outcome

While some pathways were associated with survival outcome in one or more datasets, they showed no or opposite result in another dataset. To estimate the overall survival effect of a given pathway, a similar meta-analysis approach was performed to estimate the overall

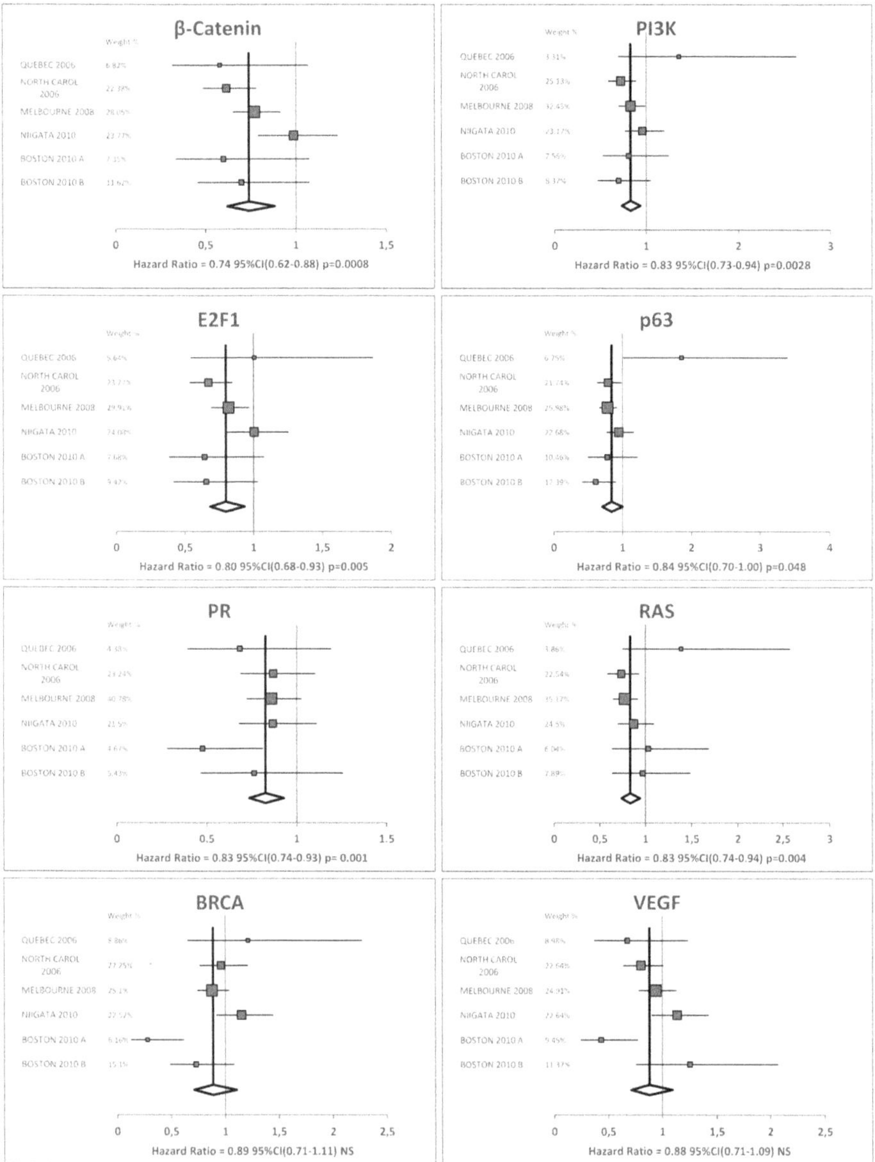

Fig. 3. Forest plots of meta-analysis using a random effects model of the β-Catenin BRCA, E2F1, p63, PR, PI3K, RAS and VEGF pathway.

effect of pathway activation using a random effects model. After this analysis, the β-Catenin, E2F1, PR, p63 PI3K and RAS pathway activation showed a significant association with clinical outcome. Considering the overall effect by means of Hazard Ratios, the β-Catenin pathway showed the most prominent effect after meta-analysis (HR= 0.74; 95%CI [0.62-0.88]). The survival analysis showed that the higher the activation of the β-Catenin pathway, the better the outcome was. Also for PR, E2F1, RAS, PI3K and p63 increased activation of respective pathway was associated with more favourable survival.

Because of these rather unexpected results, we calculated the activation scores of selected discovered pathways in other independent datasets as additional quality control to confirm whether the directions of the activation scores were certainly correct. For β-Catenin the

For the 3 prognostic signatures there was a tendency that a prognostic worse outcome predicted by IGS, WHR and GGI showed an unexpected higher probability of better clinical survival outcome. Further analysis in the Québec dataset showed that chemoresistant patients showed significant lower scores than chemosensitive patients and therefore may explain this finding.

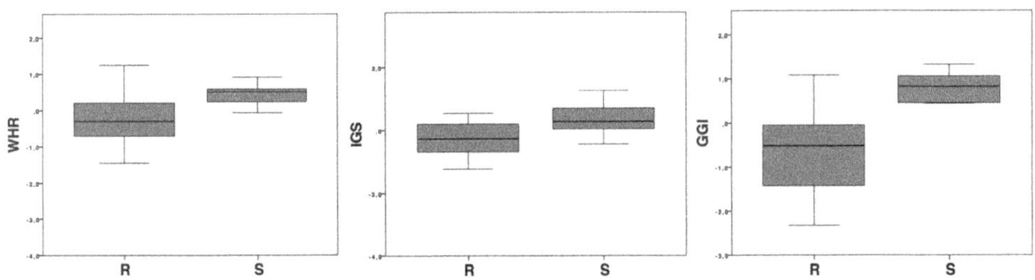

Fig. 4. In the Québec dataset sensitive (S) patients showed a higher genomic grade index (GGI) compared to chemoresistant patients (R) (p=0.002). Similarly chemosensitive patients showed a higher wound healing response score (p=0.02) and a higher invasiveness gene signature score (IGS) (p=0.06).

6. Discussion

Our initial analysis consisted of two datasets. The initial design was to use one dataset, as a discovery dataset while the other one would serve as a validation set. Since bioinformatical mislabelling errors/reproducibility issues have lead to withdrawal of papers of the same research group from which one dataset originated, we sought additional datasets to confirm our findings and render more power and reliability. (Bonnefoi et al., 2011; Potti et al., 2011) Furthermore, this research group and critical review by another research group have confirmed that the dataset that was used in the present meta-analysis was indeed correctly annotated. (Baggerly, Coombes, & Neeley, 2008; Dressman et al., 2007) With the availability of more datasets, we noticed variation among pathway's association with survival outcome. We therefore used a meta-analysis approach to estimate the overall effect. The advantage is that several studies can be combined despite differences in platforms and methodologies. This overall effect estimation takes into account the number of patients of each separate dataset and confidence interval in the estimation of correlation coefficient of survival hazard ratios. The heterogeneity among datasets (e.g. different patient selection criteria) may partly explain some opposite findings. The Québec dataset is different from others because this specifically selected patients to study differential expression between chemosensitive versus chemoresistant tumours. (Bachvarov et al., 2006) This dataset therefore may represent the extremities of this disease. Interestingly this dataset showed clearly that chemosensitive patients had tumours that were more likely to be of unfavourable outcome estimated by WHR/IGS/GGI. This contradictory finding may be explained by the finding that these three prognostic signatures are all primarily associated with increased proliferation. (Wirapati et al., 2008) It is known that chemosensitive tumours have higher tumour cell proliferation indexes in serous ovarian cancer. (Itamochi et al., 2002; Têtu et al., 2008) The estimated prognostic values in this survival analysis therefore seems strongly oppositely confounded by the predictive value for platinum/taxane-based chemotherapy.

Despite the heterogeneity in datasets and confounding of predictive value versus prognostic value, the E2F1, β-Catenin and the PI3K activation scores showed overall association with survival outcome ($p<0.01$) and consistent significant correlations with three prognostic signatures.

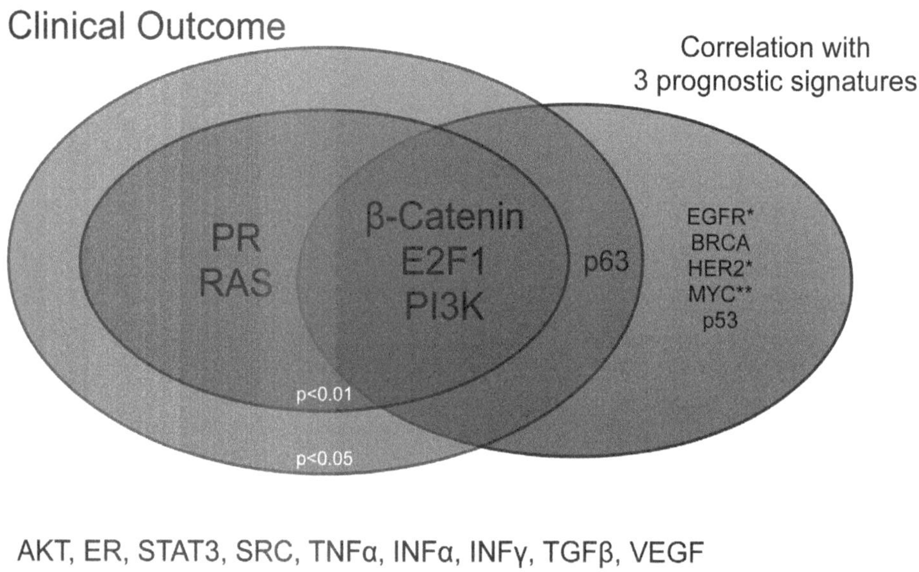

Fig. 5. A Venn diagram is showing combined results of the meta-analysis: β-Catenin, E2F1, p63 and PI3K activation scores showed significant association with survival and were significantly correlated with all three prognostic signatures (WHR/IGS/GGI) after meta-analysis. PR and RAS activation scores were associated with clinical outcome, but did not consistently correlate with prognostic signatures. *Negative correlation coefficient **borderline significance with clinical outcome

The E2F1 pathway a critical role in proliferation and apoptosis. It has been shown that transcription factor E2F1 interacts with the p53 and PI3K pathway. (Hallstrom, Mori, & Nevins, 2008; Reimer et al., 2006; 2007) Its role in ovarian cancer has been unclear, as other research groups have found similar favourable survival with increased E2F1 pathway activation (Hallstrom et al., 2008), while other findings have shown favourable survival with decreased *E2F1* gene expression by RT-PCR. (Reimer et al., 2006; 2007) It must be remarked that the latter study included an overrepresentation of patients with clear cell carcinomas (42.9%) and may be less informative here.

The β-Catenin protein is a multifunctional protein. It was originally discovered as a protein that is associated with the cytoplasmatic region of E-cadherin. E-cadherin is a transmembrane protein that is involved in cell-cell contact and cell's adhesive functions. Furthermore, β-Catenin is involved in Wnt signalling as a nuclear transcription factor and is believed to play a role in cancer stem cells. (Nusse, 2008) Loss of its membranous function or a higher nuclear presence has been linked with poor survival in several studies in ovarian cancer based upon immunohistochemical studies. (Faleiro-Rodrigues et al., 2004; Faleiro-Rodrigues, Macedo-Pinto, Pereira, & Lopes, 2004; Irving et al., 2005; 2005; Rosen et al., 2010; 2010; Stawerski et al., 2008; Stawerski, Wagrowska-Danilewicz, Stasikowska, Gottwald, & Danilewicz, 2008; Voutilainen et al., 2006; 2006) In addition, a correlation of β-Catenin protein expression has been described with tumour grade and Ki-67 expression. (Stawerski et al., 2008; Voutilainen et al., 2006) Present results are thus confirmative of earlier findings that β-Catenin is associated with survival outcome. The consideration must be made whether this effect is not attributed to its predictive value to platinum-taxane chemotherapy rather than its prognostic value. In present study, β-Catenin had strong and consistent correlation with IGS/WHR/GGI. Although these signatures were constructed based upon different oncogenic biological processes (wound healing, stem cell phenotype, grade), their major common force has been proven to be cell proliferation. (Wirapati et al., 2008) The observation that chemosensitive patients in present analysis showed significantly higher values of GGI, WHR and IGS renders credibility to this statement.

Similarly, the unexpected findings that increased activation of PI3K-, and RAS- pathways are more favourable for survival may be explained by their predictive value for chemotherapy. This hypothetically may have clinical consequences. Several compounds target the PI3K pathway or downstream effectors (e.g. mTOR) and are under early clinical development in epithelial ovarian cancer. Other compounds have inhibitory effects on the RAS pathway, e.g lonafarnib (a farnesyltransferase inhibitor). Recent findings of a randomised phase II trial (IGCS meeting 2010, W. Meier et al.) showed that the concomitant addition to standard chemotherapy (first line) and 6-month continuation of lonafarnib in primary epithelial ovarian cancer stage IIB-IV (n=105) resulted in borderline poorer outcome for the experimental- lonafarnib arm (overall survival HR=0.62 95CI%(0.36-1.06) p=0.08) or even resulted in significant unexpected worse outcome (p=0.01) in the experimental stratum of patients with suboptimal debulking. This finding may be relevant in the context of our results. Since increased activation of pathways as RAS and PI3K have been found to be favourable for survival outcome, the question should be asked whether inhibition of one of these pathways concomitant with chemotherapy is desirable. These pathways are driving forces of proliferation, which is an important factor in the efficacy of standard chemotherapeutics. We hypothesize that inhibition of these pathways may therefore also negatively affect the efficacy of these chemotherapies and theoretically induce chemoresistance. This would possibly be an explanation for the recent unexpected findings of lonafarnib in ovarian cancer. Hence, we theorize that these agents may have their potential in ovarian cancer in a sequential adjuvant setting rather than its concomitant combination with chemotherapy.

The PR pathway did not show any relevant association with IGS or GGI. It did show high significant association with survival outcome and WHR. Other immunohistochemical studies have shown that the PR protein expression has predictive of prognostic value, more than the expression of ER. (Hah et al., 2011; Høgdall et al., 2007; Tangjitgamol, Manusirivithaya, Khunnarong, Jesadapatarakul, & Tanwanich, 2009; X.-Y. Yang, Xi, K.-X. Yang, & Yu, 2009) Since PR expression is a downstream target of the ER pathway, this finding may indicate that an active ER pathway, rather than the expression of ER by itself may be of importance. Anti-hormonal therapies have shown anti-tumoural activity in relapsed/refractory ovarian cancer in phase II studies. (del Carmen et al., 2003; Papadimitriou et al., 2004; Smyth et al., 2007; C. J. Williams, 2001; C. Williams, Simera, & Bryant, 2010) Biomarker studies have shown that increasing ER expression was associated with increasing CA125 response rate. (Smyth et al., 2007) We suggest that further studies are needed to study if PR expression may add value as a suitable biomarker to select patients for anti-hormonal therapy in ovarian cancer.

7. Conclusions

To conclude, oncogenic pathway profiling of advanced serous ovarian tumours revealed that it is difficult to estimate the true prognostic value of a pathway since there seems confounding of predictive factors. Despite these biases, with a meta-analysis approach of 6 independent datasets generated on different micro-array platforms, we found that a PR and RAS activation score was associated with clinical outcome. Activation scores for β-Catenin, p63, E2F1 and PI3K were also associated with survival and were consistently correlated with three prognostic gene signatures.

8. References

Audeh, M. W., Carmichael, J., Penson, R. T., Friedlander, M., Powell, B., Bell-McGuinn, K. M., Scott, C., et al. (2010). Oral poly(ADP-ribose) polymerase inhibitor olaparib in patients with BRCA1 or BRCA2 mutations and recurrent ovarian cancer: a proof-of-concept trial *Lancet*, *376*(9737), 245–251. doi:10.1016/S0140-6736(10)60893-8

Bachvarov, D., L'esperance, S., Popa, I., Bachvarova, M., Plante, M., & Têtu, B. (2006). Gene expression patterns of chemoresistant and chemosensitive serous epithelial ovarian tumors with possible predictive value in response to initial chemotherapy *International journal of oncology*, *29*(4), 919–933.

Baggerly, K. A., Coombes, K. R., & Neeley, E. S. (2008). Run batch effects potentially compromise the usefulness of genomic signatures for ovarian cancer *Journal of clinical oncology : official journal of the American Society of Clinical Oncology*, *26*(7), 1186–7; author reply 1187–8. doi:10.1200/JCO.2007.15.1951

Bild, A. H., Yao, G., Chang, J. T., Wang, Q., Potti, A., Chasse, D., Joshi, M.-B., et al. (2006). Oncogenic pathway signatures in human cancers as a guide to targeted therapies. *Nature*, *439*(7074), 353–357. doi:10.1038/nature04296

Bonnefoi, H., Potti, A., Delorenzi, M., Mauriac, L., Campone, M., Tubiana-Hulin, M., Petit, T., et al. (2011). Retraction--Validation of gene signatures that predict the response of breast cancer to neoadjuvant chemotherapy: a substudy of the EORTC 10994/BIG 00-01 clinical trial *The lancet oncology*, *12*(2), 116. doi:10.1016/S1470-2045(11)70011-0

Burger, R. A., Brady, M. F., Bookman, M. A., Walker, J. L., Homesley, H. D., Fowler, J., Monk, B. J., et al. (2010). Phase III trial of bevacizumab (BEV) in the primary treatment of advanced epithelial ovarian cancer (EOC), primary peritoneal cancer (PPC), or fallopian tube cancer (FTC): A Gynecologic Oncology Group study. - ASCO. *Journal of Clinical Oncology, 28*(18s), suppl; abstr LBA1.

Cannistra, S. A. (2004). Cancer of the ovary. *The New England journal of medicine, 351*(24), 2519–2529. doi:10.1056/NEJMra041842

Chang, H. Y., Nuyten, D. S. A., Sneddon, J. B., Hastie, T., Tibshirani, R., Sørlie, T., Dai, H., et al. (2005). Robustness, scalability, and integration of a wound-response gene expression signature in predicting breast cancer survival. *Proceedings of the National Academy of Sciences of the United States of America, 102*(10), 3738–3743. doi:10.1073/pnas.0409462102

del Carmen, M. G., Fuller, A. F., Matulonis, U., Horick, N. K., Goodman, A., Duska, L. R., Penson, R., et al. (2003). Phase II trial of anastrozole in women with asymptomatic müllerian cancer *Gynecologic oncology, 91*(3), 596–602.

Dressman, H. K., Berchuck, A., Chan, G., Zhai, J., Bild, A., Sayer, R., Cragun, J., et al. (2007). An integrated genomic-based approach to individualized treatment of patients with advanced-stage ovarian cancer. *Journal of clinical oncology : official journal of the American Society of Clinical Oncology, 25*(5), 517–525. doi:10.1200/JCO.2006.06.3743

Faleiro-Rodrigues, C., Macedo-Pinto, I., Pereira, D., & Lopes, C. S. (2004). Loss of beta-catenin is associated with poor survival in ovarian carcinomas *International journal of gynecological pathology : official journal of the International Society of Gynecological Pathologists, 23*(4), 337–346.

Fong, P. C., Boss, D. S., Yap, T. A., Tutt, A., Wu, P., Mergui-Roelvink, M., Mortimer, P., et al. (2009). Inhibition of poly(ADP-ribose) polymerase in tumors from BRCA mutation carriers *The New England journal of medicine, 361*(2), 123–134. doi:10.1056/NEJMoa0900212

Fong, P. C., Yap, T. A., Boss, D. S., Carden, C. P., Mergui-Roelvink, M., Gourley, C., De Greve, J., et al. (2010). Poly(ADP)-ribose polymerase inhibition: frequent durable responses in BRCA carrier ovarian cancer correlating with platinum-free interval *Journal of clinical oncology : official journal of the American Society of Clinical Oncology, 28*(15), 2512–2519. doi:10.1200/JCO.2009.26.9589

Gatza, M. L., Lucas, J. E., Barry, W. T., Kim, J. W., Wang, Q., Crawford, M. D., Datto, M. B., et al. (2010). A pathway-based classification of human breast cancer. *Proceedings of the National Academy of Sciences, 107*(15), 6994–6999. doi:10.1073/pnas.0912708107

Hah, N., Danko, C. G., Core, L., Waterfall, J. J., Siepel, A., Lis, J. T., & Kraus, W. L. (2011). A Rapid, Extensive, and Transient Transcriptional Response to Estrogen Signaling in Breast Cancer Cells. *Cell, 145*(4), 622–634. Elsevier Inc. doi:10.1016/j.cell.2011.03.042

Hallstrom, T. C., Mori, S., & Nevins, J. R. (2008). An E2F1-dependent gene expression program that determines the balance between proliferation and cell death *Cancer cell, 13*(1), 11–22. doi:10.1016/j.ccr.2007.11.031

Hu, Z., Fan, C., Livasy, C., He, X., Oh, D. S., Ewend, M. G., Carey, L. A., et al. (2009). A compact VEGF signature associated with distant metastases and poor outcomes. *BMC medicine, 7*, 9. doi:10.1186/1741-7015-7-9

Høgdall, E. V. S., Christensen, L., Høgdall, C. K., Blaakaer, J., Gayther, S., Jacobs, I. J., Christensen, I. J., et al. (2007). Prognostic value of estrogen receptor and progesterone receptor tumor expression in Danish ovarian cancer patients: from the "MALOVA" ovarian cancer study *Oncology reports, 18*(5), 1051–1059.

Irving, J. A., Catasús, L., Gallardo, A., Bussaglia, E., Romero, M., Matias-Guiu, X., & Prat, J. (2005). Synchronous endometrioid carcinomas of the uterine corpus and ovary: alterations in the beta-catenin (CTNNB1) pathway are associated with independent primary tumors and favorable prognosis *Human pathology, 36*(6), 605–619. doi:10.1016/j.humpath.2005.03.005

Itamochi, H., Kigawa, J., Sugiyama, T., Kikuchi, Y., Suzuki, M., & Terakawa, N. (2002). Low proliferation activity may be associated with chemoresistance in clear cell carcinoma of the ovary *Obstetrics and gynecology, 100*(2), 281–287.

Konstantinopoulos, P. A., Spentzos, D., Karlan, B. Y., Taniguchi, T., Fountzilas, E., Francoeur, N., Levine, D. A., et al. (2010). Gene expression profile of BRCAness that correlates with responsiveness to chemotherapy and with outcome in patients with epithelial ovarian cancer. *Journal of clinical oncology : official journal of the American Society of Clinical Oncology, 28*(22), 3555–3561. doi:10.1200/JCO.2009.27.5719

Lauss, M., Ringnér, M., & Höglund, M. (2010). Prediction of stage, grade, and survival in bladder cancer using genome-wide expression data: a validation study. *Clinical cancer research : an official journal of the American Association for Cancer Research, 16*(17), 4421–4433. doi:10.1158/1078-0432.CCR-10-0606

Liu, R., Wang, X., Chen, G. Y., Dalerba, P., Gurney, A., Hoey, T., Sherlock, G., et al. (2007). The prognostic role of a gene signature from tumorigenic breast-cancer cells. *The New England journal of medicine, 356*(3), 217–226. doi:10.1056/NEJMoa063994

Mostertz, W., Stevenson, M., Acharya, C., Chan, I., Walters, K., Lamlertthon, W., Barry, W., et al. (2010). Age- and sex-specific genomic profiles in non-small cell lung cancer. *JAMA : the journal of the American Medical Association, 303*(6), 535–543. doi:10.1001/jama.2010.80

Nusse, R. (2008). Wnt signaling and stem cell control *Cell research, 18*(5), 523–527. doi:10.1038/cr.2008.47

Papadimitriou, C. A., Markaki, S., Siapkaras, J., Vlachos, G., Efstathiou, E., Grimani, I., Hamilos, G., et al. (2004). Hormonal therapy with letrozole for relapsed epithelial ovarian cancer. Long-term results of a phase II study *Oncology, 66*(2), 112–117. doi:10.1159/000077436

Potti, A., Dressman, H. K., Bild, A., Riedel, R. F., Chan, G., Sayer, R., Cragun, J., et al. (2011). Retraction: Genomic signatures to guide the use of chemotherapeutics *Nature medicine, 17*(1), 135. doi:10.1038/nm0111-135

Reimer, D., Sadr, S., Wiedemair, A., Goebel, G., Concin, N., Hofstetter, G., Marth, C., et al. (2006). Expression of the E2F family of transcription factors and its clinical relevance in ovarian cancer *Annals of the New York Academy of Sciences, 1091*, 270–281. doi:10.1196/annals.1378.073

Reimer, D., Sadr, S., Wiedemair, A., Stadlmann, S., Concin, N., Hofstetter, G., Müller-Holzner, E., et al. (2007). Clinical relevance of E2F family members in ovarian cancer--an evaluation in a training set of 77 patients *Clinical cancer research : an official journal of the American Association for Cancer Research, 13*(1), 144–151. doi:10.1158/1078-0432.CCR-06-0780

Rosen, D. G., Zhang, Z., Chang, B., Wang, X., Lin, E., & Liu, J. (2010). Low membranous expression of beta-catenin and high mitotic count predict poor prognosis in endometrioid carcinoma of the ovary *Modern pathology : an official journal of the*

United States and Canadian Academy of Pathology, Inc, *23*(1), 113–122. doi:10.1038/modpathol.2009.141

Smyth, J. F., Gourley, C., Walker, G., MacKean, M. J., Stevenson, A., Williams, A. R. W., Nafussi, A. A., et al. (2007). Antiestrogen therapy is active in selected ovarian cancer cases: the use of letrozole in estrogen receptor-positive patients *Clinical cancer research : an official journal of the American Association for Cancer Research*, *13*(12), 3617–3622. doi:10.1158/1078-0432.CCR-06-2878

Sotiriou, C., Wirapati, P., Loi, S., Harris, A., Fox, S., Smeds, J., Nordgren, H., et al. (2006). Gene expression profiling in breast cancer: understanding the molecular basis of histologic grade to improve prognosis *Journal of the National Cancer Institute*, *98*(4), 262–272. doi:10.1093/jnci/djj052

Stawerski, P., Wagrowska-Danilewicz, M., Stasikowska, O., Gottwald, L., & Danilewicz, M. (2008). Immunoexpression of beta-catenin--E-cadherin complex in primary serous ovarian tumors *Polish journal of pathology : official journal of the Polish Society of Pathologists*, *59*(1), 27–32.

Tangjitgamol, S., Manusirivithaya, S., Khunnarong, J., Jesadapatarakul, S., & Tanwanich, S. (2009). Expressions of estrogen and progesterone receptors in epithelial ovarian cancer: a clinicopathologic study *International journal of gynecological cancer : official journal of the International Gynecological Cancer Society*, *19*(4), 620–627. doi:10.1111/IGC.0b013e3181a44b62

Têtu, B., Popa, I., Bairati, I., L'esperance, S., Bachvarova, M., Plante, M., Harel, F., et al. (2008). Immunohistochemical analysis of possible chemoresistance markers identified by micro-arrays on serous ovarian carcinomas *Modern pathology : an official journal of the United States and Canadian Academy of Pathology, Inc*, *21*(8), 1002–1010. doi:10.1038/modpathol.2008.80

Tothill, R. W., Tinker, A. V., George, J., Brown, R., Fox, S. B., Lade, S., Johnson, D. S., et al. (2008). Novel molecular subtypes of serous and endometrioid ovarian cancer linked to clinical outcome. *Clinical cancer research : an official journal of the American Association for Cancer Research*, *14*(16), 5198–5208. doi:10.1158/1078-0432.CCR-08-0196

Trinh, X. B., Tjalma, W. A. A., Dirix, L. Y., Vermeulen, P. B., Peeters, D. J., Bachvarov, D., Plante, M., et al. (2011). Microarray-Based Oncogenic Pathway Profiling in Advanced Serous Papillary Ovarian Carcinoma. (S. K. Batra, Ed.)*PLoS ONE*, *6*(7), e22469. doi:10.1371/journal.pone.0022469.t003

Voutilainen, K. A., Anttila, M. A., Sillanpää, S. M., Ropponen, K. M., Saarikoski, S. V., Juhola, M. T., & Kosma, V.-M. (2006). Prognostic significance of E-cadherin-catenin complex in epithelial ovarian cancer *Journal of Clinical Pathology*, *59*(5), 460–467. doi:10.1136/jcp.2005.029876

Williams, C. J. (2001). Tamoxifen for relapse of ovarian cancer *Cochrane database of systematic reviews (Online)*, (1), CD001034. doi:10.1002/14651858.CD001034

Williams, C., Simera, I., & Bryant, A. (2010). Tamoxifen for relapse of ovarian cancer *Cochrane database of systematic reviews (Online)*, (3), CD001034. doi:10.1002/14651858.CD001034.pub2

Wirapati, P., Sotiriou, C., Kunkel, S., Farmer, P., Pradervand, S., Haibe-Kains, B., Desmedt, C., et al. (2008). Meta-analysis of gene expression profiles in breast cancer: toward a unified understanding of breast cancer subtyping and prognosis signatures *Breast cancer research : BCR*, *10*(4), R65. doi:10.1186/bcr2124

Yang, X.-Y., Xi, M.-R., Yang, K.-X., & Yu, H. (2009). Prognostic value of estrogen receptor and progesterone receptor status in young Chinese ovarian carcinoma patients *Gynecologic oncology*, *113*(1), 99–104. doi:10.1016/j.ygyno.2008.12.018

Yoshihara, K., Tajima, A., Yahata, T., Kodama, S., Fujiwara, H., Suzuki, M., Onishi, Y., et al. (2010). Gene expression profile for predicting survival in advanced-stage serous ovarian cancer across two independent datasets. *PLoS ONE*, *5*(3), e9615. doi:10.1371/journal.pone.0009615

9

Sensitive Detection of Epithelial Ovarian Cancer Biomarkers Using Tag-Laser Induced Breakdown Spectroscopy

Yuri Markushin and Noureddine Melikechi*
Optical Science Center for Applied Research,
Delaware State University
USA

1. Introduction

Epithelial ovarian cancer (EOC) is the 5th leading cause of death from cancer in women and the main cause of death from gynecological cancer (Barber, 1986). Women have a lifetime risk of ovarian cancer of around 1.5%, which makes it the second most common gynecologic malignancy after breast cancer. Ovarian cancer is often referred to as 'the silent killer' because it frequently causes non-specific symptoms, which contribute to diagnostic delay, diagnosis in a late stage and a poor prognosis. This is one of the reasons for the relatively low, approximately 40%, 5-year survival rate for women diagnosed with advanced EOC. However, when EOC is diagnosed at an early stage this rate increases up to 95% (McGuire *et al.*, 2000). This enhancement demonstrates that early detection of EOC is crucial and it is vital to develop novel diagnostic methods for higher throughput screening of human samples and new biomarkers discovery.
One of the important and promising strategies for early cancer diagnosis relies on the development of approaches that can provide accurate detection and identification of specific protein-biomarkers in the serum. These protein-biomarkers would be measured and monitored to yield specific signatures that can be used for the early detection of the disease. Recently, numerous reports demonstrated that a *single* biomarker (example: CA 125, biomarker of ovarian cancer) approach is highly unlikely to yield results that can accurately distinguish cancer samples from healthy ones. This led researchers to explore the idea of using a *basket* of biomarkers (Petricoin *et al.*, 2002; Mor *et al.*, 2005) with the expectation that this approach may yield increased specificity and sensitivity for cancer detection. Using this approach, G. Mor *et al.* reported 95% efficiency discrimination between disease-free and EOC patients, including patients diagnosed with stage I and II disease (Mor *et al.*, 2005). These authors used a blood test, based on the simultaneous identification of four biomarkers: leptin, prolactin, osteopontin, and insulin-like growth factor-II. Petricoin *et al.* reported the use of mass spectroscopy to develop a classifier that could identify serum from patients with ovarian cancer with 100% sensitivity and 95% specificity (Petricoin *et al.*, 2002). In a follow up study, Zhu *et al.* reported similar results (Zhu, 2003). However, questions were raised about tests reproducibility and reliability (Wagner, 2003; Garber,

* Corresponding Author

2004). Despite this roller coaster, the need for the development of high-throughput methods and multiplexing assays for the simultaneous detection of multiple analytes is real (Rubenstein, 2010).

Several approaches addressing the development of multiplexing assays have been reported in recent years. C.A. Mirkin *et al.* proposed using oligonucleotides as barcodes (DNA barcode) and nano-particles aggregates that can alter their physical properties (e.g. optical, electrical, mechanical) upon aggregation (Mirkin *et al.*, 2005). The simultaneous measurement of serum proteins and sequence-specific oligonucleotide probes by employing 16 sets of fluorescent microspheres and a flow cytometer has been demonstrated (Fulton *et al.*, 1997). Recently, flow injection inductively coupled plasma mass-spectrometry and macrocyclic metal chelate complexes loaded with different lanthanides have also been used to detect several model peptides and protein (Ahrends *et al.*, 2007). Further, application of multicolor quantum dots for molecular diagnostics of cancer was reported (Smith *et al.*, 2006) and barcodes striped metal nanoparticles were used to provide multiplexed data in various bioassays (Freeman *et al.*, 2005).

Many of the multiplex assays developed recently are based on antigen induced particle aggregation (Gosling *et al.*, 1990). Therefore, it is important to strive to better understand the aggregation mechanism. Various systems have been employed to study the aggregation process. Examples include lipid vesicles (Farbman-Yogev *et al.*, 1998) and metal/metalloid particles (Freeman *et al.*, 2005; Smith *et al.*, 2006). A simplified vesicle aggregation theory was developed (Farbman-Yogev *et al.*, 1998). This theory deals primarily with vesicles made of biotinylated lipid molecules. The presence of streptavidin molecules induces aggregation (flocculation). The vesicles are made of amphiphilic molecules combined to form shell-like bilayer structures. Therefore, the bonds between lipids and vesicles can be weaker than bonds between biotins on lipids and streptavidin molecules in a solution. This theory predicts the dissociation of initial cross-linked molecules from the vesicles and their re-aggregation into preferably smaller aggregates (Farbman-Yogev *et al.*, 1998).

Particle based immuno-assays have been reviewed in a number of publications (Gosling *et al.*, 1990; Smith *et al.*, 2006). Metal and metalloid particles are typically modified with the IgG molecules, which are strongly (irreversibly) attached to the surface. The presence of antigen molecules induces aggregation. In contrast to lipid vesicles, solid-state particles are unlikely to lose the cross-linked molecules and the particle aggregates are more stable (Farbman-Yogev *et al.*, 1998). From this perspective, the metal and metalloid nano- and micro-particles seem more appropriate for developing effective immuno-assays.

2. Tagging specific proteins: Multi-element coded nano- and micro-particle assay

As discussed above, multiplexing combined with particle-based assay provides an effective and promising approach for developing diagnostics. After thorough consideration of advantages and disadvantages of the existing technologies briefly described above, we present a novel type of assay on a base of multi-element coded nano- and micro-particle tags and Laser-Induced Breakdown Spectroscopy (LIBS) as a detection method (Meelikechi and Markushin, patent pending). This approach, developed in our laboratory, relies on the use of nano- and micro-particles composed of different chemical elements to yield single and multi-element code for labeling of the molecules of interest.

To illustrate this approach, we show in Figure 1 a schematic of the multi-element coded nano- and micro-particle based assay composed of *2 elements: Si and Fe*. To perform immunoassay we used ovarian cancer biomarkers *Leptin and CA 125* with pairs of relevant monoclonal antibodies. Monoclonal antibodies were biotinylated prior to performing the assay. To mimic blood conditions, all buffers contained about 5% of bovine serum albumin (BSA) (Majoor, 1946). For separation of single and aggregated particles we used test tubes equipped with 5 µm pore size filters or magnetizing.

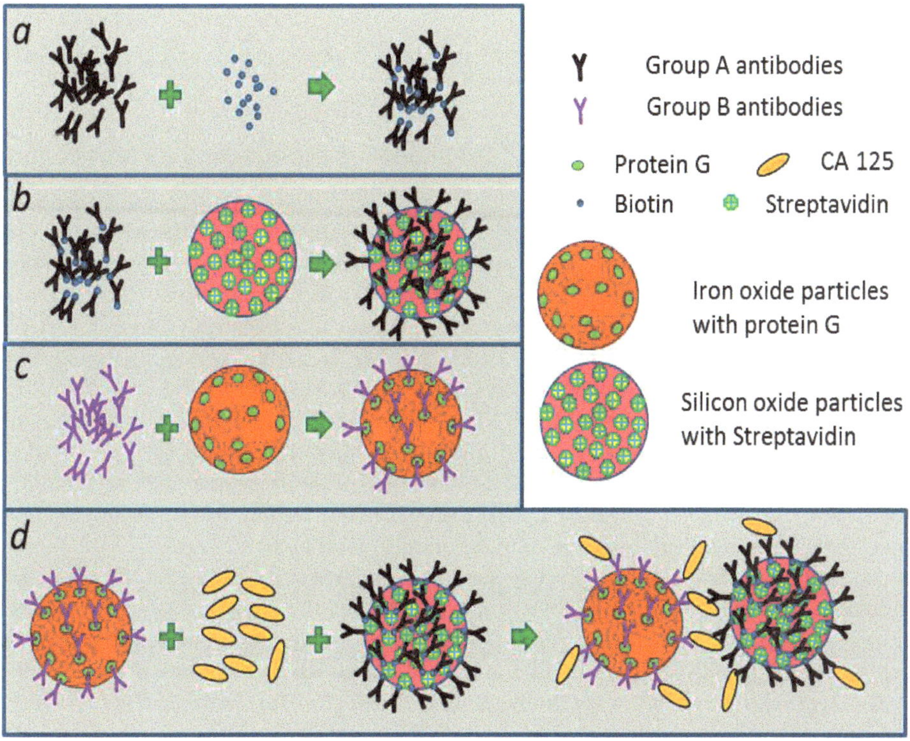

Fig. 1. Tag-LIBS experimental schematics. **Step a** – biotinylation of the group A antibodies (M86429M); **step b** – attaching biotinylated group A antibodies (M86429M) to silicon oxide particles modified with streptavidin (suspension B); **step c** – attaching of the group B antibodies (M86306M) to iron oxide particles modified with protein G (suspension A); **step d** - incubation (following by magnetizing and washing) of the mixture of suspensions A and B with various concentrations of CA 125.

Many optical detection techniques developed to perform assays are based on the use of fluorescent tags (Zal and Gascoignea, 2004). Although these techniques have many advantages, they often suffer from photo bleaching and it is therefore advantageous and useful to explore the development of approaches that do not suffer from such a limitation. To do this, it is useful to note that there is a broad class of materials (metals and non-metals), which are neither fluorescent nor effectively chemically active. These materials can be combined to yield composites that can also be used as tags. This provides a large number of possibilities: combining only 11 of such materials (i.e. iron, gold, silver, platinum, aluminum, copper, titanium, nickel, zinc, tin and copper) into micro- and nano-particles can yield more than 1000 types of different composite particles, some of which are well known alloys such as brass (copper and zinc), bronze (copper and tin), and duralumin (aluminum and copper). Each of these alloys and composites is unique by chemical content and potentially can be used as micro-tags for labeling and detection of ovarian cancer biomarkers.

Below we provide examples of the use of the multi-element coded particle assay for the detection of analytes.

3. Reading the tags: Laser induced-breakdown spectroscopy for early cancer diagnosis

Following the sample preparation described in the previous section, we focus our discussion on the detection of the micro- and/or nano-particles attached to the specific biomarkers of interest. To perform this step, we use an all-optical technique widely used in many applications ranging from space exploration to quality control but only rarely for medical applications. This technique, known as Laser Induced Breakdown Spectroscopy (LIBS) is well described in the literature and only a brief description is provided in this chapter. For more information, we refer the reader to the excellent body of literature available (Cremers and Radziemski, 2006, Miziolek *et al.* 2006, and Markushin *et al.*, 2009).

LIBS is an analytical technique based on the use of laser pulses intense enough to breakdown the chemical bonds of the constituents of a sample to be interrogated. The experimental arrangement used in our laboratory is shown in Figure 2. By focusing nanosecond long laser pulses onto a sample, a short-lived plasma of the sample is generated. These laser pulses ablate a small quantity of the sample - a few hundreds of nanograms - located on an automated 3-D translational stage. Light emitted by the plasma during cooling is collected by a bundle of optical fibers, which transmits it to a 7-channel Ocean Optics LIBS HR2000+ spectrometer (190 - 970 nm) for analysis. The 10 nsec Q-switched Nd-YAG laser (BM Industries Serie 5000) operating at 1064 nm was used for the sample ablation. About 100 laser shots on 100 different spots on a filter were used to collect the LIBS spectra. For the purpose of this investigation, we used average laser pulse energies of about 70 mJ/pulse, a double convex BK7 focusing lens with a focal length of 70 mm and antireflection coating for 1064 nm was positioned at about 61.7 mm distance from the surface of the filter. LIBS spectra were obtained at ambient atmospheric conditions. To identify the measured atomic and ionic lines, we use the LIBS spectral database developed by our group (OSCAR website, n.d., Rock *et al.*, 2008). Potentially, the multi-element coded assay is able to detect and identify numerous analytes in parallel with minimum interference. This method has the added advantage of requiring as little as a few micro liters of serum specimen. More details of the experiment can be found elsewhere (Markushin *et al.*, 2009, Rock *et al.*, 2008).

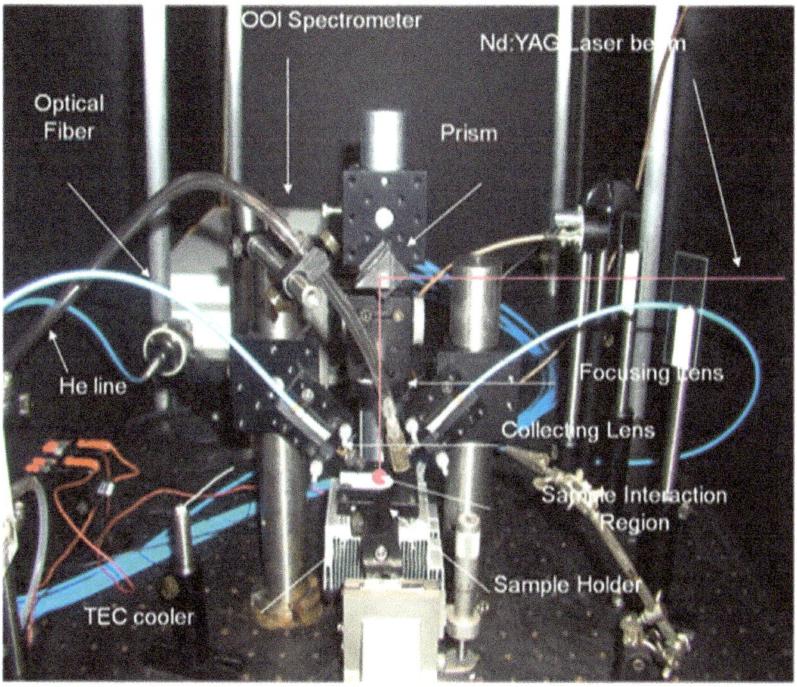

Fig. 2. LIBS experimental set-up consisting of a Nd-YAG Laser pulse laser, prism, focusing lens, bundle of light collecting optical fibers, thermoelectric cooler (TEC), a Helium line and the Ocean Optics 7-channel spectrometer (OOI spectrometer).

To implement the multi-element coded approach and demonstrate its potential, we prepared and analyzed two-element composite particles (Markushin *et al.*, 2009). We used 1.5 μm iron oxide biotinylated particles and 3 μm silicon particles with attached avidin. First, two types of control experiments (experiments #1 and # 3) were performed. In control experiments we checked for the possibility of nonspecific binding of iron oxide biotinylated particles to the plastic lab ware components (LIBS spectrum of experiment # 1 on Fig. 3a, 3b). Nonspecific binding was found to be insignificant. In another control experiment, # 3, (Fig. 3a, 3b) iron oxide biotinylated particles were pre-incubated with an excess of avidin molecules that allowed neutralizing the biotin groups of iron oxide particles with avidin. The following incubation of the neutralized iron oxide particles with Si-avidin particles and LIBS analysis demonstrates that nonspecific interactions between both types of micro-particles are limited. Some portion of silicon particles with probably bigger than the 3 μm particle size can be trapped by 5 μm pore size filter (short-dashed line on Fig. 3a, 3b). This was confirmed by additional control experiment with filtering of the 3μm size silicon particles over 5 μm pore size filters (data not shown).

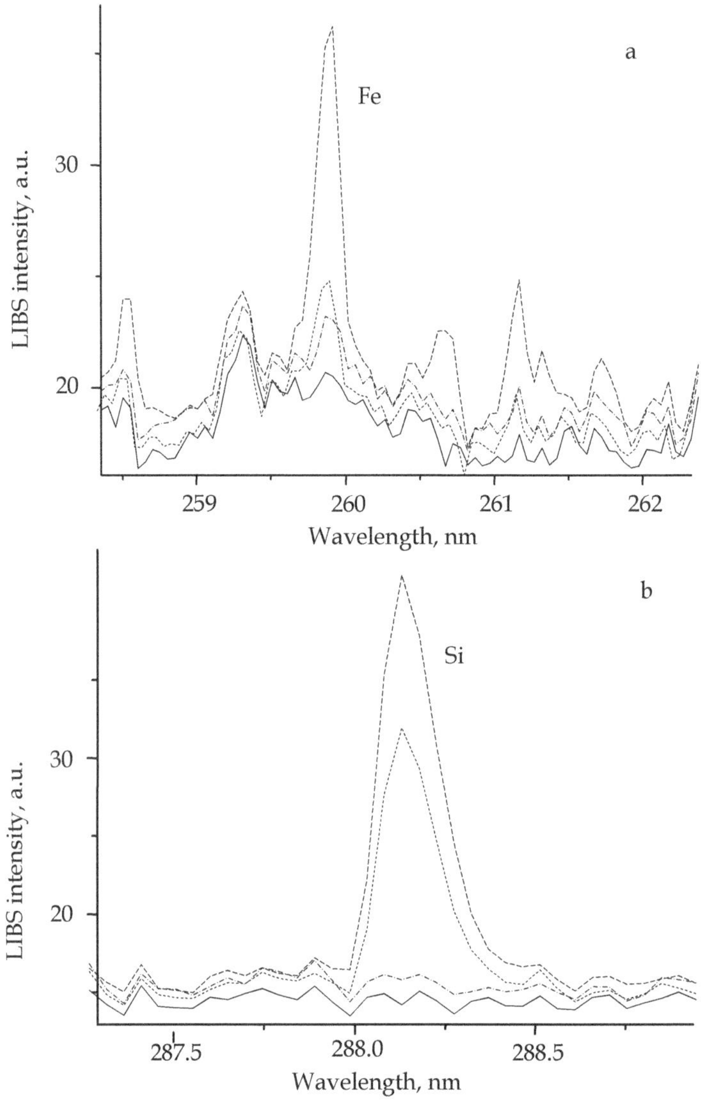

Fig. 3. LIBS based identification of two-element Fe-Si composite micro-particles. The fragment of the LIBS spectrum around 288.1 nm Si line (a). The fragment of the LIBS spectrum around 259.9 mn Fe line (b). Solid line – empty filter, dot-dashed line - experiment # 1, dashed line - experiment # 2, short-dashed lines - experiment # 3 (adapted from (Markushin *et al.*, 2009))

The two-element coded composite micro-particles were prepared by allowing the iron oxide biotinylated particles to interact with the silicon particles modified by avidin (experiment # 2). We monitored the amount of aggregates by taking 140 laser shots at the surface of 5 μm pore size centrifuge filters. After overnight incubation the filtrate with unbound micro-particles was removed by centrifuging over 5 μm pore size filters, then the top part of the test tube was cut off and the bottom part with the particles being left on a filter (residue particles) was checked by LIBS for the presence of Fe and Si elements (dashed line on Fig. 3a, 3b). The presence of both Fe (259.9 nm) and Si (288.1 nm) emission lines in the same sample proves that we generated the two-element coded composite micro-particles. Thus, the ability of LIBS to detect the presence and composition of the micro-particles is demonstrated. Further, we suggest that this technique can be employed as a detection method for the future element coded assay development.

Sensitivity is a key factor of any analytical method. To determine the sensitivity of the element-coded approach, we used the model protein avidin. We performed detection and quantification of avidin molecules using LIBS based iron oxide micro-particle assay (Fig. 4). The details of the experiment can be found elsewhere (Markushin *et al.*, 2009, Rock *et al.*, 2008). 1.5 μm iron oxide micro-particles coated with biotin were purchased from Bangs Laboratories and their aggregation was induced upon the addition of avidin. We monitored the amount of aggregates by using 140 laser shots at the surface of 5 μm pore size centrifuge filters after removing the filtrate with non-bound micro-particles. Figure 4 shows the avidin concentration dependence of the LIBS based intensity of Fe emission line at 259.9 nm integrated over the filter surface. The iron oxide micro-particle assay demonstrated limit-of-detection about 30 ppb of avidin. This Figure has a significant maximum at about 155 ppb and is discussed below.

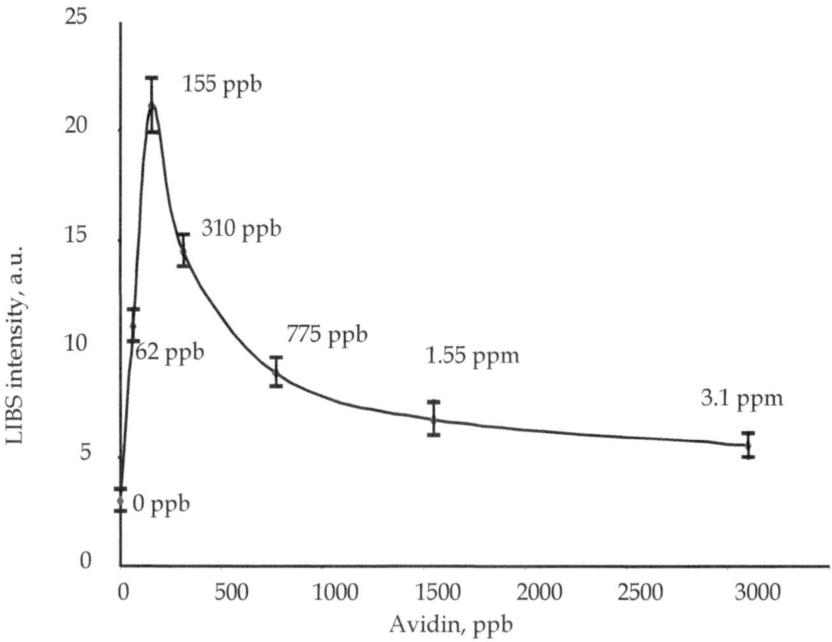

Fig. 4. Avidin concentration dependence of the micro- particles aggregation (adapted from (Markushin *et al.*, 2009))

We employed the element coded LIBS based approach for the detection of biomarker CA 125. For this particular measurement, we express the concentration of CA 125 in International Units (IU or U) per milliliter. Typically these units are used for quantification of biologically active substances (e.g. CA 125) instead of grams or moles (World Health Organization (WHO) Expert Committee on Biological Standardization, n.d.) According to the WHO Expert Committee on Biological Standardization, an International Unit is the specific biological activity of a substance, i.e. the quantity of a biologically active molecules required to produce a defined response. The use of such internationally accepted units ensures that biologically active substances with the same measured response will contain the same quantity expressed in International Units.

We also used the two-element micro-particle coding method to detect ovarian cancer biomarker CA 125. To do this, we prepared two bio-suspensions for groups A and B IgG antibody tagging (Fig. 1). In suspension B the biotinylated group A antibodies were immobilized to the silicon oxide micro particles with streptavidin. In suspension A the group B antibodies were immobilized through their Fc (fragment crystallizable region) fragments to iron oxide micro particles modified with immunoglobulin-binding protein G. Protein G mediates attachment of antibodies to the micro-particles and ensures the proper orientation of IgG molecules for the better immuno-assay efficiency (Bjorck & Kronvall, 1984). The buffer used contained 5% of BSA to mimic blood conditions (Majoor, 1946).

The following is a step-by-step description of the two-element micro-particle coding assay. To perform the analysis on the presence of CA 125 in a solution we follow the following procedure:

Step 1. the monoclonal antibodies M86429M were biotinylated prior to doing assay. EZ-Link Sulfo-NHS-Biotinylation Kit (Pierce Biotechnology, Inc.) was used for this purpose. PBS buffer used for dilutions contained 5% of BSA to mimic blood conditions (Fig 1 a).

Step 2. we prepared suspension B: the 1 μm silicon oxide particles (Bangs Laboratories, Inc.) modified with streptavidin were added to the biotinylated monoclonal antibodies M86429M solution for overnight incubation at 4° C (Fig 1 b). Following incubation, unbound IgG molecules were washed away by three wash-centrifugation cycles using spin-filters with a pore size about 100 nm (Millipore).

Step 3. we prepared suspension A by adding the 1.5 μm iron oxide particles (Polysciences, Inc.) modified with protein G to the monoclonal antibodies M86306M solution for overnight incubation at 4° C (Fig 1 c).

Step 4. CA 125 solutions of defined concentrations were added to mixtures of suspension A and suspension B taken in equal volumes and were incubated and shaken 4 hours at room temperature and overnight at 4° C, then were stored at 4° C. For the control experiment the PBS buffer with 5% of BSA (no CA 125) was added to a mixture of suspension A and suspension B and were incubated and shaken 4 hours at room temperature and overnight at 4°C then were stored at 4° C.

Unbound silicon oxide particles and dissolved CA 125 molecules were separated from unbound iron oxide particles and aggregates of iron oxide and silicon oxide particles by using strong magnets (residual flux density about 14.5-14.8 KGs (K&J Magnetics, Inc. website, n.d.). The separation-washing cycles were repeated 3 times.

After completing magnetizing and pipetting, the top part of the test tubes was cut off and the bottom filters with particles deposited on it (residue particles) were checked by LIBS for the presence of Si elements.

To obtain better sensitivity, we employed the magnetizing type of assay. In this approach, following the incubation, the unbound molecules, the single silicon particles, the single iron oxide particles and particle aggregates were separated using strong magnets. After completing steps of magnetizing and pipetting, the residue particles left on the filters were analyzed using LIBS for the presence of silicon. Fig. 5 shows the fragment of LIBS spectra around 288.1 nm silicon emission line obtained by the two-element (Si and Fe) Tag-LIBS assay for detection of CA 125 biomarker. The control lowest black line on Fig. 5 was obtained from the empty filter. The red line curve is a LIBS spectrum of control sample where instead of CA 125 the buffer was added. Other lines represent various concentrations of CA 125 in a solution (see Fig. 5). The presence of some Si in the control sample is possibly caused by non-specific interaction of micro-particles.

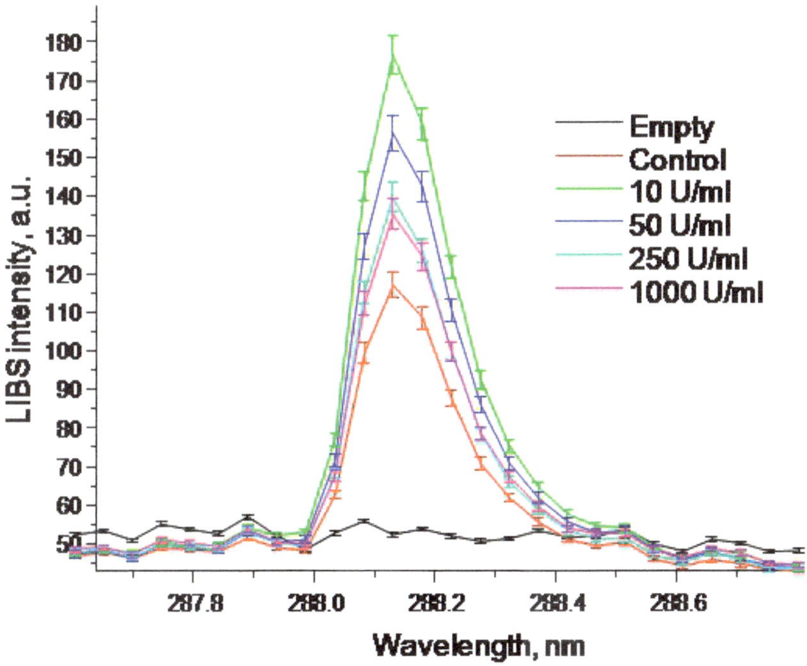

Fig. 5. The fragment of LIBS spectra around 288.1 nm silicon emission line in the two-element (Si and Fe) Tag-LIBS assay for detection of CA 125. The black line represents LIBS of the empty filter. Other lines represent various concentrations of CA 125 in a solution: red line - control sample with no CA 125, green line - 10 U/ml, blue line - 50 U/ml, light blue line - 250 U/ml, pink line - 1000 U/ml.

Figure 6 shows the experimental results of the ovarian biomarker CA 125 detection by the two-element (Fe and Si) Tag-LIBS assay in a blood mimicking PBS buffer. The curve on Fig. 6 represents the CA 125 concentration dependence of the intensity of Si emission line at about 288.1 nm obtained by Tag-LIBS assay. The experimental curve has a maximum at about 10 U/ml and will be discussed later in comparison with results of other experiments.

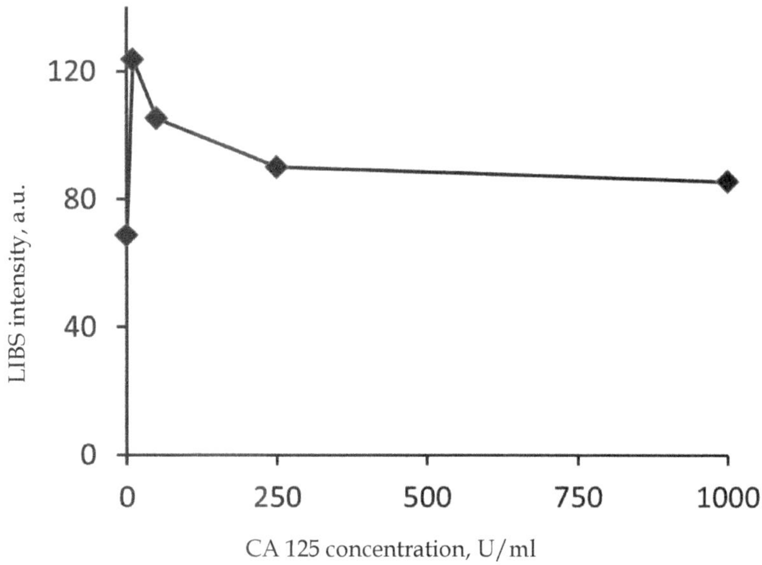

Fig. 6. Detection of ovarian cancer biomarker CA 125 by two-element (Si and Fe) micro-particle Tag-LIBS assay. The curve represents the LIBS intensity of Si emission line in the two-element Tag-LIBS assay at the various concentrations of CA 125.

The two-element (Si-Fe) coded Tag-LIBS assay has been used to analyze the ovarian cancer biomarker Leptin. Leptin, IgG monoclonal antibodies H86901M (Group A) and IgG H86412M (Group B) monoclonal antibodies to Leptin were purchased from Biodesign International. Monoclonal antibodies H86901M and H86412M were biotinylated prior to doing assay. EZ-Link Sulfo-NHS-Biotinylation Kit (Pierce Biotechnology, Inc.) was used for this purpose.

Equal amount of 3 μm silicon oxide particles (Kisker Biotech GmbH) and 1.5 μm iron oxide particles (Bangs Laboratories, Inc.) were added to pre-mixed solution of defined concentration of Leptin and equal concentrations of IgG monoclonal antibodies H86901M and IgG monoclonal antibodies H86412M for 3 hour incubation at room temperature and overnight at 4° C. Using strong magnets and residual particles on filters assayed, single and aggregated particles were separated. We monitored the amount of aggregates in a similar way like it was described earlier.

The intensity of the silicon emission line at about 288.1 nm as a function of the concentration of Leptin is shown in Fig. 7 for two independent Tag-LIBS experiments (marked with squares and diamonds) performed over with a one-month interval. The reproducibility is about 20-30%. The trend line of linear least-square approximation is shown on the figure and so is the R-squared coefficient, which is about 0.949. The ascending part of the Tag-LIBS assay curve was from 10 to ~ 400 μg/ml. In contrast with CA 125 Tag-LIBS assay (Fig. 6) the local maximum feature of the calibration curve for Leptin assay has not been determined in the range of concentrations investigated. The presence of Leptin at the level of 11μg/ml has been detected by Tag-LIBS approach.

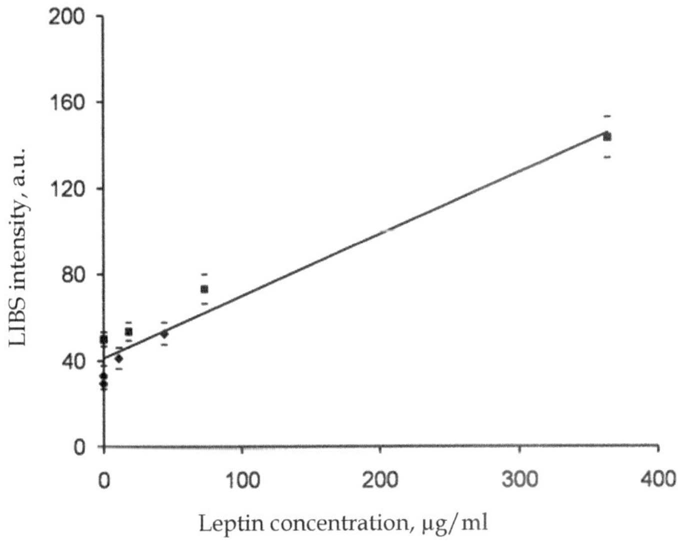

Fig. 7. Detection of ovarian cancer biomarker Leptin by two-element (Si and Fe) micro-particle Tag-LIBS assay in two independent experiments (squares and diamonds) with an interval of one month. Solid line is obtained by the linear least squares approximation.

To ensure the applicability of the Tag-LIBS approach to the clinical environment the human fluid with bio-molecules of interest has to be checked. Blood is an extremely complex solution composed of plasma with dissolved proteins and blood cells (Cohn, 1948). Therefore, human blood plasma and model molecular pair avidin-biotin were chosen to test the Tag-LIBS approach for future clinical applications. To maintain homogeneity and equivalent conditions for all samples the human blood plasma after thawing has been filtered over centrifugal filter with relatively big pore size about 5 μm.

Two types of particles were used for the assay, i.e. 50 nm gold nano-particles and 1.5 μm iron oxide micro-particles. Due to significant differences in size and taking into account the densities of gold and iron (we used density of iron instead of combined iron and iron oxide density of particle for simplicity), every microgram of gold particles counted for approximately $1.4 \cdot 10^9$ nano-particles and every microgram of iron oxide particles included about $1.8 \cdot 10^5$ micro-particles. Furthermore, the total surface area of 1 μg of gold particles was about $6.2 \cdot 10^6$ μm^2 in comparison with about $7.1 \cdot 10^5$ μm^2 total surface area of 1 μg of iron oxide particles. Thus, to balance the surface areas of the two types of particles, we took about 10 times more iron oxide particles (by weight) than gold particles. In addition, the concentration of biotin molecules attached to the nano-particles was chosen to be greater than the concentration of avidin. Under these conditions, the molecules of avidin are less likely to compete for the binding sites, which yields enhanced detection limit.

Results shown in Fig. 8 demonstrate the ability of the Tag-LIBS approach to detect model molecules avidin in human blood plasma. Tag-LIBS analysis has been performed with a series of dilutions with the following final concentrations of avidin: 0 ppb, 6 ppb, 64 ppb, 322 ppb, 644 ppb, 1483 ppb, 2321 ppb, 3224 ppb, and 6448 ppb (curves 0 - 8, Fig. 8). The spectrum of the empty filter was subtracted from the sample spectra. To enhance the clarity and viewing of the gold emission peak intensities at 280.2 nm, the sample spectra are slightly shifted along the Y-axis (Fig. 8). Data of three Tag-LIBS experiments were averaged to plot the control curve (curve 0, Fig. 8). The lowest 6 ppb concentration of model protein avidin was measured by Tag-LIBS approach in human blood plasma with about 8:1 signal-to-noise ratio (curve 1, Fig. 8).

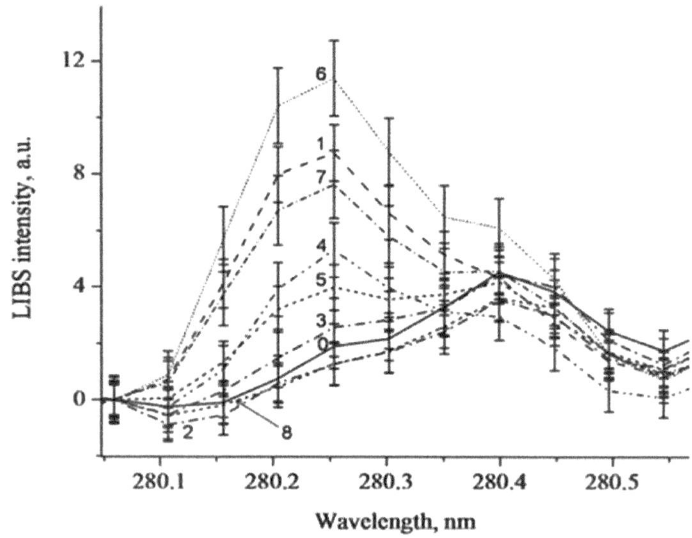

Fig. 8. The fragment of background subtracted LIBS spectra around 280.2 nm Gold emission line in the two-element (Au and Fe) Tag-LIBS assay for detection of avidin in human blood plasma. Concentration of avidin: 0 - 0 ppb (control sample), 1 - 6 ppb, 2 - 64 ppb, 3 - 322 ppb, 4 - 644 ppb, 5 - 1483 ppb, 6 - 2321 ppb, 7 - 3224 ppb, 8 - 6448 ppb.

Clearly it is important to maintain, and possibly enhance, the analytical sensitivity of an assay while at the same time obtain detection limits that are comparable or better than the current attainable. For the CA 125 biomarker the normal level has been previously determined, e.g. Niloff *et al.* (Niloff *et al.*, 1985) have demonstrated that the elevation of serum CA 125 concentration over 35 Units/ml (the upper limit of normal) correlates with cancer disease progression. For the Leptin biomarker the level below 2.5 ng/ml (the lower limit of normal) typically correlates with the presence of cancer (Mor *et al.*, 2005).

In the proof-of-principle experiments with ovarian cancer biomarkers we **achieved about 1 U/ml detection limit for CA 125 and about 11μg/ml for Leptin**. The typical minimum detectable concentration of C A125 for solid phase enzyme-linked immunosorbent assays (ELISA) was estimated to be from 5 U/ml (Alpha Diagnostic Intl. instruction manual, n.d.) to 7 U/ml (Thomas *et al.*, 1995). Therefore, the current Tag-LIBS sensitivity for CA 125 is comparable to existing commercial ELISA assays. For ovarian biomarker Leptin more work has to be done to improve sensitivity of the current method up to necessary for clinical applications level 2.5 ng/ml. To achieve the goal we plan to use more sensitive gated spectrometer (Andor ME 5000 Echelle Spectrograph) with a better spectral resolution. Preliminary experiments (data not shown) demonstrated about 20 times improved sensitivity for detection of iron oxide micro-particles. Thus, we can expect significant improvement of the Tag-LIBS detection limits for biomarkers.

Figures 4, 6 and 7 show that the binding curves have a local maximum on the calibration curves for avidin (Fig. 4) and CA 125 (Fig. 6), but has not been observed for Leptin (Fig. 7). In these experiments, three different proteins and protein molecules were investigated. These have different molecular weights (mw). The molecule avidin is a tetrameric biotin-binding protein with molecular weight about 67 KD (UniProt protein database, n.d., a), ovarian cancer biomarker CA 125 (also known as mucin 16 or MUC16 (HUGO Gene Nomenclature Committee database, n.d.)) has a molecular weight about 2,353 KD (UniProt protein database, n.d., b), and Leptin has molecular weight about 18.6 KD (UniProt protein database, n.d., c). Proteins with higher molecular weight usually have bigger size (i.e. hydrodynamic radius) (Armstrong *et al.*, 2004). Therefore, during the cross-linking process the bigger proteins may occupy larger areas and steric effects may take place especially for larger proteins (Connolly *et al.*, 2001). This is in agreement with observed Tag-LIBS data (Fig. 4, 6, and 7). The presence of local maximum on the calibration curves detected for molecules with bigger molecular weight avidin and CA 125 but not for Leptin might be in part the result of steric effects and constraints of bio-molecule access to unbound binding sites on micro-particles (Connolly *et al.*, 2001) or due to the cross linking critical concentration of protein molecules in a solution (Heidelberger, 1933). It is also possible that the differences in the experimental protocols (see description above) used for different proteins played some role. It is important to mention that the matrix effects accompanying LIBS may play a role (Cremers & Radziemski, 2006, B). Further studies are currently ongoing.

Laser-induced breakdown spectroscopy yields integrated data about atomic composition of a sample. LIBS can yield more than ten thousand spectral data points for each sample. Several methods do exist to reduce the massive amount of data up to the reasonable point. The traditional way of analysis involves taking into account the emission spectral amplitudes (or areas under the spectral lines) related to few chosen elements of interest omitting all other spectral data (Cremers & Radziemski, 2006, B). This leads to plotting standard calibration curves to be compared with unknown sample. Another way to reduce the amount of experimental data involves the use of the principal component analysis (PCA) (Labbe *et al.*, 2008). PCA converts the multi-dimensional set of experimental data into the new typically less dimensional set of principal components with higher variance. Several classification algorithms such as k-Nearest Neighbor and Support vector machines can be further employed (Vance *et al.*, 2010).

4. Conclusions

Clearly, it is important to develop novel diagnostic methods for higher throughput screening of human samples. Known types of assays for detection of the disease biomarkers include enzyme, fluorescence, chemiluminescence, nephelometric and radio- immunoassays (Koivunen & Krogsrud, 2006). Encoded particle assays are attracting more attention due to their inherent ability for easier scaling-up from the single analyte to highly parallel multi-analyte systems (Rubenstein, 2010). Such particle based assays are sometimes called virtual arrays to be distinguished from more conventional positional arrays (Rubenstein, 2010). For capture entities, the currently employed encoded particle assays use typically antibodies or oligo-nucleotides coded by nucleotide sequences or set of dyes (Rubenstein, 2010). Metals, non-metals, their alloys and composites have not been used extensively despite the fact that they can offer some advantages over traditional coding entities. First, they are chemically and biologically inert. They are stable, not harmful for patients, have longer shelf-time and relatively easier to handle.

The choice of proteins to detect is paramount to the diagnostic of cancers (Petricoin *et al.*, 2002; Mor *et al.*, 2005; Wagner, 2003; Garber, 2004). By employing the multi-element coded technique, we offer a novel approach to **detect many proteins in serum simultaneously**. The fundamental question that needs careful attention is: which proteins should be detected and monitored? Therefore, the screening for the potential cancer markers becomes crucial for the successful diagnostic development. The use of multi-element micro- and nano-particles labels for possible biomarkers can help in the multiplex biomarker panel development.

Compared with the numerous elemental analytical techniques available, LIBS provides many advantages. LIBS method requires much smaller sample volumes and minimal sample preparation. It provides real-time spectra, does not require the use of time-of-flight devices and is easy to implement. In addition, elements analyzed by LIBS have extremely narrow emission bandwidths and characterization of each chemical element, as defined by a unique series of emission lines, is highly specific. As a result, LIBS is one of the most effective techniques for multi-element analysis of samples. For the Tag-LIBS application the identification code is the multi-elemental composition of nano- and micro-particles.

Using micro-particles for the detection of biomarkers has several advantages compared to ELISA micro-titer plates type assays. First, the throughput of the particle assay can be greater because of the larger surface-to-volume ratio. Second, the use of mixtures particles coated by individual capture molecules allows development of multi-analyte assays. Nontoxic and inexpensive labels with minimal interference of background signal and improved specific activity, with unique signature appeared to be the most desirable label technologies from the viewpoint of industry and academia (Harma, 2002).

We suggest that the use of LIBS after tagging specific proteins provides a novel approach for inexpensive, robust and accurate diagnosis of EOC. In principle, the proposed method is applicable for different types of cancer (i.e. ovarian, prostate or lung cancer (Brambilla *et al.*, 2003)) provided we can identify specific biomarkers.

5. Acknowledgments

This research was supported by the Center for Research and Education in Optical Sciences and Applications funded by a National Science Foundation Center of Research Excellence in Science and Technology (award # 0630388). We thank Dr. D. Connolly of the Fox Chase Cancer Center, PA for numerous discussions and the Blood Bank of Delmarva for providing human blood plasma for research.

6. References

Ahrends, R.; Pieper, S.; Kuhn, A.; Weisshoff, H.; Hamester, M.; Lindemann, T.; Scheler, C.; Lehmann, K.; Taubner, K. & Linscheid, M.W. (2007). A metal-coded affinity tag approach to quantitative proteomics. *Molecular & Cellular Proteomics,* Vol.6, No.11, (November 2007), pp. 1907 - 1916

Alpha Diagnostic International. (n.d.). Instruction manual No. M-1820, In: *Alpha Diagnostic International.* 02.03.2011, Available from http://www.4adi.com/objects/catalog/product/extras/1820.pdf

Aragon, C.; Aguilera, J.A. & Penalba, F. (1999). Improvements in Quantitative Analysis of Steel Composition by Laser-Induced Breakdown Spectroscopy at Atmospheric Pressure Using an Infrared Nd:YAG Laser. *Applied Spectroscopy* Vol. 53, No.10, (October 1999), pp. 1259-1267

Armstrong, J.K.; Wenby, R.B.; Meiselman, H.J. & Fisher, T.C. (2004). The hydrodynamic radii of macromolecules and their effect on red blood cell aggregation. *Biophysical Journal, Vol.* 87, No.6, (December 2004), pp. 4259–4270

Barber, H.R.K. (1986). Ovarian cancer. *Cancer Journal for Clinicians,* Vol. 36, No.3, (May-June 1986), pp. 149-184

Bjorck, L. & Kronvall, G. (1984). Purification and some properties of streptococcal protein G, a novel IgG-binding reagent. *Journal of Immunology,* Vol.133, No.2, (August 1984), pp. 969-974

Brambilla, C.; Fievet, F.; Jeanmart, M.; de Fraipont, F.; Lantuejoul, S.; Frappat, V.; Ferretti, G.; Brichon, P.Y. & Moro-Sibilot, D. (2003). Early detection of lung cancer: role of biomarkers. *Europian Respiratory Journal,* Vol.21, (January 2003), pp. 36s-44s

Cohn, E.J. (1948). The chemical specificity of the interaction of diverse human plasma proteins. *Blood,* Vol.3, No.5, (May 1948), pp. 471 - 485

Connolly, S.; Cobbe, S. & Fitzmaurice, D. (2001). Effects of Ligand−Receptor Geometry and Stoichiometry on Protein-Induced Aggregation of Biotin-Modified Colloidal Gold. *Journal of Physical Chemistry B,* Vol. 105, No.11, (February 2001), pp. 2222-2226

Cremers, B. D. & Radziemski, L. J. (2006). A. In: *Handbook of Laser-Induced Breakdown Spectroscopy,* B. D. Cremers & L. J. Radziemski, 23-168, Wiley, New York

Cremers, D.A. & Radziemski, L.J. (2006). B. History and fundamentals of LIBS. In: In: *Laser-induced breakdown spectroscopy (LIBS): fundamentals and applications,* A. Miziolek, V. Palleschi, & I. Schechter (Eds.), 1-39. University Press, Cambridge

Empirical LIBS database. (n.d.) Laser-Induced Breakdown Spectroscopy Elemental Spectra. In: *OSCAR website.* 07.13.2011. Available from http://www.creosa.desu.edu/resources/libs.html

Farbman-Yogev, I.; Bohbot-Raviv, Y. & Ben-Shaul, A. (1998). A Statistical Thermodynamic Model for Cross-Bridge Mediated Condensation of Vesicles. *Journal of Physical Chemistry A,* Vol.102, No.47, (September 1998), pp. 9586-9592

Freeman, R.G.; Raju, P.A.; Norton, S.M.; Walton, I.D.; Smith, P.C.; He, L.; Natan, M.J.; Sha, M.Y. & Penn, S.G. (2005). Use of Nanobarcodes Particles in Bioassays. In: *Methods in Molecular Biology,* S.J. Rosenthal, D.W. Wright (Eds.), 73-84, Humana Press Inc, Totowa

Fulton, R.J.; McDade, R.L.; Smith, P.L.; Kienker, L.J. & Kettman, J.R. Jr. (1997). Advanced multiplexed analysis with the FlowMetrix system. *Clinical Chemistry,* Vol.43, (September 1997), No.9, pp. 1749–1756

Garber, K. (2004) Debate Rages Over Proteomic Patterns. *Journal of the National Cancer Institute,* Vol.96, No.11, (June 2004), pp. 816-818

Gosling, J.P. (1990). A decade of development in immunoassay methodology. *Clinical Chemistry*, Vol.36, No.8, (August 1990), pp. 1408-1427

Harma, H. (2002). 02.03.2011. Particle technologies in diagnostics. In: *Tekes. National Technology Agency. Technology Review 126/2002.* Available from www.tekes.fi/fi/document/43342/particle_pdf

Heidelberger, M.; Kendall, F.E. & Soo Hoo, C.M. (1933). Quantitative Studies on the Precipitin Reaction: Antibody Production in Rabbits Injected with an Azo Protein. *Journal of Experimental Medicine* 58, No. 2, (July 1933), pp. 137-152

Hugo Gene Nomenclature Committee database. (n.d.) MUC16. In: *HUGO Gene Nomenclature Committee database*, 02.03.2011. Available from http://www.genenames.org/data/hgnc_data.php?hgnc_id=15582

Ingraham, F.S. & Wooley, D. F. (1964) Polyvinyldene fluoride. *Industrial and Engineering Chemistry*, Vol.56, No.9, (September, 1964), pp. 53–55

K&J Magnetics, Inc. website. (n.d.) In: *K&J Magnetics, Inc. website.* 02.07.2011. Available from http://www.kjmagnetics.com/specs.asp

Koivunen, M.E. & Krogsrud, R.L. (2006). Principles of Immunochemical Techniques Used in Clinical Laboratories. *Labmedicine*, Vol.37, No.8, (August 2006), pp.490-497

Labbe, N.; Swamidoss, I.M.; Andre, N.; Martin, M.Z.; Young, T.M.; & Rials, T.G. (2008). Extraction of information from laser-induced breakdown spectroscopy spectral data by multivariate analysis. *Applied Optics*, Vol.47, No.31, (November 2008), pp. G158-G165

Majoor, C.L.H. (1946). The possibility of detecting individual proteins in blood serum by differentiation of solubility curves in concentrated sodium sulfate solutions. *Yale Journal of Biology and Medicine*, Vol. 18, (May 1946), pp. 419–441

Markushin Y., Marcano A., Rock S. & Melikechi N. (2010). Determination of protein hydrogen composition by laser-induced breakdown spectroscopy. *Journal of Analytical Atomic Spectrometry*, Vol.25, No.2, (December 2010), pp. 148-149

Markushin, Y.; Melikechi, N.; Marcano, A.; Rock, S.; Henderson, E. & Connolly, D. (2009). LIBS-based multi-element coded assay for ovarian cancer application, *Proceedings of the Society of Photographic Instrumentation Engineers (SPIE)*, Vol. 7190, (January 2009), pp. 719015-1-719015-6, 07.13.2011. Available from http://dx.doi.org/10.1117/12.810247

McGuire, V.; Whittemore, A.S.; Norris, R. & Oakley-Girvan, I. (2000). Survival in epithelial ovarian cancer patients with prior breast cancer. *American Journal of Epidemiology*, Vol.152, No.6, (September 2000), pp. 528-532

Melikechi, N; and Markushin, Y, (2011) Mono and Multi Coded LIBS Assays and methods, US patent US20110171636 (pending)

Mirkin, C.A.; Jwa-Min Nam & Thaxon, S. (2005). Bio-barcode based detection of target analytes. In: *United States patent # US2005/0037397 A1. 07.13.2011.* Available from http://www.freepatentsonline.com/y2005/0037397.html

Miziolek, A.W., Palleschi, V., Schechter, I., *Laser-induced breakdown spectroscopy: fundamentals and applications*, Cambridge University Press, 2006

Mor, G.; Visintin, I.; Lai, Y.; Zhao, H.; Schwartz, P.; Rutherford, T.; Yue, L.; Bray-Ward, P. & Ward, D.C. (2005). Serum protein markers for early detection of ovarian cancer.

Proceedings of the National Academy of Sciences of the United States of America, Vol.102, No.21, (May 2005), pp. 7677-7682

Niloff, J.M.; Bast, R.C.; Schaetzl, E.M. & Knapp, R.C. (1985). Predictive value of CA 125 antigen levels in second-look procedures for ovarian cancer. *American Journal of Obstetrics & Gynecology*, Vol.151, No.7, (April 1985), pp. 981-986

OSCAR website. (n.d.) Optical Science Center for Applied Research at Delaware State University. In: *OSCAR website*. 07.12.2011. Available from http://www.creosa.desu.edu/

Petricoin, E.F.; Ardekani, A.M.; Hitt, B.A.; Levine, P.J.; Fusaro, V.A.; Steinberg, S.M.; Mills, G.B.; Simone, C.; Fishman, D.A.; Kohn, E.C. & Liotta L.A. (2002). Use of proteomic patterns in serum to identify ovarian cancer. *The Lancet*, Vol. 359, (February, 2002), pp. 572-577

Rock, S.; Marcano, A.; Markushin, Y.; Sabanayagam, C. & Melikechi, N. (2008). Elemental analysis of laser induced breakdown spectroscopy aided by an empirical spectral database. *Applied Optics*, Vol.47, No.31, (September 2008), pp. G99-G104

Rubenstein, K. (2010). Multiplex Assays: Evolving Technologies, Applications and Future Directions. In: *Insight Pharma Reports*, 07.13.2010. Available from http://www.insightpharmareports.com/uploadedFiles/Reports/Reports/Multiplex_Assays/Sample_Pages.pdf

Smith, A.M.; Dave, S.; Nie, S.; True, L. & Gao, X. (2006). Multicolor quantum dots for molecular diagnostics of cancer. *Expert Review of Molecular Diagnostics*, Vol.6, No.2, (March 2006), pp. 231-244

Thomas, C.M.; Massuger, L.F.; Segers, M.F.; Schijf, C.P.; Doesburg, W.H. & Wobbes, T. (1995). Analytical and clinical performance of improved Abbott IMx CA 125 assay: comparison with Abbott CA 125 RIA. *Clinical Chemistry*, Vol.41, No.2, (February 1995), pp. 211-216

UniProtKB/Swiss-Prot. protein database. A. (n.d.). P02701, In: *Protein Knowledgebase (UniProtKB)*. 07.05.2011. Available from http://www.uniprot.org/uniprot/P02701

UniProtKB/Swiss-Prot. protein database. B. (n.d.). Q8WXI7, In: *Protein Knowledgebase (UniProtKB)*. 07.05.2011. Available from http://www.uniprot.org/uniprot/Q8WXI7

UniProtKB/Swiss-Prot. protein database. C. (n.d.). P41159, In: *Protein Knowledgebase (UniProtKB)*. 07.05.2011. Available from http://www.uniprot.org/uniprot/P41159

Vance, T.; Pokrajac, D.; Lazarevic, A.; Marcano, A.; Markushin, Y.; McDaniel, S. & Melikechi, N. (2010) Classification of LIBS Protein Spectra Using Multilayer Perceptrons. *Transactions on Mass-Data Analysis of Images and Signals*, Vol.2, No.1, (September 2010), pp. 96-111

Wagner, L., (2003) A test before its time? FDA stalls distribution process of proteomic test. *Journal of the National Cancer Institute*, Vol.96, No.7, (April 2003), pp.500-501

WHO Expert Committee on Biological Standardization. (n.d.). Biological methods. In: *Antibiotics-microbiological assay*. 07.12.2011. Available from http://whqlibdoc.who.int/publications/1979/9241541504_p143-223.pdf

Zal, T, & Gascoignea, N.R. (2004). Photobleaching-Corrected FRET Efficiency Imaging of Live Cells. *Biophysical Journal*, Vol.86, No.6, (June 2004), pp. 3923-3939

Zhu, W.; Wang, X.; Ma, Y.; Rao, M.; Glimm, J. & Kovach, J.S. (2003). Detection of cancer-specific markers amid massive mass spectral data. *Proceedings of the National Academy of Sciences of the United States of America*, Vol.100, No.25, (December, 2003) pp. 14666–14671

10

Potential Tumor Biomarkers for Ovarian Cancer

Ryan Serio and Blase Billack
St. John's University, Department of Pharmaceutical Sciences
USA

1. Introduction

In the United States, invasive ovarian cancer is the 5th most deadly malignancy in females, accounting for an estimated 13,850 deaths in 2010 (Ahmad, 2011; American Cancer Society, 2010). The risk of dying from ovarian cancer depends on staging and varies greatly. Ovarian cancer patients diagnosed at the localized stage exhibit a 5 year survival rate of 94%. This rate is 73% when diagnosed at the regional stage following local dissemination and drops to 28% when a patient is diagnosed at the distant stage with metastasis to organs outside the pelvis. Overall, the combined 5 year survival rate for all ovarian cancer patients is an unmanageable 46% (American Cancer Society, 2010).

Upon histological evaluation, most ovarian cancers are found to be epithelial in nature and are collectively referred to as ovarian epithelial cancers (OEC). The most common OEC subtypes include, in decreasing order of frequency, serous adenocarcinomas, followed by endometrioid, and smaller subsets of mucinous, clear cell, transitional, and undifferentiated carcinomas (Tavassoli and Devilee, 2003).

The typical progression of invasive ovarian cancer is dissemination from the primary site into the peritoneal mesothelium. The close proximity of the ovary to the mesothelium explains the high incidence of peritoneal dissemination observed in nearly all cases of ovarian cancer. Tumors are thought to arise either from implanted cells from the fringe of the fallopian tube (Jarboe et al, 2008) or from dysplastic inclusion cysts which develop out of the mesothelial-like ovarian surface epithelium (OSE). As the tumor progresses, cells shed into the peritoneal fluid, escape apoptotic mechanisms, and begin to attach to their surrounding mesothelium via integrin-mediated interactions with extracellular matrix components (Ahmed et al, 2005; Cannistra et al., 1995; Yokoyama et al., 2007). Unlike most malignancies, ovarian cancers rarely metastasize through the hematogenous route until the advanced stages (Rose et al., 1989). Approximately 62% of cases of ovarian cancer are diagnosed at the distant stage (American Cancer Society, 2010) and the clinical prognosis for such patients is poor.

The high mortality associated with ovarian cancer stems, in part, from late detection and underpins the exigent need to identify predictive and early stage diagnostic biomarkers. The task is not an easy one. Difficulty in the validation of current screening tests is mainly attributed to the lack of uniformity in clinical presentation of the disease, which varies with epithelial cell morphology, depending on whether the carcinoma is of a serous, clear cell, mucinous, or endometrioid type. To the present date, blood concentration measurements of CA125 (mucin-16), in conjunction with ultrasonography, have been used to screen for ovarian cancer. However, it has been found that detection of serum CA125 alone is inadequate for reliably detecting ovarian cancer for a number of reasons. These include a lack of specificity, questionable prognostic ability, frequent false positive readings, liver clearance of circulating antigen, and elevation associated more often with progression in late rather than early stages (Helzlsouer et al., 1993; Jacobs and Bast, 1989; Maggino et al, 1994). These confounds have hindered the diagnostic potential of CA125 for detecting OEC in stage I or II, when the disease shows much a much higher cure rate. Moreover, annual screening with CA125 and ultrasonography fails to reduce mortality and deleterious complications may arise from surgical interventions in women exhibiting false positive results (Buys et al, 2011). Clearly, efforts to identify better diagnostic markers are warranted.

2. Carbohydrate biomarkers

A major benefit of using carbohydrates as tumor biomarkers comes as a result of both their abundance and importance in shaping and maintaining the tumor microenvironment (Fukuda, 1996). Cellular communication, adhesion, and trafficking are all major functions of carbohydrate polymers, or glycans, which constitute a significant portion of glycoconjugates (Li et al., 2010a; Ohtsubo and Marth, 2006; Varki et al., 2009). Glycosylation, the formation of a linkage of a glycan with a protein, a lipid, or other organic molecule, greatly increases the complexity of those latter molecules and, resultantly, the potential for information storage. Altered protein glycosylation is believed to be an early event in tumorigenesis which contributes to invasion and metastasis of tumor cells (Chiang et al., 2010; Dall'Olio and Chiricolo, 2001; Hakomori, 1996; Hakomori, 2002; Varki et al, 1969; Kuzmanov et al., 2009; Meezan et al., 1969; Saldova et al, 2008; Yogeeswaran and Salk, 1981). Many prominent proteins in OEC pathophysiology, such as integrins and the receptor for epidermal growth factor (EGFR), are found to be heavily glycosylated (Stroop et al, 2000; Gu and Taniguchi, 2004).

Some important factors in cancer are the percentage of glycosylated proteins, the degree of branching versus linear polymers, the preponderance of specific chemical groups added to glycans, and the type, or "signature," of glycosylation observed. Proteins in cancer are generally highly glycosylated compared to non-malignant phenotypes, particularly on the cell surface and on proteins with a secretory function (Hakomori, 2002), suggesting an active role in establishing the extracellular tumor microenvironment. Varying conformations associated with differential glycan arrangements serve as molecular switches which can alter protein functions. Frequent protein modifications observed in cancer cells include alterations in core and terminal fucosylation, changes in sulfation and sialylation patterns, increased glycan branching, and alterations in Lewis isotopes (Varki et al, 2009). Lewis isotopes are glycoprotein antigens confined to red blood cells and epithelial secretions that belong to the Lewis blood group system.

Growing knowledge of the changing glycosylation patterns of small, soluble glycoproteins specific for certain cancers have made the possibility for developing novel diagnostic serum and even urine tests using protein markers with aberrantly expressed glycosylation patterns an endeavor worthy of pursuit. Some of the changes in glycosylation observed in OEC are described below, with potential tumor markers revealed.

2.1 Fucosylation

Addition of the five carbon sugar, fucose, to glycans reduces flexibility around glycosidic linkages of branching point antennae to enhance selectivity for ligands and increase molecular stability of the glycoconjugate. Unlike most other carbohydrate moieties, fucose contains only one free hydroxyl group available for hydrogen bonding. This feature restricts rotational freedom and enhances stability. The presence of bulky terminal fucose groups in a glycoconjugate restricts access to galactose residues. These moieties are normally recognized by asialoglycoproteins that target the molecules for degradation. This inevitably leads to lifespan extension of the modified glycoconjugate. Changes in structure/function mechanics are attributed to core fucosylation as well. Core fucosylation of the innermost residue in the chain greatly affects ligand specificity of glycoproteins by providing an extended conformation with altered binding affinity (Stubbs et al., 1996).

A glycoprotein that has thus far become a legitimate candidate as a potential biomarker is thrombospondin 1 (THBS-1). THBS-1 is released by platelets to negatively regulate angiogenesis by disrupting vascular endothelial growth factor (VEGF) signaling (Zaslavsky et al, 2010). A four-fold increase in expression levels of this protein has been observed in serum of ovarian cancer patients, and shows considerable core fucosylation not seen in healthy patients as determined by reactivity with the Aleuria aurantia lectin (AAL), which preferentially binds most strongly with core fucose-containing glycoconjugates (Abbott et al, 2010, Yamashita et al, 1985). Abbott et al (2010) also identified a second marker, periostin (POSTN), that exhibited altered glycosylation in the form of increased bisecting N-acetylglucosamine (GlcNAc) in serum from ovarian cancer compared to sera from healthy controls (Abbott et al, 2010). These modifications were examined only in endometrioid OEC cases (Abbott et al, 2010). THBS-1 and POSTN are known to be highly expressed in other subtypes (Kodama et al, 2001, Zhu et al, 2010); though POSTN is associated more with late stages (Zhu et al, 2010). Core fucosylation patterns have not yet been described for ovarian cancers displaying non-endometrioid histology. If tumor-specific alterations in fucosylation patterns are replicated in other types of ovarian cancers, particularly in the prevalent serous phenotype, this glycan-modified cancer marker may be a useful diagnostic indicator in the future.

Fucosylation affects OEC physiology in additional ways. For instance, the difucosylated oligosaccharide, Le^Y (CD174), is often highly expressed on mucins 1 and 16 (Yin et al, 1996). Mucins are large glycoproteins that are widely expressed in a number of carcinomas, including OEC. Their ability to contribute to disease pathogenesis by a variety of mechanisms is well-documented (Bafna et al, 2010; Thériault et al, 2011). Increased Le^Y antigens have been correlated with a number of tumorigenic effects, such as enhanced binding to mesothelial CD44, stimulation of $\alpha_5\beta_1$ signaling, increased expression of MMP-2/9, and down-regulation of inhibitory TIMP-1/2 (Gao et al, 2011; Li et al, 2010b; Yan et al, 2010). A positive effect on growth factor activation has additionally been observed, as Le^Y participates in EGFR signaling and aids in the secretion of the angiogenic factors VEGF and basic FGF (Basu et al, 1987; Li et al, 2010b).

Le^Y displays specificity for epithelium-derived cancers, and is present in 70-90% of malignancies with this provenance (Chhieng et al, 2003). This Lewis antigen is most frequently active during embryonic development, and its expression in adults is limited solely to epithelial cells and granulocytes (Li et al, 2010b). Specificity is somewhat diminished by its appearance in certain non-malignant conditions, such as in ovarian cysts (Yang et al, 2009). The Le^Y antigen is not expressed in normal OSE, however, and is expressed in only 25% of benign tumors compared to 81% of malignant and 52% of borderline tumors (Wang et al, 2011). Based on these data, Le^Y is a promising potential biomarker for OEC and its value in the recognition of specific cancer stages awaits further studies.

2.2 Sulfation

Enhanced adhesion of heparin-binding epidermal growth factor–like growth factor (HB-EGF) to heparan sulfate proteoglycans (HSPGs), and subsequent activation in OEC, is attributed to changes in sulfation patterns of these cell surface molecules (Shipp and Hsieh-Wilson, 2007). As HSPG sulfation increases, potential for interaction with HB-EGF also rises (Lai et al, 2003). Increased sulfation of glycosaminoglycan chains on HSPGs is a common feature in many epithelial cancers, including breast, kidney, hepatocellular, and ovarian cancers (Bret et al, 2011; Lai et al., 2003). A major mechanism by which this is achieved is through the down-regulation of HSulf-1. This enzyme is an arylsulfatase that degrades heparin preferentially at the C-6 position of glucosamine within specific subregions of the heparin molecule (Morimoto-Tomita et al, 2002). It is expressed ubiquitously in nonlymphoid tissue but significantly reduced in many epithelial cancers, including ovarian cancer.

Loss of HSulf-1 leads to increased sulfation of cell surface HSPGs and an expansion in the number of binding sites with HB-EGF. HB-EGF promotes transcoelomic metastasis in ovarian cancer through its involvement in epithelial-mesenchymal transition (EMT) (Yagi et al., 2008). Re-expression of the enzyme *in vitro* has been shown to diminish downstream signaling of HB-EGF, as demonstrated by reduction of ERK activity and abrogation of EGFR phosphorylation (Lai et al, 2003). Loss of HSulf-1 and the resultant hypersulfated state also modulates angiogenesis via binding of a VEGF isoform through its heparin-binding domain (Narita et al, 2006). Evidence suggests HSulf-1 down-regulation is an early event in tumorigenesis, as total inactivation of this enzyme was observed in fibrocystic breast cells with a normal phenotype while 80% of stage I/II ovarian cancer tumors exhibited barely detectable mRNA levels (Lai et al, 2003). Interestingly, the same study reported that >75% of ovarian tumors lacked HSulf-1 expression (Lai et al., 2003). Taken together, these observations suggest that loss of HSulf-1 could serve as an early biomarker for upcoming EMT events.

Down-regulation of HSulf-1 is a finding consistent with many epithelium-derived malignancies, and thus might not be highly effective as a stand-alone diagnostic marker for ovarian cancer. Its presence in serum may prove to be indicative of a cancerous state when concomitantly evaluated alongside additional markers. Further assessment of effects on specific HSPG substrates, such as the highly expressed proteoglycan, syndecan-1 (SDC1), may raise the value of HSulf-1 in OEC tumor diagnosis. The combination of HSulf-1 inhibition and SDC1 expression may be more specific for OEC than abrogation of HSulf-1 alone. SDC1 is a type of HSPG that is not expressed in normal OSE but quotidian to ovarian tumor tissue (Davies et al, 2004). In contrast, other HSPGs studied are found to be ubiquitously expressed in normal and diseased ovaries (Davies et al, 2004). Furthermore, the presence of SDC1 in serum as circulating CD138 antigen makes it relatively simple to detect in a noninvasive manner.

2.3 Sialylation

Over 50 types of neuraminic acid-derived monosaccharides have been described and are collectively referred to as sialic acids (Varki and Schauer, 2009). Sialic acids have been found to exhibit numerous cellular functions, examples of which include the stabilization of molecules and cell membranes, the enhancement of mucin viscosity, the protection of molecules and cells from degradation and the modulation of cellular interactions with the microenvironment (Varki and Schauer, 2009). The contribution of sialylation per se to increased tumorigenesis rests in its ability to allow permissive regulation of cellular interactions. The strong negative charge resulting from the low acid-base dissociation constant of sialic acids produces a charge repulsion effect. This, in addition to prominent hydration and conformational instability give heavily sialylated glycans a slippery effect to substantially reduce cell-cell interactions (Dall'Olio and Chiricolo, 2001; Schauer et al, 2011). As a result, adhesion and differentiation effects are not favored, and metastatic characteristics of migration and invasion become exacerbated when sialylation becomes enhanced by constituents of the microenvironment. The presence of sialic acids can also mask antigenic sites and, in this regard, thwart the activity of immune cells (Schauer, 2000). Finally, through their ability to avoid recognition by immune cells, highly sialylated cancer cells can efficiently evade tumor surveillance mechanisms, further promoting the malignant phenotype (Schauer et al, 2011).

The most abundant sialic acid in human cells is Neu5Ac, in which the C-5 is substituted with an N-acetyl group. Other mammals mainly produce Neu5Gc, in which the substituted N-acetyl group is hydroxylated to form an N-glycol substituent. This latter modification of neuraminic acid can be acquired by humans through diet and, following absorption, can generate an antigenic inflammatory response (Hedlund et al, 2008; Tangvoranuntakul et al., 2003). While tumor tissue and serum samples have been found to contain secreted Neu5Gc (Higashi et al, 1984; Siskos and Spyridaki, 1999), the potential association between Neu5Gc intake from the diet and ovarian cancer risk requires further study. Evidence supporting a major role for Neu5Gc in OEC was discovered in the ovarian cancer cell line JHOC-5, where secreted sialoglycoproteins, and especially mucin-like proteins, exhibited up to 40% representation of total sialic acid content by this exogenous carbohydrate moiety (Inoue et al, 2010). These data suggest a possible role for Neu5Gc as a predictive biomarker for ovarian cancer.

Under usual circumstances, sialic acid is attached to substrates such as glycosphingolipids and N- or O-linked glycans as single molecules or short oligomers. The attachment of longer chains of sialic acids, known as polysialic acids, to substrates is less common. Sialic acids are normally removed from substrates through the activity of another class of enzymes known as the sialidases. The neuronal cell adhesion molecule (NCAM, CD56) is, however, a noteworthy exception which is modified post-translationally via polysialylation, particularly during embryonic development and then downregulated shortly thereafter (Rutishauser and Landmesser, 1996). The reappearance of polysialylated NCAM has been observed in some forms of cancer, such as malignant neuroblastomas and rhabdomyosarcomas (Daniel et al., 2001; Fukuda, 1996; Gluer et al., 1998a; Gluer et al, 1998b; Jensen and Berthold, 2007) and correlates with increased metastatic potential and poor clinical outcome (Seidenfaden et al., 2003). Recently, NCAM expression has been studied in serous ovarian tumors and found to correlate with greater peritoneal dissemination and larger tumor volume following surgical debulking (Zueva et al, 2010). Sialylation status of NCAM in ovarian cancer is yet to be deciphered.

Glycan branching in cancers inhibits molecular clustering and cell adhesion while increasing the number of available sialylation sites and facilitating migratory potential (André et al, 2009), so it is not surprising that ovarian cancer is associated with increased α2,6 branched sialyl expression and decreased α2,3 linear sialylation (Wang et al, 2005). A major sialyltransferase responsible for branched sialylation of glycans is ST6Gal-I, which is abundantly expressed in OEC (Christie et al, 2008; Wang et al, 2005). Elevated ST3Gal-I and reduced levels of ST3Gal-III, ST3Gal-IV, and ST3Gal-VI have also been observed (Wang et al, 2005). A major function of ST6Gal-I in ovarian cancer is the sialylation of β_1 integrins (Wang et al, 2005). Sialylation enhances integrin-mediated signaling in cancers, leading to increased migration and invasiveness in the extracellular matrix (ECM) (Chiang et al, 2010). ST6Gal-I responds to a variety of genetic, inflammatory, and hormonal signals. Some triggers of ST6Gal-I overexpression that may be relevant to OEC are high IL-6 activity, Ras signaling (from either mutations or overexpression), and ER-α mutations (Hanasaki et al, 1994; Lau et al, 1999; Seales et al, 2003). The presence of serum cancer-specific markers synthesized by ST6Gal-I may adumbrate tumorigenic events if detected sufficiently early. Due to the documented high ST6Gal-I activity in OEC, it would be expected that β_1 integrins are hypersialylated. Determining alterations in sialylation patterns compared to controls may be useful in the quest for biomarker identification as these abundantly expressed integrins so crucial to early epithelial-to-mesenchymal transition (EMT) events are detectable in serum (Liu et al, 2005).

The presence of only one glycosylation site makes a candidate marker more amenable to testing than glycoconjugates with more convoluted patterns due to ease of identification with less confounding variables. Cancer-specific aberrations in the glycosylation signature of a macromolecule with a lone glycan moiety would improve sensitivity and specificity of a candidate biomarker. A tumor marker that has garnered much attention in ovarian cancer diagnosis is kallikrein-like peptidase-6 (KLK6) (Bast et al, 2005; El Sherbini et al, 2011; White et al, 2009). This protein is a trypsin-like serine protease consisting of a single N-glycosylation site. When juxtaposed against the same protein derived from a non-malignant site, only KLK6 taken from ovarian cancer ascitic fluid displayed α2,6 branched sialylation (Kuzmanov et al, 2009). KLK6 is also a serum marker and these results may translate to this less invasive approach. Recognition of this specific isoform can only improve the status of KLK6 as a marker for ovarian cancer. KLK6 is up-regulated in most ovarian cancer tumors (Shan et al, 2007). Sensitivity of the marker for early detection does not exceed that of CA125 (El Sherbini et al, 2011), although the combination was shown to improve sensitivity by 10-30% (Diamandis et al, 2003). Screening for the robust sialylated isoform of KLK6 in OEC tumors may possibly improve accuracy of detection.

There are several other abnormally sialylated molecules that may serve as molecular markers for ovarian cancer. Sialylated Lewis x (sLe^x) is a terminal glycan epitope that is positioned on the surface of cells attached to glycoconjugates and is preferentially recognized by endothelial selectins to promote cell migration. The sLe^x epitope of the Lewis blood group is composed of Neu5Ac in an α2,3 linkage to a galactose sugar. Following sialylation of Le^x, fucosylation occurs via the action of α(1,3/1,4) fucosyltransferases (Aubert et al, 2000). SLe^x has been identified in ovarian cancer on the surface of the acute phase proteins α_1-acid glycoprotein (AGP), α_1-antichymotrypsin, and haptoglobin (Hp) β-chain (Saldova et al, 2007) (See Table 1). The acute phase response is initiated during times of trauma, inflammation, and infection, and provides an environment to keep cells alive during these crisis situations. The combination of sialylation and fucosylation on acute phase proteins has been shown to prolong half-life and reduce apoptosis (Saldova et al, 2008). Sialylation is sometimes combined with sulfation as well. Ovarian cancers of mucinous, papillary serous, and clear cell subtypes often present with increased levels of N-acetylglucosamine 6-O-sulfotransferase 2 (GlcNAc6ST-2), which catalyzes formation of a 6-sulfo-sLe^x group on L-selectin ligands (Kanoh et al, 2006). 6-sulfo-sLe^x (CD15su) is readily detectable in serum and thus may be conducive to analysis as a potential ovarian cancer biomarker.

Glycoprotein	Type of Modification	Modified Group
AGP	sialylation	sLe(x)
Hp β-chain	sialylation	sLe(x)
α_1-antichymotrypsin	sialylation	sLe(x)
CA15-3 (Muc1)	sialylation oligosaccharide replacement	sTn Tn
CA15-3	asialylation oligosaccharide replacement	TF
CA15-3	fucosylation	Le(y)
CA125	fucosylation	Le(y)
THBS1	fucosylation	core fucose
CD138 (SDC1)	hypersulfation	GAG chain
β_1 integrin	sialylation	α2,6 sialic acid
L-selectin ligands	sialylation sulfation	6-sulfo-sLe(x)
POSTN	β1,4 branching	bisecting GlcNAc
KLK6	sialylation	α2,6 sialic acid

Table 1. Carbohydrate Modifications as Potential Biomarkers for Ovarian Cancer.

2.4 Altered glycosylation of epithelial mucins

O-glycans which are covalently α-linked via an N-acetylgalactosamine (GalNAc) moiety to the -OH of serine or threonine by an O-glycosidic bond are designated mucin O-glycans or, for short, mucins (Brockhausen et al., 2009). It is common to find the GalNAc further extended with galactose, N-acetylglucosamine, fucose, or sialic acid; alterations which give rise to different core structures (Brockhausen et al., 2009). These core mucin structures can be modified further with carbohydrate substituents, and can also be branched (Brockhausen et al., 2009). Due to the nature and complexity of their respective structures, mucins tend to be high molecular weight glycoproteins that are heterogeneous and heavily glycosylated. Mucins are synthesized by epithelial cells in various tissues, including the genitourinary epithelium. Mucin-1 (MUC-1) was the first mucin gene to have been identified and, to date, there are about 19 others known to exist (Brockhausen et al., 2009; Spurr-Michaud et al., 2007).

Two general categories of mucins include those which are secreted, to protect epithelial surfaces against damage and infection by pathogens, and those which span the plasma membrane and are involved in cell adhesion (van Klinken et al., 1995; Fukuda, 2002) or cell signaling (Hartel-Schenk et al., 2001). Transmembrane mucins are positioned for mediation of communication between the extracellular milieu and the interior of cells. It has recently been proposed that the mucin covering of epithelia may be compromised when exposed to certain triggers, such as during processes involving elevated stress or remodeling (Kufe, 2009; Zhao et al, 2009), providing greater invasive potential. In this manner, a chronic inflammatory condition can theoretically turn the effects of transmembrane mucins against the cells they normally protect. Evidence supporting this assertion can be observed in a number of adenocarcinomas, where specific transmembrane mucins are often overexpressed (Jonckheere and Van Seuningen, 2010). The usual protective effects of mucins in epithelial cells with normal physiologic adhesion patterns become reversed in cancers by a perturbed glycosylation signature.

2.5 The role of hypoglycosylated mucins in cancer

The serum test for MUC1, also known as carcinoma antigen 15-3 (CA 15-3), has been validated for breast cancer diagnosis. High levels of the splice variant muc-1C have been associated with enhanced growth receptor signaling and activation of NFκβ in breast carcinoma (Ahmad et al, 2009). MUC1 is a potential indicator for OEC as well, as its expression soared from 5% to 90% in a comparison between paraffin-embedded sections of tissue from normal ovarian epithelia and cancerous lesions (Wang et al, 2007). In contrast, muc-16 (CA125), the only antigen FDA approved for diagnosis of ovarian cancer, is expressed in 80% of OEC tissue (Bast et al, 1981). MUC1 is detectable in ascitic fluid and serum in addition to tissue (Tuzun et al, 2009). In a study evaluating 49 biomarkers for ovarian cancer, MUC1 was ranked among the top five best candidates in terms of specificity and sensitivity (Cramer et al, 2011). It has been assessed as an early biomarker for stage I ovarian cancer and has demonstrated improved accuracy in tumor diagnosis as part of a four-marker composite test (Zhang et al, 2007).

A prime feature of mucins is the presence of 10-81 amino acid-comprised tandem repeats of proline-threonine-serine (PTS) in which O-glycosylation occurs at a high rate (Fontenot et al, 1993). In ovarian cancer, and possibly other cancers derived from a glandular origin, there is aberrant hypoglycosylation of mucins evinced by high levels of splice variants lacking the tandem repeat sites. This loss of structural integrity of these towering glycoproteins leading to exposure of the protein core is likely a reason for compromised protection. Smaller hypoglycosylated variants appear to provide better access to epithelium for a number of diverse molecules that would otherwise be thwarted from engaging in cell surface interactions (Zhao et al, 2009). MUC1 additionally promotes EGFR activation by inhibiting its degradation (Pochampalli et al, 2007). High expression of MUC1/Y, MUC1/Z, and, to a lesser extent, MUC1/X, have been demonstrated in ovarian cancer (Obermair et al, 2002). These three variants all lack the signature tandem repeat domain. Elevation of the former two variants has also been shown in prostate cancer, another glandular carcinoma (Schut et al, 2003). Aberrantly glycosylated muc-1 variants identified by glycoforms exhibiting short Tn/sTn oligosaccharides in place of the complex O-glycans that form on PTS repeat sites showed a strong correlation with all forms of ovarian cancer, being exhibited in 84% and 85% of primary tumors and metastatic lesions, respectively (Van Elssen et al, 2010).

The Thomsen-Friedenreich (TF) antigen is an additional short oligosaccharide presenting on a large number of hypoglycosylated epithelial cells. Sialylated TF is commonly found in hematopoietic and somatic cells, but the oligosaccharide is rarely observed in normal cells lacking sialyl groups (Schauer et al., 2011). In its desialylated form, this antigen is thought to be involved in triggering metastasis by stimulating interaction with galactoside-binding galectin-3 and exposing endothelial binding sites to cancer cells (Zhao et al, 2009).

2.6 Mucin-16 as a biomarker: Strengths and weaknesses

Mucin-16 (muc-16, CA125) is another type of transmembrane mucin that mediates adhesive interactions in ovarian cancer. Adhesion of ovarian cancer cells to the peritoneum is in part facilitated by the binding of cleaved cell surface MUC16 to mesothelin (Rump et al, 2004). Muc-16 additionally dampens immune response by binding to the inhibitory siglec-9 receptor on a wide range of cells involved in both innate and adaptive immunity, allowing growing tumors to evade immune system surveillance (Belisle et al, 2010).

The CA125 assay displays a superior sensitivity of 95% in tumors positive for the cell surface antigen in human serum (Cramer et al, 2011). Muc-16 becomes increasingly elevated with progression of OEC, and is expressed in approximately 80% of patients. Stage I tumors have much lower concentrations of muc-16, expressing the mucin at only a 58% rate (Jacobs and Bast, 1989). In addition, sonography is inefficient for detecting tumors that have not yet developed into a large mass. The CA125 assay has very low specificity, as this mucin is often expressed in additional cancers or inflammatory diseases. As a result, the current diagnosis strategy is highly inadequate for early tumor detection.

Despite inefficiency in early detection, the mainstay of ovarian cancer diagnosis continues to be muc-16 detection combined with ultrasonography. Recently, this has been challenged as a prospective study monitoring over 78,000 women showed that mortality was not decreased in women annually screened via this combination (Buys et al, 2011). In addition, surgical follow-up for false positive readings occurred unnecessarily in 1080 women, with 15% experiencing one or more serious complications (Buys et al, 2011).

Because CA125 alone is insufficient for early tumor detection, the focus of much research is the improvement of assay sensitivity by combining this mucin marker with one or more additional indicators. This practice has not yet led to the validation of a composite assay for ovarian cancer diagnosis, mainly because of the tradeoff in specificity encountered when increasing sensitivity via use of multiple agents (Florkowski, 2008). Ideally, a powerful diagnostic assay should consist of the minimum number of test agents possible for this reason. Combining CA125 with a marker that is not only highly expressed in OEC but is replete with a unique glycosylation signature specific for the disease is one viable option for optimizing sensitivity and specificity. The combination of CA125 with other protein markers occasionally yields productive data as well. Improved sensitivity in detecting early ovarian cancer has been observed when CA125 measurement was combined with mesothelin detection (McIntosh et al, 2004). In addition, combination of CA125 with the T-cell expressed B7-H4 protein was demonstrated to improve early detection by 13% over CA125 alone (Simon et al, 2006). Although current guidelines recommend CA125 measurement as the sole biomarker criterion for ovarian cancer diagnosis, it is likely that more powerful assays will develop from its use in combination with one or more highly specific agents. Novel discoveries from the increased use of proteomic and glycomic approaches will assuredly allow for the search for quality biomarkers to continue unabated.

3. Epigenetic modifications as tumor markers

Epigenetics is a branch of science which has for its purpose the study of heritable changes in gene function that do not occur as the result of changes in DNA sequence (Wu and Morris, 2001). In addition, chromatin architecture is affected by epigenetic mechanisms (Zaina et al., 2010). An "epigenetic pathway" involving three components has recently been proposed. In this pathway, a signal is received from the external environment, after which an epigenetic initiator determines the precise chromatin location to be affected, called the mark, and an epigenetic maintainer works to sustain the changed chromatin environment (Berger et al., 2009). Whereas epigenetic initiators include DNA binding factors and non-coding RNAs, epigenetic maintainers include modifiers of histone proteins and histone variants and DNA modifiers, such as DNA methyltransferases (DNMTs) (Berger et al., 2009). The role of RNAs in epigenetic initiation, particularly with respect to marking targeted regions and silencing them via RNA-associated silencing, is also an area of intense study (Malecova and Morris, 2010; Zhou et al., 2010).

There are many examples of epigenetic deregulation in ovarian cancer, which include alterations in patterns of DNA methylation (Makarla et al, 2005; Rathi et al, 2002), histone modifications (Caslini et al, 2006), and microRNA (miRNA) expression (Li et al, 2010c; Wyman et al, 2009). Changes in histone modifications currently have little diagnostic value, due to low sensitivity and the need for obtaining tissue samples. Detection of hyper- and hypomethylation patterns of DNA proffers several advantages in the quest for quality biomarkers for early OEC diagnosis. Testing would be minimally invasive since DNA is easily accessible from the bloodstream and peritoneal fluid that is not quantitatively different from DNA in cells directly extracted from tumors (Asadollahi et al, 2010; Maradeo and Cairns, 2011). The regions of the genomes of cells in serum analyzed are often confined to specific locations, such as the CpG islands of promoter regions of specific genes. Once isolated, the DNA can then be amplified readily using methylation-specific PCR, ensuring high sensitivity (Cairns, 2007). Other advantages include stability of the portent indicators, via their resistance to degradation, and cost-effectiveness. A major limitation, however, is that different phenotypes lead to disparate methylation profiles because of the heterogeneous presentation of ovarian cancer. There is hope that, in time, selection of a combination of aberrantly methylated genes may serve as a composite marker specific for a general OEC phenotype, with certain markers serving as red flags for aggressive forms of cancer. As promoter methylation is a frequent early event in cancers, the ability to detect and analyze patterns consistent with malignancy in ovarian tumors may provide an opportunity for more accurate early detection.

3.1 Altered DNA methylation profiles

Cells from invasive tumors have widespread hypomethylation of repetitive elements with frequent hypermethylation of CpG dinucleotide-containing promoter regions of genes with tumor suppressive function (Balch et al, 2009). DNA methylation patterns reflect the stage and degree of tumor progression in ovarian cancer (Shih et al, 2010; Yang et al, 2006). Invasive tumors display a much larger set of genes whose methylation patterns are affected, with mean methylation index increasing threefold or higher compared with low malignancy tumors (Makarla et al, 2005). These differences reflect the category of tumor; whether the disease results from an accruement of gradual changes (low grade) or a sudden and more invasive phenotype from widespread chromosomal instability (CIN) (high grade). The latter is more prevalent, occurring in the majority of cases, including approximately 75% of serous carcinoma cases (Shih and Kurman, 2004). These tumors have recently been classified as CpG island methylator phenotype (CIMP) cancers, and are characterized by a rapid inactivation of a large number of genes, often by hypermethylation due to alterations in expression of DNMTs. Inactivation of *TP53* by mutation is a frequent result of CIN and accounted for in 96% of high grade serous ovarian carcinomas (Bell et al, 2011). In addition to the critical effects p53 maintains in cell cycle regulation, its inhibition is thought to play a role in the large scale hypermethylation of tumor suppressor genes, as its abrogation is associated with activation of DNMT1 via PI3K/Akt signaling (Cheng et al, 2011). Upregulated expression of DNMTs occurs frequently in ovarian cancer (Ahluwalia et al, 2001). Complete inactivation of *TP53* by mutation is the most common mutational event in aggressive high grade OEC (Singer et al, 2005, Bell et al, 2011). In contrast, low-grade OEC is characterized instead by mutations in *KRAS/BRAF/ERBB2*. It is not associated with the sudden, highly invasive phenotype observed in high-grade disease but rather via a slow, indolent progression (Singer et al, 2005). Methylation patterns in low-grade tumors are closer to those of the benign cystadenomas that may develop into them, although more pronounced, reflecting their gradual progression (Shih et al, 2010).

The inhibitory effects of p53 on the cell adhesion protein, E-cadherin, are multifaceted. E-cadherin can either be transcriptionally repressed by the absence of p53 through Twist activation (Yang et al, 2004), or be silenced by promoter methylation by DNMT1 (Cheng et al, 2011). Benign adenomas exhibit promoter hypermethylation at a 13% rate. The percentage is increased to 17% in low malignancy tumors and 26% in invasive tumors, showing an increase with increasing malignancy potential (Makarla et al, 2005). The steady increase from benign to low-malignancy-potential adenomas appear to reflect the step-by-step progression observed in low grade ovarian tumors unrelated to *TP53* mutation, while widespread CIN coupled with *TP53* inactivation are believed to account for the higher percentage of methylation in high grade tumors. Because loss of E-cadherin is essential in precipitating EMT in certain subsets of OEC (Patel et al, 2003) , it may be speculated that p53 down-regulation as a result of CIN caused by aneuploidy from extensive remodeling of the ECM may have major effects on hypermethylation of tumor suppressor promoters from a fairly early stage (Cheng et al, 2011). In contrast, despite the hereditary involvement of BRCA1/2, aneuploidy and CIN are involved in all cases of serous OEC studied, regardless of BRCA status (Pradhan et al, 2010). In sporadic but not hereditary OEC, *BRCA1* is highly methylated (Bol et al, 2010). Therefore, inactivation of the *BRCA1* gene through either mutation, loss of heterozygosity or promoter hypermethylation may be implicated in maintaining the tumor promoting environment, while *TP53* inactivation may affect gene expression in a more direct manner through its effect on DNMT1 as well as its other effects on cell cycle regulation and DNA damage repair.

While thousands of genes may have their methylation patterns altered, several common genes repressed by promoter methylation in ovarian cancer that may be useful as part of a methylation biomarker panel are listed in Table 2. These include a number of genes involved in tumor suppression, apoptosis, and cell adhesion. Although these genes are frequently silenced by epigenetic dysregulation, a number of them can also be inactivated through other mechanisms, such as loss of heterozygosity, imprinting, mutation, or transcriptional downregulation. Most hypermethylated genes observed in ovarian tumor tissue are detectable in blood via methylation-specific PCR analysis, and various combinations can be tested for utility as composite serum markers for diagnostic screening with high sensitivity (Melnikov et al, 2009).

Global hypomethylation of genes and repetitive elements is also a frequent finding in OEC, with extent correlating with increasing invasiveness (Shih et al, 2010). Repetitive elements have lost function over the course of evolution, so sudden loss of methylation on DNA components silenced for thousands or millions of years may be a critical factor in the disruption of chromosomal integrity observed in invasive carcinomas (Eden et al, 2003). Hypomethylation of LINE1 transposons and Sat2/Satα repeats commonly occurs in ovarian cancer (Widschwendter et al, 2004). LINE1 elements contain many splice sites that, when activated, could cause hybrid splicing events with closely positioned genes to alter their translational products in cancer (Belancio et al, 2006). Satellite repeats in heterochromatic regions of chromosome 1 have been observed to lose methylation status in proportion to

Gene	Functions	UniProt/Swiss-Prot ID
APC	Cell adhesion, Wnt inhibition, pro-apoptotic	P25054
ARHI	P21/p27 induction, STAT3 inhibition, pro-autophagic	O95661
BRCA1	DNA damage response, transcription regulation	P38398
DAPK	Pro-apoptotic	P53355
E-cadherin	Contact inhibition, p27 expression	P12830
GSTP1	Xenobiotic detoxification	P09211
H-cadherin	Contact inhibition, p21 expression	P55290
HIC1	Cooperative role with p53 via SIRT1 inhibition	Q14526
HSulf1	Inhibition of GF binding to HSPGs	Q8IWU6
ICAM1	Cell/matrix adhesion in immune/endothelial cells	P05362
IGFBP3	Inhibition of proliferation and invasion, pro-apoptotic	P17936
MCJ	MDR transporter inhibition	Q9Y5T4
MGMT	O6-MeG removal from damaged DNA	P16455
MLH1	DNA mismatch repair	P40692
OPCML	Cell adhesion, Ras inhibition	Q14982
PALB2	Colocalization with BRCA2 in damage response	Q86YC2
PAX5	B-cell differentiation	Q02548
PEG3	Re-localization of pro-apoptotic agents to favor apoptosis	Q9GZU2
PGR	Progesterone binding and signaling	P06401
PLAGL1	Inhibition of proliferation, pro-apoptotic	Q9UM63
PTEN	Inhibition of PI3K/Akt signaling, cell polarity establishment	P60484
P16	Cell cycle regulator, maintenance of senescence	Q8N726
RASSF1A	Ras inhibition, cyclin D1 inhibition, microtubule stabilization	Q9NS23
SPARC	LPA inhibition, prevention of GF-receptor binding, repression of VEGF-integrin-MMP axis	P09486
TCEAL7	NFκβ inhibition, apoptotic regulation	Q9BRU2
THBS1	Cell/matrix adhesion, platelet aggregation	P07996
14-3-3 sigma	Stabilization of p53	P31947

Table 2. Common Genes Repressed by Promoter Methylation in Ovarian Cancer.

tumor grade, and may help to differentiate between ovarian cancers of varying malignant potential as a result (Qu et al, 1999). Several oncogene promoters are hypomethylated as well in OEC, including synuclein-γ(*SNCG*), claudin-4 (*CLDN4*) and insulin-like growth factor-2 (*IGF2*), further contributing to the tumorigenic phenotype (Balch et al, 2009). These compounds have all been investigated as ovarian cancer biomarkers (Hibbs et al, 2004; Palmer et al, 2008), so identification of those genes displaying diminished methylation status may enhance their specificity for the disease.

3.2 miRNAs in ovarian cancer

miRNA signatures are 22-23 nucleotides in length once processed from precursor transcripts, and are being actively pursued as composite diagnostic markers for OEC. They can be analyzed in body fluids and show greater stability than mRNAs due to their greater resistance to RNase (Mitchell et al, 2008). Several miRNAs have been shown to be up-regulated in repeated experiments, and many have oncogenic potential by either inhibiting translation of tumor suppressors when up-regulated or facilitating unimpeded expression of oncogenes when down-regulated (Calin and Croce, 2006).

Common miRNAs frequently overexpressed in ovarian cancer include miR-93, miR-106b, miR-155, miR-200a/b/c, miR-221/222, and miR-372/373; underexpressed miRNAs include miR-15/16, miR-34b*/c, miR-125b1, miR-140, miR-145, and let-7i (Balch et al, 2009; Maradeo and Cairns, 2011). Increased neovascularization has been associated with high expression of miR-93, which may serve as an early indicator of tumor growth and angiogenesis (Fang et al, 2011). Other miRNAs, such as miR-106b and miR-221, target cell cycle inhibitors p21 and p27, respectively (le Sage et al, 2007; Li et al, 2011). Down-regulation of miR-34b*/c has been correlated with progression to advanced disease (Corney et al, 2010).

Some miRNAs may be up- or downregulated in the same tumor based on differentiation status of cells constituting the mass. Under the regulatory command of Twist, decreased miR-214 and miR-199a were observed in CD44+ OEC cells that were greatly dedifferentiated, while their normally differentiated CD44- counterparts exhibited higher concentrations of these non-coding RNAs (Yin et al, 2010). Low expression levels of these miRNAs, which silence PTEN and IKKβ/NF-κβ pathways, respectively, may have prognostic value, as the CD44+ cells studied displayed stem-like qualities and constitutively active inflammatory signaling (Chen et al, 2007). Additional clues for OEC characterization and prognosis will be provided as more miRNA markers are revealed and their functions elucidated. Along with evaluation of methylation signatures, miRNA signature analysis offers a promising non-invasive technique in the diagnosis and characterization of ovarian cancer adjuvant to traditional methods.

To recapitulate, epigenetic markers are gaining favor as diagnostic biomarkers for ovarian cancer because of their expression early in disease pathogenesis and the fact that most are amenable to the use of serum as a source. The types of methylation profiles vary based on malignancy potential and tumor source, so a panel of commonly expressed methylation markers could essentially help to differentiate between the multitudes of forms characterized by this heterogeneous cancer. Although it is far from an exhaustive list, Table 2 lists some of the more frequently hypermethylated genes frequently observed in ovarian cancer after over a decade of detailed analysis. Concomitant ongoing studies on miRNA profiles in ovarian cancer provide an alternate epigenetic approach for early detection. As patterns of epigenetic alterations are better clarified, panels consisting of the most sensitive and specific of these markers identified will likely be developed for further testing and possible validation.

4. HE4 as a potential early marker

A promising protein marker receiving much attention for its potential role in the early diagnosis of ovarian cancer is human epididymis secretory protein 4 (HE4). This protein is a member of the whey acidic four-disulfide core (WFDC) family, which includes secretory leukocyte protease inhibitor (SLPI) and elafin. Its function has not yet been elucidated, although it does not appear to exhibit protease inhibitor activity like most other members of the WFDC family. HE4 was first identified in human epididymis epithelium (Kirchhoff et al, 1991). Since its discovery, HE4 has been found in some other tissues as well, including the respiratory tract and nasopharynx. It is a frequently expressed selective early marker for this disease. While normal OSE does not express HE4, the protein can be detected in sera of patients diagnosed with the most prevalent forms of OEC, and is detectable even in inclusion cysts that may precede tumor formation (Drapkin et al, 2005).

Finding a protein biomarker to rival CA125 in sensitivity and specificity has posed a major challenge. Despite the failure of CA125 to accurately predict early disease, this marker has alone displayed the greatest overall diagnostic ability in repeated studies (Canney et al, 1984; Cramer et al, 2011; Medeiros et al, 2009). However, detection of HE4 holds some advantages over CA125, and its use in combination with the mucin marker is currently being evaluated. Overall specificity for HE4 is comparable to CA125 with greater discriminatory ability for the detection of early disease in patients with a pelvic mass (Hellstrom and Hellstrom, 2011; Montagnana et al, 2009; Nolen et al, 2010). Detection of HE4 has displayed a better ability to differentiate between benign and malignant disease, as the sensitivity was 56.7% for HE4 compared to 10.8% with CA125 at high specificity (Hellstrom et al, 2003). Receiver operator characteristic (ROC) curves, which plot changes in sensitivity in relation to specificity, were used to ascertain information on the usefulness of both markers in a head-to-head comparison. The AUC values of ROC curves generated for both HE4 and CA125 showed comparable rates for early detection, with HE4 exhibiting slightly higher values. Comparison of ROC curves for all cases yielded superior detection rates for CA125. Similar results from ROC-AUC analyses were reproduced elsewhere (Anastasi et al, 2010; Montagnana et al, 2009). However, ROC curves are not used as diagnostic criteria for ovarian cancer detection. The major benefit of serum HE4 testing observed in the study by Hellstrom et al (2003) was that there were significantly less false positive readings than with CA125.

In a retrospective study comparing CA125 and two different HE4 assays, the HE4 assays showed better sensitivity (Ruggeri et al, 2011). At 95% specificity, sensitivity was 83.3% and 84.4% for HE4 compared to 76% for CA125, and as the specificity increased to 99%, the difference increased further, with a 79.2% sensitivity for both HE4 assays and a 59.4% sensitivity for the CA125 assay.

An additional benefit of HE4 lies in its ability to be quantified in not only serum and ascitic fluid but urine as well. Specificity and sensitivity rates for urine samples were demonstrated to be comparable to serum concentrations, displaying results of 94.4% and 86.6%, respectively, for stage I/II cancers (Hellstrom et al, 2010). These data allow for the possibility of a noninvasive urine test adjuvant to other diagnostic criteria for ovarian cancer if this can be reproduced in larger studies. Measurement of serum HE4 is also effective for predicting early recurrence of ovarian cancer, as expression of HE4 increases an average of 5-8 months prior to a rise in CA125 in relapsing tumors (Anastasi et al, 2010).

Whereas CA125 is a better biomarker for overall ovarian cancer detection than HE4 based on multiple comparative studies (Cramer et al, 2011; Medeiros et al, 2009; Van Gorp et al, 2011), a composite assay measuring concentrations of both proteins may be ideal for enabling early detection. This could potentially translate into higher survival rates as the differences in mortality between early and late stage ovarian cancer are considerable. For this reason, combinatory testing has been explored in several prospective and retrospective studies (Andersen et al, 2010; Jacob et al, 2011; Shah et al, 2009; Van Gorp et al, 2011). The results thus far have been mixed, with naysayers arguing that the benefit of testing for HE4 in addition to CA125 is not sufficient to warrant clinical use.

In a prospective study of 389 patients with a pelvic mass of ovarian origin, ROC-AUC values showed only a slight advantage for HE4 testing in premenopausal patients compared to CA125 (Van Gorp et al, 2011). The CA125 assay was superior for postmenopausal patients, although a Risk of Ovarian Malignancy Algorithm (ROMA) based on a logarithmic formula of HE4 concentrations with menopausal status did improve detection ability in post-menopausal women. Unlike previous studies, sensitivity and specificity for HE4 were poor. Sensitivity was 74.5% at a specificity of 83.3%. In contrast, a case control study that included a large number of early stage patients demonstrated 77% sensitivity for HE4 detection at 94.9% specificity (Andersen et al, 2010). Overall sensitivity was slightly higher for CA125 (81%), but combining the two markers led to a significant increase in sensitivity without a major tradeoff in specificity. HE4 better detected early disease, and high risk patients were identified at 100% sensitivity compared to only 78.6% for CA125 at 95% specificity (Andersen et al, 2010). Shah and colleagues (2009) showed a benefit of HE4 over CA125 in discriminating between risk-matched healthy controls and cases in high risk groups. At a specificity of 95%, sensitivity in these cases was 87.8% for HE4 versus 82.9% for CA125. A cohort study of 160 subjects with mixed phenotypes (18% OEC) reproduced beneficial results for HE4 in early stage cancer detection, as well as a greater propensity for discriminating between borderline and malignant tumors (Jacob et al, 2011). High cost of HE4 screening caused the authors to caution against using the combination, however, as the overall benefits were minimal. Finally, a four marker panel consisting of HE4 and CA125 along with two additional markers (VCAM-1 and CEA) observed a 86% sensitivity at a high specificity of 98% (Yurkovetsky et al, 2010).

Although the advantages of combination testing with CA125 and HE4 biomarkers have been below expectations, the ability of HE4 to effectively diagnose early disease, identify disease in high risk patients for which screening is essential, and differentiate between borderline and malignant disease have increased its value as a diagnostic indicator. While data from older, post-menopausal women are subpar (Van Gorp et al, 2011), composite testing of CA125 and HE4 may be valuable for certain groups with further investigation, such as premenopausal women at high risk for disease.

5. Inherited mutations as biomarkers for ovarian cancer

There are several hereditary syndromes which increase the likelihood of ovarian cancer in a patient. Examples of such include hereditary breast and ovarian cancer (HBOC), hereditary nonpolyposis colorectal cancer (HNPCC), site-specific ovarian cancer (SSOC), Gorlin's syndrome, and Peutz-Jeghers syndrome (Russo et al., 2009). Of these, HBOC, HNPCC and

SSOC comprise about 99% of hereditary ovarian cancers. However, it is important to note that 10-13% of all ovarian cancer cases can be classified as hereditary and linked to the inherited mutations described below (Pal et al., 2005; Risch, 2001; Stratton JF, 1999; Sowter and Ashworth, 2005). In sporadic cancers, the mutational activation of oncogenes, coupled with non-mutational inactivation of tumor suppressor genes, is often observed (Kenemans et al., 2004). In hereditary cancers, germline mutations in a single allele confer an elevated risk for cancer development (Radice, 2002). Therefore, while genetic screening to identify at risk individuals is highly desirable in patients with a family history of breast, ovarian or colon cancer, the potential biomarkers described below may or may not be applicable for the detection of sporadic ovarian cancers.

5.1 Human MutS homolog 2 (*hMSH2*) and Human MutL homolog 1 (*hMLH1*)

Ovarian carcinomas in patients from HNPCC families typically present as early-onset, non-serous epithelial tumors (Ketabi et al., 2011). *hMSH2* and *hMLH1* are the two most frequently mutated genes in this syndrome and confer a 9-12% lifetime risk of ovarian cancer (Aarnio et al., 1995; Brown et al., 2001; Kasprzak et al., 1999; Russo et al., 2009). The hMSH2 and hMLH1 proteins are the fundamental components of DNA mismatch repair (MMR) (Kolodner et al., 1994) and defects in these genes significantly increase the rate of mutation, which is believed to contribute to cancer development (Loeb, 2011; Valeri et al., 2010). In particular, microsatellite instability (MSI) has been observed in tumors from HNPCC patients (Dietmaier et al., 1997) and stems, at least in part, from a mutation or inherited epigenetic inactivation of hMLH1 (Gazzoli et al., 2002; Goecke et al., 2006; Hitchins et al, 2007; Kane et al., 1997). Interestingly, Valeri and colleagues (2010) reported that a non-coding miRNA designated as miR-155 is significantly overexpressed in human colorectal cancers and that an inverse correlation exists between the expression of miR-155 and the expression of hMLH1 or hMSH2 proteins in these tissues. miR-155 has been detected in blood samples derived from patients with ovarian cancer, though the sensitivity is still too low to be used as a reliable and predictive indicator of disease progression (Hausler et al., 2010). miR-155 has been put forth as a potential biomarker for the detection of early pancreatic neoplasia (Habbe et al., 2009).

Screening for mutations in genes important to MMR, such as *hMSH2* and *hMLH1*, and for epigenetic changes relevant to MMR such as hMLH1 promoter methylation, should prove to be an effective strategy for identifying patients in HNPCC families who may also be at risk for developing ovarian cancer. Moreover, screening for the upregulation of the noncoding RNA miR-155 may also prove to be effective in this regard. Important questions concerning the latter remain to be answered; including whether miR-155 upregulation is involved with sporadic ovarian cancers and if this noncoding RNA can be used as an early diagnostic marker.

5.2 Breast Cancer Susceptibility Genes (*BRCA1* and *BRCA2*)

BRCA1 and BRCA2 are large nuclear proteins which act as tumor suppressors and contribute to genetic stability and DNA damage repair (Arai et al., 2004; Meindl et al., 2011; van der Groep et al., 2011). Whereas numerous biochemical and molecular functions have been described for both proteins (reviewed in Narod & Foulkes, 2004; Venkitaraman, 2002), they have both been implicated in the repair of double-strand breaks (DSBs) by homologous recombination (HR) (Badie et al., 2010; Boulton, 2006; Moynahan et al., 1999; Moynahan et al., 2001; Murphy and Moynahan, 2010; Shrivastav et al., 2008; Venkitaraman, 2003).

Approximately half of high grade serous carcinomas exhibit defects in HR, solidifying the importance of this process in its implications for disease pathology extending beyond the presence of germline mutations (Bell et al., 2011).

The risk of ovarian cancer is about 40% in carriers with BRCA1 mutations (Antoniou et al., 2003; Ford et al., 1994). BRCA1 is composed of 1863 amino acids and possesses a N-terminal RING domain and and two C-terminal BRCT domains, present in tandem, at its C-terminus. The RING domain is protein-protein interaction motif which mediates the binding of BRCA1 to its obligate partner BARD1 (Meza et al., 1999; Wu et al., 1996). The BRCA1:BARD1 complex possesses ubiquitin ligase activity (Starita et al., 2004) while the BRCT domains of BRCA1 serve as sites of numerous protein-protein interactions, regulate transcription, and possess the ability to bind to phosphopeptides (reviewed in Narod and Foulkes, 2004; Starita and Parvin, 2003; Manke et al., 2003). Numerous cancer-associated missense mutations which disrupt interactions with putative binding partners have been described in the RING and BRCT domains of BRCA1 (reviewed in Carvalho et al., 2007; Morris and Solomon, 2004; Szabo et al., 2004).

The risk of ovarian cancer is about 25% in patients with *BRCA2* mutations (Ford et al., 1998). BRCA2 is composed of 3418 amino acids and possesses two distinct classes of BRC repeats which interact with the RAD51 protein, the mammalian homolog of *Escherichia coli* RecA (Carreira and Kowalczykowski, 2011). In addition, the C-terminal region of BRCA2, TR2, interacts with RAD51 (van der Groep et al., 2011). A major mechanism by which RAD51 is recruited to damaged DNA is via its interaction with BRCA2 and, along with the latter, plays a critical role in homologous recombination (Badie et al., 2010; Davies et al., 2001; Jensen et al., 2010). Cancer associated point mutations on BRC repeats which disrupt interaction of BRCA2 with RAD51 have been reported (Venkitaraman, 2009). Based on the observation that BRC repeats bind distinct regions of RAD51 and are not equal in their mode of interaction, it was hypothesized that a mutation within even one of the eight BRC repeats in this region could be sufficient to affect the way that BRCA2 interacts with RAD51, and lead to an increased risk of cancer (Galkin et al., 2005). Interestingly, certain families exhibit *BRCA2* mutations which appear to predispose carriers to ovarian cancer and which are located within exon 11 (Gayther et al., 1997; Lubinski et al., 2004; Petrucelli et al., 2002; Thompson et al., 2001). While this area is generally referred to as the ovarian cancer cluster region, Al-Saffar and Foulkes (2002) proposed that this region of exon 11 be known as the diminished breast cancer risk region.

Ovarian tumors in women carrying mutations in *BRCA1* or *BRCA2* are generally serous carcinomas and tend to be of high grade when diagnosed (Sowter and Ashworth, 2005). High grade serous carcinomas associated with *BRCA* mutations are believed to arise from the distal fallopian tube (Crum, 2009; Piek et al., 2003) and are frequently accompanied by mutations in *TP53* (Ahmed et al., 2010; Milner et al, 1993; reviewed in Hall et al., 2004). A comprehensive model for the development of high grade serous ovarian cancer has been put forth by Bowtell (2010) in which the loss of p53 and BRCA disrupts the HR repair of damaged DNA and, in turn, leads to CIN and carcinogenesis. A link between ovarian inclusion cysts and serous carcinomas has been proposed (Sowter and Ashworth, 2005) and may be explained by a mechanism in which cells from the fimbria travel to inclusion cysts and there become transformed and malignant via endometriosis or a series of mitogenic events and malignant (Crum, 2009). Alternatively, high grade serous carcinomas may be derived from stem-like ovarian cancer cells which have been dysregulated due, at least in part, to *BRCA* inactivation (Foulkes, 2004; Yin et al., 2010). Other hypotheses to explain the tissue specific cancers observed in mutant *BRCA* carriers have also been reviewed elsewhere

(Billack and Monteiro, 2005). It is interesting to note that while epigenetic silencing of *BRCA1* in high grade tumors has been reported (Wilson et al., 1999), somatic mutations in *BRCA1* and *BRCA2* are rare in sporadic breast and ovarian cancers (Futreal et al., 1994; Lancaster et al., 1996).

While DNA testing for *BRCA* mutations is becoming more common, not all women will obtain a clear cut result. One possible outcome of *BRCA* genetic testing is the finding that the patient possesses a *BRCA* variant of uncertain significance for which there is no clinical information regarding its cancer association. Methods have been developed to assess the cancer risk of unclassified *BRCA* variants which involve the use of functional assays (Carvalho et al., 2007; Lee et al., 2010) and structure-based supervised learning computation models (Karchin et al., 2007). One example of how functional assays and computational models can be used to characterize rare *BRCA* alleles was recently described in a collaborative study involving our lab (Carvalho et al., 2009). In that study, a Swedish kindred L1383 revealed a proband with ovarian cancer at age 59 (Figure 1A, arrow). The proband's mother also had ovarian cancer while the proband's grandmother died from rectal cancer. Upon analysis it was found that this patient had a rare variant of *BRCA1* denoted as 5673insC which codes for an insertion of a cytosine at nt5673 in exon 24. The cytosine insertion produces a frameshift in which the last 12 amino acids of the protein are changed to a modified 15-amino acid segment. Functional growth assays utilizing a reporter gene driven by LexA were carried out to examine the effect of this insertion. Yeast transformed with fusion constructs coding for either wildtype (W) or mutated BRCA1 (5673insC) fused to a LexA DNA binding domain revealed that the mutant failed to activate the reporter gene, resulting in a significantly reduced growth compared to yeast expressing the wildtype construct (Figure 1B). Use of computational structural modeling suggested that the insertion could generate a novel 13-residue α-helix that might modify the binding of phosphopeptide to the BRCT binding pocket (Figure 1C, golden helix). Taken together, the functional data and the structure prediction suggest that the insertion leads to an impact on protein function. Despite the wealth of information generated via these functional and computational approaches, clinical validation is difficult to obtain due to the rarity of most uncharacterized *BRCA* variants. Moreover, the complexity of this approach makes high throughput analyses cumbersome. Nevertheless, the more information available for genetic counseling purposes the better.

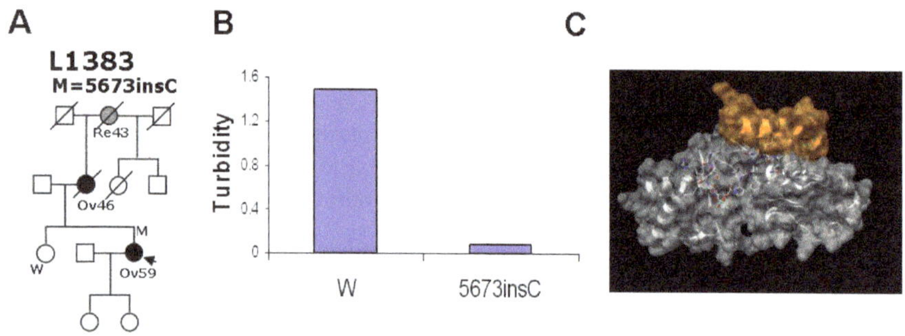

Fig. 1. Use of family history (Panel A), functional analysis (Panel B) and structure-based supervised learning computation models (Panel C) to assess uncharacterized variants of BRCA1. Reprinted from Carvalho et al., 2009, with permission from Elsevier.

There are medical options for a woman with a strong family history of cancer and altered *BRCA* status. In particular, a woman with a highly penetrant cancer-associated *BRCA* mutation who undergoes a prophylactic bilateral salpingo-oophorectomy decreases her risk of ovarian cancer by 80% (Brown and Parker, 2011; Finch et al., 2006). A decreased risk of ovarian cancer has been observed in carriers of *BRCA* mutations who undergo tubal ligation, though it should be noted that this procedure is not as effective as removal of the ovaries (Brown and Parker, 2011). About 2-5% of patients who undergo the prophylactic oophorectomy procedure exhibit an occult cancer of the ovaries upon histological examination (Lu et al., 2000; Schrag et al., 1997). Based on these observations, prophylactic oophorectomy for BRCA1 or BRCA2 mutation carriers appears to be the more effective method of reducing cancer risk, particularly if reproduction and child rearing has occurred (Olopade and Artioli, 2004; Salhab et al., 2010). It is also worthy to note that ovarian cancer patients with traditional *BRCA* mutations have been found to show better survival rates than those with hypermethylation silencing (Bell et al., 2011). It is therefore imperative to identify at risk patients harboring cancer predisposing and inherited mutations in *BRCA1* and *BRCA2*.

6. Sporadic ovarian cancer and new genetic markers

PCR-based technologies have the potential to allow for the rapid identification of patients who exhibit genetic variations within gene sequences, introns, promoters and other important regions of DNA, such as cancer susceptibility loci. Genetic variations associated with the androgen receptor have been observed to increase the risk of sporadic ovarian cancer in both Caucasian (Ludwig, 2009) and African-American (Schilkdkraut, 2007) populations. Furthermore, single nucleotide polymorphisms (SNPs) have been identified in several genes which are likely or very likely to associate with ovarian cancer including *CCND1* (Quaye et al., 2009), *MRPL23* (Quaye et al., 2009), *CDKN1B* (Goode et al., 2009), *CDKN2A/2B* (Goode et al., 2009) and *RB1* (Song et al., 2006; Braem et al., 2011). Aside from these SNPs in specific genes, several ovarian cancer susceptibility loci have been identified and analyzed using genome wide association studies. These studies have been reviewed by Braem and colleagues (2011), who conclude that there is strong evidence to establish a correlation between ovarian cancer and SNPs on chromosomes 9p22.2, 2q31, 8q24, and 3q25. Taken together, these studies point to several genes and susceptibility loci which may be amenable to high throughput screening and may help to identify ovarian cancer before it begins or in early stages, when survival is highest.

7. Summary and future directions

Understanding of the landscape of ovarian cancer pathogenesis has evolved over recent years, and with it, strategies for patient care. Early detection continues to be a top priority to diagnose this pernicious disease when it is still highly responsive to treatment. Novel discoveries in genomics, epigenetics, proteomics, and functional glycomics have rapidly expanded the number of potential tumor markers available. To make better sense of which candidate markers have the greatest significance, several strategies have been employed. Identification of cancer-specific alterations in glycosylation signatures and development of composite epigenetic serum panels are two minimally invasive approaches that may, in time, allow for more accurate early detection of ovarian cancer.

Aside from CA125, which currently remains the sole validated ovarian cancer biomarker, other serum markers may be comparable or superior for early detection. Among these, HE4 appears especially promising, and the use of CA125 testing with HE4 or other emerging markers may prove to be clinically useful. In addition, better identification of women with greatest genetic risk may help to isolate a small subset of the population that requires the closest monitoring. By employing strategies such as those described above, it is hopeful that ovarian cancer mortality rates, which have remained intractably high over the past several decades, will finally begin to decline.

8. Acknowledgements

We gratefully appreciate the efforts of the following colleagues who provided helpful comments during the preparation of this chapter: Drs. C. Lau-Cam and L. Schramm (St. John's University, Jamaica, NY), Dr. Dong-Hua Yang (Fox Chase Cancer Center, Philadelphia, PA), Dr. Alvaro Monteiro (Moffitt Cancer Center, Tampa, FL) and Dr. X.X. Xu (University of Miami Miller School of Medicine, Miami, FL).

9. Dedication

This chapter is dedicated to all women who are living with and those who have died from ovarian cancer.

10. References

Aarnio M. et al. (1995) Life-time risk of different cancers in hereditary non-polyposis colorectal cancer (HNPCC) syndrome. *Int.J.Cancer.* 64, 430-433.

Abbott K.L. et al. (2010) Identification of candidate biomarkers with cancer-specific glycosylation in the tissue and serum of endometrioid ovarian cancer patients by glycoproteomic analysis. *Proteomics.* 10, 470-481.

Ahluwalia A. et al. (2001) DNA methylation in ovarian cancer. II. Expression of DNA methyltransferases in ovarian cancer cell lines and normal ovarian epithelial cells. *Gynecol.Oncol.* 82, 299-304.

Ahmad R. et al. (2009) MUC1-C oncoprotein functions as a direct activator of the nuclear factor-kappaB p65 transcription factor. *Cancer Res.* 69, 7013-7021.

Ahmad S. (2011) Advances in ovarian cancer screening: health and medicine for women: a multidisciplinary, evidence-based review of mid-life health concerns. *Yale J.Biol.Med.* 84, 47-49.

Ahmed A.A. et al. (2010) Driver mutations in TP53 are ubiquitous in high grade serous carcinoma of the ovary. *J.Pathol.* 221, 49-56.

Ahmed N. et al. (2005) Role of integrin receptors for fibronectin, collagen and laminin in the regulation of ovarian carcinoma functions in response to a matrix microenvironment. *Clin.Exp.Metastasis.* 22, 391-402.

Al-Saffar M. & Foulkes W.D. (2002). Hereditary ovarian cancer resulting from a non-ovarian cancer cluster region (OCCR) BRCA2 mutation: is the OCCR useful clinically? *J. Med. Genet.* 39, e68.

Anastasi E. et al. (2010) HE4: a new potential early biomarker for the recurrence of ovarian cancer. *Tumour.Biol.* 31, 113-119.

Andersen M.R. et al. (2010) Use of a Symptom Index, CA125, and HE4 to predict ovarian cancer. *Gynecol.Oncol.* 116, 378-383.

Andre S. et al. (2009) From structural to functional glycomics: core substitutions as molecular switches for shape and lectin affinity of N-glycans. *Biol.Chem.* 390, 557-565.

Antoniou A. et al. (2003) Average risks of breast and ovarian cancer associated with BRCA1 or BRCA2 mutations detected in case Series unselected for family history: a combined analysis of 22 studies. *Am.J.Hum.Genet.* 72, 1117-1130.

Arai M., Utsunomiya J., & Miki Y. (2004) Familial breast and ovarian cancers. *Int.J.Clin.Oncol.* 9, 270-282.

Asadollahi R., Hyde C.A., & Zhong X.Y. (2010) Epigenetics of ovarian cancer: from the lab to the clinic. *Gynecol.Oncol.* 118, 81-87.

Aubert M. et al. (2000) Peritoneal colonization by human pancreatic cancer cells is inhibited by antisense FUT3 sequence. *Int.J.Cancer.* 88, 558-565.

Badie S. et al. (2010) BRCA2 acts as a RAD51 loader to facilitate telomere replication and capping. *Nat.Struct.Mol.Biol.* 17, 1461-1469.

Bafna S., Kaur S., & Batra S.K. (2010) Membrane-bound mucins: the mechanistic basis for alterations in the growth and survival of cancer cells. *Oncogene.* 20;29, 2893-2904.

Balch C. et al. (2009) Minireview: epigenetic changes in ovarian cancer. *Endocrinology.* 150, 4003-4011.

Bast R.C., Jr. et al. (1981) Reactivity of a monoclonal antibody with human ovarian carcinoma. *J.Clin.Invest.* 68, 1331-1337.

Bast R.C., Jr. et al. (2005) New tumor markers: CA125 and beyond. *Int.J.Gynecol.Cancer.* 15 Suppl 3:274-81., 274-281.

Basu A. et al. (1987) Presence of tumor-associated antigens in epidermal growth factor receptors from different human carcinomas. *Cancer Res.* 47, 2531-2536.

Belancio V.P., Hedges D.J., & Deininger P. (2006) LINE-1 RNA splicing and influences on mammalian gene expression. *Nucleic Acids Res.* 34, 1512-1521.

Belisle J.A. et al. (2010) Identification of Siglec-9 as the receptor for MUC16 on human NK cells, B cells, and monocytes. *Mol.Cancer.* 9:118., 118.

Bell D. (2011) Integrated genomic analyses of ovarian carcinoma. *Nature.* 474, 609-615.

Berger S.L. et al. (2009) An operational definition of epigenetics. *Genes Dev.* 23, 781-783.

Billack B. & Monteiro A.N. (2005) BRCA1 in breast and ovarian cancer predisposition. *Cancer Lett.* 227, 1-7.

Bol G.M. et al. (2010) Methylation profiles of hereditary and sporadic ovarian cancer. *Histopathology.* 57, 363-370.

Boulton S.J. (2006) Cellular functions of the BRCA tumour-suppressor proteins. *Biochem.Soc.Trans.* 34, 633-645.

Bowtell D.D. (2010) The genesis and evolution of high-grade serous ovarian cancer. *Nat.Rev.Cancer.* 10, 803-808.

Braem M.G. et al. (2011). Genetic susceptibility to sporadic ovarian cancer: A systematic review. *Biochem. Biophys. Acta* 1816, 132-146.

Bret C. et al. (2011) SULFs in human neoplasia: implication as progression and prognosis factors. *J.Transl.Med.* 9:72., 72.

Brockhausen I, Schachter H, Stanley P. O-GalNAc Glycans. In: Varki A, Cummings RD, Esko JD, Freeze HH, Stanley P, Bertozzi CR, Hart GW, Etzler ME, editors.

Essentials of Glycobiology. 2nd edition. Cold Spring Harbor (NY): Cold Spring Harbor Laboratory Press; 2009. Chapter 9.

Brown G.J. et al. (2001) Cancer risk in young women at risk of hereditary nonpolyposis colorectal cancer: implications for gynecologic surveillance. *Gynecol.Oncol.* 80, 346-349.

Brown K.R., Parker, L.P. (2011). Hereditary Ovarian Cancer and Other Gynecologic Malignancies. In: Ellis CN, editor. Inherited Cancer Syndromes: Current Clinical Management.. 2nd edition. Springer Science Press (NY); Chapter 10.

Buys S.S. et al. (2011) Effect of screening on ovarian cancer mortality: the Prostate, Lung, Colorectal and Ovarian (PLCO) Cancer Screening Randomized Controlled Trial. *JAMA.* 305, 2295-2303.

Cairns P. (2007) Gene methylation and early detection of genitourinary cancer: the road ahead. *Nat.Rev.Cancer.* 7, 531-543.

Calin G.A. & Croce C.M. (2006) MicroRNA-cancer connection: the beginning of a new tale. *Cancer Res.* 66, 7390-7394.

Canney P.A. et al. (1984) Ovarian cancer antigen CA125: a prospective clinical assessment of its role as a tumour marker. *Br.J.Cancer.* 50, 765-769.

Cannistra S.A. et al. (1995) Expression and function of beta 1 and alpha v beta 3 integrins in ovarian cancer. *Gynecol.Oncol.* 58, 216-225.

Carreira A. & Kowalczykowski S.C. (2011) Two classes of BRC repeats in BRCA2 promote RAD51 nucleoprotein filament function by distinct mechanisms. *Proc.Natl.Acad.Sci.U.S.A.*

Carvalho M. et al. (2009) Analysis of a set of missense, frameshift, and in-frame deletion variants of BRCA1. *Mutat.Res.* 660, 1-11.

Carvalho M.A., Couch F.J., & Monteiro A.N. (2007) Functional assays for BRCA1 and BRCA2. *Int.J.Biochem.Cell Biol.* 39, 298-310.

Caslini C. et al. (2006) Histone modifications silence the GATA transcription factor genes in ovarian cancer. *Oncogene.* 25, 5446-5461.

Chen R. et al. (2007) Inflammation, cancer and chemoresistance: taking advantage of the toll-like receptor signaling pathway. *Am.J.Reprod.Immunol.* 57, 93-107.

Cheng J.C., Auersperg N., & Leung P.C. (2011) Inhibition of p53 represses E-cadherin expression by increasing DNA methyltransferase-1 and promoter methylation in serous borderline ovarian tumor cells. *Oncogene.*

Chhieng D.C. et al. (2003) Expression of CEA, Tag-72, and Lewis-Y antigen in primary and metastatic lesions of ovarian carcinoma. *Hum.Pathol.* 34, 1016-1021.

Chiang C.H. et al. (2010) A novel sialyltransferase inhibitor AL10 suppresses invasion and metastasis of lung cancer cells by inhibiting integrin-mediated signaling. *J.Cell Physiol.* 223, 492-499.

Christie D.R. et al. (2008) ST6Gal-I expression in ovarian cancer cells promotes an invasive phenotype by altering integrin glycosylation and function. *J.Ovarian.Res.* 1, 3.

Corney D.C. et al. (2010) Frequent downregulation of miR-34 family in human ovarian cancers. *Clin.Cancer Res.* 16, 1119-1128.

Cramer D.W. et al. (2011) Ovarian cancer biomarker performance in prostate, lung, colorectal, and ovarian cancer screening trial specimens. *Cancer Prev.Res.(Phila).* 4, 365-374.

Crum C.P. (2009) Intercepting pelvic cancer in the distal fallopian tube: theories and realities. *Mol.Oncol.* 3, 165-170.

Dall'Olio F. & Chiricolo M. (2001) Sialyltransferases in cancer. *Glycoconj.J.* 18, 841-850.

Daniel L. et al. (2001) A nude mice model of human rhabdomyosarcoma lung metastases for evaluating the role of polysialic acids in the metastatic process. *Oncogene.* 20, 997-1004.

Davies A.A. et al. (2001) Role of BRCA2 in control of the RAD51 recombination and DNA repair protein. *Mol.Cell.* 7, 273-282.

Davies E.J. et al. (2004) Distribution and clinical significance of heparan sulfate proteoglycans in ovarian cancer. *Clin.Cancer Res.* 10, 5178-5186.

Diamandis E.P. et al. (2003) Human kallikrein 6 (hK6): a new potential serum biomarker for diagnosis and prognosis of ovarian carcinoma. *J.Clin.Oncol.* 21, 1035-1043.

Dietmaier W. et al. (1997) Diagnostic microsatellite instability: definition and correlation with mismatch repair protein expression. *Cancer Res.* 57, 4749-4756.

Drapkin R. et al. (2005) Human epididymis protein 4 (HE4) is a secreted glycoprotein that is overexpressed by serous and endometrioid ovarian carcinomas. *Cancer Res.* 65, 2162-2169.

Eden A. et al. (2003) Chromosomal instability and tumors promoted by DNA hypomethylation. *Science.* 300, 455.

El Sherbini M.A. et al. (2011) Diagnostic value of serum kallikrein-related peptidases 6 and 10 versus CA125 in ovarian cancer. *Int.J.Gynecol.Cancer.* 21, 625-632.

Fang L. et al. (2011) MicroRNA miR-93 promotes tumor growth and angiogenesis by targeting integrin-beta8. *Oncogene.* 30, 806-821.

Finch A. et al. (2006) Salpingo-oophorectomy and the risk of ovarian, fallopian tube, and peritoneal cancers in women with a BRCA1 or BRCA2 Mutation. *JAMA.* 296, 185-192.

Florkowski C.M. (2008) Sensitivity, specificity, receiver-operating characteristic (ROC) curves and likelihood ratios: communicating the performance of diagnostic tests. *Clin.Biochem.Rev.* 29 Suppl 1: S83-S87.

Fontenot J.D. et al. (1993) Biophysical characterization of one-, two-, and three-tandem repeats of human mucin (muc-1) protein core. *Cancer Res.* 53, 5386-5394.

Ford D. et al. (1994) Risks of cancer in BRCA1-mutation carriers. Breast Cancer Linkage Consortium. *Lancet.* 19;343, 692-695.

Ford D. et al. (1998) Genetic heterogeneity and penetrance analysis of the BRCA1 and BRCA2 genes in breast cancer families. The Breast Cancer Linkage Consortium. *Am.J.Hum.Genet.* 62, 676-689.

Foulkes W.D. (2004) BRCA1 functions as a breast stem cell regulator. *J.Med.Genet.* 41, 1-5.

Fukuda M. (1996) Possible roles of tumor-associated carbohydrate antigens. *Cancer Res.* 56, 2237-2244.

Fukuda M. (2002) Roles of mucin-type O-glycans in cell adhesion. *Biochim.Biophys.Acta.* 19;1573, 394-405.

Futreal P.A. et al. (1994) BRCA1 mutations in primary breast and ovarian carcinomas. *Science.* 266, 120-122.

Galkin V.E. et al. (2005) BRCA2 BRC motifs bind RAD51-DNA filaments. *Proc.Natl.Acad.Sci.U.S.A.* 102, 8537-8542.

Gao L. et al. (2011) Enhancive effects of Lewis y antigen on CD44-mediated adhesion and spreading of human ovarian cancer cell line RMG-I. *J.Exp.Clin.Cancer Res.* 30:15., 15.

Gayther S.A. et al. (1997) Variation of risks of breast and ovarian cancer associated with different germline mutations of the BRCA2 gene. *Nat.Genet.* 15, 103-105.

Gazzoli I. et al. (2002) A hereditary nonpolyposis colorectal carcinoma case associated with hypermethylation of the MLH1 gene in normal tissue and loss of heterozygosity of the unmethylated allele in the resulting microsatellite instability-high tumor. *Cancer Res.* 62, 3925-3928.

Gluer S. et al. (1998a) Serum polysialylated neural cell adhesion molecule in childhood neuroblastoma. *Br.J.Cancer.* 78, 106-110.

Gluer S. et al. (1998b) Polysialylated neural cell adhesion molecule in childhood rhabdomyosarcoma. *Pediatr.Res.* 43, 145-147.

Goecke T. et al. (2006) Genotype-phenotype comparison of German MLH1 and MSH2 mutation carriers clinically affected with Lynch syndrome: a report by the German HNPCC Consortium. *J.Clin.Oncol.* 24, 4285-4292.

Goode E.L. et al. (2009) Candidate gene analysis using imputed genotypes: cell cycle single-nucleotide polymorphisms and ovarian cancer risk. *Cancer Epidemiol.Biomarkers Prev.* 18, 935-944.

Gu J. & Taniguchi N. (2004) Regulation of integrin functions by N-glycans. *Glycoconj.J.* 21, 9-15.

Habbe N. et al. (2009) MicroRNA miR-155 is a biomarker of early pancreatic neoplasia. *Cancer Biol.Ther.* 8, 340-346.

Hakomori S. (1996) Tumor malignancy defined by aberrant glycosylation and sphingo(glyco)lipid metabolism. *Cancer Res.* 56, 5309-5318.

Hakomori S. (2002) Glycosylation defining cancer malignancy: new wine in an old bottle. *Proc.Natl.Acad.Sci.U.S.A.* 99, 10231-10233.

Hall J., Paul J., & Brown R. (2004) Critical evaluation of p53 as a prognostic marker in ovarian cancer. *Expert.Rev.Mol.Med.* 6, 1-20.

Hanasaki K. et al. (1994) Cytokine-induced beta-galactoside alpha-2,6-sialyltransferase in human endothelial cells mediates alpha 2,6-sialylation of adhesion molecules and CD22 ligands. *J.Biol.Chem.* 269, 10637-10643.

Hartel-Schenk S. et al. (2001) Novel adapter protein AP162 connects a sialyl-Le(x)-positive mucin with an apoptotic signal transduction pathway. *Glycoconj.J.* 18, 915-923.

Hausler S.F. et al. (2010) Whole blood-derived miRNA profiles as potential new tools for ovarian cancer screening. *Br.J.Cancer.* 103, 693-700.

Hedlund M. et al. (2008) Evidence for a human-specific mechanism for diet and antibody-mediated inflammation in carcinoma progression. *Proc.Natl.Acad.Sci.U.S.A.* 105, 18936-18941.

Hellstrom I. et al. (2003) The HE4 (WFDC2) protein is a biomarker for ovarian carcinoma. *Cancer Res.* 63, 3695-3700.

Hellstrom I. et al. (2010) Detection of the HE4 protein in urine as a biomarker for ovarian neoplasms. *Cancer Lett.* 296, 43-48.

Hellstrom I. & Hellstrom K.E. (2011) Two novel biomarkers, mesothelin and HE4, for diagnosis of ovarian carcinoma. *Expert.Opin.Med.Diagn.* 5, 227-240.

Helzlsouer K.J. et al. (1993) Prospective study of serum CA-125 levels as markers of ovarian cancer. *JAMA.* 269, 1123-1126.

Hibbs K. et al. (2004) Differential gene expression in ovarian carcinoma: identification of potential biomarkers. *Am.J.Pathol.* 165, 397-414.

Higashi H. et al. (1984) Tumor-associated expression of glycosphingolipid Hanganutziu-Deicher antigen in human cancers. *Gann.* 75, 1025-1029.

Hitchins M.P. et al. (2007) Inheritance of a cancer-associated MLH1 germ-line epimutation. *N.Engl.J.Med.* 356, 697-705.

Inoue S., Sato C., & Kitajima K. (2010) Extensive enrichment of N-glycolylneuraminic acid in extracellular sialoglycoproteins abundantly synthesized and secreted by human cancer cells. *Glycobiology.* 20, 752-762.

Jacob F. et al. (2011) No benefit from combining HE4 and CA125 as ovarian tumor markers in a clinical setting. *Gynecol.Oncol.* 121, 487-491.

Jacobs I. & Bast R.C., Jr. (1989) The CA 125 tumour-associated antigen: a review of the literature. *Hum.Reprod.* 4, 1-12.

Jarboe E. et al. (2008) Serous carcinogenesis in the fallopian tube: a descriptive classification. *Int.J.Gynecol.Pathol.* 27, 1-9.

Jensen M. & Berthold F. (2007) Targeting the neural cell adhesion molecule in cancer. *Cancer Lett.* 258, 9-21.

Jensen R.B., Carreira A., & Kowalczykowski S.C. (2010) Purified human BRCA2 stimulates RAD51-mediated recombination. *Nature.* 467, 678-683.

Jonckheere N. & Van Seuningen, I (2010) The membrane-bound mucins: From cell signalling to transcriptional regulation and expression in epithelial cancers. *Biochimie.* 92, 1-11.

Kane M.F. et al. (1997) Methylation of the hMLH1 promoter correlates with lack of expression of hMLH1 in sporadic colon tumors and mismatch repair-defective human tumor cell lines. *Cancer Res.* 57, 808-811.

Kanoh A. et al. (2006) Ectopic expression of N-acetylglucosamine 6-O-sulfotransferase 2 in chemotherapy-resistant ovarian adenocarcinomas. *Glycoconj.J.* 23, 453-460.

Karchin R. et al. (2007) Functional impact of missense variants in BRCA1 predicted by supervised learning. *PLoS.Comput.Biol.* 3, e26.

Kasprzak L., Foulkes W.D., & Shelling A.N. (1999) Forth nightly review: hereditary ovarian carcinoma. *BMJ.* 20;318, 786-789.

Kenemans P., Verstraeten R.A., & Verheijen R.H. (2004) Oncogenic pathways in hereditary and sporadic breast cancer. *Maturitas.* 49, 34-43.

Ketabi Z. et al. (2011) Ovarian cancer linked to lynch syndrome typically presents as early-onset, non-serous epithelial tumors. *Gynecol.Oncol.* 121, 462-465.

Kirchhoff C. et al. (1991) A major human epididymis-specific cDNA encodes a protein with sequence homology to extracellular proteinase inhibitors. *Biol.Reprod.* 45, 350-357.

Kodama J. et al. (2001) Thrombospondin-1 and -2 messenger RNA expression in epithelial ovarian tumor. *Anticancer Res.* 21, 2983-2987.

Kolodner R.D. et al. (1994) Structure of the human MSH2 locus and analysis of two Muir-Torre kindreds for msh2 mutations. *Genomics.* 24, 516-526.

Kufe D.W. (2009) Mucins in cancer: function, prognosis and therapy. *Nat.Rev.Cancer.* 9, 874-885.

Kuzmanov U. et al. (2009) Differential N-glycosylation of kallikrein 6 derived from ovarian cancer cells or the central nervous system. *Mol.Cell Proteomics.* 8, 791-798.

Lai J. et al. (2003) Loss of HSulf-1 up-regulates heparin-binding growth factor signaling in cancer. *J.Biol.Chem.* 20;278, 23107-23117.

Lancaster J.M. et al. (1996) BRCA2 mutations in primary breast and ovarian cancers. *Nat.Genet.* 13, 238-240.

Lau K.M., Mok S.C., & Ho S.M. (1999) Expression of human estrogen receptor-alpha and -beta, progesterone receptor, and androgen receptor mRNA in normal and malignant ovarian epithelial cells. *Proc.Natl.Acad.Sci.U.S.A.* 96, 5722-5727.

le Sage C. et al. (2007) Regulation of the p27(Kip1) tumor suppressor by miR-221 and miR-222 promotes cancer cell proliferation. *EMBO J.* 26, 3699-3708.

Lee M.S. et al. (2010) Comprehensive analysis of missense variations in the BRCT domain of BRCA1 by structural and functional assays. *Cancer Res.* 70, 4880-4890.

Li B. et al. (2011) Down-regulation of microRNA 106b is involved in p21-mediated cell cycle arrest in response to radiation in prostate cancer cells. *Prostate.* 71, 567-574.

Li M., Song L., & Qin X. (2010a) Glycan changes: cancer metastasis and anti-cancer vaccines. *J.Biosci.* 35, 665-673.

Li Q. et al. (2010b) Expression and correlation of Lewis y antigen and integrins alpha5 and beta1 in ovarian serous and mucinous carcinoma. *Int.J.Gynecol.Cancer.* 20, 1482-1489.

Li S.D. et al. (2010c) The role of microRNAs in ovarian cancer initiation and progression. *J.Cell Mol.Med.* 14, 2240-2249.

Liu T. et al. (2005) Human plasma N-glycoproteome analysis by immunoaffinity subtraction, hydrazide chemistry, and mass spectrometry. *J.Proteome.Res.* 4, 2070-2080.

Loeb L.A. (2011) Human cancers express mutator phenotypes: origin, consequences and targeting. *Nat.Rev.Cancer.* 11, 450-457.

Lu K.H. et al. (2000) Occult ovarian tumors in women with BRCA1 or BRCA2 mutations undergoing prophylactic oophorectomy. *J.Clin.Oncol.* 18, 2728-2732.

Lubinski J. et al. (2004) Cancer variation associated with the position of the mutation in the BRCA2 gene. *Fam.Cancer.* 3, 1-10.

Ludwig A.H. et al. (2009) Androgen, progesterone, and FSH receptor polymorphisms in ovarian cancer risk and outcome. *Endocr.Relat Cancer.* 16, 1005-1016.

Maggino T. et al. (1994) Prospective multicenter study on CA 125 in postmenopausal pelvic masses. *Gynecol.Oncol.* 54, 117-123.

Makarla P.B. et al. (2005) Promoter hypermethylation profile of ovarian epithelial neoplasms. *Clin.Cancer Res.* 11, 5365-5369.

Malecova B. & Morris K.V. (2010) Transcriptional gene silencing through epigenetic changes mediated by non-coding RNAs. *Curr.Opin.Mol.Ther.* 12, 214-222.

Manke I.A. et al. (2003) BRCT repeats as phosphopeptide-binding modules involved in protein targeting. *Science.* 302, 636-639.

Maradeo M.E. & Cairns P. (2011) Translational application of epigenetic alterations: Ovarian cancer as a model. *FEBS Lett.* 585, 2112-2120.

McIntosh M.W. et al. (2004) Combining CA 125 and SMR serum markers for diagnosis and early detection of ovarian carcinoma. *Gynecol.Oncol.* 95 , 9-15.

Medeiros L.R. et al. (2009) Accuracy of CA 125 in the diagnosis of ovarian tumors: a quantitative systematic review. *Eur.J.Obstet.Gynecol.Reprod.Biol.* 142, 99-105.

Meindl A. et al. (2011) Hereditary breast and ovarian cancer: new genes, new treatments, new concepts. *Dtsch.Arztebl.Int.* 108, 323-330.

Melnikov A. et al. (2009) Differential methylation profile of ovarian cancer in tissues and plasma. *J.Mol.Diagn.* 11, 60-65.

Meza J.E. et al. (1999) Mapping the functional domains of BRCA1. Interaction of the ring finger domains of BRCA1 and BARD1. *J.Biol.Chem.* 274, 5659-5665.

Milner B.J. et al. (1993) p53 mutation is a common genetic event in ovarian carcinoma. *Cancer Res.* 53, 2128-2132.

Mitchell P.S. et al. (2008) Circulating microRNAs as stable blood-based markers for cancer detection. *Proc.Natl.Acad.Sci.U.S.A.* 105, 10513-10518.

Montagnana M. et al. (2009) The utility of serum human epididymis protein 4 (HE4) in patients with a pelvic mass. *J.Clin.Lab Anal.* 23, 331-335.

Morimoto-Tomita M. et al. (2002) Cloning and characterization of two extracellular heparin-degrading endosulfatases in mice and humans. *J.Biol.Chem.* 20;277, 49175-49185.

Morris J.R. & Solomon E. (2004) BRCA1 : BARD1 induces the formation of conjugated ubiquitin structures, dependent on K6 of ubiquitin, in cells during DNA replication and repair. *Hum.Mol.Genet.* 13 , 807-817.

Moynahan M.E. et al. (1999) Brca1 controls homology-directed DNA repair. *Mol.Cell.* 4, 511-518.

Moynahan M.E., Pierce A.J., & Jasin M. (2001) BRCA2 is required for homology-directed repair of chromosomal breaks. *Mol.Cell.* 7, 263-272.

Murphy C.G. & Moynahan M.E. (2010) BRCA gene structure and function in tumor suppression: a repair-centric perspective. *Cancer J.* 16, 39-47.

Narita K. et al. (2006) HSulf-1 inhibits angiogenesis and tumorigenesis in vivo. *Cancer Res.* 66, 6025-6032.

Narod S.A. & Foulkes W.D. (2004) BRCA1 and BRCA2: 1994 and beyond. *Nat.Rev.Cancer.* 4, 665-676.

Nolen B. et al. (2010) Serum biomarker panels for the discrimination of benign from malignant cases in patients with an adnexal mass. *Gynecol.Oncol.* 117, 440-445.

Obermair A. et al. (2002) Expression of MUC1 splice variants in benign and malignant ovarian tumours. *Int.J.Cancer.* 100, 166-171.

Ohtsubo K. & Marth J.D. (2006) Glycosylation in cellular mechanisms of health and disease. *Cell.* 126, 855-867.

Olopade O.I. & Artioli G. (2004) Efficacy of risk-reducing salpingo-oophorectomy in women with BRCA-1 and BRCA-2 mutations. *Breast J.* 10 Suppl 1:S5-9., S5-S9.

Pal T. et al. (2005) BRCA1 and BRCA2 mutations account for a large proportion of ovarian carcinoma cases. *Cancer.* 104, 2807-2816.

Palmer C. et al. (2008) Systematic evaluation of candidate blood markers for detecting ovarian cancer. *PLoS.One.* 3, e2633.

Patel I.S. et al. (2003) Cadherin switching in ovarian cancer progression. *Int.J.Cancer.* 20;106, 172-177.

Petrucelli et al. (2002) Clinical interpretation and recommendations for patients with a variant of uncertain significance in BRCA1 or BRCA2: a survey of genetic counseling practice. Genet Test. 2002 6:107-13.

Piek J.M. et al. (2003) Histopathological characteristics of BRCA1- and BRCA2-associated intraperitoneal cancer: a clinic-based study. *Fam.Cancer.* 2, 73-78.

Pochampalli M.R., el Bejjani R.M., & Schroeder J.A. (2007) MUC1 is a novel regulator of ErbB1 receptor trafficking. *Oncogene.* 26, 1693-1701.

Pradhan M. et al. (2010) Gross genomic alterations and gene expression profiles of high-grade serous carcinoma of the ovary with and without BRCA1 inactivation. *BMC.Cancer.* 10:493., 493.

Qu G. et al. (1999) Satellite DNA hypomethylation vs. overall genomic hypomethylation in ovarian epithelial tumors of different malignant potential. *Mutat.Res.* 423, 91-101.

Quaye L. et al. (2009) Tagging single-nucleotide polymorphisms in candidate oncogenes and susceptibility to ovarian cancer. *Br.J.Cancer.* 100, 993-1001.

Radice P. (2002) Mutations of BRCA genes in hereditary breast and ovarian cancer. *J.Exp.Clin.Cancer Res.* 21, 9-12.

Rathi A. et al. (2002) Methylation profiles of sporadic ovarian tumors and nonmalignant ovaries from high-risk women. *Clin.Cancer Res.* 8, 3324-3331.

Risch H.A. et al. (2001) Prevalence and penetrance of germline BRCA1 and BRCA2 mutations in a population series of 649 women with ovarian cancer. *Am.J.Hum.Genet.* 68, 700-710.

Rose P.G. et al. (1989) Metastatic patterns in histologic variants of ovarian cancer. An autopsy study. *Cancer.* 64, 1508-1513.

Ruggeri G. et al. (2011) HE4 and epithelial ovarian cancer: Comparison and clinical evaluation of two immunoassays and a combination algorithm. *Clin.Chim.Acta.* 412, 1447-1453.

Rump A. et al. (2004) Binding of ovarian cancer antigen CA125/MUC16 to mesothelin mediates cell adhesion. *J.Biol.Chem.* 279, 9190-9198.

Russo A. et al. (2009) Hereditary ovarian cancer. *Crit Rev.Oncol.Hematol.* 69, 28-44.

Rutishauser U. & Landmesser L. (1996) Polysialic acid in the vertebrate nervous system: a promoter of plasticity in cell-cell interactions. *Trends Neurosci.* 19, 422-427.

Saldova R. et al. (2007) Ovarian cancer is associated with changes in glycosylation in both acute-phase proteins and IgG. *Glycobiology.* 17, 1344-1356.

Saldova R. et al. (2008) Glycosylation changes on serum glycoproteins in ovarian cancer may contribute to disease pathogenesis. *Dis.Markers.* 25, 219-232.

Salhab M., Bismohun S., & Mokbel K. (2010) Risk-reducing strategies for women carrying BRCA1/2 mutations with a focus on prophylactic surgery. *BMC.Womens Health.* 10:28., 28.

Schauer R. (2000) Achievements and challenges of sialic acid research. *Glycoconj.J.* 17, 485-499.

Schauer R. et al. (2011) O-acetylated sialic acids and their role in immune defense. *Adv.Exp.Med.Biol.* 705:525-48., 525-548.

Schildkraut J.M. et al. (2007) Trinucleotide repeat polymorphisms in the androgen receptor gene and risk of ovarian cancer. *Cancer Epidemiol.Biomarkers Prev.* 16, 473-480.

Schrag D. et al. (1997) Decision analysis--effects of prophylactic mastectomy and oophorectomy on life expectancy among women with BRCA1 or BRCA2 mutations. *N.Engl.J.Med.* 336, 1465-1471.

Schut I.C. et al. (2003) MUC1 expression, splice variant and short form transcription (MUC1/Z, MUC1/Y) in prostate cell lines and tissue. *BJU.Int.* 91, 278-283.

Seales E.C. et al. (2003) Ras oncogene directs expression of a differentially sialylated, functionally altered beta1 integrin. *Oncogene.* 22, 7137-7145.

Seidenfaden R. et al. (2003) Polysialic acid directs tumor cell growth by controlling heterophilic neural cell adhesion molecule interactions. *Mol.Cell Biol.* 23, 5908-5918.

Shah C.A. et al. (2009) Influence of ovarian cancer risk status on the diagnostic performance of the serum biomarkers mesothelin, HE4, and CA125. *Cancer Epidemiol.Biomarkers Prev.* 18, 1365-1372.

Shan S.J. et al. (2007) Transcriptional upregulation of human tissue kallikrein 6 in ovarian cancer: clinical and mechanistic aspects. *Br.J.Cancer.* 96, 362-372.

Shih I. & Kurman R.J. (2004) Ovarian tumorigenesis: a proposed model based on morphological and molecular genetic analysis. *Am.J.Pathol.* 164, 1511-1518.

Shih I. et al. (2010) Distinct DNA methylation profiles in ovarian serous neoplasms and their implications in ovarian carcinogenesis. *Am.J.Obstet.Gynecol.* 203, 584-22.

Shipp E.L. & Hsieh-Wilson L.C. (2007) Profiling the sulfation specificities of glycosaminoglycan interactions with growth factors and chemotactic proteins using microarrays. *Chem.Biol.* 14, 195-208.

Shrivastav M., De Haro L.P., & Nickoloff J.A. (2008) Regulation of DNA double-strand break repair pathway choice. *Cell Res.* 18, 134-147.

Simon I. et al. (2006) B7-h4 is a novel membrane-bound protein and a candidate serum and tissue biomarker for ovarian cancer. *Cancer Res.* 66, 1570-1575.

Singer G. et al. (2005) Patterns of p53 mutations separate ovarian serous borderline tumors and low- and high-grade carcinomas and provide support for a new model of ovarian carcinogenesis: a mutational analysis with immunohistochemical correlation. *Am.J.Surg.Pathol.* 29, 218-224.

Siskos P.A. & Spyridaki M.H. (1999) Determination of sialic acids in biological fluids using reversed-phase ion-pair high-performance liquid chromatography. *J.Chromatogr.B Biomed.Sci.Appl.* 724, 205-212.

Song H. et al. (2006) Common variants in RB1 gene and risk of invasive ovarian cancer. *Cancer Res.* 66, 10220-10226.

Sowter H.M. & Ashworth A. (2005) BRCA1 and BRCA2 as ovarian cancer susceptibility genes. *Carcinogenesis.* 26, 1651-1656.

Spurr-Michaud S., Argueso P., & Gipson I. (2007) Assay of mucins in human tear fluid. *Exp.Eye Res.* 84, 939-950.

Starita L.M. & Parvin J.D. (2003) The multiple nuclear functions of BRCA1: transcription, ubiquitination and DNA repair. *Curr.Opin.Cell Biol.* 15, 345-350.

Starita L.M. et al. (2004) BRCA1-dependent ubiquitination of gamma-tubulin regulates centrosome number. *Mol.Cell Biol.* 24, 8457-8466.

Stratton J.F. et al. (1999) The genetic epidemiology of early-onset epithelial ovarian cancer: a population-based study. *Am.J.Hum.Genet.* 65, 1725-1732.

Stroop C.J. et al. (2000) Characterization of the carbohydrate chains of the secreted form of the human epidermal growth factor receptor. *Glycobiology.* 10, 901-917.

Stubbs H.J. et al. (1996) Influence of core fucosylation on the flexibility of a biantennary N-linked oligosaccharide. *Biochemistry.* 35, 937-947.

Szabo C.I., Worley T., & Monteiro A.N. (2004) Understanding germ-line mutations in BRCA1. *Cancer Biol.Ther.* 3, 515-520.

Tangvoranuntakul P. et al. (2003) Human uptake and incorporation of an immunogenic nonhuman dietary sialic acid. *Proc.Natl.Acad.Sci.U.S.A.* 100 , 12045-12050.

Tavassoli FA, Devilee P (2003) Pathology and genetics of tumors of the breast and female genital organs. In: World Health Organization Classification of Tumors. Lyon, France: IARC,113–145.

Theriault C. et al. (2011) MUC16 (CA125) regulates epithelial ovarian cancer cell growth, tumorigenesis and metastasis. *Gynecol.Oncol.* 121, 434-443.

Thompson D. & Easton D. (2001) Variation in cancer risks, by mutation position, in BRCA2 mutation carriers. *Am.J.Hum.Genet.* 68, 410-419.

Tuzun Y. et al. (2009) Correlation of tumour markers in ascitic fluid and serum: are measurements of ascitic tumour markers a futile attempt? *J.Int.Med.Res.* 37, 79-86.

Valeri N. et al. (2010) Modulation of mismatch repair and genomic stability by miR-155. *Proc.Natl.Acad.Sci.U.S.A.* 107, 6982-6987.

Van der Groep P., van der W.E., & van Diest P.J. (2011) Pathology of hereditary breast cancer. *Cell Oncol.(Dordr.).* 34, 71-88.

Van Elssen C.H. et al. (2010) Expression of aberrantly glycosylated Mucin-1 in ovarian cancer. *Histopathology.* 57, 597-606.

Van Gorp T. et al. (2011) HE4 and CA125 as a diagnostic test in ovarian cancer: prospective validation of the Risk of Ovarian Malignancy Algorithm. *Br.J.Cancer.* 104, 863-870.

Van Klinken B.J. et al. (1995) Mucin gene structure and expression: protection vs. adhesion. *Am.J.Physiol.* 269, G613-G627.

Varki A. et al. (1969) Glycosylation Changes in Cancer: Comparative studies on the carbohydrate-containing membrane components of normal and virus-transformed mouse fibroblasts. II. Separation of glycoproteins and glycopeptides by sephadex chromatography. *Biochemistry.* 8, 2518-2524.

Varki A. (2001) N-glycolylneuraminic acid deficiency in humans. *Biochimie.* 83, 615-622.

Varki A., Schauer R., & Schauer R. (2009) Sialic Acids: Sialic acids as regulators of molecular and cellular interactions. *Curr.Opin.Struct.Biol.* 19, 507-514.

Varki A, Schauer R. (2009). Sialic acids. In: Varki A, Cummings RD, Esko JD, Freeze HH, Stanley P, Bertozzi CR, Hart GW, Etzler ME, editors. Essentials of Glycobiology. 2nd edition. Cold Spring Harbor (NY): Cold Spring Harbor Laboratory Press; Chapter 14.

Varki A, Kannagi R, Toole BP. Glycosylation changes in cancer. In: Varki A, Cummings RD, Esko JD, et al., editors (2009) Essentials of Glycobiology. 2nd ed. New York, Cold Spring Harbor University Press, Ch. 44

Venkitaraman A.R. (2002) Cancer susceptibility and the functions of BRCA1 and BRCA2. *Cell.* 108, 171-182.

Venkitaraman A.R. (2003) A growing network of cancer-susceptibility genes. *N.Engl.J.Med.* 348, 1917-1919.

Venkitaraman A.R. (2009) Linking the cellular functions of BRCA genes to cancer pathogenesis and treatment. *Annu.Rev.Pathol.* 4:461-87., 461-487.

Wang L. et al. (2007) Expression of MUC1 in primary and metastatic human epithelial ovarian cancer and its therapeutic significance. *Gynecol.Oncol.* 105, 695-702.

Wang P.H. et al. (2005) Altered mRNA expressions of sialyltransferases in ovarian cancers. *Gynecol.Oncol.* 99, 631-639.

Wang Y. et al. (2011) Study on the Expression and Clinical Significances of Lewis y Antigen and Integrin alphav, beta3 in Epithelial Ovarian Tumors. *Int.J.Mol.Sci.* 12, 3409-3421.

White N.M. et al. (2009) Human kallikrein related peptidases 6 and 13 in combination with CA125 is a more sensitive test for ovarian cancer than CA125 alone. *Cancer Biomark.* 5, 279-287.

Widschwendter M. et al. (2004) DNA hypomethylation and ovarian cancer biology. *Cancer Res.* 64, 4472-4480.

Wilson C.A. et al. (1999) Localization of human BRCA1 and its loss in high-grade, non-inherited breast carcinomas. *Nat.Genet.* 21, 236-240.

Wu C. & Morris J.R. (2001) Genes, genetics, and epigenetics: a correspondence. *Science.* 293, 1103-1105.

Wu L.C. et al. (1996) Identification of a RING protein that can interact in vivo with the BRCA1 gene product. *Nat.Genet.* 14, 430-440.

Wyman S.K. et al. (2009) Repertoire of microRNAs in epithelial ovarian cancer as determined by next generation sequencing of small RNA cDNA libraries. *PLoS.One.* 4, e5311.

Yagi H., Yotsumoto F., & Miyamoto S. (2008) Heparin-binding epidermal growth factor-like growth factor promotes transcoelomic metastasis in ovarian cancer through epithelial-mesenchymal transition. *Mol.Cancer Ther.* 7, 3441-3451.

Yamashita K. et al. (1985) Fractionation of L-fucose-containing oligosaccharides on immobilized Aleuria aurantia lectin. *J.Biol.Chem.* 260, 4688-4693.

Yan L. et al. (2010) Lewis (y) Antigen Overexpression Increases the Expression of MMP-2 and MMP-9 and Invasion of Human Ovarian Cancer Cells. *Int.J.Mol.Sci.* 11, 4441-4452.

Yang H.J. et al. (2006) Differential DNA methylation profiles in gynecological cancers and correlation with clinico-pathological data. *BMC.Cancer.* 6:212., 212.

Yang J. et al. (2004) Twist, a master regulator of morphogenesis, plays an essential role in tumor metastasis. *Cell.* 117, 927-939.

Yang Z. et al. (2009) Expression of sialyl Lex, sialyl Lea, Lex and Ley glycotopes in secreted human ovarian cyst glycoproteins. *Biochimie.* 91 , 423-433.

Yin B.W. et al. (1996) Serological and immunochemical analysis of Lewis y (Ley) blood group antigen expression in epithelial ovarian cancer. *Int.J.Cancer.* 65, 406-412.

Yin G. et al. (2010) TWISTing stemness, inflammation and proliferation of epithelial ovarian cancer cells through MIR199A2/214. *Oncogene.* 29, 3545-3553.

Yogeeswaran G. & Salk P.L. (1981) Metastatic potential is positively correlated with cell surface sialylation of cultured murine tumor cell lines. *Science.* 212, 1514-1516.

Yokoyama Y., Sedgewick G., & Ramakrishnan S. (2007) Endostatin binding to ovarian cancer cells inhibits peritoneal attachment and dissemination. *Cancer Res.* 67, 10813-10822.

Yurkovetsky et al. (2010) Development of a multimarker assay for early detection of ovarian cancer. J Clin Oncol. 2010 May 1;28(13):2159-66

Zaina S., Perez-Luque E.L., & Lund G. (2010) Genetics talks to epigenetics? The interplay between sequence variants and chromatin structure. *Curr.Genomics.* 11, 359-367.

Zaslavsky A. et al. (2010) Platelet-derived thrombospondin-1 is a critical negative regulator and potential biomarker of angiogenesis. *Blood.* 115, 4605-4613.

Zhang Z. et al. (2007) Combining multiple serum tumor markers improves detection of stage I epithelial ovarian cancer. *Gynecol.Oncol.* 107, 526-531.

Zhao Q. et al. (2009) Circulating galectin-3 promotes metastasis by modifying MUC1 localization on cancer cell surface. *Cancer Res.* 69, 6799-6806.

Zhou H., Hu H., & Lai M. (2010) Non-coding RNAs and their epigenetic regulatory mechanisms. *Biol.Cell.* 102, 645-655.

Zhu M. et al. (2010) Periostin promotes ovarian cancer angiogenesis and metastasis. *Gynecol.Oncol.* 119, 337-344.

Zueva E.V. et al. (2010) Immunological peculiarities of CD-56-positive serous ovarian adenocarcinoma. *Bull.Exp.Biol.Med.* 149, 604-608.

11

P53 Network in Ovarian Cancer

Fabiola Moretti and Francesca Mancini
Institute of Cell Biology and Neurobiology
National Research Council of Italy (CNR)
Italy

1. Introduction

P53 (Tp53, tumor protein p53) is one of the most relevant human oncosuppressor genes. Accordingly, inactivation of p53 by direct mutation of the gene is one of the most frequent genetic lesions in human tumors.

In Ovarian Carcinoma (OC), p53 is altered in 30–80% of cases. Molecular and genetic studies have further confirmed the relevance of p53 in the development and progression of OC. Several studied have attempted to establish the p53 status as a marker of clinicopathological features. However, the predictive value of p53 alterations is still ambiguous, suggesting that multiple factors contribute to define p53 function. One of these factors may be related to the recent discovery of p53 variants in OC that may modulate, or even antagonize wild-type p53 function (Hofstetter et al., 2010).

Additional studies in molecular oncology have revealed alternative routes of p53 inactivation through deregulation of its negative regulators, MDM2 and MDM4. MDM family members are key regulators of p53 activity and levels, by acting as repressors of p53 transcriptional function and as a complex for the degradation of p53 protein. Their overexpression has been observed in many human tumors characterized by wild-type p53 status, supporting the model of multiple ways of p53 inactivation in tumor cells. In fact, p53 dysfunction measured as pathogenic mutations or altered copy number of MDM2 and MDM4, approaches 100% of confirmed high-grade serous carcinoma (Ahmed et al., 2010).

Recent data, also from our group, have contributed to define an even higher level of complexity in the p53 network. Indeed, it has been shown that the canonical inhibitors MDM2 and MDM4 may actually exhibit a dual mode of action (Shmueli & Oren, 2007; Mancini et al., 2009a). Particularly, following DNA damage, MDM4 functions as a cooperative factor in p53 apoptosis and promotes cell death in cisplatinum-treated ovarian cancer cells. Accordingly, MDM4 levels/p53 status correlates significantly with chemosensitivity of OC (Mancini et al., 2009b).

Interestingly, various studies have evidenced that the estrogen signalling pathway has a profound impact on the activity of MDM2/MDM4/p53 network (Bond & Levine, 2007) suggesting the relevance of hormonal status too in the prediction of p53 function.

Overall, these data suggest that a combined signature of p53 network may be a better prognostic factor for clinicopathological properties of ovarian cancer in agreement to what it has been recently published (Kalloger et al., 2011).

In this chapter, we will summarize all these data and try to compose potential scenario for novel predicting properties of p53 network in ovarian cancer.

2. P53

P53 is a central hub in the cellular response to a variety of stress signals, including DNA damage, hypoxia and aberrant proliferative signals, such as oncogene activation. Its activation results in the fulfillment of key cellular processes as cell-cycle arrest, senescence and, most importantly for tumor clearance, apoptosis.
P53 is a transcriptional factor able to bind specific DNA sequences and to modulate transcription of several targets by its transactivation domain. P53 transcriptional activities are mediated by its oligomerization (Figure 1).

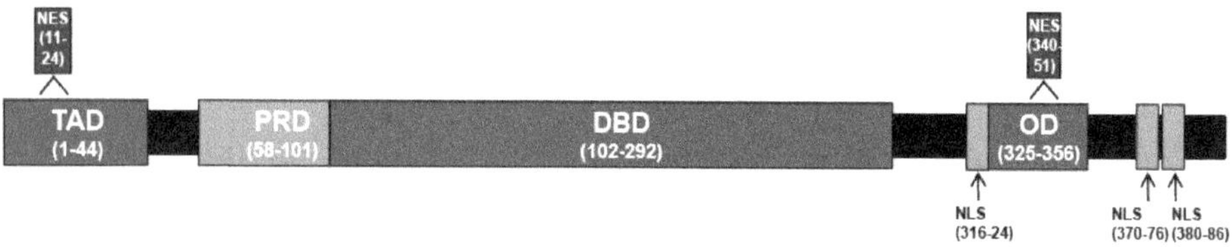
NES (11-24)
TAD (1-44)
PRD (58-101)
DBD (102-292)
NES (340-51)
OD (325-356)
NLS (316-24)
NLS (370-76)
NLS (380-86)

Fig. 1. P53 protein domains. TAD=Trans-Activation domain; PRD=Proline-Rich domain; DBD=DNA-binding domain; OD=Oligomerization domain; NES=Nuclear export signal; NLS=Nuclear localization signal.

The traditional view describing p53 activation in response to cellular stress comprises three basic steps: stabilization of p53, sequence-specific DNA binding, and transcriptional activation of target genes (Yee & Vousden, 2005). Promoter selection is dictated by numerous factors, including posttranslational modifications of p53 that can influence the recruitment of p53 binding proteins to specific promoters.
In addition to these nuclear activities, p53 possesses also cytosolic activities that can induce apoptosis in a transcription-independent manner (Green & Kroemer, 2009). Specifically, in response to various cell death signals, such as ionizing radiation, p53 rapidly localizes to the mitochondria where induces mitochondrial outer membrane permeabilization (MOMP) leading to the release of pro-apoptotic factors.
The relevance of this function in the tumor suppression has been demonstrated by mouse models expressing mitochondrial-targeted p53 variants (Galluzzi et al., 2008).
Because of its potent tumor suppressive activity, it is widely assumed that the complete molecular understanding of p53 action will produce fundamental insights into the natural processes that limit tumorigenesis and will contribute to identify key molecular targets for therapeutic intervention.

2.1 P53 role in ovarian cancer

Most of the epithelial ovarian cancers (EOC) are thought to arise from a single cell of the ovarian surface epithelium (OSE) which accumulates different genetic and epigenetic alterations which in turn lead to the malignant phenotype. The molecular events underlying this transformation are poorly understood. The inactivation of p53 oncosuppressor function seems to be an early event in the induction of hereditary ovarian cancer characterized by germ-line mutations of the BRCA1 tumor suppressor (Werness et al., 2000), suggesting that the loss of p53 function is required for a transformed cell to tolerate the loss of the BRCA1 function. Consistent with this, familial ovarian cancers have high frequency of p53 mutations (Ramus et al., 1999).

The cooperative action of p53 in BRCA1-driven tumorigenesis and in the induction of hereditary ovarian cancer is further strengthened by the phenotype of knock-out mice. *Brca1*$^{-/-}$ mouse embryos are embryonic lethal at embryonic day 6.5; if embryos are deleted simultaneously for both *Brca1* and *p53*, the embryonic lethality is delayed (Scully & Livingston, 2000). This suggests that p53 function antagonizes genome instability induced by BRCA1 loss, causing embryo lethality. Therefore, in order to promote tumor development, p53 activity must be lost so that the cell transformation process can go on easily.

According to this model, in ovaries removed prophylactically from women heterozygote for BRCA1, alteration of p53 was observed in all early stage I serous carcinomas as well as in the adjacent dysplastic surface epithelium (Pothuir et al., 2001). Although sporadic ovarian carcinomas were not analyzed in this study, the clinical and pathological features of BRCA-associated ovarian carcinomas and their sporadic counterparts are indistinguishable, suggesting that their histogenesis may be similar.

Overall, these observations support a general model in which *p53* inactivation is required not only for tumor progression but also for the early development of OC.

2.2 P53 mutation and ovarian cancer

Alterations of p53 pathway are one of the most frequent events in sporadic epithelial ovarian cancer (EOC). The majority of p53 mutations at its locus 17p13.1 are missense mutations that cause single residue changes, largely occurring in the DNA binding domain (Figure 1) (Sigal & Rotter, 2000). The p53 Web Site (http://p53.free.fr/index.html) reports that the most representative mutations found in ovarian cancers occur in the canonical hot spots of p53 gene, namely residues 273, 248, and 175 (ranging from 8% to 5%).

Although p53 mutations have been detected in all histological types of EOC, they are more strongly associated with high grade serous carcinomas then with low grade or borderline serous carcinomas (Kupryjanczyk et al., 1993; Kupryjanczyk et al., 1995; Skomedal et al., 1997; Zheng et al., 1995). The percentage of p53 gene mutations was reported to be lower also in others tumor types as endometrioid, mucinous, and clear-cell ovarian tumors (28%, 16%, and 10%, respectively) (Skilling et al., 1996).

The pathogenesis of ovarian carcinoma lacks of a defined tumor progression model. According to Kurman and Shih, the surface epithelial tumors are divided into two categories designated type I and type II tumors that correspond to two main pathways of tumorigenesis. Type I tumors tend to be low-grade neoplasms that arise in a stepwise manner from borderline tumors whereas type II tumors are high-grade neoplasms for which morphologically recognizable precursor lesions have not been identified (*de novo* development). According to this classification, high-grade serous carcinoma is the prototypic type II tumor whereas low-grade serous carcinoma and all other histological types are the prototypic type I tumor. Importantly, p53 gene mutation is the most common single genetic alteration observed in high-grade serous carcinomas, clinically the most important histological subtype of ovarian cancer (Kurman & Shih, 2011).

Recently, The Cancer Genome Atlas project has evidenced the presence of p53 mutations in almost all analyzed high-grade serous ovarian adenocarcinomas (96%) (Cancer Genome Atlas Research Network, 2011). Similarly, Ahmed et al., reported the presence of p53 mutation in 96.7% of high-grade serous carcinoma. Interestingly, molecular and pathological review of mutation-negative cases showed in these cases copy number gain of

MDM2 or MDM4, confirming the potential role of p53 network in contributing to p53 dysfunction (Ahmed et al., 2010). In this tumor context, therefore p53 mutation appears to be a driver pathogenetic event.

2.3 P53 predictive value in ovarian cancer

According to previous observations, several studies have tried to define the association of p53 with clinicopathological features of the OC. Because p53 mutation is almost invariably present in high-grade serous carcinoma, it is not of substantial prognostic or predictive significance in this tumor type.

On the contrary, considering the tumor stage, the prevalence of p53 genetic alterations appears to rise with increasing stage. Indeed, p53 gene mutations occur more often in stage III and IV ovarian cancers when compared to stage I and II, i.e., 58% versus 37% respectively (reviewed by Shelling et al., 1995), suggesting a positive selection of p53 mutation along tumor progression.

In the same direction, Bernardini et al. evidenced a correlation of the type of p53 mutation with the stage of the tumor. Early stage cancers have a significantly higher rate of null mutations (frameshift or chain terminating mutations that cause the lack of p53 protein) in comparison to late stage disease (38% vs. 8%) (Bernardini et al., 2010). These data suggest that along tumor progression p53 missense mutations are positively selected compared to null mutation, probably due to the "gain of function" of some p53 mutants that promote cell proliferation, tumor formation and invasion.

Accordingly, p53 overexpression (a specific feature of mutant p53 protein in cancer cells), has been associated with poor prognosis, poor overall survival and altered sensitivity to chemotherapy in patients with ovarian cancer (Fujita et al., 1994; Ferrandina et al., 1999; Sengupta et al., 2000; Reles et al., 2001; Hashiguchi et al., 2001; Tachibana et al., 2003; Bali et al., 2004; Bartel et al., 2008; Bernardini et al., 2010; Lee et al., 2011). However, others studies showed that overexpression of p53 is not associated with patient outcome (Havrilesky et al., 2003), has no prognostic value (Laframboise et al., 2000; Fallows et al., 2001) and is not predictive for responsiveness to platinum-based chemotherapy (Bauerschlag et al., 2010). Recently, a meta-analysis of studies on the prognostic value of p53 expression, showed that aberrant p53 status is associated only with poor overall survival (de Graeffet al., 2009), although there was ample heterogeneity among studies.

A number of factors can affect the predictive value of p53 alterations in OC. At first, it is increasingly evident that the overexpression of p53 protein, as usually detected by immunohistochemistry, is not strictly linked to its mutation. Indeed, Bartel et al. described a group of patients with p53 overexpression in which 49% of samples retain wild-type p53 (Bartel et al., 2008).

Moreover, the mere expression of p53 protein or its mutational status could not be sufficient to explain its behavior in the tumor context. P53 regulators, such as MDM2 and MDM4, can be altered (by overexpression or mutation) and differently modulate p53 wild-type functions (see next paragraphs).

Moreover, besides p53 regulators, other p53 alterations, as p53 alternative splicing (see next paragraph) can affect p53 function and, of note, create false results depending on the methodology of p53 detection. Particularly, immunohistochemical analysis cannot easily distinguish the protein form and the genetic status of a positive p53 staining.

All these data underline the necessity to assess the global functionality of p53 pathway and to distinguish the p53 genetic status in order to improve its prediction sensitivity in OC.

2.4 P53 splicing variants and p53 targets

Many cancer-associated genes, including the tumor suppressor p53, exhibit alternative pre-mRNA splicing. These variants may derive from canonical splice sites or by mutations that introduce new aberrant splicing sites.

In ovarian cancers cell lines and in primary ovarian cancers, different p53 splice variants were recently identified, some of them previously reported and others as novel cancer-specific forms (Hofstetter et al., 2010) (Figure 2).

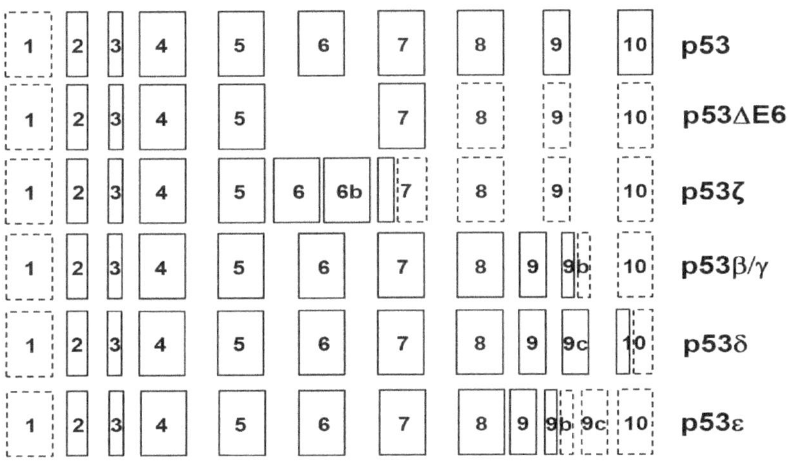

Fig. 2. Exon structure of the human p53 gene and p53 splice variants encoding C-terminally truncated proteins. Coding sequence (continuous lines); non-coding sequence (dashed lines).

Alternative splicing at the C terminus gives rise to p53β, containing 133 additional base pairs (bp) from intron 9 (exon 9b), and p53γ, retaining the distal 58 bp of exon 9b. These insertions result in a frameshift that introduces a premature termination codon. The p53β and p53γ proteins lack the basic regulatory domain and most of the oligomerization domain (OD) and possess unique short C-terminal tails of 10 and 15 new residues, respectively. Another splice variant, p53ΔE6, is missing exon 6 and encodes a C-terminally truncated p53 protein that lacks part of the DNA binding domain and the entire OD (Jolly et al., 1994). The three novel p53 splice variants identified in OC are p53ζ, p53δ and p53ε, arising from alternative splicing of exon 6 or intron 9. P53 splice variants were present in 18 of 34 ovarian cancer cell lines analysed (52.9%) and 134 of 245 primary ovarian cancers (54.7%). In this study, p53δ expression was associated with impaired response to primary platinum-based chemotherapy and its expression constituted an independent prognostic marker for recurrence-free and overall survival. P53β expression was associated with adverse clinicopathologic markers, that is, serous and poorly differentiated cancers and correlated with worse recurrence-free survival in patients exhibiting functionally active p53 (Hofstetter et al., 2010). The other p53 splice variants differ in their clinical relevance, implicating that they possess different functions in vivo. The exact molecular function of these variants has not been completely ascertained; however, it has been hypothesized that they can modulate wild-type p53 function as well as be endowed of autonomous activity.

Overall, the discovery of the high frequency of p53 splice variants in ovarian cancer increases the complexity of the deregulation of p53 pathway in OC and therefore the understanding of p53 contribution to the pathogenesis of ovarian carcinoma.

Another layer of complexity in the prediction of p53 function, is represented by the analysis of some p53 targets. One of the most relevant and more studied is p21waf1/cip1. It is a cyclin-dependent kinase inhibitor that is usually induced through a p53-related pathway. P21waf1/cip1 has been shown to be integral to the control of the cell cycle after DNA damage. Indeed, up-regulation of p21waf1/cip1 by p53 is essential to sustain cell cycle arrest after DNA damage.

Although p21waf1/cip1 has been studied in EOC, the role of this protein as a prognostic indicator is still controversial (Sengupta et al., 2000; Geisler et al., 2001). Some studies confirm the importance of the combination of p21 and p53 staining in determining EOC prognosis. Indeed, expression of p53 protein in the absence of p21waf1/cip1 was a better marker of poor prognosis than either p53 or p21waf1/cip1 expression alone (Bali et al., 2004; Geisler et al., 2001; Werness et al., 1999).

Cai et al. suggested that since p21 expression may be an indicator of wild-type p53 function, lack of p21 in the presence of p53 expression may be predictive of an inactivated status of p53. Given that p53 inactivation precedes morphological transformation of the ovarian surface epithelium in most cases, the double analysis of these proteins might constitute an early marker of pre-neoplastic lesions (Cai et al., 2009).

Another important group of p53 targets involved in ovarian cancer was recently identified in the MicroRNAs molecules. MicroRNAs (miRNA) are a recently discovered class of noncoding RNAs that negatively regulate gene expression. Evidence indicates that miRNAs play an important role in cancer development. MiR-34b and miR-34c are the miRNAs most significantly affected by p53 and have been shown to cooperate in suppressing proliferation and transformation of neoplastic epithelial ovarian cells (Corney et al., 2007). Analyzing a group of EOC, Corney et al., showed that miR-34b/c expression is decreased in 72% of tumors with p53 mutation. Furthermore, expression of miR-34b/c is significantly reduced in stage IV tumors compared to stage III. These data suggest that miR-34 family plays an important role in EOC pathogenesis and that reduced expression of miR-34b/c may be particularly important for tumor progression to the most advanced stages (Corney et al., 2010).

Overall, these data highlight the importance of the analysis of p53 and of its targets as a tool with improved prediction properties in OC.

3. MDM2

MDM2 (for transformed mouse 3T3 cell double minute 2) is the first and best known negative regulator of p53. It has been isolated from a spontaneous transformed BALB/c 3T3 mouse cell line in 1992.

MDM2 interacts physically with p53 and brings this oncosuppressor to degradation besides to inhibit its transcriptional function masking the p53 activation domain. Molecular and genetic studies have confirmed the crucial role of MDM2 in the inhibition of p53 function, leading to the concept that MDM2 overexpression may be an alternative way of p53 inactivation in human tumors (Marine & Lozano, 2010). Accordingly, MDM2 overexpression has been observed in many human cancers (Momand et al., 1998). Recent data have led to reconsider MDM2 not only as a p53 inhibitor but also as a modifier of p53 response. Indeed, after stress, MDM2 contributes to lower the protein levels of some proapoptotic factors (i.e. HIPK2, TIP60) that assist p53 in activating its apoptotic function. Therefore, increase or decline of MDM2 levels would affect p53 choice between growth arrest and apoptosis respectively (Shmueli & Oren., 2007). The relevance of this model in the oncosuppressive activity of p53 as well as in its role in chemosensitivity remains to be elucidated.

3.1 MDM2 alterations and ovarian cancer

MDM2 aberrant expression has been reported in human tumors, including ovarian cancer. Several ways of MDM2 aberrant expression have been recognized. The first way is the amplification of the gene. The human MDM2 gene (also HDM2) resides on chromosome 12q13-14 and is amplified in a large cohort of human tumors (about 7% in a survey of 28 tumor types). MDM2 overall amplification frequency in all ovarian cancer was reported to be 3.1% (Momand, 1998). However, analysing specific tumor subtype, MDM2 amplification has been recognized in 80% of serous borderline tumors (Mayr and al., 2006) often associated to co-expression of p21WAF1/CIP1 suggesting that in this histotype these cell cycle control proteins might be important for cancer phenotype (Palazzo et al., 2000).
In addition, MDM2 levels can be upregulated independently of gene amplification. Both enhanced MDM2 protein levels as well as high levels of MDM2 transcripts have been reported in different tumor histotypes although the molecular mechanisms that underlie such alterations have not been completely characterized. In OC, MDM2 overexpression has been reported by various reports (varying among 17%, 33%, and 47, 5%) (Baekelandt et al., 1999; Dogan et al., 2005; Cho et al., 2006). In one study, it has been demonstrated the independency from amplification events (Foulkes et al., 1995) confirming the existence of mechanism of MDM2 stabilization in the ovarian cancer too.
More recently, two single nucleotide polymorphisms (SNP) in the P2 promoter of the MDM2 gene able to modify MDM2 levels have been identified. The first one, at the 309th nucleotide in the first intron, alters the affinity of the transcriptional activator Sp1 resulting in different levels of MDM2 mRNA and protein. Particularly, the T to G nucleotide change extends the length of one Sp1 DNA binding site, increasing the transcription of the MDM2 gene. This in turn results in attenuation of the p53 activity and accelerated tumor formation (Bond et al., 2004). The presence of this polymorphism has been considered an oncogenic predisposing factor. Indeed the authors found out a significant correlation of SNP309G with earlier age of onset in a group of sporadic soft tissue sarcoma. Subsequently, the SNP309G effects appeared to be mediated by the hormonal status, being effective in the presence of an active estrogen signalling pathway (Bond & Levine, 2007). Therefore, the role of this polymorphism has been especially studied in breast and ovarian cancer. However, relative studies have reported controversial results indicating both association between SNP309G and OC risk (Yarden et al., 2008) or earlier age of onset in estrogen receptor-overexpressing FIGO stage III patients (Bartel et al., 2008) as well as the lack of its association with OC (Campbell et al., 2006) or cancer risk (Krekac et a., 2008). Recently, an important study has solved these controversies. It has been identified an additional SNP (at nucleotide 285)

whose activity profoundly impacts on the activity of SNP309G. In vitro, SNP285C strongly reduces the Sp1 binding to MDM2 promoter therefore counteracting the inhibitory activity of SNP309 towards p53 pathway. Indeed, the authors demonstrated that the presence of SNP285C antagonizes the activity of the SNP309G lowering the risk and the age of appearance of ovarian cancer. Interestingly, SNP285C has been evidenced in Caucasian individuals only, while being absent in Chinese population (Knappskog et al., 2011).
An additional way of MDM2 deregulation is the expression of MDM2 splicing variants. Indeed, besides full-length (fl) mRNA, more than 40 different splice variants of MDM2 transcripts have been identified in normal tissues and tumors including OC (Sigalas et al., 1996; Bartel et al., 2002), and tumorigenicity of some of these variants has been in vivo and in vitro assessed. Although the specific role of MDM2 variants in OC has not been studied, their presence may lead to a misinterpretation of MDM2 expression in tumor samples. Indeed, MDM2 detection by immunohistochemistry often lacks the sufficient specificity to distinguish wild type protein from splicing forms. This is of relevance taking into consideration the fact that many of these variants show a p53-independent function as they have lost, at least in part, the p53-binding domain. Therefore, their presence should be clearly ascertained when considering the p53 network.

3.2 MDM2 predictive value in ovarian cancer

Given the frequent alteration of MDM2 in OC, several studies have investigated the association of its expression with ovarian carcinoma properties. Conflicting results have been reported, suggesting that the analysis of sole MDM2 as well as of sole p53 are not good predictors. A recent study has supported this hypothesis demonstrating that a 9 marker set (including MDM2, CDKN2A, DKK1, HNF1B, PGR, TFF3, TP53, VIM and WT1) is the most predictive factor of ovarian cancer subtype (high-grade serous, clear cell, endometrioid, mucinous and low-grade serous) in a 322 archival ovarian carcinoma by tissue microarrays (Kalloger et al., 2011). Validation of this panel in two independent series of 81 cases demonstrated good to excellent ability to predict subtype (k=0.85 and 0.78). These data point to multiple immunohistochemical analysis as the gold standard for diagnostic accuracy in the future.

4. MDM4

Murine Mdm4 (for transformed mouse 3T3 cell double minute 4, also Mdmx) and human ortholog MDM4 (also HDMX) have been identified as the closest analogues of Mdm2 in 1996 (Marine et al., 2007).
Similarly to MDM2, MDM4 inhibits p53 transcriptional function although less efficiently than MDM2. However, at variance with MDM2, MDM4 is unable to degrade p53 protein or other targets. In the human cell, MDM4 heterodimerizes with MDM2 and their complex is considered the effective controller of p53 activity. In agreement with its inhibitory function, MDM4 overexpression has been observed in some human cancer, in some cases associated to simultaneous MDM2 overexpression (Macchiarulo et al., 2011).
However, recent evidence indicates that, in analogy to MDM2, MDM4 is not only a p53 inhibitor. It has been demonstrated that upon stress, MDM4 contributes to p53 activation by stabilizing its levels and promoting the mitochondrial apoptotic response (Mancini et al., 2009a). Noteworthy, this MDM4 activity is able to modify chemosensitivity of cancer cell

lines by altering the p53 apoptotic response. This scenario is even more complicated by the observation that under stress, MDM2 may degrade MDM4 and therefore inhibit MDM4-mediated proapoptotic function. These molecular data lead to a reconsideration of the role of MDM4 and/or MDM2 in p53 suppression. Their relative balance rather than the single molecules could be relevant for their function in the regulation of p53 (Mancini et al., 2010). Interestingly, a recent mathematical model provided support for this hypothesis: it shows that MDM4 may stabilize or even amplify DNA damage-induced p53 response, depending on the balance with MDM2, the main regulator of MDM4 levels (Kim et al., 2010) (Figure 3).

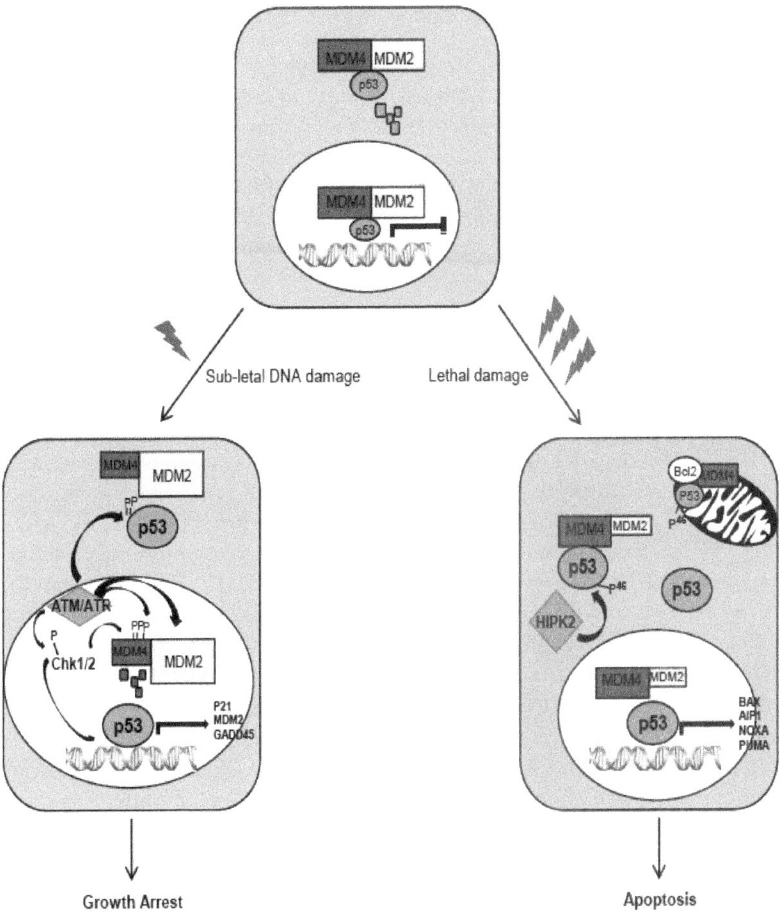

Fig. 3. P53 network following different DNA damages.

4.1 MDM4 and ovarian cancer

To date, MDM4 overexpression or amplification have not been reported in OC. On the contrary, a significant downregulation of MDM4 mRNA and protein levels has been observed in a group of wt-p53 carrying OC characterized by resistance to platinum-derived therapy in comparison to the responsive ones (Mancini et al., 2009b). These data have been correlated to the ability of MDM4 to promote p53-dependent mitochondrial apoptosis. Although few data have been reported on the role of mitochondrial apoptosis in the sensitivity to particular chemotherapeutic drugs, it has been shown that the expression of mitochondrial proteins BCL2 (antiapoptotic) and BAX (proapoptotic) have predictive value in ovarian cancer patients treated with platinum-based chemotherapy (Kupryjańczyk et al., 2003), confirming that the mitochondrial pathway may have a relevant function in the response to this chemotherapy in these tumors. Of note, these data may contribute to explain the difficulties to correlate p53 status with chemotherapy response. Indeed, not only p53 status but also the status of its regulators may profoundly affect the chemosensitivity of ovarian cancer.

These findings are supported by evidence that in other human tumours MDM4 levels are significantly downregulated in association with more aggressive features (Prodosmo et al., 2008) and that in breast cancer MDM4 presence is considered a positive prognostic factor (Abdel-Fatah et al., 2010).

Further studies about the role of MDM4 in OC have highlighted that the estrogen pathway is an important modifier, in analogy to what observed for MDM2. Indeed, it has been recognized a SNP at position 34091 in the 3′ untranslated region (UTR) of MDM4, just 32 nucleotides downstream of the stop codon. SNP34091C introduces an illegitimate binding site for a miRNA, miR-191, that is ubiquitously expressed in human normal and cancer tissues.

The presence of SNP34091C is correlated to a decrease in the MDM4 levels. Interestingly, SNP34091A correlates with increased MDM4 expression in a group of 66 primary ovarian carcinomas and with significant decreased overall survival and increased risk of tumor-related death (Wynendaele et al., 2010). Noteworthy, this occurs only in patients negative for estrogen receptor (ER) expression suggesting the MDM4 oncogenic function is modified by ER signalling pathway although no ER binding sites are present in the MDM4 gene. Intriguingly, ER status affects MDM4 and MDM2 in an opposite way. It counteracts oncogenic activity of MDM4 while potentiates that of MDM2. The understanding of the molecular mechanism underlying these effects will further clarify the role of these proteins in the development and progression of ovarian cancer. It has to be emphasized that SNP34091A does not correlate with p53 status suggesting that MDM4 may exert oncogenic function independently of p53 too (Wynendaele et al., 2010).

In a second genetic study, the authors identified additional SNP that confer an earlier age of onset of familial and sporadic OC in 3 different populations of Caucasian of different ethnic background and in 1 population of African Americans. However, the effects of these SNP on MDM4 levels and/or activity were not identified as well as any relationship with estrogen signalling (Atwal et al., 2009).

Finally, in analogy to MDM2, alternative splicing of MDM4 has been described as well (Mancini et al., 2009c). Particularly, a tumor-specific form, MDM4-211, derived from an aberrant splicing between exon 2 and exon 11, is frequently present in OC (unpublished data). This form lacks the p53-binding domain and therefore cannot directly modulate p53 function. However, it can stabilize MDM2 and in turn inhibit p53 function (Giglio et al., 2006). The relevance of this variant in OC features remains to be elucidated. However, as previously described, the presence of these variants suggests measures of caution in the interpretation of MDM4 IHC positive results.

5. Conclusion

P53 is a central hub in the stress response and its function plays a major role in human oncogenesis.

In ovarian cancer, it seems to be a key determinant in the appearance as well as in the progression of the tumor. In addition, its status affects the response to the chemotherapy.

Despite this, the numerous studies aimed to use p53 detection as a marker for prediction of clinicopathological features of OC have provided some conflicting results. Accordingly, clinical trials based on the status of p53 are not currently in progress. Increasing evidence from literature suggests that the assessment of p53 function and therefore its predictive/diagnostic value might be foreseen more effectively by the analysis of its network, particularly of its regulators MDM4 and MDM2 and of some of its targets, as p21 and Bcl2. The recent work by Kalloger (Kalloger et al., 2011) using tissue microarray gave strong support to this hypothesis. Moreover, it is assuming increased relevance integrated genomic analyses for simultaneous analysis of mRNA, miRNA and promoter methylation to delineate transcriptional subtype associated to clinicopathological properties of tumor (Cancer Genome Atlas Research Network, 2011).

In the future, the integration of disease-specific transcriptional profile analysis and protein detection could represent the optimum for patient diagnosis and cure.

6. References

Abdel-Fatah, TM., Powe, DG., Agboola, J., Adamowicz-Brice, M., Blamey, RW., Lopez-Garcia, MA., Green, AR., Reis-Filho, JS. & Ellis, IO. (2010). The biological, clinical and prognostic implications of p53 transcriptional pathways in breast cancers. *J Pathol.* 220: 419-34.

Ahmed, AA., Etemadmoghadam, D., Temple, J., Lynch, AG., Riad, M., Sharma, R., Stewart, C., Fereday, S., Caldas, C., Defazio, A., Bowtell, D. & Brenton, JD. (2010). Driver mutations in TP53 are ubiquitous in high grade serous carcinoma of the ovary. *J Pathol.* 221:49-56.

Atwal, GS., Kirchhoff, T., Bond, EE., Montagna, M., Menin, C., Bertorelle, R., Scaini, MC., Bartel, F., Böhnke, A., Pempe, C., Gradhand, E., Hauptmann, S., Offit, K., Levine, AJ. & Bond, GL. (2009). Altered tumor formation and evolutionary selection of genetic variants in the human MDM4 oncogene. *Proc Natl Acad Sci U S A* 106: 10236-41.

Baekelandt, M., Kristensen, GB., Nesland, JM., Tropé, CG. & Holm, R. (1999) Clinical significance of apoptosis-related factors p53, Mdm2, and Bcl-2 in advanced ovarian cancer. J Clin Oncol. 17: 2061.

Bali, A., O'Brien, PM., Edwards, LS., Sutherland, RL., Hacker, NF. & Henshall, SM. (2004). Cyclin D1, p53, and p21Waf1/Cip1 expression is predictive of poor clinical outcome in serous epithelial ovarian cancer. Clin Cancer Res 10:5168–5177.

Bartel, F., Taubert, H. & Harris, LC. (2002). Alternative and aberrant splicing of MDM2 mRNA in human cancer. Cancer Cell 2: 9-15.

Bartel, F., Jung, J., Böhnke, A., Gradhand, E., Zeng, K., Thomssen, C. & Hauptmann, S. (2008). Both germ line and somatic genetics of the p53 pathway affect ovarian cancer incidence and survival. Clin Cancer Res. 14:89-96.

Bauerschlag, DO., Schem, C., Weigel, MT., Von Kaisenberg, C., Strauss, A., Bauknecht, T., Maass, N. & Meinhold-Heerlein I. (2010). The role of p53 as a surrogate marker for chemotherapeutical responsiveness in ovarian cancer. J Cancer Res Clin Oncol. 136:79-88.

Bernardini, MQ., Baba, T., Lee, PS., Barnett, JC., Sfakianos, GP., Secord, AA., Murphy, SK., Iversen, E., Marks, JR. & Berchuck, A. (2010). Expression signatures of TP53 mutations in serous ovarian cancers. BMC Cancer. 10: 237.

Bond, GL., Hu, W., Bond, EE., Robins, H., Lutzker, SG., Arva, NC., Bargonetti, J., Bartel, F., Taubert, H., Wuerl, P., Onel, K., Yip, L., Hwang, SJ., Strong, LC., Lozano, G. & Levine, AJ. (2004). A single nucleotide polymorphism in the MDM2 promoter attenuates the p53 tumor suppressor pathway and accelerates tumor formation in humans. Cell 119: 591-602.

Bond, GL. & Levine, AJ. (2007). A single nucleotide polymorphism in the p53 pathway interacts with gender, environmental stresses and tumor genetics to influence cancer in humans. Oncogene. 26:1317-23.

Cai, KQ., Wu, H., Klein-Szanto, AJ. & Xu, XX. (2009). Acquisition of a second mutation of the Tp53 alleles immediately precedes epithelial morphological transformation in ovarian tumorigenicity. Gynecol Oncol. 114:18-25.

Campbell, IG., Eccles, DM. & Choong, DY. (2006). No association of the MDM2 SNP309 polymorphism with risk of breast or ovarian cancer. Cancer Lett. 240:195-7.

Cancer Genome Atlas Research Network (2011). Integrated genomic analyses of ovarian carcinoma. Nature 474:609-15.

Cho, EY., Choi, YL., Chae, SW., Sohn, JH. & Ahn, GH. (2006). Relationship between p53-associated proteins and estrogen receptor status in ovarian serous neoplasms. Int J Gynecol Cancer. 16: 1000-6.

Corney, DC., Flesken-Nikitin, A., Godwin, AK., Wang, W. & Nikitin, AY. (2007). MicroRNA-34b and MicroRNA-34c are targets of p53 and cooperate in control of cell proliferation and adhesion-independent growth. Cancer Res. 67: 8433-8.

Corney, DC., Hwang, CI., Matoso, A., Vogt, M., Flesken-Nikitin, A., Godwin, AK., Kamat, AA., Sood, AK., Ellenson, LH., Hermeking, H. & Nikitin, AY. (2010). Frequent downregulation of miR-34 family in human ovarian cancers. Clin Cancer Res. 16: 1119-28.

de Graeff, P., Crijns, AP., de Jong, S., Boezen, M., Post, WJ., de Vries, EG., van der Zee, AG. & de Bock, GH. (2009). Modest effect of p53, EGFR and HER-2/neu on prognosis in epithelial ovarian cancer: a meta-analysis. Br J Cancer. 101: 149-59.

Dogan, E., Saygili, U., Tuna, B., Gol, M., Gürel, D., Acar, B. & Koyuncuoğlu, M. (2005). p53 and mdm2 as prognostic indicators in patients with epithelial ovarian cancer: a multivariate analysis. Gynecol Oncol. 97: 46-52.

Fallows, S., Price, J., Atkinson, RJ., Johnston, PG., Hickey, I. & Russell, SE. (2001). P53 mutation does not affect prognosis in ovarian epithelial malignancies. J Pathol. 194: 68-75.

Ferrandina, G., Fagotti, A., Salerno, MG., Natali, PG., Mottolese, M., Maneschi, F., De Pasqua, A., Benedetti-Panici, P., Mancuso, S. & Scambia, G. (1999). p53 overexpression is associated with cyto-reduction and response to chemotherapy in ovarian cancer. Br J Cancer 81: 733–740.

Foulkes, WD., Stamp, GW., Afzal, S., Lalani, N., McFarlane, CP., Trowsdale, J. & Campbell, IG. (1995). MDM2 overexpression is rare in ovarian carcinoma irrespective of TP53 mutation status. Br J Cancer. 72: 883-8.

Fujita, M., Enomoto, T., Inoue, M., Tanizawa, O., Ozaki, M., Rice, JM. & Nomura, T. (1994). Alteration of the p53 tumor suppressor gene occurs independently of K-ras activation and more frequently in serous adenocarcinomas than in other common epithelial tumors of the human ovary. Jpn J Cancer Res 85:1247–1256.

Galluzzi, L., Morselli, E., Kepp, O., Tajeddine, N. & Kroemer, G. (2008). Targeting p53 to mitochondria for cancer therapy. Cell Cycle 7: 1949-55.

Geisler, HE., Geisler, JP., Miller, GA., Geisler, MJ., Wiemann, MC., Zhou, Z. & Crabtree, W. (2001) p21 and p53 in ovarian carcinoma: their combined staining is more valuable than either alone. Cancer 92:781–6.

Giglio, S., Mancini, F., Gentiletti, F., Sparaco, G., Felicioni, L., Barassi, F., Martella, C., Prodosmo, A., Iacovelli, S., Buttitta, F., Farsetti, A., Soddu, S., Marchetti, A., Sacchi, A., Pontecorvi, A. & Moretti F. (2005). Identification of an aberrantly spliced form of HDMX in human tumors: a new mechanism for HDM2 stabilization. Cancer Res. 65: 9687-94.

Green, DR. & Kroemer, G. (2009). Cytoplasmic functions of the tumour suppressor p53. Nature 458: 1127-30.

Hashiguchi, Y., Tsuda, H., Yamamoto, K., Inoue, T., Ishiko, O. & Ogita, S. (2001). Combined analysis of p53 and RB pathways in epithelial ovarian cancer. Hum Pathol. 32: 988–996.

Havrilesky, L., Darcy, M., Hamdan, H., Priore, RL., Leon, J., Bell, J. & Berchuck, A. (2003). Prognostic significance of p53 mutation and p53 overexpression in advanced epithelial ovarian cancer: a Gynecologic Oncology Group Study. J Clin Oncol. 21: 3814-25.

Hofstetter, G., Berger, A., Fiegl, H., Slade, N., Zorić, A., Holzer, B., Schuster, E., Mobus, VJ., Reimer, D., Daxenbichler, G., Marth, C., Zeimet, AG., Concin, N. & Zeillinger, R. (2010). Alternative splicing of p53 and p73: the novel p53 splice variant p53delta is an independent prognostic marker in ovarian cancer. Oncogene. 29: 1997-2004.

Kalloger, SE., Köbel, M., Leung, S., Mehl, E., Gao, D., Marcon, KM., Chow, C., Clarke, BA., Huntsman, DG. & Gilks, CB. (2011). Calculator for ovarian carcinoma subtype prediction. Mod Pathol. 24: 512-21.

Kim, S., Aladjem, MI., McFadden, GB. & Kohn, KW. (2010). Predicted functions of MdmX in fine-tuning the response of p53 to DNA damage. PLoS Comput Biol. 6: e1000665.

Knappskog, S., Bjørnslett, M., Myklebust, LM., Huijts, PE., Vreeswijk, MP., Edvardsen, H., Guo, Y., Zhang, X., Yang, M., Ylisaukko-Oja, SK., Alhopuro, P., Arola, J., Tollenaar, RA., van Asperen, CJ., Seynaeve, C., Staalesen, V., Chrisanthar, R., Løkkevik, E., Salvesen, HB., Evans, DG., Newman, WG., Lin, D., Aaltonen, LA., Børresen-Dale, AL. Tell, GS. Stoltenberg, C. Romundstad, P. Hveem, K. Lillehaug, JR., Vatten, L., Devilee, P., Dørum, A. & Lønning, PE. (2011). The MDM2 promoter SNP285C/309G haplotype diminishes Sp1 transcription factor binding and reduces risk for breast and ovarian cancer in Caucasians. Cancer Cell 19: 273-82.

Krekac, D., Brozkova, K., Knoflickova, D., Hrstka, R., Muller, P., Nenutil, R. & Vojtesek, B. (2008). MDM2SNP309 does not associate with elevated MDM2 protein expression or breast cancer risk. Oncology 74: 84-7.

Kupryjanczyk, J., Thor, AD., Beauchamp, R., Merritt, V., Edgerton, SM., Bell, DA. & Yandell, DW. (1993). p53 gene mutations and protein accumulation in human ovarian cancer. Proc Natl Acad Sci U S A. 90: 4961-4965.

Kupryjanczyk, J., Bell, DA., Dimeo, D., Beauchamp, R., Thor, AD. & Yandell, DW. (1995). p53 gene analysis of ovarian borderline tumors and stage I carcinomas. Hum Pathol. 26: 387-392.

Kupryjańczyk, J., Szymańska, T., Madry, R., Timorek, A., Stelmachów, J., Karpińska, G., Rembiszewska, A., Ziółkowska, I., Kraszewska, E., Debniak, J., Emerich, J., Ułańska, M., Płuzańska, A., Jedryka, M., Goluda, M., Chudecka-Głaz, A., Rzepka-Górska, I., Klimek, M., Urbański, K., Breborowicz, J., Zieliński, J. & Markowska J. (2003). Evaluation of clinical significance of TP53, BCL-2, BAX and MEK1 expression in 229 ovarian carcinomas treated with platinum-based regimen. Br J Cancer 88: 848-54.

Kurman, RJ. & Shih, IeM. (2011). Molecular pathogenesis and extraovarian origin of epithelial ovarian cancer-Shifting the paradigm. Hum Pathol. 42:918-31.

Laframboise, S., Chapman, W., McLaughlin, J. & Andrulis, IL. (2000). p53 mutations in epithelial ovarian cancers: possible role in predicting chemoresistance. Cancer J. 6: 302-8.

Lee, YH., Heo, JH., Kim, TH., Kang, H., Kim, G., Kim, J., Cho, SH. & An, HJ. (2011). Significance of cell cycle regulatory proteins as malignant and prognostic biomarkers in ovarian epithelial tumors. Int J Gynecol Pathol. 30: 205-17.

Macchiarulo, A., Giacchè, N., Carotti, A., Moretti, F. & Pellicciari, R. (2011) Expanding the Horizon of Chemotherapeutic Targets: From MDM2 to MDMX (MDM4). Med Chem Commun. 2: 455-465.

Mancini, F. & Moretti, F. (2009a). Mitochondrial MDM4 (MDMX): an unpredicted role in the p53-mediated intrinsic apoptotic pathway. Cell Cycle 8:3854-9.

Mancini, F., Di Conza, G., Pellegrino, M., Rinaldo, C., Prodosmo, A., Giglio, S., D'Agnano, I., Florenzano, F., Felicioni, L., Buttitta, F., Marchetti, A., Sacchi, A., Pontecorvi, A., Soddu, S. & Moretti, F. (2009b). MDM4 (MDMX) localizes at the mitochondria and facilitates the p53-mediated intrinsic-apoptotic pathway. EMBO J. 28: 1926-39.

Mancini, F., Di Conza, G. & Moretti, F. (2009c). MDM4 (MDMX) and its Transcript Variants. Curr Genomics 10: 42-50.

Mancini, F., Di Conza, G., Monti, O., Macchiarulo, A., Pellicciari, R., Pontecorvi, A. & Moretti F. (2010). Puzzling over MDM4-p53 network. Int J Biochem Cell Biol. 42: 1080-3.

Marine, JC., Dyer, MA. & Jochemsen, AG. (2007). MDMX: from bench to bedside. J Cell Sci. 120: 371-8.

Marine, JC. & Lozano, G. (2010). Mdm2-mediated ubiquitylation: p53 and beyond. Cell Death Differ. 17: 93-102.

Mayr, D., Kanitz, V., Anderegg, B., Luthardt, B., Engel, J., Löhrs, U., Amann, G. & Diebold J. (2006). Analysis of gene amplification and prognostic markers in ovarian cancer using comparative genomic hybridization for microarrays and immunohistochemical analysis for tissue microarrays. Am J Clin Pathol.126: 101-9.

Momand, J., Jung, D., Wilczynski, S. & Niland, J. (1998). The MDM2 gene amplification database. Nucleic Acids Res. 26: 3453-9.

Palazzo, JP., Monzon, F., Burke, M., Hyslop, T., Dunton, C., Barusevicius, A., Capuzzi, D. & Kovatich, AJ. (2000). Overexpression of p21WAF1/CIP1 and MDM2 characterizes serous borderline ovarian tumors. Hum Pathol. 31: 698-704.

Pothuir, B., Leitao, M., Barakat, R., Akram, M., Bogomolniy, F., Olvera, N. & Lin, O. (2001). Genetic analysis of ovarian carcinoma histogenesis. Society of Gynecologic Oncologists 32nd Annual Meeting.

Prodosmo, A., Giglio, S., Moretti, S., Mancini, F., Barbi, F., Avenia, N., Di Conza, G., Schünemann, HJ., Pistola, L., Ludovini, V., Sacchi, A., Pontecorvi, A., Puxeddu, E. & Moretti, F. (2008). Analysis of human MDM4 variants in papillary thyroid carcinomas reveals new potential markers of cancer properties. J Mol Med. 86: 585-96.

Ramus, SJ., Bobrow, LG., Pharoah, PD., Finnigan, DS., Fishman, A., Altaras, M., Harrington, PA., Gayther, SA., Ponder, BA. & Friedman, LS. (1999). Increased frequency of TP53 mutations in BRCA1 and BRCA2 ovarian tumours. Genes Chromosomes Cancer 25: 91-6.

Reles, A., Wen, WH., Schmider, A., Gee, C., Runnebaum, IB., Kilian, U., Jones, LA., El-Nagga,r A., Minguillon, C., Schönborn, I., Reich, O., Kreienberg, R., Lichtenegger, W. & Press, MF. (2001). Correlation of p53 mutations with resistance to platinum-based chemotherapy and shortened survival in ovarian cancer. Clin Cancer Res. 7: 2984-97.

Scully, R. & Livingston, DM. (2000). In search of the tumour-suppressor functions of BRCA1 and BRCA2. Nature 408: 429–432.

Sengupta, PS., McGown, AT., Bajaj, V., Blackhall, F., Swindell, R., Bromley, M., Shanks, JH., Ward, T., Buckley, CH., Reynolds, K., Slade, RJ. & Jayson, GC. (2000). p53 and related proteins in epithelial ovarian cancer. Eur J Cancer 36: 2317–28.

Shelling, AN., Cooke, IE. & Ganesan, TS. (1995). The genetic analysis of ovarian cancer. Br J Cancer. 72: 521-7.

Shmueli, A. & Oren, M. (2007). Mdm2: p53's lifesaver? Mol Cell. 25:794-6.

Sigal, A. & Rotter, V. (2000). Oncogenic mutations of the p53 tumor suppressor: the demons of the guardian of the genome. Cancer Res. 60: 6788–6793.

Sigalas, I., Calvert, AH., Anderson, JJ., Neal, DE. & Lunec J. (1996) Alternatively spliced mdm2 transcripts with loss of p53 binding domain sequences: transforming ability and frequent detection in human cancer. Nat Med. 2: 912-7.

Skilling, JS., Sood, A., Niemann, T., Lager, DJ. & Buller, RE. (1996). An abundance of p53 null mutations in ovarian carcinoma. Oncogene 13: 117-23.

Skomedal, H., Kristensen, GB., Abeler, VM., Borresen-Dale, AL., Trope, C. & Holm, R. (1997). TP53 protein accumulation and gene mutation in relation to overexpression of MDM2 protein in ovarian borderline tumours and stage I carcinomas. J Pathol. 181: 158–165.

Tachibana, M., Watanabe, J., Matsushima, Y., Nishida, K., Kobayashi, Y., Fujimura, M. & Shiromizu, K. (2003). Independence of the prognostic value of tumor suppressor protein expression in ovarian adenocarcinomas: A multivariate analysis of expression of p53, retinoblastoma, and related proteins. Int J Gynecol Cancer 13: 598–606.

Werness, BA., Freedman, AN., Piver, MS., Romero-Gutierrez, M. & Petrow, E. (1999). Prognostic significance of p53 and p21(waf1/cip1) immunoreactivity in epithelialcancers of the ovary. Gynecol Oncol. 75: 413–8.

Werness, BA., Parvatiyar, P., Ramus, SJ., Whittemore, AS., Garlinghouse-Jones, K., Oakley-Girvan, I., DiCioccio, RA., Wiest, J., Tsukada, Y., Ponder, BA. & Piver, MS. (2000). Ovarian carcinoma in situ with germline BRCA1 mutation and loss of heterozygosity at BRCA1 and TP53. J Natl Cancer Inst. 92: 1088–1091.

Wynendaele, J., Böhnke, A., Leucci, E., Nielsen, SJ., Lambertz, I., Hammer, S., Sbrzesny, N., Kubitza, D., Wolf, A., Gradhand, E., Balschun,K., Braicu, I., Sehouli, J., Darb-Esfahani, S., Denkert, C. Thomssen, C., Hauptmann, S., Lund, A., Marine, JC. & Bartel, F. (2010). An illegitimate microRNA target site within the 3' UTR of MDM4 affects ovarian cancer progression and chemosensitivity. Cancer Res. 70: 9641-9.

Yarden, RI., Friedman, E., Metsuyanim, S., Olender, T., Ben-Asher, E. & Papa, MZ. (2008). MDM2 SNP309 accelerates breast and ovarian carcinogenesis in BRCA1 and BRCA2 carriers of Jewish-Ashkenazi descent. Breast Cancer Res Treat. 111:497-504.

Yee, KS. & Vousden, KH. (2005). Complicating the complexity of p53. Carcinogenesis 26: 1317-22.

Zheng, J., Benedict, WF., Xu, HJ., Hu, SX., Kim, TM., Velicescu, M., Wan, M., Cofer, KF. & Dubeau, L. (1995). Genetic disparity between morphologically benign cysts contiguous to ovarian carcinomas and solitary cystadenomas. J Natl Cancer Inst. 87: 1146–1153.

12

Homeobox Genes and Their Functional Significance in Ovarian Tumorigenesis

Bon Quy Trinh and Honami Naora
University of Texas MD Anderson Cancer Center
USA

1. Introduction

It is widely recognized that many pathways that control normal embryonic patterning are deregulated in human cancers. Mutations or aberrant expression of components of the Wnt, Hedgehog and Notch signaling pathways have been demonstrated to play pivotal roles in tumorigenesis. Homeobox genes constitute an evolutionarily conserved gene super-family that represents another important class of patterning regulators. These genes encode transcription factors that are essential for controlling cell differentiation and specification of the body plan during embryonic development. Although many homeobox genes have been reported to be aberrantly expressed in ovarian cancer, the functional significance of these genes in ovarian tumorigenesis has only emerged in recent years. This chapter discusses recent research studies that demonstrate that homeobox genes have diverse functions in the biology of ovarian cancer. These functions include specifying patterns of histologic differentiation of ovarian cancers, controlling growth and survival of tumor cells, and promoting tumor angiogenesis, cell-cell interactions and tumor cell invasiveness. This chapter discusses how studies of homeobox genes provide insights into our understanding of the cell-of-origin of ovarian cancers, the striking morphologic heterogeneity of these tumors, and the unique clinical behavior of ovarian cancer.

2. Overview of homeobox genes

Homeobox genes were first discovered in *Drosophila* by their mutations that caused homeotic transformation, a phenomenon in which body segments form in inappropriate locations (Gehring & Hiromi, 1986; McGinnis & Krumlauf, 1992). A classic example of a homeotic transformation in *Drosophila* is the formation of legs rather than antennae caused by ectopic expression of the *Antennapedia* gene (Schneuwly et al., 1987). Homeobox genes play essential roles in defining the unique identities of specific organs and body regions during embryonic development. Distinct sets of homeobox genes control skeletal patterning, limb formation, craniofacial morphogenesis, development of the central nervous system and other organ systems including the gastrointestinal tract and urogenital organs (Capecchi, 1997; Beck, 2002; Panganiban & Rubenstein, 2002; Christensen et al., 2008). Homeobox genes also control cell renewal and tissue regeneration processes in adults such as hematopoiesis, angiogenesis, spermatogenesis and endometrial remodeling (Gorski & Walsh, 2000; Argiropoulos & Humphries, 2007; Vitiello et al., 2007; Maclean & Wilkinson, 2010).

Mutations in homeobox genes cause a spectrum of complex developmental disorders. For example, mutations in the *HOXA13* gene cause hand-foot-genital syndrome, an autosomal dominant trait characterized by distal limb and genitourinary malformations (Mortlock & Innis, 1997). *SIX1* mutations cause branchio-oto-renal syndrome, a disorder characterized by hearing loss and renal abnormalities (Ruf et al., 2004).

2.1 Organization of mammalian homeobox genes

There are approximately 200 homeobox genes in the human genome (Tupler et al., 2001) and these are categorized into several different families named after their homologs in the fly (Banerjee-Basu & Baxevanis, 2001). For example, members of the mammalian *PAX, MSX* and *CDX* gene families are related to the *Drosophila* genes *paired, muscle segment* and *caudal,* respectively. Whereas most homeobox genes are scattered throughout the genome, the members of the mammalian *HOX* and *DLX* gene families are organized in clusters. The *HOX* family is related to the *Drosophila HOM-C* cluster and comprises 39 genes. *HOX* genes are organized in four clusters located on different chromosomes and are aligned into 13 paralogous groups (Figure 1). The six members of the *DLX* family are related to the *Drosophila distal-less* (*dll*) gene and are organized in bigene clusters located upstream of *HOX* clusters (Figure 1). These gene clusters are thought to have arisen from gene duplication during evolution (Sumiyama et al., 2003; Lemons & McGinnis, 2006). A striking feature of *HOX* genes is their temporal and spatial colinearity. This phenomenon describes the coupling of the timing and location of expression of *HOX* genes along the anterior-posterior body axis to their relative position in the gene clusters. *HOX* genes that are located at the 3′ end of the clusters tend to be expressed early in development and in anterior body regions, whereas those at the 5′ end of clusters are generally expressed later and in more posterior body regions (McGinnis & Krumlauf, 1992; Pearson et al., 2005) (Figure 1).

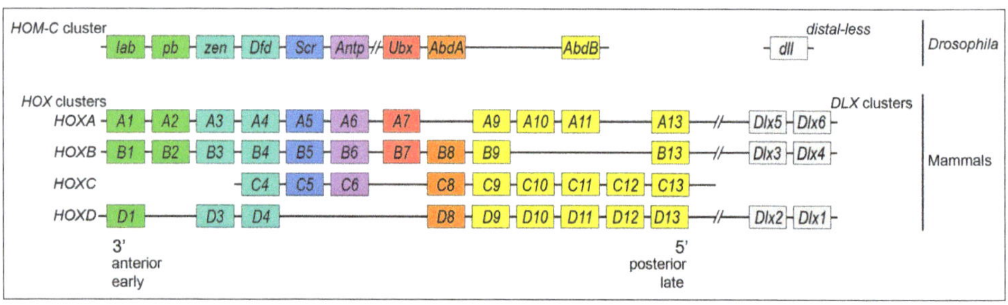

Fig. 1. Organization of *HOX* and *DLX* gene clusters in *Drosophila* and mammals.

2.2 Structural features and mechanisms

Homeobox genes encode transcription factors, often called 'homeoproteins' that are characterized by a 61 amino acid DNA-binding domain termed the homeodomain. The homeodomain forms a helix-turn-helix structure that binds DNA elements containing a TAAT core motif (Gehring et al., 1994). Although the three-dimensional structure of the homeodomain is highly conserved among homeoproteins, diversity in the amino acid residues gives rise to different DNA-binding specificities (Gehring et al., 1994; Biggin & McGinnis, 1997). Binding affinity and selectivity of homeoproteins for target gene promoters are also mediated by additional conserved motifs that are present in the different families. PAX proteins contain an additional DNA-binding domain called the paired box (Robson et al., 2006). HOX proteins contain a hexapeptide motif that mediates interactions with PBX co-factors (Chang et al., 1995). MEIS proteins also act as co-factors for HOX proteins (Shanmugam et al., 1999). Furthermore, target specificity and functional diversity of homeoproteins are achieved via interactions with other transcription factors (Chariot et al., 1999). Whereas homeoproteins have highly selective functions *in vivo*, they exhibit relatively promiscuous DNA-binding *in vitro* (Biggin & McGinnis, 1997). As a consequence, only few *bona fide* target genes have been identified. Several homeoproteins also have intriguing non-transcriptional functions. The *Drosophila* homeoprotein Bicoid represses translation of *caudal* mRNA by directly binding to the 3′ untranslated region of *caudal* mRNA (Dubnau & Struhl, 1996). HOXA9 has been reported to bind the translation initiation factor eIF4E and to stimulate eIF4E-dependent export of *cyclin D1* mRNA (Topisirovic et al., 2005). HOXB7 binds Ku proteins and stimulates DNA repair (Rubin et al., 2007).

2.3 Misexpression of homeobox genes in tumors

In the past 15 years, there has been increasing evidence that many homeobox genes are aberrantly expressed in a variety of malignancies. Much of the pioneering work has come from the hematopoietic field, where overexpression of various *HOX* genes has been found to promote leukemogenesis (Thorsteinsdottir et al., 1997; Kroon et al., 1998; Fischbach et al., 2005). Expression patterns of homeobox genes in solid tumors can be divided into three broad categories (Abate-Shen, 2002; Samuel & Naora, 2005). Firstly, homeobox genes that are normally expressed in differentiated adult tissues are often down-regulated in tumors. Two examples are *NKX3.1* and *HOXA10* that control morphogenesis of the prostate and uterus respectively, and are expressed in these tissues during development and in the adult (Bhatia-Gaur et al., 1999; Benson et al., 1996). *NKX3.1* is frequently deleted in prostate cancers (He et al., 1997), whereas *HOXA10* is often silenced by methylation in high-grade endometrial cancers (Yoshida et al., 2006). Secondly, homeobox genes can be re-expressed in tumors derived from tissues in which these genes are normally expressed during embryonic development. *PAX2,* a regulator of urogenital patterning, is normally expressed in the developing kidney and is reactivated in renal cancers (Dressler et al., 1990; Gnarra & Dressler, 1995). A third, less common, category includes homeobox genes that are expressed in tumors derived from a lineage in which the particular gene is not expressed during development. An example is *PAX5* that is expressed in medulloblastoma but not in neonatal cerebellum (Kozmik et al., 1995). Loss or gain of homeobox gene expression in tumors therefore often reflects an inappropriate recapitulation of embryonic pathways and, in many but not all cases, this misexpression can be indicative of the cell-of-origin of the tumor.

3. Homeobox genes and the origin of ovarian cancers

Whereas other types of tumors often exhibit 'loss' of the specialized features of the tissue from which they derive, many ovarian cancers exhibit specialized features of non-ovarian lineages. Epithelial ovarian cancers have been thought to originate from the simple monolayered epithelium that lines the ovarian surface (OSE) or from post-ovulatory inclusion cysts that arise from invaginations of the ovarian surface (Feeley & Wells, 2001). However, the major subtypes of ovarian cancer (serous, endometrioid, mucinous) exhibit morphologic features that resemble those of the epithelia of the reproductive tract that derive from the Müllerian ducts (*viz.* fallopian tube, endometrium, endocervix, respectively). Mucinous ovarian cancers also exhibit intestinal-like features. The OSE origin has been supported by several mouse genetic models in which tumors were induced by introducing specific oncogenic alterations into the OSE (Orsulic et al., 2002; Connolly et al., 2003; Wu et al., 2007). On the other hand, various histopathologic and genetic studies have supported origins in primary Müllerian derivatives such as the tubal fimbria (Lee et al., 2007) and in secondary Müllerian structures such as endometriosis (Prowse et al., 2006). Detailed discussions of these studies are beyond the scope of this chapter and these are elegantly reviewed in several articles (Dubeau, 2008; Jarboe et al., 2008; Cho & Shih, 2009).

3.1 *HOX* genes and the Müllerian phenotype

One argument against the OSE as the origin of ovarian cancers has been the lack of evidence that demonstrates the capability of OSE cells to differentiate along multiple Müllerian lineages. Differentiation of the Müllerian ducts is controlled by several sets of homeobox genes. These include the tandemly arranged *Hoxa9, Hoxa10, Hoxa11* and *Hoxa13* genes that are related to the *Drosophila* abdominal patterning gene *Abdominal-B* (*AbdB*) (Benson et al., 1996; Hsieh-Li et al., 1995; Zhao & Potter, 2001) (Figure 1). Targeted mutagenesis of *AbdB HOX* genes results in region-specific defects along the reproductive tract. For example, *Hoxa10*-deficient female mice exhibit homeotic transformation of the anterior segment of the uterus into oviductal-like structures (Benson et al., 1996). Replacement of the homeobox of the *Hoxa11* gene with that of *Hoxa13* in mice causes homeotic transformation of the uterus into cervical/vaginal-like structures (Zhao & Potter, 2001). The *AbdB HOX* genes are uniformly expressed along the axis of the Müllerian ducts early in embryonic development. As the ducts differentiate, *Hoxa9, Hoxa10, Hoxa11* and *Hoxa13* become expressed in the primordia of the fallopian tubes, uterus, lower uterine segment/cervix, and upper vagina, respectively (Taylor et al., 1997). This colinear *HOX* expression is maintained in the adult tract with sharply defined anterior boundaries of expression and tapered posterior expression. We have found that the *AbdB HOX* genes are not expressed in normal human OSE whereas their colinear expression patterns in Müllerian epithelia are recapitulated in the major subtypes of ovarian cancers according to the pattern of Müllerian-like differentiation of these tumors (Cheng et al., 2005). HOXA9 was found to be expressed in serous tumors and also in endometrioid and mucinous tumors. In contrast, HOXA10 was strongly expressed in endometrioid and mucinous but not serous tumors, whereas HOXA11 was mostly restricted to mucinous tumors (Table 1). Clear-cell ovarian carcinomas have features that overlap with those of serous and endometrioid tumors, and were found to express HOXA9 and HOXA10. This recapitulation of the *AbdB HOX* gene program in ovarian cancers could be interpreted to reflect Müllerian origins. However, by ectopically expressing *AbdB HOX* genes in undifferentiated, transformed mouse OSE cells and propagating transfected cells in the peritoneum of female mice, we demonstrated that OSE-derived cells acquire features of different Müllerian lineages. Mouse OSE cells that expressed *Hoxa9* formed papillary tumors that resembled high-grade serous ovarian carcinoma, whereas expression of *Hoxa10* and *Hoxa11* induced formation of high-grade endometrioid-like and mucinous-like tumors, respectively (Cheng et al., 2005). We also found that the *Hoxa7* gene, located 3′ of *Hoxa9*, is expressed in normal Müllerian epithelia and in differentiated ovarian tumors irrespective of their histologic subtype. Expression of

Hoxa7 in transformed mouse OSE cells promoted the abilities of *Hoxa9, Hoxa10* and *Hoxa11* to induce tumor differentiation along their respective pathways (Cheng et al., 2005).
The study of Cheng *et al* (2005) cannot be interpreted to conclusively demonstrate that the OSE is the cell-of-origin of ovarian cancers. However, the findings of this study suggest an intriguing model in which OSE-derived tumors acquire Müllerian phenotypes through homeotic transformation. The finding that colinearity of *AbdB HOX* expression (i.e. HOXA9, HOXA10, HOXA11) is recapitulated in ovarian cancers is striking, as it might explain the relative abundance of the ovarian cancer subtypes (i.e. serous> endometrioid> mucinous). The capability of OSE cells to acquire features of different lineages could stem from the intrinsically 'uncommitted' or embryonic-like phenotype of adult OSE cells (Auersperg et al., 2001; Naora, 2007). Unlike most other adult epithelia, the OSE lacks specialized features and expresses little or no E-cadherin (Maines-Bandiera & Auersperg, 1997). The OSE expresses both fibroblast markers and markers characteristic of simple epithelium (Auersperg et al., 1994), and also highly expresses stem cell maintenance genes (Bowen et al., 2009). This plasticity of the OSE is likely to be important for post-ovulatory repair (Auersperg et al., 2001). Both the OSE and Müllerian ducts derive from the coelomic epithelium, and the predominance of Müllerian phenotypes in ovarian cancers could reflect the close primordial relationship between the OSE and Müllerian ducts (Auersperg et al., 2001). More recently, it has been reported that the OSE and tubal fimbria are anatomically contiguous and that these tissues are parts of a transitional epithelium (Auersperg, 2011). On the other hand, less common subtypes of ovarian cancers such as clear-cell and transitional-cell tumors have features resembling those of renal and urothelial tissues whose embryonic relationship to the OSE is more distant.

3.2 PAX expression and differential diagnosis

More recently, expression of other homeobox genes that control urogenital patterning has been studied in ovarian cancers. *Pax2* is expressed in the developing kidneys, Wolffian ducts and Müllerian ducts (Dressler et al., 1990; Torres et al., 1995). *Pax8* is also expressed in the developing kidney and Müllerian ducts (Plachov et al., 1990). Female *Pax2* homozygous mutant mice lack the entire reproductive tract (Torres et al., 1995). Female *Pax8* null mice do not develop a functional uterus whereas development of the oviduct, cervix and vagina is unaffected (Mittag et al., 2007). PAX2 and PAX8 are normally expressed in tubal, endometrial and endocervical epithelia (Tong et al., 2007; Tong et al., 2011). PAX2 has also been detected in secondary Müllerian structures such as endometriosis, endosalpingiosis and rete ovarii (Tong et al., 2007). PAX2 and PAX8 have been detected in 64 to 100% of non-mucinous ovarian cancers, and in 74 to 90% of primary and metastatic renal cell carcinomas (Bowen et al., 2007; Tong et al., 2007; Nonaka et al., 2008; Chivukula et al., 2009; Zhai et al., 2010; Laury et al., 2011; Tacha et al., 2011). The absence or rareness of PAX2 and PAX8 in many other types of cancers such as colorectal carcinomas and mesotheliomas has raised the possibility that these proteins could be useful markers for differential diagnosis (Tong et al., 2007; Zhai et al., 2010; Laury et al., 2011; Tacha et al., 2011), but this depends on the appropriate setting. Ovarian metastasis from renal cell carcinoma and renal metastasis from ovarian carcinoma are rare. However, ovarian cancer commonly involves the uterus and omentum. PAX2 and PAX8 are frequently expressed in endometrial carcinomas (56 to 98%) (Sharma et al., 2010; Laury et al., 2011; Tacha et al., 2011), but have been detected at low frequency (<10%) in mucinous ovarian cancers that closely resemble colorectal carcinomas (Muratovska et al., 2003; Bowen et al., 2007; Nonaka et al., 2008). On the other hand, PAX8 has been reported to have comparable sensitivity to the Wilms tumor gene product WT1 in detecting serous ovarian cancer cells in fluid cytologic specimens and superior specificity to WT1 in distinguishing tumor cells from mesothelial cells (McKnight et al., 2010).

One interpretation of the frequency of PAX2 and PAX8 expression in ovarian cancers is that it implicates Müllerian origins of these tumors (Tong et al., 2007; Tong et al., 2011). However, there are several observations that challenge this notion. Whereas most studies have not detected PAX2 or PAX8 in normal OSE, these proteins have been detected in inclusion cysts (Bowen et al., 2007; Chivukula et al., 2009; Zhai et al., 2010; Auersperg, 2011). PAX8 has also been detected in peritoneal serous carcinomas (Tong et al., 2011). These tumors originate from the peritoneal mesothelium, a coelomic epithelial derivative to which the OSE is very closely related. Furthermore, PAX2 and PAX8 have been detected in tumors derived from non-urogenital lineages such as Kaposi's sarcoma (Buttiglieri et al., 2004) and thymic tumors (Laury et al., 2011). These cases might fall within the third category of anomalously expressed homeobox genes described above.

3.3 *CDX2* and the intestinal phenotype

Another homeoprotein that has been extensively studied in differential diagnosis is CDX2. *Cdx2* controls intestinal differentiation and is expressed in the gut during development and in the adult (James et al., 1994). In contrast to PAX2 and PAX8, CDX2 is more frequently detected in mucinous ovarian carcinomas (64 to 93%) than in non-mucinous subtypes (0 to 7%) (Fraggetta et al., 2003; Werling et al., 2003; Groisman et al., 2004). CDX2 has been detected at lower frequency in mucinous ovarian cystadenomas and borderline tumors in keeping with the decreased prevalence of intestinal differentiation in these tumors (Werling et al., 2003). The most common secondary tumor to mimic an ovarian primary tumor is metastatic colorectal adenocarcinoma. Distinguishing primary mucinous ovarian carcinoma from metastatic colorectal adenocarcinoma is essential for clinical management but can be very difficult given their similar morphologic features. CDX2 alone is unsuitable for distinguishing primary from secondary mucinous ovarian tumors, as it is expressed in 90% of colorectal carcinomas metastatic to the ovary (Tornillo et al., 2004). However, several studies have reported promising predictive values when CDX2 is combined with other markers. These include cytokeratin 7 and mucin 5AC that are more frequently expressed in cancers of ovarian rather than lower gastrointestinal origin, and mucin 2 and carcinoembryonic antigen that are more frequently expressed in cancers of gastrointestinal rather than ovarian origin (Groisman et al., 2004; Park et al., 2007).

3.4 Other diagnostic applications of homeoproteins

The studies discussed above indicate that expression of several homeobox genes in ovarian cancers is associated with specific patterns of differentiation (Table 1), and raise the possibility that homeoproteins could serve as markers for differential diagnosis when used in appropriate settings and in combination with other tissue-specific markers. Misexpressed homeoproteins might also be useful for early detection. A significant limitation of assaying molecules that are shed by tumor cells is that their levels might not be detected in body fluids particularly when tumors are small. On the other hand, cancer patients often generate antibodies to molecules that are expressed in tumors and not in normal tissues and to self-antigens that are overexpressed in tumors. These circulating antibodies can be regarded as 'signals' that are amplified by the immune system and could serve as biomarkers for early cancer detection. One approach of identifying tumor antigens is to screen tumor cDNA expression libraries with cancer patient sera and has been termed SEREX (serologic identification of antigens by recombinant expression cloning) (Sahin et al., 1995). We have identified the HOXA7 and HOXB7 homeoproteins as ovarian tumor antigens by using the SEREX approach (Naora et al., 2001a, 2001b). Serum antibodies to HOXA7 were detected in 16 of 24 (67%) patients with differentiated ovarian carcinomas and in 0/30 (0%) healthy women (Naora et al., 2001a). Antibodies to HOXA7 were also detected in 13 of 19 (68%) women with cystadenomas, but in only one of 24 (4%) patients with poorly differentiated ovarian carcinoma (Naora et al., 2001a). This serologic reactivity reflected the prevalence of HOXA7 expression in cystadenomas and differentiated ovarian carcinomas as compared to poorly differentiated carcinomas (Naora et al., 2001a). Whereas HOXA7 is absent from normal OSE, HOXB7 was detected in normal OSE and at higher levels in ovarian carcinomas irrespective of the type or degree of differentiation (Naora et al., 2001b). Serum antibodies to HOXB7 were detected in only one of 29 (3%) healthy women and in 13 of 39 (33%) ovarian cancer patients (Naora et al., 2001b). Although this frequency is not high, the application of Bayesian modeling to multiplexed assays of serum antibodies to multiple ovarian tumor antigens has found that assaying serum antibodies to HOXB7, p53 and the antigen NY-CO-8 is the most effective combination for discriminating between ovarian cancer patients and healthy women (Erkanli et al., 2006). Widschwendter *et al.* (2009) reported that methylation of the *HOXA9* and *HOXA11* genes in normal endometrium can discriminate between premenopausal women with ovarian cancer and age-matched healthy women. Although the biological significance of these findings is unclear, this study raises the intriguing possibility that the methylation status of specific *HOX* genes in the endometrium might be useful for predicting risk of ovarian cancer.

	HOXA7*	HOXA9	HOXA10	HOXA11	PAX2	PAX8	CDX2
serous	+	+	-	-	+	+	-
endometrioid	+	+	+	-/+	-	+	-
mucinous	+	+	+	+	-	-/+	+
clear-cell	+	+	+	-	+	+	?

(* mostly restricted to differentiated tumors)

Table 1. Homeobox gene expression in histologic subtypes of ovarian cancer.

4. Homeobox genes and the hallmarks of cancer

Given their essential developmental functions, it is not surprising that many homeobox genes are misexpressed in different types of cancers. In some cases, this aberrant expression reflects changes in cell differentiation in tumors and could occur as a consequence of tumorigenesis. On the other hand, there is increasing evidence that anomalous expression of homeobox genes plays causal roles in tumorigenesis (Abate-Shen, 2002; Samuel & Naora, 2005; Robson et al., 2006). Overexpression of several *HOX* genes in bone marrow cells leads to acute myeloid leukemia (Thorsteinsdottir et al., 1997; Kroon et al., 1998; Fischbach et al., 2005). Conversely, loss or down-regulation of a homeobox gene that is normally expressed in adult tissues can predispose cells for transformation. Inactivation of *Nkx3.1* in mice leads to the development of lesions that resemble prostate intraepithelial neoplasia (Kim et al.,

2002a). Inactivation of *Nkx3.1* cooperates with loss-of-function of *Pten* to induce carcinoma (Kim et al., 2002b). *Cdx2* heterozygous mutant mice develop adenomatous intestinal polyps (Chawengsaksophak et al., 1997). *Cdx2* inactivation enhances the sensitivity of mice to chemically induced colon carcinogenesis (Bonhomme et al., 2003). Re-expression of *Nkx3.1* and *Cdx2* in prostate and colon cancer cells, respectively, inhibits cell proliferation (Kim et al., 2002a; Mallo et al., 1998). On the other hand, re-expression of *Hoxa10* in endometrial cancer cells does not alter proliferation but inhibits invasive behavior (Yoshida et al., 2006). Up- or down- regulation of homeobox genes in tumors, depending on their context, can therefore significantly modulate different hallmark capabilities of cancer.

4.1 Sustained proliferative signaling

A well-established hallmark of cancer cells is their ability to sustain chronic proliferation (Hanahan and Weinberg, 2000). One important growth factor that promotes autocrine cell growth and that is frequently overexpressed in ovarian cancers is fibroblast growth factor-2 (FGF-2) (Le Page et al., 2006). The *FGF-2* gene is a transcriptional target of HOXB7 (Caré et al., 1996). Enforced expression of *HOXB7* in OSE cells induces FGF-2 expression and cell proliferation (Naora et al., 2001b). The homeoprotein DLX4 is absent from most normal adult tissues and is expressed in >50% of ovarian cancers (Hara et al., 2007). We have found that overexpression of DLX4 in ovarian cancer cells induces FGF-2 expression, increases clonogenicity *in vitro* and promotes tumor growth *in vivo* (Hara et al., 2007), but it is not known whether DLX4 directly activates *FGF-2* transcription. We recently found that DLX4 also induces expression of c-Myc (Trinh et al., 2011). This induction occurs by two mechanisms. We identified that DLX4 prevents transforming growth factor-β (TGF-β)-mediated repression of c-*myc* transcription, and also induces c-*myc* promoter activity independently of TGF-β/Smad signaling (Trinh et al., 2011). DLX5, another member of the *DLX* family, has also been found to directly activate c-*myc* transcription in lung cancer cells (Xu and Testa, 2009). It has been reported that DLX5 is overexpressed in ovarian cancers and that inhibiting DLX5 expression by RNA interference attenuates AKT signaling and inhibits growth of ovarian cancer cells (Tan et al., 2010). Furthermore, *DLX5* cooperates with activated *HRAS* in transformation of human OSE cells. This growth-stimulatory effect of DLX5 has been attributed in part to its ability to activate transcription of the gene encoding insulin receptor substrate 2, an oncogenic signaling adaptor protein (Tan et al., 2010).

The studies discussed above demonstrate that activation of specific sets of homeobox genes in ovarian cancers drives tumor cell proliferation by inducing transcription of genes that encode multiple, different components of signaling pathways. In several cases, a homeobox gene promotes proliferation by the same mechanism in cells of different lineages. HOXB7 induces FGF-2 expression in OSE cells, breast cancers and melanomas, and stimulates growth of these cell types (Caré et al., 1996; 1998; Naora et al., 2001b). Overexpression of *SIX1* stimulates proliferation of breast and ovarian cancer cells by inducing cyclin A1 expression (Coletta et al., 2004; Behbakht et al., 2007). On the other hand, the effect of a homeobox gene can be cell type-specific. For example, overexpression of HOXA10 in myelomonocytic cells activates transcription of the gene encoding the cyclin-dependent kinase inhibitor $p21^{WAF1/Cip1}$ and induces cell cycle arrest in G_1 phase (Bromleigh & Freedman, 2000). In contrast, we have found that overexpression of HOXA10 in OSE-derived cells has no effect on cell proliferation (Ko et al., 2010). Because homeoproteins of a given family share regions of extensive homology, it is not surprising that family members have overlapping functions. For example, both DLX4 and DLX5 induce c-Myc expression (Xu and Testa 2009; Trinh et al., 2011). On the other hand, MSX1 induces expression of growth arrest genes such as GADD153 and inhibits proliferation of ovarian cancer cells (Park et al., 2001), whereas MSX2 promotes ovarian cancer growth (Zhai et al., 2011). As discussed earlier, diversity in amino acid residues in the homeodomain and other motifs of family members gives rise to different DNA-binding specificities and can result in different phenotypes. The function or mechanism of a homeoprotein cannot therefore be inferred from studies of its related family members.

4.2 Evasion of growth-suppressors

A second important hallmark of cancer cells is their ability to circumvent signals that inhibit cell growth (Hanahan & Weinberg, 2000). Whereas TGF-β induces G_1 arrest in most types of normal cells, many tumors are resistant to the anti-proliferative effect of TGF-β (Siegel & Massagué, 2003). The gene responses that are central to the TGF-β cytostatic program are activation of the cyclin-dependent kinase inhibitors $p15^{Ink4B}$ and $p21^{WAF1/Cip1}$ and repression of c-myc and ID transcription factors. This cytostatic program is tightly regulated by a network of transcription factors that include Smad proteins, Sp1 and c-myc (Feng et al., 2000; 2002; Gartel et al., 2001). Resistance to the anti-proliferative effect of TGF-β has been attributed to TGF-β receptor or Smad4 mutations in several types of tumors, particularly those of gastrointestinal origin (Markowitz et al., 1995; Hahn et al., 1996). TGF-β receptor mutations have been detected in 12 to 31% of ovarian cancers, but many TGF-β-resistant ovarian cancers have been found to express functional receptors and rarely have Smad4 mutations (Yamada et al., 1999; Wang et al., 2000; Francis-Thickpenny et al., 2001). We have found that DLX4 blocks the anti-proliferative effect of TGF-β by inactivating transcriptional control of the TGF-β cytostatic program through three distinct but integrated mechanisms (Trinh et al., 2011). Firstly, DLX4 directly binds Smad4 and prevents Smad4 from forming transcriptional complexes with Smad2 and Smad3. Secondly, DLX4 binds the DNA-binding domain of Sp1 and impairs the DNA-binding ability of Sp1. In addition, DLX4 induces expression of c-Myc, a repressor of $p15^{Ink4B}$ and $p21^{WAF1/Cip1}$ transcription (Trinh et al., 2011). An important outcome of our finding that DLX4 disables key transcriptional control mechanisms of the TGF-β cytostatic program is that it explains why tumors that lack TGF-β receptor or Smad mutations become resistant to the anti-proliferative effect of TGF-β.

4.3 Resistance to cell death

Cancer cells encounter many physiologic stresses that trigger cell death and have evolved adaptive strategies to circumvent cell death programs. One important selective advantage is evasion of anoikis. A significant proportion of ovarian cancer cells in ascites exist as multicellular aggregates (Burleson et al., 2004). We have found that overexpression of HOXA10 in OSE-derived cells promotes homophilic cell adhesion and enables these cells to escape anoikis (Ko et al., 2010). Another selective advantage is the ability to survive under conditions where levels of growth factors are limited. We have found that DLX4 enables ovarian cancer cells to escape apoptosis induced by withdrawal of exogenous growth factors. This effect was due at least in part to induction of FGF-2 expression by DLX4 in tumor cells (Hara et al., 2007). In addition, DLX4 (also known as BP1 and DLX7) has been reported to induce bcl-2 and GATA-1 expression and to promote survival of leukemic and breast cancer cells (Shimamoto et al., 1997; Stevenson et al., 2007). PAX2 has also been reported to promote survival of ovarian cancer cells and various other cell types such as bladder cancer cells, Kaposi's sarcoma and renal cell carcinoma cells (Gnarra & Dressler, 1995; Muratovska et al., 2003; Buttiglieri et al., 2004), but the underlying mechanism of the anti-apoptotic effect of PAX2 is not known.

Chemoresistance is a major challenge in the clinical management of ovarian cancer. *BARX2* is a homeobox gene that has been strongly implicated in modulating sensitivity of tumor cells to platinum. A study by Sellar *et al.* (2002) investigated isogenic ovarian cancer cell lines that were established from patients' tumors before and after platinum therapy. It was found that *BARX2* expression was down-regulated in tumor cell lines that were established upon tumor recurrence after platinum therapy and that transfection of *BARX2* into platinum-resistant cells reversed platinum-resistance. There has been significant interest in studying platinum-resistance in stem cell-like cell populations in ovarian cancers, and the homeoprotein Nanog has been used as a stem cell marker in these studies (Zhang et al., 2008). Furthermore, some homeobox genes confer resistance to cell death induced by other agents or signals. Expression of *HOXB13* in ovarian cancer cells has been reported to confer resistance to tamoxifen-mediated apoptosis (Miao et al., 2007). On the other hand, *SIX1* overexpression renders ovarian cancer cells resistant to tumor necrosis factor-related apoptosis inducing ligand (TRAIL)-mediated apoptosis (Behbakht et al., 2007).

4.4 DNA repair and genomic instability

Most agents that are commonly used to treat ovarian cancer induce cell death by causing DNA damage. The DNA double-strand break (DSB) is the most dangerous type of DNA damage. DSBs are induced by ionizing radiation and topoisomerase II inhibitors such as etoposide (Helleday et al., 2008). The inability of a cell to properly respond to DSBs leads to genomic instability. Genomic instability has been described as an 'enabling' characteristic of cancer cells (Hanahan & Weinberg, 2011). The primary mechanisms that repair DSBs are homologous recombination (HR) and non-homologous end-joining (NHEJ). The latter is the dominant DSB repair pathway in mammalian cells and is error-prone (Lieber et al., 2003). Both deficiencies and increases in NHEJ activity contribute to DNA repair infidelity and genomic instability (Difilippantonio et al., 2000; Brady et al., 2003). Several homeoproteins have been implicated in DNA repair and genomic instability. HOXB7 has been reported to stimulate NHEJ-mediated DNA repair and to confer resistance to ionizing radiation (Rubin et al., 2007). This activity was associated with the ability of HOXB7 to bind Ku proteins. Ku proteins form a complex that binds to the ends of DSBs (Lieber et al., 2003). On the other hand, DLX4 has been reported to inhibit expression of BRCA1, a component of the HR-mediated DNA repair pathway (Kluk et al., 2010). Overexpression of SIX1 has been found to lead to genomic instability by attenuating the G_2-M DNA damage checkpoint (Coletta et al., 2008). In these studies, the functions of HOXB7, DLX4 and SIX1 were studied in breast cancer cells. However, these homeoproteins are also overexpressed in ovarian cancers (Naora et al., 2001b, Hara et al., 2007; Behbakht et al., 2007), and might potentially contribute to DNA repair infidelity and genomic instability in ovarian cancer cells.

4.5 Invasion and metastasis

The ability of tumor cells to invade adjacent tissues and colonize distant sites is another well-established hallmark of cancer (Hanahan & Weinberg, 2000). The lethality of ovarian cancer stems from its propensity for aggressive intraperitoneal dissemination, with 70% of patients presenting with advanced-stage disease. FGF-2 stimulates cell migration, and advanced-stage ovarian cancers express a gene signature associated with FGF-2 signaling (De Cecco et al., 2004). HOXB7 induces FGF-2 expression in OSE-derived cells (Naora et al., 2001b) and inhibiting *HOXB7* expression in ovarian cancer cells inhibits invasiveness (Yamashita et al., 2006). Invasiveness of ovarian cancer cells is also inhibited when *HOXB13* expression is suppressed (Yamashita et al., 2006). Overexpression of *SIX1* increases metastasis of rhabdomyosarcoma by inducing expression of the cytoskeletal protein ezrin (Yu et al., 2004), but it is not known whether *SIX1* promotes ovarian cancer dissemination by the same mechanism. Conversely, *BARX2* inhibits invasiveness of ovarian cancer cells and loss of *BARX2* in ovarian cancers is associated with adverse survival (Sellar et al., 2001). The tumor-suppressive property of *BARX2* has been attributed in part to its ability to induce expression of the cell adhesion molecule cadherin-6 (Sellar et al., 2001).

Functions of several other homeobox genes that have been implicated in ovarian tumor progression are more complex. In addition to its anti-proliferative effect, TGF-β is well-known to induce epithelial-to-mesenchymal transition (EMT) and metastasis (Siegel and Massagué, 2003). We have found that DLX4 not only blocks the anti-proliferative effect of TGF-β by sequestering Smad4, but also partially inhibits TGF-β-induced EMT (Trinh et al., 2011). The ability of DLX4 to inhibit TGF-β-induced EMT could explain the reported association of DLX4 with favorable prognosis in lung cancer patients and its metastasis-suppressive activity (Tomida et al., 2007). On the other hand, we have found that DLX4 expression in ovarian cancers is strongly associated with disease progression (Hara et al., 2007). This association is likely to be due to the ability of DLX4 to stimulate other tumor-promoting processes via its induction of c-Myc, FGF-2 and vascular endothelial growth factor (VEGF) (Hara et al., 2007; Trinh et al., 2011). Another example of a homeobox gene with paradoxical functions is *HOXA4*. Whereas *HOXA4* is more highly expressed in invasive than in non-invasive ovarian cancers, *HOXA4* inhibits ovarian cancer cell migration (Klausen et al., 2009). These authors have speculated that increased *HOXA4* expression in invasive cancers might constitute a homeostatic response.

In contrast to many other types of cancers, ovarian cancer rarely spreads by hematogenous routes. Ovarian cancer cells typically disseminate by intraperitoneal 'seeding' whereby exfoliated tumor cells are transported throughout the pelvic cavity by the peritoneal fluid and frequently implant onto the mesothelial linings of the cavity wall and omentum (Naora & Montell, 2005). Attachment of ovarian cancer cells to mesothelial surfaces is mediated in part by interactions between ECM proteins and integrins (Heyman et al., 2008). We have found that HOXA10 stimulates attachment of OSE-derived cells to omental mesothelial cells by inducing expression of αvβ3 integrin (Ko et al., 2010). The *ITGB3* gene that encodes β3 integrin has also been reported to be a transcriptional target of HOXA10 in endometrial cells (Daftary et al., 2002). However, comparison of our studies of HOXA10 in ovarian and endometrial cancers reveals striking differences as well as similarities. We have found that gain of *HOXA10* expression in endometrioid ovarian carcinomas is associated with endometrial-like differentiation (Cheng et al., 2005), whereas *HOXA10* down-regulation in endometrial carcinomas correlates with loss of glandular differentiation (Yoshida et al., 2006). Consistent with these observations, *HOXA10* promoted homophilic cell adhesion in both endometrial cancer cells and OSE-derived cells (Yoshida et al., 2006; Ko et al., 2010). However, whereas *HOXA10* expression in endometrial cancer cells inhibited invasiveness and metastasis (Yoshida et al., 2006), *HOXA10* activation in OSE-derived tumor cells lead to increased numbers of peritoneal implants by enabling tumor cells to escape anoikis and stimulating their attachment to mesothelial surfaces (Ko et al., 2010). These studies indicate that cellular behavior induced by a homeobox gene can differ depending on the cell type and context, and highlight fundamental differences between intraperitoneal seeding of ovarian cancer and 'classic' metastasis of endometrial and many other types of carcinomas.

4.6 Angiogenesis

Angiogenesis is a well-established hallmark of cancer that has been extensively studied in ovarian cancer. The angiogenic factors VEGF, FGF-2 and IL-8 are overexpressed in ovarian cancers and tumor microvessel density is a strong predictor of outcomes (Hollingsworth et al., 1995; Yoneda et al., 1998). VEGF is also the causative factor of ascites (Zhang et al., 2002). We have found that DLX4 expression in ovarian cancers is strongly associated with ascites and reduced overall survival in patients (Hara et al., 2007). Furthermore, we have demonstrated that overexpression of DLX4 in ovarian cancer cells promotes ascites and increases tumor microvessel density in mouse xenograft models. This activity of DLX4 was attributed to its induction of FGF-2 and VEGF expression (Hara et al., 2007). HOXB7 has also been found to induce FGF-2 and VEGF expression in breast cancer cells (Caré et al., 2001), and might stimulate angiogenesis in ovarian cancer by the same mechanism.

4.7 Implications for therapy

To date, functions of homeobox genes have not been described in replicative immortality or in emerging hallmarks and enabling characteristics of cancer such as deregulated cellular energetics, inflammation and evasion of immune destruction (Hanahan & Weinberg, 2011). Because homeoproteins control expression of numerous genes in different cell types and in response to different cellular signals, it is likely that misexpressed homeoproteins also modulate tumor pathogenesis by regulating one or more of these other hallmark capabilities. One central finding that has emerged from recent studies is that misexpression of an individual homeoprotein can promote multiple hallmark capabilities (Table 2).

	DLX4 ↑	DLX5 ↑	HOXB7 ↑	HOXB13 ↑	HOXA10 ↑	SIX1 ↑	PAX2 ↑	MSX2 ↑	BARX2 ↓
Sustained proliferative signaling	+	+	+			+		+	
Evasion of growth suppressors	+								
Resistance to cell death	+			+	+	+	+		+
DNA repair / Genomic instability			+			+			
Invasion / Metastasis	?		+	+		?			+
Angiogenesis	+		+						

Table 2. Implicated functions of up- (↑) and down- (↓) regulated homeobox genes in ovarian cancer.

This raises the possibility that homeoproteins could be attractive therapeutic targets. The most significant challenge to effectively inhibiting an overexpressed homeoprotein in tumors is specificity. As discussed earlier, different homeoproteins particularly within a family have highly conserved domains. One approach by which HOX protein activity can be inhibited in cells is by using a cell-penetrating peptide that blocks interactions between HOX and PBX proteins. This peptide has been reported to inhibit growth of ovarian cancer cells (Morgan et al., 2010). However, it should be noted that many different HOX proteins are expressed in normal cells as well as in tumors and utilize PBX proteins as co-factors (Chang et al., 1995; Shanmugam et al., 1999). On the other hand, the studies to date indicate that distinct sets of homeoproteins control cell cycle progression and cell survival. Homeoproteins might therefore be useful as markers for predicting responsiveness to chemotherapeutic agents.

5. Mechanisms of homeobox gene deregulation in tumors

As discussed above, studies of *NKX3.1* and *CDX2* have demonstrated that misexpression of homeobox genes can induce pre-neoplastic lesions or predispose cells to transformation (Kim et al., 2002a; 2002b; Chawengsaksophak et al., 1997). Studying how homeobox genes are deregulated in tumors could therefore provide important insights into cancer risk. However, the mechanisms that cause aberrant expression of homeobox genes in solid tumors are poorly understood. Mutations in homeobox genes are associated with many developmental abnormalities (Mortlock and Innis, 1997; Ruf et al., 2004), but have rarely been detected in solid tumors. Deregulation of many *HOX* genes in leukemias and some *PAX* genes in sarcomas has been attributed to chromosomal translocations (Samuel & Naora, 2005; Argiropoulos & Humphries, 2007). A few homeobox genes localize to 'hot-spots' that undergo loss of heterozygosity (LOH) or are amplified in tumors. The *HOXB* gene cluster and *DLX4* map to the 17q21.3-q22 region, a 'hot-spot' that is amplified in ~10% of breast and ovarian cancers (Watanabe et al., 2001; Hyman et al., 2002; Hirasawa et al., 2003). However, overexpression of *HOXB7* and *DLX4* occurs in >50% of breast and ovarian cancers (Naora et al., 2001b; Man et al., 2005; Wu et al., 2006; Hara et al., 2007), indicating that gene amplification is not the sole mechanism underlying the overexpression of these genes. On the other hand, *NKX3.1* maps to 8p21, a region that is deleted in ~80% of prostate cancers (He et al., 1997). *BARX2* is located at 11q24-q25, within a minimal region that is associated with frequent LOH and adverse survival in ovarian cancer (Gabra et al., 1996). It is interesting to note that *BARX2* is the only homeobox gene with tumor-suppressive properties that has been identified to be lost in ovarian cancer. In contrast, other homeobox genes have been found to be overexpressed in ovarian cancers (Table 2). In this regard, the pattern of misexpression of homeobox genes in ovarian cancers is remarkably more similar to that in hematologic malignancies rather than in other solid tumors.

5.1 Developmental signals

Little is known about the signaling pathways that control expression of homeobox genes in tumors. However, studies from the developmental biology field can provide important insights. Cross-regulatory interactions have been reported between bone morphogenetic proteins (BMPs) and *DLX* genes during normal cell differentiation. For example, BMP-2 activates *Dlx3* transcription (Park & Morasso, 2002), whereas Smad6, an antagonist of BMP signaling, inhibits DLX3 transcriptional activity (Berghorn et al., 2006). We have observed that levels of DLX4 protein decrease in cells following TGF-β stimulation (Trinh et al., 2011). This raises the possibility that DLX4 is a component of a regulatory loop that blocks TGF-β signaling and is conversely regulated by TGF-β. There is considerable evidence that patterning of the reproductive tract is controlled by a regulatory network of distinct sets of Wnts and homeobox genes (Kobayashi & Behringer, 2003). *MSX2* is a transcriptional target of β-catenin/TCF and *MSX2* expression is increased in endometrioid ovarian carcinomas with deregulated β-catenin (Zhai et al., 2011). Expression of *AbdB HOX* genes in the endometrium is also tightly regulated by estrogen and progesterone (Ma et al., 1998). WT1 is a transcription factor that is used as a marker of serous ovarian cancer and reportedly represses *HOXA10* expression (Andikyan & Taylor, 2009). WT1-mediated repression could explain why many serous ovarian cancers do not express *HOXA10* (Cheng et al., 2005).

5.2 Epigenetic mechanisms

DNA methylation is the most commonly identified mechanism that silences expression of homeobox genes in solid tumors such as breast and lung cancers (Novak et al., 2006; Rauch et al., 2007). We have found that *HOXA10* down-regulation in high-grade endometrial carcinomas is due to promoter methylation (Yoshida et al., 2006). DNA methyltransferases that methylate DNA are recruited by Polycomb repressive complexes (Mills, 2010). Polycomb and Trithorax group proteins form multi-protein complexes that contain histone methyltransferase activity and dynamically alter chromatin structure by modifying specific residues in histone tails. Polycomb group proteins keep *HOX* genes repressed, whereas Trithorax group proteins counteract Polycomb-mediated silencing and maintain *HOX* expression (Soshnikova & Duboule, 2009). Polycomb and Trithorax group proteins are aberrantly expressed in different types of cancers (Mills, 2010), but it is unclear whether altered expression of these proteins causes *HOX* activation in ovarian cancers. A striking aspect of *HOX* gene clusters is the presence of long noncoding RNAs and microRNAs in the intergenic regions. These non-coding RNAs control transcription of *HOX* genes through a variety of *cis-* and *trans-* acting mechanisms (Lemons & McGinnis, 2006; Yekta et al., 2008). One intriguing example is the long non-coding RNA *HOTAIR*. *HOTAIR* is located in the *HOXC* locus and interacts with and targets the Polycomb repressive complex 2 (PRC2) to the *HOXD* locus located on a different chromosome (Rinn et al., 2007). *HOTAIR* expression in primary breast tumors has been found to be a strong predictor of metastasis (Gupta et al., 2010). Enforced expression of *HOTAIR* in cancer cells increased metastasis by inducing genome-wide re-targeting of PRC2 to an occupancy pattern that resemble that of embryonic fibroblasts (Gupta et al., 2010). Almost all homeobox genes that have been studied in ovarian cancer are overexpressed (Tables I,II), and their activation in tumors might arise from down-regulation of non-coding RNAs. Indeed, microRNA-185 has been reported to target *Six1* and is expressed at decreased levels in ovarian cancers (Imam et al., 2010).

6. Conclusions

In conclusion, the functional significance of homeobox genes in ovarian cancer is rapidly emerging as an intriguing research area that provides new molecular insights into the histogenesis of the different subtypes of ovarian cancer and the progression of this disease. The studies to date raise the possibility that specific sets of homeoproteins might serve as diagnostic or predictive markers in the appropriate settings and in combination with other markers. However, more mechanistic studies are essential to further develop our understanding of the functions of homeobox genes in ovarian cancer biology and to translate this research into clinical applications. In particular, the target genes of homeoproteins and the mechanisms that cause aberrant homeobox gene expression in tumors need to be identified. It is also important to determine whether a given homeobox gene controls a cellular process by the same mechanism in cells of different lineages, or has cell type-specific effects. Studies from the developmental biology field have provided powerful insights into the regulation, functions and mechanisms of homeobox genes in human cancers. Stronger integration between the developmental and cancer biology fields will be instrumental for furthering our understanding of the functional significance of homeobox genes in ovarian cancer.

7. Acknowledgement

Studies by H. Naora are supported by a grant from the National Institutes of Health (R01 CA141078) and by a University of Texas MD Anderson Cancer Center Institutional Research Grant. Our work is dedicated to the memory of Sean Patrick.

8. References

Abate-Shen, C. (2002) Deregulated homeobox gene expression in cancer: cause or consequence? *Nat Rev Cancer,* Vol. 2, No. 10, pp. 777-785, ISSN 1474-175X.

Andikyan V. & Taylor H.S. (2009) WT1 represses *HOX* gene expression in the regulation of gynaecologic tumour histologic type. *J Cell Mol Med,* Vol. 13, No. 11-12, pp. 4522-4531, ISSN 1582-1838.

Argiropoulos, B. & Humphries, R.K. (2007) *Hox* genes in hematopoiesis and leukemogenesis. *Oncogene,* Vol. 26, No. 47, pp. 6766-6776, ISSN 0950-9232.

Auersperg, N., Maines-Bandiera, S.L., Dyck, H.G., Kruk, P.A. (1994) Characterization of cultured human ovarian surface epithelial cells: phenotypic plasticity and premalignant changes. *Lab Invest,* Vol. 71, No. 4, pp. 510-518, ISSN 0023-6837.

Auersperg, N., Wong, A.S., Choi, K.C., Kang, S.K., Leung, P.C. (2001) Ovarian surface epithelium: biology, endocrinology, and pathology. *Endocr Rev,* Vol. 22, No. 2, pp. 255-288, ISSN 0163-769X.

Auersperg, N. (2011) The origin of ovarian carcinomas: A unifying hypothesis. *Int J Gynecol Pathol,* Vol. 30, No. 1, pp. 12–21, ISSN 0277-1691.

Banerjee-Basu, S. & Baxevanis, A.D. (2001) Molecular evolution of the homeodomain family of transcription factors. *Nucl Acids Res,* Vol. 29, No. 15, pp. 3258-3269, ISSN 0305-1048.

Beck, F. (2002) Homeobox genes in gut development. *Gut,* Vol. 51, No. 3, pp. 450-454, ISSN 0017-5749.

Behbakht, K., Qamar, L., Aldridge, C.S., Coletta, R.D., Davidson, S.A., Thorburn, A., Ford, H.L. (2007) Six1 overexpression in ovarian carcinoma causes resistance to TRAIL-mediated apoptosis and is associated with poor survival. *Cancer Res,* Vol. 67, No. 7, pp. 3036-3042, ISSN 0008-5472.

Benson, G.V., Lim, H., Paria, B.C., Satokata, I., Dey, S.K., Maas, R.L. (1996) Mechanisms of reduced fertility in *Hoxa-10* mutant mice: uterine homeosis and loss of maternal *Hoxa-10* expression. *Development,* Vol. 122, No. 9, pp. 2687-2696, ISSN 0950-1991.

Berghorn, K.A., Clark-Campbell, P.A., Han, L., McGrattan, M., Weiss, R.S., Roberson, M.S. (2006) Smad6 represses Dlx3 transcriptional activity through inhibition of DNA binding. *J Biol Chem,* Vol. 281, No. 29, pp. 20357-20367, ISSN 0021-9258.

Bhatia-Gaur, R., Donjacour, A.A., Sciavolino, P.J., Kim, M., Desai, N., Young, P., Norton, C.R., Gridley, T., Cardiff, R.D., Cunha, G.R., Abate-Shen, C., Shen, M.M. (1999) Roles for *Nkx3.1* in prostate development and cancer. *Genes Dev,* Vol. 13, No. 8, pp. 966-977, ISSN 0890-9369.

Biggin, M.D. & McGinnis, W. (1997) Regulation of segmentation and segmental identity by *Drosophila* homeoproteins: the role of DNA binding in functional activity and specificity. *Development,* Vol. 124, No. 22, pp. 4425-4433, ISSN 0950-1991.

Bonhomme, C., Duluc, I., Martin, E., Chawengsaksophak, K., Chenard, M.P., Kedinger, M., Beck, F., Freund, J.N., Domon-Dell, C. (2003) The *Cdx2* homeobox gene has a tumour suppressor function in the distal colon in addition to a homeotic role during gut development. *Gut,* Vol. 52, No. 10, pp. 1465–1471, ISSN 0017-5749.

Bowen, N.J., Logani, S., Dickerson, E.B., Kapa, L.B., Akhtar, M., Benigno, B.B., McDonald, J.F. (2007) Emerging roles for PAX8 in ovarian cancer and endosalpingeal development. *Gynecol Oncol.* Vol. 104, No. 2, pp. 331-337, ISSN 0090-8258.

Bowen N.J., Walker L.D., Matyunina L.V., Logani S., Totten K.A., Benigno B.B., McDonald J.F. (2009) Gene expression profiling supports the hypothesis that human ovarian surface epithelia are multipotential and capable of serving as ovarian cancer initiating cells. *BMC Med Genomics,* Vol. 2, pp. 71–85, ISSN 1755-8794.

Brady, N., Gaymes, T.J., Cheung, M., Mufti, G.J., Rassool, F.V. (2003) Increased error-prone NHEJ activity in myeloid leukemias is associated with DNA damage at sites that recruit key nonhomologous end-joining proteins. *Cancer Res,* Vol. 63, No. 8, pp. 1798-1805, ISSN 0008-5472.

Bromleigh, V.C. & Freedman, L.P. (2000) *p21* is a transcriptional target of HOXA10 in differentiating myelomonocytic cells. *Genes Dev,* Vol. 14, No. 20, pp. 2581-2586, ISSN 0890-9369.

Burleson, K.M., Casey, R.C., Skubitz, K.M., Pambuccian, S.E., Oegema, T.R., Skubitz, A.P. (2004) Ovarian carcinoma ascites spheroids adhere to extracellular matrix components and mesothelial cell monolayers. *Gynecol Oncol,* Vol. 93, No. 1, pp. 170–181, ISSN 0090-8258.

Buttiglieri, S., Deregibus, M.C., Bravo, S., Cassoni, P., Chiarle, R., Bussolati, B., Camussi, G. (2004) Role of Pax2 in apoptosis resistance and proinvasive phenotype of Kaposi's sarcoma cells. *J Biol Chem,* Vol. 279, No. 6, pp. 4136–4143, ISSN 0021-9258.

Capecchi, M.R. (1997) *Hox* genes and mammalian development. *Cold Spring Harb Symp Quant Biol,* Vol. 62, pp. 273-281, ISSN 0091-7451.

Caré, A., Silvani, A., Meccia, E., Mattia, G., Stoppacciaro, A., Parmiani, G., Peschle, C., Colombo, M.P. (1996) HOXB7 constitutively activates basic fibroblast growth factor in melanomas. *Mol Cell Biol,* Vol. 16, No. 9, pp. 4842–4851, ISSN 0270-7306.

Caré, A., Silvani, A., Meccia, E., Mattia, G., Peschle, C., Colombo, M.P. (1998) Transduction of the SkBr3 breast carcinoma cell line with the *HOXB7* gene induces bFGF expression, increases cell proliferation and reduces growth factor dependence. *Oncogene,* Vol. 16, No. 25, pp. 3285–3289, ISSN 0950-9232.

Caré, A., Felicetti, F., Meccia, E., Bottero, L., Parenza, M., Stoppacciaro, A., Peschle, C., Colombo, M.P. (2001) HOXB7: a key factor for tumor-associated angiogenic switch. *Cancer Res,* Vol. 61, No. 17, pp. 6532–6539, ISSN 0008-5472

Chang, C.-P., Shen, W-F., Rozenfeld, S., Lawrence, H.J., Largman, C., Cleary, M.L. (1995) Pbx proteins display hexapeptide-dependent cooperative DNA binding with a subset of Hox proteins. *Genes Dev*, Vol. 9, No. 6, pp. 663–674, ISSN 0890-9369.

Chariot, A., Gielen, J., Merville, M.P., Bours, V. (1999) The homeodomain-containing proteins. An update on their interacting partners. *Biochem Pharmacol,* Vol. 58, No. 12, pp. 1851-1857, ISSN 0006-2952.

Chawengsaksophak, K., James, R., Hammond, V.E., Kontgen, F., Beck F. (1997) Homeosis and intestinal tumours in *Cdx2* mutant mice. *Nature,* Vol. 386, No. 6620, pp. 84–87, ISSN 0028-0836.

Cheng, W., Liu, J., Yoshida, H., Rosen, D., Naora, H. (2005) Lineage infidelity of epithelial ovarian cancers is controlled by *HOX* genes that specify regional identity in the reproductive tract. *Nat Med,* Vol. 11, No. 5, pp. 531-537, ISSN 1078-8956.

Chivukula, M., Dabbs, D.J., O'Connor, S., Bhargava, R. (2009) PAX 2: a novel Müllerian marker for serous papillary carcinomas to differentiate from micropapillary breast carcinoma. *Int J Gynecol Pathol,* Vol. 28, No. 6, pp. 570-578, ISSN 0277-1691.

Cho, K.R. & Shih, I.M. (2009) Ovarian cancer. *Annu Rev Pathol,* Vol. 4, pp. 287-313, ISSN 1553-4006.

Christensen, K.L., Patrick, A.N., McCoy, E.L., Ford, H.L. (2008) The *Six* family of homeobox genes in development and cancer. *Adv Cancer Res,* Vol. 101, pp. 93-126, ISSN 0065-230X.

Coletta, R.D., Christensen, K., Reichenberger, K.J., Lamb, J., Micomonaco, D., Huang, L., Wolf, D.M., Müller-Tidow, C., Golub, T.R., Kawakami, K., Ford, H.L. (2004) The Six1 homeoprotein stimulates tumorigenesis by reactivation of cyclin A1. *Proc Natl Acad Sci USA,* Vol. 101, No. 17, pp. 6478-6483, ISSN 0027-8424.

Coletta, R.D., Christensen, K.L., Micalizzi, D.S., Jedlicka, P., Varella-Garcia, M., Ford, H.L. (2008) Six1 overexpression in mammary cells induces genomic instability and is sufficient for malignant transformation. *Cancer Res,* Vol. 68, No. 7, pp. 2204-2213, ISSN 0008-5472.

Connolly, D.C., Bao, R., Nikitin, A.Y., Stephens, K.C., Poole, T.W., Hua, X., Harris, S.S., Vanderhyden, B.C., Hamilton, T.C. (2003) Female mice chimeric for expression of the simian virus 40 TAg under control of the MISIIR promoter develop epithelial ovarian cancer. *Cancer Res,* Vol. 63, No. 6, pp. 1389-1397, ISSN 0008-5472.

Daftary, G.S., Troy, P.J., Bagot, C.N., Young, S.L., Taylor, H.S. (2002) Direct regulation of beta3-integrin subunit gene expression by HOXA10 in endometrial cells. *Mol Endocrinol,* Vol. 16, No. 3, pp. 571-579, ISSN 0888-8809.

De Cecco, L., Marchionni, L., Gariboldi, M., Reid, J.F., Lagonigro, M.S., Caramuta, S., Ferrario, C., Bussani, E., Mezzanzanica, D., Turatti, F., Delia, D., Daidone, M.G., Oggionni, M., Bertuletti, N., Ditto, A., Raspagliesi, F., Pilotti, S., Pierotti, M.A., Canevari, S., Schneider, C. (2004) Gene expression profiling of advanced ovarian cancer: characterization of a molecular signature involving fibroblast growth factor 2. *Oncogene,* Vol. 23, No. 49, pp. 8171-8183, ISSN 0950-9232.

Difilippantonio, M.J., Zhu, J., Chen, H.T., Meffre, E., Nussenzweig, M.C., Max, E.E., Ried, T., Nussenzweig, A. (2000) DNA repair protein Ku80 suppresses chromosomal aberrations and malignant transformation. *Nature,* Vol. 404, No. 6777, pp. 510-514, ISSN 0028-0836.

Dressler, G.R., Deutsch, U., Chowdhury, K., Nornes, H.O., Gruss, P. (1990) *Pax2,* a new murine paired-box-containing gene and its expression in the developing excretory system. *Development,* No. 109, No. 4, pp. 787-795, ISSN 0950-1991.

Dubeau, L. (2008) The cell of origin of ovarian epithelial tumors. *Lancet Oncol,* Vol. 9, No. 12, pp. 1191-1197, ISSN 1470-2045.

Dubnau, J. & Struhl, G. (1996) RNA recognition and translational regulation by a homeodomain protein. *Nature,* Vol. 379, No. 6567, pp. 694-699, ISSN 0028-0836.

Erkanli, A., Taylor, D.D., Dean, D., Eksir, F., Egger, D., Geyer, J., Nelson, B.H., Stone, B., Fritsche, H.A., Roden, R.B. (2006) Application of Bayesian modeling of autologous antibody responses against ovarian tumor-associated antigens to cancer detection. *Cancer Res,* Vol. 66, No. 3, pp. 1792-1798, ISSN 0008-5472.

Feeley, K.M. & Wells, M. (2001) Precursor lesions of ovarian epithelial malignancy. *Histopathology,* Vol. 38, No. 2, pp. 87-95, ISSN 0309-0167.

Feng, X.H., Lin, X., Derynck, R. (2000) Smad2, Smad3 and Smad4 cooperate with Sp1 to induce $p15^{Ink4B}$ transcription in response to TGF-β. *EMBO J,* Vol. 19, No. 19, pp. 5178-5193, ISSN 0261-4189.

Feng, X.H., Liang, Y.Y., Liang, M., Zhai, W., Lin, X. (2002) Direct interaction of c-Myc with Smad2 and Smad3 to inhibit TGF-β-mediated induction of the CDK inhibitor $p15^{Ink4B}$. *Mol Cell,* Vol. 9, No. 1, pp. 133-143, ISSN 1097-2765.

Fischbach, N.A., Rozenfeld, S., Shen, W., Fong, S., Chrobak, D., Ginzinger, D., Kogan, S.C., Radhakrishnan, A., Le Beau, M.M., Largman, C., Lawrence, H.J. (2005) *HOXB6* overexpression in murine bone marrow immortalizes a myelomonocytic precursor *in vitro* and causes hematopoietic stem cell expansion and acute myeloid leukemia *in vivo. Blood,* Vol. 105, No. 4, pp. 1456-1466, ISSN 0006-4971.

Fraggetta, F., Pelosi, G., Cafici, A., Scollo, P., Nuciforo, P., Viale, G. (2003) CDX2 immunoreactivity in primary and metastatic ovarian mucinous tumours. *Virchows Arch,* Vol. 443, No. 6, pp. 782-786, ISSN 0945-6317.

Francis-Thickpenny, K.M., Richardson, D.M., van Ee, C.C., Love, D.R., Winship, I.M., Baguley, B.C., Chenevix-Trench, G., Shelling, A.N. (2001) Analysis of the TGF-β functional pathway in epithelial ovarian carcinoma. *Br J Cancer,* Vol. 85, No. 5, pp. 687-691, ISSN 0007-0920.

Gabra, H., Watson, J.E., Taylor, K.J., Mackay, J., Leonard, R.C., Steel, C.M., Porteous, D.J., Smyth, J.F. (1996) Definition and refinement of a region of loss of heterozygosity at 11q23.3-q24.3 in epithelial ovarian cancer associated with poor prognosis. *Cancer Res,* Vol. 56, No. 5, pp. 950–954, ISSN 0008-5472.

Gartel, A.L., Ye, X., Goufman, E., Shianov, P., Hay, N., Najmabadi, F., Tyner, A.L. (2001) Myc represses the $p21^{WAF1/Cip1}$ promoter and interacts with Sp1/Sp3. *Proc Natl Acad Sci USA,* Vol. 98, No. 8, pp. 4510-4515, ISSN 0027-8424.

Gehring, W.J. & Hiromi, Y. (1986) Homeotic genes and the homeobox. *Annu Rev Genet,* Vol. 20, pp. 147-173, ISSN 0066-4197.

Gehring, W.J., Qian, Y.Q., Billeter, M., Furukubo-Tokunaga, K., Schier, A.F., Resendez-Perez, D., Affolter, M., Otting, G., Wüthrich, K. (1994) Homeodomain-DNA recognition. *Cell,* Vol. 78, No. 2, pp. 211-223, ISSN 0092-8674.

Gnarra, J.R. & Dressler, G.R. (1995) Expression of Pax-2 in human renal cell carcinoma and growth inhibition by antisense oligonucleotides. *Cancer Res,* Vol. 55, No. 18, pp. 4092–4098, ISSN 0008-5472.

Gorski, D.H. & Walsh, K. (2000). The role of homeobox genes in vascular remodeling and angiogenesis. *Circ Res*, Vol. 87, No. 10, pp. 865-872, ISSN 0009-7330.

Groisman, G.M., Meir, A., Sabo, E. (2004) The value of Cdx2 immunostaining in differentiating primary ovarian carcinomas from colonic carcinomas metastatic to the ovaries. *Int J Gynecol Pathol*, Vol. 23, No. 1, pp. 52-57, ISSN 0277-1691.

Gupta, R.A., Shah, N., Wang, K.C., Kim, J., Horlings, H.M., Wong, D.J., Tsai, M.C., Hung, T., Argani, P., Rinn, J.L., Wang, Y., Brzoska, P., Kong, B., Li, R., West, R.B., van de Vijver, M.J., Sukumar, S., Chang, H.Y. (2010) Long non-coding RNA *HOTAIR* reprograms chromatin state to promote cancer metastasis. *Nature*, Vol. 464, No. 7291, pp. 1071-1076, ISSN 0028-0836.

Hahn, S.A., Schutte, M., Hoque, A.T., Moskaluk, C.A., da Costa, L.T., Rozenblum, E., Weinstein, C.L., Fischer, A., Yeo, C.J., Hruban, R.H., Kern, S.E. (1996) *DPC4*, a candidate tumor suppressor at human chromosome 18q21.1. *Science*, Vol. 271, No. 5247, pp. 350-353, ISSN 0036-8075.

Hanahan, D. & Weinberg, R.A. (2000) The hallmarks of cancer. *Cell*, Vol. 100, No. 1, pp. 57-70, ISSN 0092-8674.

Hanahan, D. & Weinberg, R.A. (2011) Hallmarks of cancer: The next generation. *Cell*, Vol. 144, No. 5, pp. 646-674, ISSN 0092-8674.

Hara, F., Samuel, S., Liu, J., Rosen, D., Langley, R.R., Naora, H. (2007) A homeobox gene related to *Drosophila Distal-less* promotes ovarian tumorigenicity by inducing expression of vascular endothelial growth factor and fibroblast growth factor-2. *Am J Pathol*, Vol . 170, No. 5, pp. 1594-1606, ISSN 0002-9440.

He, W.W., Sciavolino, P.J., Wing, J., Augustus, M., Hudson, P., Meissner, P.S., Curtis, R.T., Shell, B.K., Bostwick, D.G., Tindall, D.J., Gelmann, E.P., Abate-Shen, C., Carter, K.C. (1997) A novel human prostate-specific, androgen-regulated homeobox gene (*NKX3.1*) that maps to 8p21, a region frequently deleted in prostate cancer. *Genomics*, Vol. 43, No. 1, pp. 69-77, ISSN 0888-7543.

Helleday, T., Petermann, E., Lundin, C., Hodgson, B., Sharma, R.A. (2008) DNA repair pathways as targets for cancer therapy. *Nat Rev Cancer*, Vol. 8, No. 3, pp. 193-204, ISSN 1474-175X.

Heyman, L., Kellouche, S., Fernandes, J., Dutoit, S., Poulain, L., Carreiras, F. (2008) Vitronectin and its receptors partly mediate adhesion of ovarian cancer cells to peritoneal mesothelium *in vitro*. *Tumor Biol*, Vol. 29, No. 4, pp. 231-244, ISSN 1010-4283.

Hirasawa, A., Saito-Ohara, F., Inoue, J., Aoki, D., Susumu, N., Yokoyama, T., Nozawa, S., Inazawa, J., Imoto, I. (2003) Association of 17q21-q24 gain in ovarian clear cell adenocarcinomas with poor prognosis and identification of *PPM1D* and *APPBP2* as likely amplification targets. *Clin Cancer Res*, Vol. 9, No. 6, pp. 1995-2004, ISSN 1078-0432.

Hollingsworth, H.C., Kohn, E.C., Steinberg, S.M., Rothenberg, M.L., Merino, M.J. (1995) Tumor angiogenesis in advanced stage ovarian carcinoma. *Am J Pathol*, Vol. 147, No. 1, pp. 33-41, ISSN 0002-9440.

Hsieh-Li, H.M., Witte, D.P., Weinstein, M., Branford, W., Li, H., Small, K., Potter, S.S. (1995) *Hoxa 11* structure, extensive antisense transcription, and function in male and female fertility. *Development*, Vol. 121, No. 5, pp. 1373-1385, ISSN 0950-1991.

Hyman, E., Kauraniemi, P., Hautaniemi, S., Wolf, M., Mousses, S., Rozenblum, E., Ringnér, M., Sauter, G., Monni, O., Elkahloun, A., Kallioniemi, O.P., Kallioniemi, A. (2002) Impact of DNA amplification on gene expression patterns in breast cancer. *Cancer Res*, Vol. 62, No. 21, pp. 6240-6245, ISSN 0008-5472.

Imam, J.S., Buddavarapu, K., Lee-Chang, J.S., Ganapathy, S., Camosy, C., Chen, Y., Rao, M.K. (2010) MicroRNA-185 suppresses tumor growth and progression by targeting the *Six1* oncogene in human cancers. *Oncogene*, Vol. 29, No. 35, pp. 4971–4979, ISSN 0950-9232.

James, R., Erler, T., Kazenwadel, J. (1994) Structure of the murine homeobox gene *cdx-2*. Expression in embryonic and adult intestinal epithelium. *J Biol Chem*, Vol. 269, No. 21, pp. 15229–15237, ISSN 0021-9258.

Jarboe E.A., Folkins A.K., Drapkin R., Ince T.A., Agoston E.S., Crum C.P. (2008) Tubal and ovarian pathways to pelvic epithelial cancer: a pathologic perspective. *Histopathology*, Vol. 53, No. 2, pp. 127-138, ISSN 0309-0167.

Kim, M.J., Bhatia-Gaur, R., Banach-Petrosky, W.A., Desai, N., Wang, Y., Hayward, S.W., Cunha, G.R., Cardiff, R.D., Shen, M.M., Abate-Shen, C. (2002a) *Nkx3.1* mutant mice recapitulate early stages of prostate carcinogenesis. *Cancer Res*, Vol. 62, No. 11, pp. 2999-3004, ISSN 0008-5472.

Kim M.J., Cardiff R.D., Desai N., Banach-Petrosky W.A., Parsons R., Shen M.M., Abate-Shen C. (2002b) Cooperativity of *Nkx3.1* and *Pten* loss of function in a mouse model of prostate carcinogenesis. *Proc Natl Acad Sci USA*, Vol. 99, No. 5, pp. 2884–2889, ISSN 0027-8424.

Klausen, C., Leung, P.C., Auersperg, N. (2009) Cell motility and spreading are suppressed by HOXA4 in ovarian cancer cells: possible involvement of beta1 integrin. *Mol Cancer Res*, Vol. 7, No. 9, pp. 1425-1437, ISSN 1541-7786.

Kluk, B.J., Fu, Y., Formolo, T.A., Zhang, L., Hindle, A.K., Man, Y-G., Siegel, R.S., Berg, P.E., Deng, C., McCaffey, T.A., Fu, S.W. (2010). BP1, an isoform of DLX4 homeoprotein, negatively regulates *BRCA1* in sporadic breast cancer. *Int J Biol Sci*, Vol. 6, No. 5, pp. 513-524, ISSN 1449-2288.

Ko, S.Y., Lengyel, E., Naora, H. (2010) The Müllerian *HOXA10* gene promotes growth of ovarian surface epithelial cells by stimulating epithelial-stromal interactions. *Mol Cell Endocrinol*, Vol. 317, No. 1-2, pp. 112-119, ISSN 0303-7207.

Kobayashi, A. & Behringer, R.R. (2003) Developmental genetics of the female reproductive tract in mammals. *Nat Rev Genet*, Vol. 4, No. 12, pp. 969-980, ISSN 1471-0056.

Kozmik, Z., Sure, U., Rüedi, D., Busslinger, M., Aguzzi, A. (1995). Deregulated expression of *PAX5* in medulloblastoma. *Proc Natl Acad Sci USA*, Vol. 92, No. 12, pp. 5709–5713, ISSN 0027-8424.

Kroon, E., Krosl, J., Thorsteinsdottir, U., Baban, S., Buchberg, A.M., Sauvageau, G. (1998) HoxA9 transforms primary bone marrow cells through specific collaboration with Meis1a but not Pbx1b. *EMBO J*, Vol. 17, No. 13, pp. 3714–3725, ISSN 0261-4189.

Laury, A.R., Perets, R., Piao, H., Krane, J.F., Barletta, J.A., French, C., Chirieac, L.R., Lis, R., Loda, M., Hornick, J.L., Drapkin, R., Hirsch, M.S. (2011) A comprehensive analysis of PAX8 expression in human epithelial tumors. *Am J Surg Pathol*, Vol. 35, No. 6, pp. 816-826, ISSN 0147-5185.

Lee, Y., Miron, A., Drapkin, R., Nucci, M.R., Medeiros, F., Saleemuddin, A., Garber, J., Birch, C., Mou, H., Gordon, R.W., Cramer, D.W., McKeon, F.D., Crum, C.P. (2007) A candidate precursor to serous carcinoma that originates in the distal fallopian tube. *J Pathol*, Vol. 211, No. 1, pp. 26-35, ISSN 0022-3417.

Lemons, D. & McGinnis, W. (2006) Genomic evolution of *Hox* gene clusters. *Science*, Vol. 313, No. 5795, pp. 1918-1922, ISSN 0036-8075.

Le Page, C., Ouellet, V., Madore, J., Hudson, T.J., Tonin, P.N., Provencher, D.M., Mes-Masson, A.M. (2006) From gene profiling to diagnostic markers: IL-18 and FGF-2 complement CA125 as serum-based markers in epithelial ovarian cancer. *Int J Cancer*, Vol. 118, No. 7, pp. 1750–1758, ISSN 0020-7136.

Lieber, M.R., Ma, Y., Pannicke, U., Schwarz, K. (2003) Mechanism and regulation of human non-homologous DNA end-joining. *Nat Rev Mol Cell Biol*, Vol. 4, No. 9, pp. 712-720, ISSN 1471-0072.

Ma L., Benson G.V., Lim H., Dey S.K., Maas R.L. (1998) *Abdominal B (AbdB) Hoxa* genes: regulation in adult uterus by estrogen and progesterone and repression in müllerian duct by the synthetic estrogen diethylstilbestrol (DES). *Dev Biol*, Vol. 197, No. 2, pp. 141–154, ISSN 0012-1606.

MacLean, J.A. & Wilkinson, M.F. (2010) The *Rhox* genes. *Reproduction*. 140(2), pp. 195-213, ISSN 1470-1626.

Maines-Bandiera, S.L. & Auersperg, N. (1997) Increased E-cadherin expression in ovarian surface epithelium: an early step in metaplasia and dysplasia? *Int J Gynecol Pathol*, Vol. 16, No. 3, pp. 250-255, ISSN 0277-1691.

Mallo, G.V., Soubeyran, P., Lissitzky, J.C., André, F., Farnarier, C., Marvaldi, J., Dagorn, J.C., Iovanna J.L. (1998) Expression of the *Cdx1* and *Cdx2* homeotic genes leads to reduced malignancy in colon cancer-derived cells. *J Biol Chem*, Vol. 273, No. 22, pp. 14030–14036, ISSN 0021-9258.

Man, Y.G., Fu, S.W., Schwartz, A., Pinzone, J.J., Simmens, S.J., Berg, P.E. (2005) Expression of *BP1*, a novel homeobox gene, correlates with breast cancer progression and invasion. *Breast Cancer Res Treat*, Vol. 90, No. 3, pp. 241-247, ISSN 0167-6806.

Markowitz, S., Wang, J., Myeroff, L., Parsons, R., Sun, L., Lutterbaugh, J., Fan, R.S., Zborowska, E., Kinzler, K.W., Vogelstein, B., Brattain, M., Willson, J.K. (1995) Inactivation of the type II TGF-beta receptor in colon cancer cells with microsatellite instability. *Science*, Vol. 268, No. 5215, pp. 1336-1338, ISSN 0036-8075.

McGinnis, W. & Krumlauf, R. (1992) Homeobox genes and axial patterning. *Cell*, Vol. 68, No. 2, pp. 283-302, ISSN 0092-8674.

McKnight, R., Cohen, C., Siddiqui, M.T. (2010) Utility of paired box gene 8 (PAX8) expression in fluid and fine-needle aspiration cytology: an immunohistochemical study of metastatic ovarian serous carcinoma. *Cancer Cytopathol*, Vol. 118, No. 5, pp. 298-302, ISSN 1934-662X.

Miao, J., Wang, Z., Provencher, H., Muir, B., Dahiya, S., Carney, E., Leong, C.O., Sgroi, D.C., Orsulic, S. (2007) *HOXB13* promotes ovarian cancer progression. *Proc Natl Acad Sci USA*, Vol. 104, No. 43, pp. 17093-17098, ISSN 0027-8424.

Mills, A.A. (2010) Throwing the cancer switch: reciprocal roles of polycomb and trithorax proteins. *Nat Rev Cancer*, Vol. 10, No. 10, pp. 669-682, ISSN 1474-175X.

Mittag, J., Winterhager, E., Bauer, K., Grümmer, R. (2007) Congenital hypothyroid female *Pax8*-deficient mice are infertile despite thyroid hormone replacement therapy. *Endocrinology*, Vol. 148, No. 2, pp. 719–725, ISSN 0013-7227.

Morgan, R., Plowright, L., Harrington, K.J., Michael, A., Pandha, H.S. (2010) Targeting HOX and PBX transcription factors in ovarian cancer. *BMC Cancer,* Vol. 10, No. 1, pp. 89, ISSN 1471-2407.

Mortlock, D.P. & Innis, J.W. (1997) Mutation of *HOXA13* in hand-foot-genital syndrome. *Nat Genet,* Vol. 15, No. 2, pp. 179-180, ISSN 1061-4036.

Muratovska, A., Zhou, C., He, S., Goodyer, P., Eccles, M.R. (2003) Paired-Box genes are frequently expressed in cancer and often required for cancer cell survival. *Oncogene,* Vol. 22, No. 39, pp. 7989–7997, ISSN 0950-9232.

Naora, H. & Montell, D.J. (2005) Ovarian cancer metastasis: Integrating studies from disparate model organisms. *Nat Rev Cancer,* Vol. 5, No. 5, pp. 355-366, ISSN 1474-175X.

Naora, H., Montz, F.J., Chai, C.Y., Roden, R.B. (2001a) Aberrant expression of homeobox gene *HOXA7* is associated with müllerian-like differentiation of epithelial ovarian tumors and the generation of a specific autologous antibody response. *Proc Natl Acad Sci USA,* Vol. 98, No. 26, pp. 15209-15214, ISSN 0027-8424.

Naora, H., Yang, Y.Q., Montz, F.J., Seidman, J.D., Kurman, R.J., Roden, R.B. (2001b) A serologically identified tumor antigen encoded by a homeobox gene promotes growth of ovarian epithelial cells. *Proc Natl Acad Sci USA,* Vol. 98, No. 7, pp. 4060-4065, ISSN 0027-8424.

Naora, H. (2007) The heterogeneity of epithelial ovarian cancers: reconciling old and new paradigms. *Expert Rev Mol Med,* Vol. 9, No. 13, pp. 1-12, ISSN 1462-3994.

Nonaka, D., Chiriboga, L., Soslow, R.A. (2008) Expression of pax8 as a useful marker in distinguishing ovarian carcinomas from mammary carcinomas. *Am J Surg Pathol,* Vol. 32, No. 10, pp. 1566-1571, ISSN 0147-5185.

Novak, P., Jensen, T., Oshiro, M.M., Wozniak, R.J., Nouzova, M., Watts, G.S., Klimecki, W.T., Kim, C., Futscher, B.W. (2006) Epigenetic inactivation of the *HOXA* gene cluster in breast cancer. *Cancer Res,* Vol. 66, No. 22, pp. 10664-10670, ISSN 0008-5472.

Orsulic, S., Li, Y., Soslow, R.A., Vitale-Cross, L.A., Gutkind, J.S., Varmus, H.E. (2002) Induction of ovarian cancer by defined multiple genetic changes in a mouse model system. *Cancer Cell,* Vol. 1, No. 1, pp. 53-62. ISSN 1535-6108.

Panganiban, G. & Rubenstein, J.L. (2002) Developmental functions of the *Distal-less/Dlx* homeobox genes. *Development,* Vol. 129, No. 19, pp. 4371-4386, ISSN 0950-1991.

Park, J., Park, K., Kim, S., Lee, J.H. (2001) *Msx1* gene overexpression induces G1 phase cell arrest in human ovarian cancer cell line OVCAR3. *Biochem Biophys Res Commun,* Vol. 281, No. 5, pp. 1234-1240, ISSN 0006-291X.

Park, G.T. & Morasso, M.I. (2002) Bone morphogenetic protein-2 (BMP-2) transactivates Dlx3 through Smad1 and Smad4: alternative mode for Dlx3 induction in mouse keratinocytes. *Nucl Acids Res,* Vol. 30, No. 2, pp. 515-522, ISSN 0305-1048.

Park, S.Y., Kim, B.H., Kim, J.H., Lee, S., Kang, G.H. (2007) Panels of immunohistochemical markers help determine primary sites of metastatic adenocarcinoma. *Arch Pathol Lab Med,* Vol. 131, No. 10, pp. 1561-1567, ISSN 0003-9985.

Pearson, J.C., Lemons, D., McGinnis, W. (2005) Modulating *Hox* gene functions during animal body patterning. *Nat Rev Genet,* Vol. 6, No. 12, pp. 893-904, ISSN 1471-0056.

Plachov, D., Chowdhury, K., Walther, C., Simon, D., Guenet, J.L., Gruss, P. (1990) *Pax8*, a murine paired box gene expressed in the developing excretory system and thyroid gland. *Development*, Vol. 110, No. 2, pp. 643–651, ISSN 0950-1991.

Prowse, A.H., Manek, S., Varma, R., Liu, J., Godwin, A.K., Maher, E.R., Tomlinson, I.P., Kennedy, S.H. (2006) Molecular genetic evidence that endometriosis is a precursor of ovarian cancer. *Int J Cancer*, Vol. 119, No. 3, pp. 556-562, ISSN 0020-7136.

Rauch, T., Wang, Z., Zhang, X., Zhong, X., Wu, X., Lau, S.K., Kernstine, K.H., Riggs, A.D., Pfeifer, G.P. (2007) Homeobox gene methylation in lung cancer studied by genome-wide analysis with a microarray-based methylated CpG island recovery assay. *Proc Natl Acad Sci USA*, Vol. 104, No. 13, pp. 5527-5532, ISSN 0027-8424.

Rinn, J.L., Kertesz, M., Wang, J.K., Squazzo, S.L., Xu, X., Brugmann, S.A., Goodnough, L.H., Helms, J.A., Farnham, P.J., Segal, E., Chang, H.Y. (2007) Functional demarcation of active and silent chromatin domains in human *HOX* loci by noncoding RNAs. *Cell*, Vol. 129, No. 7, pp. 1311–1323, ISSN 0092-8674.

Robson, E.J., He, S-J., Eccles, M.R. (2006) A panorama of *PAX* genes in cancer and development. *Nat Rev Cancer*, Vol. 6, No. 1, pp. 52-62, ISSN 1474-175X.

Rubin, E., Wu, X., Zhu, T., Cheung, J.C., Chen, H., Lorincz, A, Pandita, R.K., Sharma, G.G., Ha, H.C., Gasson, J., Hanakahi, L.A., Pandita, T.K., Sukumar, S. (2007) A role for the HOXB7 homeodomain protein in DNA repair. *Cancer Res*, Vol. 67, No. 4, pp. 1527-1535, ISSN 0008-5472.

Ruf, R.G., Xu, P.X., Silvius, D., Otto, E.A., Beekmann, F., Muerb, U.T., Kumar, S., Neuhaus, T.J., Kemper, M.J., Raymond, R.M., Brophy, P.D., Berkman, J., Gattas, M., Hyland, V., Ruf, E.M., Schwartz, C., Chang, E.H., Smith, R.J., Stratakis, C.A., Weil, D., Petit, C., Hildebrandt, F. (2004) *SIX1* mutations cause branchio-oto-renal syndrome by disruption of EYA1-SIX1-DNA complexes. *Proc Natl Acad Sci USA*, Vol. 101, No. 21, pp. 8090–8095, ISSN 0027-8424.

Sahin, U., Türeci, O., Schmitt, H., Cochlovius, B., Johannes, T., Schmits, R., Stenner, F., Luo, G., Schobert, I. & Pfreundschuh, M. (1995) Human neoplasms elicit multiple specific immune responses in the autologous host. *Proc Natl Acad Sci USA*, Vol. 92, No. 25, pp. 11810–11813, ISSN 0027-8424.

Samuel, S. & Naora, H. (2005). Homeobox gene expression in cancer: insights from developmental regulation and deregulation. *Eur J Cancer*, Vol. 41, No. 16, pp. 2428-2437, ISSN 0959-8049.

Schneuwly, S., Klemenz, R., Gehring, W.J. (1987). Redesigning the body plan of *Drosophila* by ectopic expression of the homeotic gene *Antennapedia*. *Nature*, Vol. 325, No. 6107, pp. 816-818, ISSN 0028-0836.

Sellar, G.C., Li., L., Watt, K.P., Nelkin, B.D., Rabiasz, G.J., Stronach, E.A., Miller, E.P., Porteous, D.J., Smyth, J.F., Gabra, H. (2001) BARX2 induces cadherin 6 expression and is a functional suppressor of ovarian cancer progression. *Cancer Res*, Vol. 61, No. 19, pp. 6977–6981, ISSN 0008-5472.

Sellar, G.C., Watt, K.P., Li, L., Nelkin, B.D., Rabiasz, G.J., Porteous, D.J., Smyth, J.F, Gabra, H. (2002) The homeobox gene *BARX2* can modulate cisplatin sensitivity in human epithelial ovarian cancer. *Int J Oncol*, Vol. 21, No. 5, pp. 929-933, ISSN 1019-6439.

Shanmugam, K., Green, N.C., Rambaldi, I., Saragovi, H.U., Featherstone, M.S. (1999) PBX and MEIS as non-DNA-binding partners in trimeric complexes with HOX proteins. *Mol Cell Biol*, Vol. 19, No. 11, pp. 7577-7588, ISSN 0270-7306.

Sharma, S.G., Gokden, M., McKenney, J.K., Phan, D.C., Cox, R.M., Kelly, T., Gokden, N. (2010) The utility of PAX-2 and renal cell carcinoma marker immunohistochemistry in distinguishing papillary renal cell carcinoma from nonrenal cell neoplasms with papillary features. *Appl Immunohistochem Mol Morphol,* Vol. 18, No. 6, pp. 494-498, ISSN 1533-4058.

Shimamoto, S., Nakamura, S., Bollekens, J., Ruddle, F.H., Takeshita, K. (1997) Inhibition of *DLX-7* homeobox gene causes decreased expression of *GATA-1* and *c-myc* genes and apoptosis. *Proc Natl Acad Sci USA,* Vol. 94, No. 7, pp. 3245-3249, ISSN 0027-8424.

Siegel, P.M. & Massagué, J. (2003) Cytostatic and apoptotic actions of TGF-β in homeostasis and cancer. *Nat Rev Cancer.* Vol. 3, No. 11, pp. 807-820, ISSN 1474-175X.

Soshnikova, N. & Duboule, D. (2009) Epigenetic regulation of vertebrate *Hox* genes. A dynamic equilibrium. *Epigenetics,* Vol. 4, No. 8, pp. 537-540, ISSN 1559-2294.

Stevenson, H.S., Fu, S.W., Pinzone, J.J., Rheey, J., Simmens, S.J., Berg, P.E. (2007) BP1 transcriptionally activates bcl-2 and inhibits TNFalpha-induced cell death in MCF7 breast cancer cells. *Breast Cancer Res,* Vol. 9, No. 5, pp. R60, ISSN 1465-5411.

Sumiyama, K., Irvine, S.Q., Ruddle, F.H. (2003) The role of gene duplication in the evolution and function of the vertebrate *Dlx/distal-less* bigene clusters. *J Struct Funct Genomics,* Vol. 3, No. 1-4, pp. 151-159, ISSN 1345-711X.

Tacha, D., Zhou, D., Cheng, L. (2011) Expression of PAX8 in normal and neoplastic tissues: A comprehensive immunohistochemical study. *Appl Immunohistochem Mol Morphol,* Vol. 19, No. 4, pp. 293-299, ISSN 1533-4058.

Tan, Y., Cheung, M., Pei, J., Menges, C.W., Godwin, A.K., Testa, J.R. (2010) Upregulation of DLX5 promotes ovarian cancer cell proliferation by enhancing IRS-2-AKT signaling. *Cancer Res,* Vol. 70, No. 22, pp. 9197–9206, ISSN 0008-5472.

Taylor, H.S., Vanden Heuvel, G.B., Igarashi, P. (1997) A conserved *Hox* axis in the mouse and human female reproductive system: late establishment and persistent adult expression of the *Hoxa* cluster genes. *Biol Reprod,* Vol. 57, No. 6, pp. 1338-1345, ISSN 0006-3363.

Thorsteinsdottir, U., Sauvageau, G., Hough, M.R., Dragowska, W., Lansdorp, P.M., Lawrence, H.J., Largman, C., Humphries, R.K. (1997) Overexpression of *HOXA10* in murine hematopoietic cells perturbs both myeloid and lymphoid differentiation and leads to acute myeloid leukemia. *Mol Cell Biol,* Vol. 17, No. 1, pp. 495–505, ISSN 0270-7306.

Tomida, S., Yanagisawa, K., Koshikawa, K., Yatabe, Y., Mitsudomi, T., Osada, H., Takahashi, T. (2007) Identification of a metastasis signature and the DLX4 homeobox protein as a regulator of metastasis by a combined transcriptome approach. *Oncogene,* Vol. 26, No. 1, pp. 4600-4608, ISSN 0950-9232.

Tong, G.X., Chiriboga, L., Hamele-Bena, D., Borczuk, A.C. (2007) Expression of PAX2 in papillary serous carcinoma of the ovary: immunohistochemical evidence of fallopian tube or secondary Müllerian system origin? *Mod Pathol,* Vol. 20, No. 8, pp. 856-863, ISSN 0893-3952.

Tong, G.X., Devaraj, K., Hamele-Bena, D., Yu, W.M., Turk, A., Chen, X., Wright, J.D., Greenebaum, E. (2011) PAX8: A marker for carcinoma of Müllerian origin in serous effusions. *Diagn Cytopathol,* Vol. 39, No. 8, pp. 567-574, ISSN 1097-0339.

Topisirovic, I., Kentsis, A., Perez, J.M., Guzman, M.L., Jordan, C.T., Borden, K.L. (2005) Eukaryotic translation initiation factor 4E activity is modulated by HOXA9 at multiple levels. *Mol Cell Biol,* Vol. 25, No. 3, pp. 1100-1112, ISSN 0270-7306.

Tornillo, L,, Moch, H., Diener, P.A., Lugli, A., Singer, G. (2004) CDX-2 immunostaining in primary and secondary ovarian carcinomas. *J Clin Pathol,* Vol. 57, No. 6, pp. 641-643, ISSN 0021-9746.

Torres, M., Gómez-Pardo, E., Dressler, G.R., Gruss, P. (1995) *Pax-2* controls multiple steps of urogeneital development. *Development,* Vol. 121, No. 12, pp. 4057-4065, ISSN 0950-1991.

Trinh, B.Q., Barengo, N., Naora, H. (2011) Homeodomain protein DLX4 counteracts key transcriptional control mechanisms of the TGF-β cytostatic program and blocks the anti-proliferative effect of TGF- β. *Oncogene,* Vol. 30, No. 24, pp. 2718–2729, ISSN 0950-9232.

Tupler, R., Perini, G., Green, M.R. (2001) Expressing the human genome. *Nature,* Vol. 409, No. 6822, pp. 832-833, ISSN 0028-0836.

Vitiello, D., Kodaman, P.H., Taylor, H.S. (2007) *HOX* genes in implantation. *Semin Reprod Med,* Vol. 25, No. 6, pp. 431-436, ISSN 1526-4564.

Wang, D., Kanuma, T., Mizunuma, H., Takama, F., Ibuki, Y., Wake, N., Mogi, A., Shitara, Y., Takenoshita, S. (2000) Analysis of specific gene mutations in the transforming growth factor-β signal transduction pathway in human ovarian cancer. *Cancer Res,* Vol. 60, No. 16, pp. 4507-4512, ISSN 0008-5472.

Watanabe, T., Imoto, I., Kosugi, Y., Ishiwata, I., Inoue, S., Takayama, M., Sato, A., Inazawa, J. (2001) A novel amplification at 17q21-23 in ovarian cancer cell lines detected by comparative genomic hybridization. *Gynecol Oncol,* Vol. 81, No. 2, pp. 172-177, ISSN 0090-8258.

Werling, R.W., Yaziji, H., Bacchi, C.E., Gown, A.M. (2003) CDX2, a highly sensitive and specific marker of adenocarcinomas of intestinal origin: an immunohistochemical survey of 476 primary and metastatic carcinomas. *Am J Surg Pathol,* Vol. 27, No. 3, pp. 303-310, ISSN 0147-5185.

Widschwendter, M., Apostolidou, S., Jones, A.A., Fourkala, E.O., Arora, R., Pearce, C.L., Frasco, M.A., Ayhan, A., Zikan, M., Cibula, D., Iyibozkurt, C.A., Yavuz, E., Hauser-Kronberger, C., Dubeau, L., Menon, U., Jacobs, I.J. (2009) *HOXA* methylation in normal endometrium from premenopausal women is associated with the presence of ovarian cancer: a proof of principle study. *Int J Cancer,* Vol. 125, No. 9, pp. 2214-2218, ISSN 0020-7136.

Wu, X., Chen, H., Parker, B., Rubin, E., Zhu, T., Lee, J.S., Argani, P., Sukumar, S. (2006) HOXB7, a homeodomain protein, is overexpressed in breast cancer and confers epithelial-mesenchymal transition. *Cancer Res,* Vol. 66, No. 19, pp. 9527-9534, ISSN 0008-5472.

Wu, R., Hendrix-Lucas, N., Kuick, R., Zhai, Y., Schwartz, D.R., Akyol, A., Hanash, S., Misek, D.E., Katabuchi, H., Williams, B.O., Fearon, E.R., Cho, K.R. (2007) Mouse model of human ovarian endometrioid adenocarcinoma based on somatic defects in the Wnt/beta-catenin and PI3K/Pten signaling pathways. *Cancer Cell,* Vol. 11, No. 4, pp. 321-333, ISSN 1535-6108.

Xu, J. & Testa, J.R. (2009) *DLX5* (distal-less homeobox 5) promotes tumor cell proliferation by transcriptionally regulating *MYC*. *J Biol Chem,* Vol. 284, No. 31, pp. 20593–20601, ISSN 0021-9258.

Yamada, S.D., Baldwin, R.L., Karlan, B.Y. (1999) Ovarian carcinoma cell cultures are resistant to TGF-β1-mediated growth inhibition despite expression of functional receptors. *Gynecol Oncol,* Vol. 75, No. 1, pp. 72-77, ISSN 0090-8258.

Yamashita, T., Tazawa, S., Yawei, Z., Katayama, H., Kato, Y., Nishiwaki, K., Yokohama, Y., Ishikawa, M. (2006) Suppression of invasive characteristics by antisense introduction of overexpressed *HOX* genes in ovarian cancer cells. *Int J Oncol,* Vol. 28, No. 4, pp. 931-938, ISSN 1019-6439.

Yekta, S., Tabin, C.J., Bartel, D.P. (2008) MicroRNAs in the *Hox* network: an apparent link to posterior prevalence. *Nat Rev Genet*, Vol. 9, No. 10, pp. 789-796, ISSN 1471-0056.

Yoneda, J., Kuniyasu, H., Crispens, M.A., Price, J.E., Bucana, C.D., Fidler, I.J. (1998) Expression of angiogenesis-related genes and progression of human ovarian carcinomas in nude mice. *J Natl Cancer Inst,* Vol. 90, No. 6, pp. 447-454, ISSN 0027-8874.

Yoshida, H., Broaddus, R., Cheng, W., Xie, S., Naora, H. (2006) Deregulation of the *HOXA10* homeobox gene in endometrial carcinoma: Role in epithelial-mesenchymal transition. *Cancer Res,* Vol. 66, No. 2, pp. 889-897, ISSN 0008-5472.

Yu Y., Khan J., Khanna C., Helman L., Meltzer P.S., Merlino G. (2004) Expression profiling identifies the cytoskeletal organizer ezrin and the developmental homeoprotein Six-1 as key metastatic regulators. *Nat Med,* Vol. 10, No. 2, pp. 175–181, ISSN 1078-8956.

Zhai, Q.J., Ozcan, A., Hamilton, C., Shen, S.S., Coffey, D., Krishnan, B., Truong, L.D. (2010) PAX-2 expression in non-neoplastic, primary neoplastic, and metastatic neoplastic tissue: A comprehensive immunohistochemical study. *Appl Immunohistochem Mol Morphol,* Vol. 18, No. 4, pp. 323-332, ISSN 1533-4058.

Zhai, Y., Iura, A., Yeasmin, S., Wiese, A.B., Wu, R., Feng, Y., Fearon, E.R., Cho, K.R. (2011) *MSX2* is an oncogenic downstream target of activated WNT signaling in ovarian endometrioid adenocarcinoma. *Oncogene,* [Epub ahead of print], ISSN 0950-9232.

Zhang L., Yang N., Garcia J.R., Mohamed A., Benencia F., Rubin S.C., Allman D., Coukos G. (2002) Generation of a syngeneic mouse model to study the effects of vascular endothelial growth factor in ovarian carcinoma. *Am J Pathol,* Vol. 161, No. 6, pp. 2295-2309, ISSN 0002-9440.

Zhang, S., Balch, C., Chan, M.W., Lai, H.C., Matei, D., Schilder, J.M., Yan, P.S., Huang, T.H., Nephew, K.P. (2008) Identification and characterization of ovarian cancer-initiating cells from primary human tumors. *Cancer Res,* Vol. 68, No. 11, pp. 4311-4320, ISSN 0008-5472.

Zhao, Y. & Potter, S. S. (2001) Functional specificity of the *Hoxa13* homeobox. *Development,* Vol. 128, No. 16, pp. 3197–3207, ISSN 0950-1991.

13

Transcriptomic Analysis of Human Ovarian Cancer Cells: Changes Mediated by Luteinizing Hormone Receptor Activation

Juan Cui[1], Ying Xu[1,2,3] and David Puett[1,*]
[1]*Department of Biochemistry and Molecular Biology*
[2]*The Institute of Bioinformatics, University of Georgia, Athens, Georgia,*
[3]*College of Computer Science and Technology, Jilin University, Changchun,*
[1,2]*USA*
[3]*China*

1. Introduction

According to the American Cancer Society (American Cancer Society, 2011), there were approximately 21,880 new cases of ovarian cancer in the US in 2010, representing ~3% of all cases of newly diagnosed cancer. It is estimated that 13,850 women died from the disease in the same year, thus ranking ovarian cancer as the fifth leading cause of cancer death in the US, only behind lung, breast, colorectal, and pancreatic. These five cancers account for over 60% of cancer deaths in the US. The high mortality rate associated with ovarian cancer is attributable largely to its diagnosis at later stages of progression (Choi et al., 2007) when treatment options are limited and often ineffectual. In the early stages of the disease, most patients are asymptomatic or exhibit rather non-specific symptoms or discomfort.

Epidemiological evidence has established that risk factors for ovarian cancer include a family history of ovarian or breast cancer, often arising from mutations in the BRCA1 or the BRCA2 gene, occurrence of breast cancer, again often due to the same mutations, high body weight, and the use of just estrogen without added progesterone for postmenopausal hormone therapy. Some protection appears to arise from oral contraceptives, pregnancy, tubal ligation, and perhaps hysterectomy (American Cancer Society, 2011).

The etiology of ovarian cancer is overall poorly understood. There is, however, a prevailing theory that the pituitary gonadotropins, luteinizing hormone (LH) and follicle-stimulating hormone (FSH), may be contributory to the development or progression of the disease. The gonadotropins are heterodimeric glycoprotein hormones characterized by a common α-subunit and a hormone specific β-subunit. Both LH and FSH have been shown to have numerous effects on cultured ovarian carcinoma cells (Choi et al., 2007; Leung & Choi, 2007; Mandai et al., 2007; Lau et al., 2010). Moreover, the G protein-coupled receptors for LH (LHR) and FSH (FSHR) are expressed in the epithelial cells of the ovary (Choi et al., 2007). In the postmenopausal years, serum concentrations of LH and FSH are high due to the lack of negative feedback to the hypothalamus and pituitary concomitant with cessation of ovarian

*Corresponding Author

function. The structural and functional aspects of gonadotropins and their receptors have been recently reviewed (Ascoli & Puett, 2009).

In contrast to the above suggestion that gonadotropins are involved in the initiation or progression of the disease, there are clinical reports showing very little evidence that the use of gonadotropins to treat infertility increases the risk of ovarian cancer (Mosgaard et al., 1997; Sanner et al., 2009). Considering the available data, including gonadotropin ablation with gonadotropin-releasing hormone (GnRH) analogs, the conclusion was reached that if gonadotropins are involved in ovarian cancer, their role is probably more important in tumorigenesis and early growth, not in later stages (Huhtaniemi, 2010).

In this controversial area surrounding gonadotropins and ovarian cancer, there are a number of mixed, often conflicting, reports on established ovarian cancer cell lines regarding the actions of gonadotropins on cell proliferation, invasion, and migration (Choi et al., 2007). Consequently, a thorough examination of LH action on gene expression may aid in determining if LH contributes to any of the essential components of cancer such as self-sufficiency in growth signals, evasion of apoptosis, bypassing growth inhibitors, sustained angiogenesis, activation of metastasis and invasion, indefinite replication, evasion of immune destruction, and altered metabolism (Hanahan & Weinberg, 2011).

There is also considerable interest in developing diagnostic biomarkers for ovarian and other cancers at early stages. We have explored a novel biomarker-search paradigm through effective combination of computational and experimental techniques to enhance biomarker discovery from the rather low-yield trial-and-error methods in current use. Our paradigm involves analysis of gene expression data for identification of differentially expressed genes in cancer *versus* controls in conjunction with prediction of proteins that can be secreted into blood and then excreted into urine. The results obtained with primary tumor tissues from patients with gastric cancer, the number two cancer killer in the world, have demonstrated the success of this approach (Cui et al., 2008, 2011a; Hong et al., 2011). In addition, considerable effort has also been invested into the use of gene expression profiling techniques by others to elucidate their utility in predicting metastasis and survivability in ovarian cancer (Lancaster et al., 2006; Sabatier et al., 2009).

Herein we focus our discussion on the *in vitro* use of an ovarian carcinoma cell line, SKOV-3 cells (Warrenfeltz et al., 2008; Puett et al., 2010; Cui et al., 2011b,c), rather than tumor tissues, in part because of the desire to work with an established cell line in which continuing studies can be performed in a controlled and reproducible manner. Such cell lines have provided an enormous wealth of information on the characteristics of ovarian cells and their responses to various inhibitors or growth factors (Choi et al., 2007; Leung & Choi, 2007; Mandai et al., 2007). The question being addressed is whether transcriptomic profiling can be used to determine if LH, acting on LHR+ cells, is stimulatory, inhibitory, or has no effect on ovarian carcinoma cells. Hence, the experimental design has been focused on LH-mediated effects on cancer cells, not if LH is involved in the transformation process of an epithelial-to-carcinoma cell. Due to a considerable interest in the development of reliable serum or urine biomarkers for early detection of ovarian cancer, the results of earlier work are also mentioned. This chapter provides a summary of those studies and links them to other related findings.

2. Properties of the SKOV-3 ovarian carcinoma cell line

The SKOV-3 human ovarian cancer cell line was selected since it does not express LHR (Parrott et al., 2001; Mandai et al., 2007; Warrenfeltz et al., 2008) and can serve as a negative control. Some lines do, however, appear to express LHR and respond to LH (Lau et al., 2010). Following transfection with a full-length human LHR-pcDNA3 or an empty vector, two sub-lines were generated, one expressing about 12,000 receptors per cell (LHR+) and the other, i.e. the mock-transfected cells, that does not express LHR (LHR-) (Warrenfeltz et al., 2008).

The LHR+ cells bound radio-labeled human chorionic gonadotropin with a Kd of 0.3 nM in saturation binding assays and an IC50 of 0.8 nM in competition binding assays. The expressed LHR was functional as determined by increased production of cyclic AMP and inositol phosphates in response to LH. The LHR- cells, in contrast, exhibited no specific binding of human chorionic gonadotropin and showed no response to LH in terms of second messengers.

Expression of LHR in the SKOV-3 cells, in the absence of LH, had no effect on cell migration or proliferation. It did, however, reduce the invasive index of the cells by a small margin. LH was found to reduce migration and proliferation of LHR+ cells but not of LHR- cells, while the invasiveness was not altered (Warrenfeltz et al., 2008).

3. The transcriptomic profile of SKOV-3 Cells: Alterations associated with LHR expression and activation

RNA was extracted from SKOV-3 cells (Warrenfeltz et al., 2008), and the resulting cDNAs were analyzed by Almac Diagnostics (Durham, NC, USA) using the Affymetrix Human U133 Plus2 Arrays (Cui et al., 2011c). In a parallel study on microRNA expression, the ovarian cancer DSA™ array (Almac Diagnostics) was used (Cui et al., 2011b). The advantages in using ovarian cancer-specific arrays include the gathering of extensive amounts of novel mRNA data that are not covered by other platforms and putting both microRNA and mRNA probes on the same chips, hence avoiding potential noise introduced during data collection on separate chips. Gene expression profiling was done on both the LHR- and the LHR+ cells, and gene-expression data were also collected on the latter at multiple time points, specifically at 1, 4, 8, and 20 h after incubation with human LH. qRT-PCR was carried out to validate a few significantly altered gene expression patterns detected through microarray data analyses (Cui et al., 2011c).

4. Altered gene expression and pathways associated with LHR expression and activation

Among the ~100,000 transcripts profiled in this study, 2,210 and 4,297 were found to show up-regulation and down-regulation with at least 2-fold changes between the LHR+ SKOV3 cells and the control cells, respectively. Most of these differentially expressed transcripts are involved in cell division and in DNA replication and transcription, while genes primarily involved in carbohydrate transport/metabolism and lipid metabolism, cell communication, and ECM interaction were only down-regulated.

When the cells were exposed to LH, 14,903 transcripts exhibited elevated expression, which extend the above functions to include posttranslational modification, RNA processing and modification, intracellular trafficking and secretion, signal transduction mechanisms, and coenzyme metabolism, while 10,389 transcripts found to be down-regulated were associated with cellular defense mechanisms based on our enrichment analyses against COG functions (Tatusov et al., 2000).

In total, 2,373 genes were differentially expressed in LHR+ cells (in the absence of LH) *versus* control (LHR- cells) or LH-treated LHR+ cells. Of these, 689 genes are cancer relevant and 265 are highly expressed in the ovary (GeneGo, 2000). These genes participate in pathways involved in the cell cycle, focal adhesion, cytokine-cytokine receptor interaction, regulation of the actin cytoskeleton, purine metabolism, and the key signaling pathways involved in cell growth, e.g. MAPK, TGF-β, p53, and Jak-STAT. Functional analysis revealed that five major families, namely growth factors, translation regulators, transporters, GPCRs, and ligand-dependent nuclear receptors, were significantly enriched (Fig. 1).

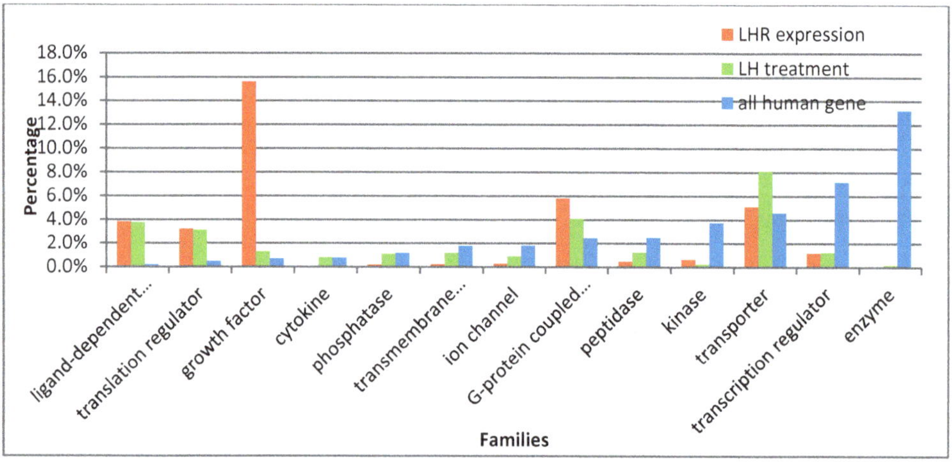

Fig. 1. Distribution of the 2,373 differentially expressed genes in SKOV-3 cells across 13 major functional families. Each red bar represents the percentage of differentially expressed genes associated with LHR expression; each green bar represents the percentage of differentially expressed genes upon incubation with LH; each blue bar is the percentage of all human genes. The y-axis represents the percentage; the x-axis denotes functional families.

Twelve gene clusters, each containing a highly co-expressed pattern, were identified among the 2,373 genes through a clustering analysis, termed a self-organizing map (SOM) (Kohonen 1982) (Table 1). On each gene cluster, Gene Ontology (GO) and pathway enrichment analyses were conducted to identify functional groups and cellular processes that are possibly affected by LHR expression and activation. The details of the findings are discussed elsewhere (Cui et al., 2011c), but the major observations are as follows: LHR expression in control SKOV-3 cells seems to have a positive impact on the activation of gap junctions and the associated growth signaling pathways, and to have moderately suppressed apoptosis, DNA mismatch repair, and the Ras-independent pathways in NK cell-mediated cytotoxicity, which are overall advantageous to cell growth; LH, subsequently, regulated expression of genes involved in the cell cycle, p53 and VEGF signaling, gap junction pathways, immune responses, and the complement and coagulation cascades, as well as a few metabolic pathways (Cui et al., 2011c).

Earlier *in vitro* studies demonstrated that LHR expression, in the absence of LH, slightly inhibited invasiveness, but had no effect on cell proliferation or migration. The addition of LH reduced the growth rate and migratory properties, but was without effect on invasiveness (Warrenfeltz et al., 2008). The current transcriptomic analysis shows that the observed expression changes in the above-mentioned pathways support the previous observations about the measured cellular properties (Warrenfeltz et al., 2008; Cui et al., 2011c).

LHR activated genes		
	Clusters LHR-,LHR+,LH 1-20h (# of genes)	**Enriched GO functions/pathways (P-value)**
LH(↑)	C1 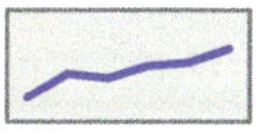 144	extracellular matrix structural constituent 6.54E-04 platelet-derived growth factor alpha-receptor activity 4.38E-03 regulation of vesicle fusion 4.38E-03 hydroxyacid-oxoacid transhydrogenase activity 4.38E-03 pathways: TCR 9.66E-0.2; EGFR1 1.68E-01; IL4 1.79E-01
	C2 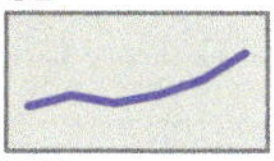 157	negative regulation of apoptosis 3.57E-04 leukocyte differentiation 5.75E-04 carboxylic acid metabolic process 7.47E-04 pathways: EGFR1 2.09E-03; TGFBR 4.94E-03; ID 9.55E-03; Kit Receptor 4.23E-02
	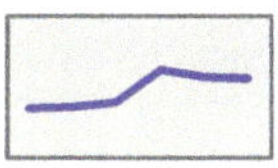 C3 152	multicellular organismal development 3.80E-06 cell proliferation 2.31E-05 cyclic-nucleotide phosphodiesterase activity 2.86E-04 regulation of transcription, DNA-dependent 3.44E-04 cell-cell signaling 4.49E-04 pathways: Hematopoietic cell lineage 1.40E-02
LH(-)	C4 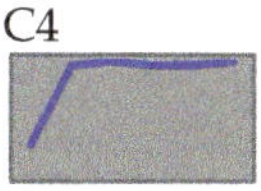 205	nervous system development 7.37E-05 neurogenesis 7.84E-04 notch binding 1.71E-03 calcium ion binding 2.16E-03 cell morphogenesis 4.22E-03 pathways: NOTCH 8.29E-02

LHR activated genes		
	Clusters LHR-,LHR+,LH 1-20h (# of genes)	**Enriched GO functions/pathways (P-value)**
LH(↓)	C5 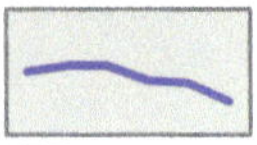 157	response to external stimulus 1.08E-04 positive regulation of cellular metabolic process 1.54E-05 pathways: Androgen Receptor 8.42E-02; EGFR1 2.32E-01
	C6 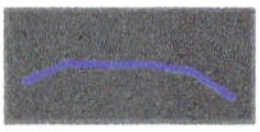 270	cadmium ion binding 1.70E-06 transcription 2.32E-04 spermidine biosynthetic process 5.52E-04 regulation of RNA metabolic process 7.51E-04 pathways: MT-Heavy Metal-Pathway 1.96E-04; TCR 2.71E-02; IL4 6.76E-02; TNF alpha/NF-kB 9.59E-02
	C7 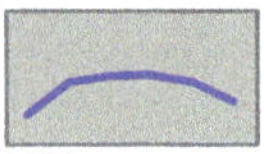 167	neutrophil chemotaxis 5.52E-06 positive regulation of heart rate 2.03E-05 calcium-mediated signaling 6.13E-05 leukocyte chemotaxis 9.57E-05 regulation of cell migration 2.02E-04 pathways: IL-7 9.19E-02; ID 1.60E-01
LHR suppressed genes		
	Clusters	**Enriched GO functions/pathways (P-value)**
LH(↑)	C8 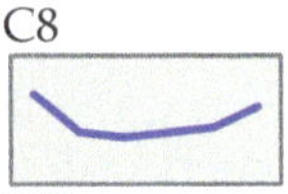 145	extracellular region 6.34E-11 collagen fibril organization 2.68E-05 complement component C3b binding 3.63e-05 fibrillar collagen 4.56E-05 inflammatory response 9.80E-05 response to external stimulus 3.44E-04 protein digestion 3.98E-04 pathways IL-7 2.84e-03; IL3 3.00E-01; Wnt 3.98e-01
	C9 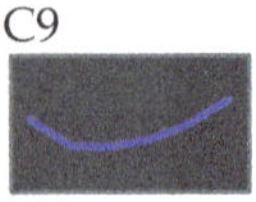 261	alpha-amylase activity 4.37E-11 amylase activity 2.61E-10 calcium ion binding 5.02E-09 homophilic cell adhesion 3.57E-07 synaptogenesis 3.67E-06 pathway: IL-7 1.16E-01; ID 2.00-01; EGFR1 3.90E-01

LHR suppressed genes		
	Clusters	**Enriched GO functions/pathways (P-value)**
LH(-)	C10 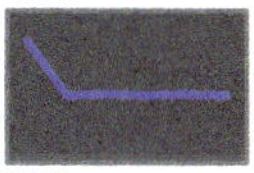 288	proteinaceous extracellular matrix 6.00E-09 polysaccharide binding 3.04e-08 glycosaminoglycan binding 2.22E-06 regulation of defense response 6.56E-06 G-protein signaling, coupled to IP3 second messenger 1.15E-05 enzyme inhibitor activity 3.59E-05 pathways: Wnt 5.23E-02; EGFR1 1.81E-01
LH(↓)	C11 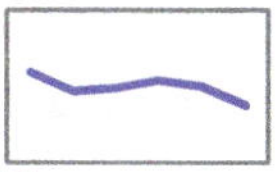 71	regulation of aldosterone metabolic process 9.16E-06 regulation of hormone metabolic process 5.93E-04 auditory receptor cell differentiation 1.36E-03 epidermis development 1.54E-03 growth factor activity 2.44E-03 pathways: NOTCH 1.58E-02; TGFBR 4.74E-02
	C12 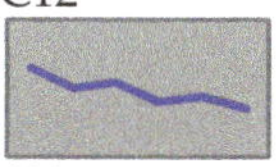 191	cell cycle phase 1.56E-43 mitosis 9.04E43 microtubule cytoskeleton 4.80E-19 pathways: BCR 5.92E-02

Table 1. Enriched GO functions and pathways in each of the 12 gene clusters identified from the differentially expressed genes (modified and extended from Cui et al., 2011c). Plots represent the expression pattern across six groups (LHR- SKOV3 control, LHR expression but with no added LH, and incubation of the LHR+ cells with LH for 1, 4, 8, and 20 h.) "↑" and "↓" denote responses of up-regulation and down-regulation of gene expression, respectively and "-" denotes no alteration of gene expression.

Some of the affected major processes related to cell growth and death (Cui et al., 2011c) have been further investigated. It was found that LHR expression in the control cells led to the up-regulation of genes involved in gap junction, purine metabolism, calcium signaling, and actin cytoskeleton regulation, indicating a possible activation of these processes at a moderate level. In particular, the up-regulation of genes involved in gap junction formation and function may indicate reduced tumor progression and metastasis (Holder et al., 1993).
LH-activated genes are involved in VEGF signaling, the Toll-like receptor signaling, and the B-cell receptor signaling pathway, as well as those involved in gap junction and Notch signaling, which may accelerate cell-cell communication and influence several key aspects of normal cell development by regulating differentiation, proliferation, and apoptosis (Sjolund et al., 2005). One particularly interesting observation was that the substantially increased expression of the tumor necrosis factor member 10 gene (*TNFSF10*), involved in natural killer cell-mediated cytotoxicity, may induce apoptosis (Pan et al., 1997). LH also led to

considerable activation of the genes for interleukin-6 (*IL-6*) and IL-8, pleiotropic cytokines, which are believed to be involved in ovarian carcinogenesis and angiogenesis (Asschert et al., 1999; Schwartz et al., 2001; Chou et al., 2005).

5. Comparative profiling between SKOV-3 cells and normal Human Ovarian Surface Epithelium (HOSE) cells, and molecular markers

The genes most highly expressed (top 5%) in SKOV-3 cells are largely different from those in the normal HOSE cells. It was found that 1,056 such genes were specific to the LHR- SKOV-3 cells, involved in regulation of translation, cell division, chromosome partitioning, post-translational modifications, protein turnover, chaperones, and signal transduction mechanisms, suggesting increased cell growth and proliferation. Another 689 genes were specific to the LH-treated cells and found to be associated with coenzyme metabolism, post-translational modifications, nucleotide transport, DNA replication and repair, intracellular trafficking, and secretion.

Two lists of genes, one with 185 up-regulated genes and the other with 248 down-regulated genes, were identified to show differential expressions between normal and cancer cells regardless of LHR expression or activation (Cui et al., 2011c). Functional analyses revealed that the up-regulated genes are involved in cell-cell communication, ECM-receptor interaction, focal adhesion, cell division and chromosome partitioning, as well as carbohydrate transport and metabolism, which are essential to cancer growth. Of interest, 106 of these genes were found to be specific to ovarian cancer, based on our analyses of their differential expression patterns in ovarian cancer *versus* those of other human diseases with available genome-scale expression data in the public database (http://bioinfosrv1.bmb.uga.edu/DMarker/).

These results engender confidence in proposing some of them as potential molecular markers for ovarian epithelial carcinoma cells *versus* normal HOSE cells. Using a prediction method that we recently developed and validated (Cui et al., 2008), 103 of these genes were predicted to have their protein products secreted into circulation, thus providing another important pool of potential serum markers for ovarian cancer (Cui et al., 2011c).

6. Known therapeutic targets involved in the cellular response to LH action

As of now, 39 genes have been proposed as therapeutic targets for ovarian cancer based on our database search against the Therapeutic Target Database (TTD) (Mandai et al., 2007). Among them, endothelin-1 (ET-1), stromal cell-derived factor 1 (SCD-1), and insulin-like growth factor II (IGF2) show the most significant expression changes associated with LH.

ET-1, acting through its receptor, ETAR, has been extensively studied in its physiological roles in vasoconstriction and proliferation of smooth muscle cells, as well as its pathophysiological role in hypertension, heart failure, and coronary vasospasms. Recently it was also identified as important in ovarian cancer initiation and progression (Bagnato & Rosano, 2008; Bhalla et al., 2009; Rosano et al., 2010). These findings have led to the development of endothelin-converting enzyme-1 inhibitors and small interfering RNAs as new therapeutic agents for ovarian cancer (Rayhman et al., 2008). LH increases gene expression of ET-1 by some 10-fold, peaking at 1 h, an observation documented by qRT-PCR

(Cui et al., 2011c). This observation, along with findings that ET_AR shows a moderate elevation in expression, while endothelin-converting enzyme-1 and the endothelin B receptor show no changes in their expression, may indicate a possible enhancement of cell proliferation in response to LH.

SCD-1 has been reported to increase the invasiveness and migration of breast cancer cells (Kang et al., 2005), and IGF2 is known to be a fetal promoter of cell proliferation in various cancers (Zaina et al., 2002). The up-regulation of these genes may suggest that LH exerts positive effects on tumor growth and metastasis. However, reduced cell growth is manifested in LH-treated cells (Warrenfeltz et al., 2008), and thus expression of the negative regulators, e.g. *c-JUN, TNFSF10,* and *MMPs* (Cui et al., 2011c), must assume a dominant role in relating gene expression and tumor cell properties.

7. MicroRNA regulation involved in LH treatment of LHR+ SKOV3 cells

In addition to the aforementioned ~100,000 protein-encoding transcripts, 132 microRNAs were selectively profiled on the DSA array. It is known that small non-coding RNAs serve in various regulatory roles in degradation of mRNAs and inhibition of translation (Bartel, 2004) in all major cellular processes, such as differentiation, apoptosis, and proliferation (Ambros, 2004; Bartel, 2004). Many microRNAs are androgen related, and their deregulation is highly correlated with initiation, progression, and prognosis of cancer (Calin et al., 2005; Yanaihara et al., 2006; Bloomston et al., 2007; Ambs et al., 2008; Garzon et al., 2008; Schetter et al., 2008; Croce, 2009; Wyman et al., 2009).

Recently, 17 microRNAs were found to be differentially expressed in LHR+ SKOV-3 cells *versus* control cells (Cui et al., 2011b), specifically: six up-regulated (miR-101-1, -101-2, -199b, -559, -573, and -7-3) and 11 down-regulated (miR-103-2, -200c, 151, 29c, 301b, 548a2, 552, 561, 566, 613, and 642). After incubation with LH, 57 microRNAs were found to be differentially expressed, including the most highly-expressed microRNAs, such as miR-21, -200c, -593, -103-1, and -124-3. Some of these microRNAs are located in the fragile sites (also called *hot spots*) in the human genome (Calin et al., 2004; Bignell et al., 2010), where genomic alternations in these regions were found to be associated with certain types of cancer. For example, the loss of 11p15 (covering miR-210) is found in ovarian cancer (Peng et al., 2000), and amplification of 17q23 (covering miR-301a and miR-21) is found in breast cancer (Barlund et al., 2000), as well as those reported (Calin et al., 2002; He et al., 2005).

The present focus is to examine LH-mediated transcriptional changes of the microRNAs, but it should be mentioned that the SKOV-3 cancer cells have probably undergone some genomic alternations, resulting in altered gene expression levels in the control cancer cells that cannot be determined by our current expression data. Collectively, 65 microRNAs have been identified to be differentially expressed in LHR+ SKOV-3 cells *versus* control. The mRNAs with which the microRNA may interact have been studied in order to infer potentially regulated processes involving the microRNAs (Cui et al., 2011b).

Specifically, Spearman correlation analysis was performed between the expression of the 65 differentially-expressed microRNAs and the expression of 60,860 well-annotated mRNAs across all sample groups under consideration, resulting in 62,150 and 931,009 microRNA-mRNA pairs with significantly correlated expressions, positive or negative, using cutoffs $|rho|>0.8$ and P-value <0.05, where rho represents the Spearman correlation coefficient. More positively correlated microRNA-mRNA pairs than negatively correlated pairs were found for the vast majority of the microRNAs, except for nine microRNAs: miR-181B2, miR-

582, miR-497, miR-559, miR-561, miR-101-1, miR-187, miR-572, and miR-301A. The prevalence in positively correlated microRNA-mRNA pairs suggests that such microRNAs are probably located in introns or 5′ untranslated regions of the corresponding mRNAs and hence are regulated by the same transcription regulators of their host genes. The negatively correlated pairs may indicate possible biochemically important interactions.

MiRanda (Miranda et al., 2006) and TargetScan (Lewis et al., 2005) were applied for microRNA target prediction. A total of 584 genes were predicted to interact with the 65 differentially expressed microRNAs. Although not all predicted pairs possess high correlations, it does show a trend that the percentage of predicted pairs decreased as the coefficients increase along its distribution. With the above cutoffs, only 155 genes were retained as highly-confident microRNA targets for further analysis. For each of the 65 microRNAs under consideration, its function was predicted through identification of the functions and pathways enriched by their target genes; the functions of 16 differentially-expressed microRNAs were so predicted (Cui et al., 2011b).

For example, miR-199b-5p is predicted to participate in angiogenesis, nucleotide excision repair, the PDGF signaling pathway, the cadherin/Wnt/integrin signaling pathway, apoptosis, and the MAPK signaling pathway. MiR-101 is predicted to be involved in the Wnt/MAPK/cadherin signaling pathway, as well as in hypertrophic cardiomyopathy, melanogenesis, the metabotropic glutamate receptor group III pathway, and ubiquitin-mediated proteolysis. In addition, it may also be involved in the regulation of the mRNAs involved in cyclic AMP regulation; cyclic AMP-specific phosphodiesterase 4D (*PDE4D*) was highly up-regulated by LH in LHR+ cells (Cui et al., 2011c). MiR-29c is predicted to regulate ECM-receptor interaction, focal adhesion, collagen α chains, and the integrin signaling pathway. It is noteworthy that several of the microRNAs are predicted to be potentially involved in regulation of various tyrosine and serine/threonine kinases (Cui et al., 2011b). The main regulation of miR-129 is that of angiogenesis, the Wnt signaling pathway, transcription regulation, and cell junction. The predicted involvement of miR-199b-5p, miR-101, and miR-129 in the Wnt pathway may suggest its possible role in ovarian tumorigenesis (Gatcliffe et al., 2008).

To affirm that some microRNAs participate in the LH regulation of cancer cells, the experimentally validated targets of the 65 differentially-expressed microRNAs were examined, and 70 such genes were extracted from miRecords (Xiao et al., 2009). Of these, 20 genes are differentially expressed in the LH-treated cells, and some are known to be involved in the regulation of cell migration and proliferation (IRS1, IRS2, IL6R, TPM1, GLI1, BMPR2, GRN), cell surface receptor-linked signal transduction (SOCS5, RAF1), anti-apoptosis (FAS, MCL1, SGK3), and transcription regulation (DNMT3B, GLI1, EZH2) (Cui et al., 2011b). Only six of the 20 genes exhibited highly correlated expression patterns with some of the 65 microRNAs (Cui et al., 2011c), namely IRS1, IRS2, and RAF1 with miR-7-1, SGK3 and MTAP with miR-21, and GRN with miR-659. The expression changes of these genes indicate that LH may impose a positive regulation of cell proliferation, nucleotide metabolic processes, and cell surface receptor-linked signal transduction, and a negative regulation of apoptosis on ovarian cancer cells through these microRNAs.

Additionally, 54 oncogene and tumor-suppressor genes (Jiang et al., 2009; Bignell et al., 2010) were examined to determine if some of the microRNAs may participate in transcriptional regulation (Cui et al., 2011b). It was found that miR-21 was up-regulated while its target, TPM1, a tumor suppressor gene, was down-regulated in response to LH, suggesting a role of miR-21 in inhibiting apoptosis and subsequently having a positive impact of LH on cancer development. However, our other observations such as up-regulation of *NF1*, *RB1*, and *SUFU* may indicate a negative effect on cancer growth, consistent with our previous report (Warrenfeltz et al., 2008).

As important gene regulators, microRNAs exhibit characteristics that allow speculation on some of the key roles they may have in regulating the downstream LHR signaling in ovarian cancer. The indicative clues of regulating apoptosis and cell proliferation may provide useful guidance for further research on the causes and treatment of ovarian cancer. It should be noted from the above analysis that detection of microRNA-mRNA pairs is a key step to understand the functions of microRNAs. All current computational programs used for predicting microRNA/mRNA interactions are mainly based on information embodied in the sequence and structure (Dai & Zhou, 2010). Yet the Argonaute (Ago) proteins have a central role in recognizing and binding to target mRNAs (Wang et al., 2010), and we thus anticipate that a method taking into consideration the sequence or structure information of AGO proteins may efficiently improve the prediction performance.

8. Conclusions

Numerous studies have appeared on the physiological roles and biochemical mechanisms of the pituitary gonadotropins, LH and FSH, in developmental and reproductive processes, as well as the pathophysiology associated with aberrant expression and mutations in the genes encoding the three gonadotropin subunits and the two gonadotropin receptors. Recent experimental findings and epidemiological evidence has arisen suggesting that the hormones and receptors are also involved in the development and/or progression of ovarian cancer. There is, however, much controversy associated with the role(s), if any, of the gonadotropins in ovarian cancer. Research undertaken in our laboratory has focused on experimental measurements of altered cellular properties and transcriptomic profiling of SKOV-3 cells in response to LH, in an effort to clarify aspects of this important area (Warrenfeltz et al., 2008; Puett et al., 2010; Cui et al., 2011a,b,c). This work has established that the expression of many genes and microRNAs is altered by LHR expression in SKOV-3 cells and by activation of the receptor with its natural ligand, LH. Some of the changes involve genes and pathways associated with cell growth, apoptosis, and many more cellular processes. Of interest was the observation that many genes had altered expression patterns upon expression of LHR in the absence of ligand. Such changes presumably arise from ligand-independent actions of LHR and from the unoccupied receptor adopting an active, or active-like, conformation periodically. Incubation of the cells with LH resulted in the expression of myriad genes (over 2,000), many of which are important in biological processes such as proliferation, apoptosis, and others. Further studies on microRNAs identified 65 that exhibited altered expression in LHR+ cells and LHR+ cells incubated with LH. Some of these microRNAs may aid in diminishing cell proliferation and possibly enhancing apoptosis. The conflicting results often obtained with transcriptomic profiling, including evidence for both positive and negative enhancement of important processes such as proliferation, apoptosis, etc., documents the need to always have experimental studies on the cellular phenotype with regard, in the present case, to LHR expression and LH-mediated LHR activation. The net effect, as determined from cell studies is a slight inhibition of proliferation, invasiveness, and migration upon LHR expression and activation. Of potential importance was the observation that some 100 genes were identified that may lead to secreted proteins, thus offering an array of possible serum biomarkers specific for ovarian cancers expressing LHR in the presence of circulating LH, often the case in post-menopausal women.

9. Acknowledgments

This research was supported by NIH (DK033973, DK069711, GM075331) and NSF (DEB-0830024, DBI-0542119). This paper is dedicated to the memory of Stacie Rosenblum who lost her valiant battle with ovarian cancer at a young age.

10. References

Ambros, V. (2004). The Functions of Animal microRNAs, *Nature,* Vol. 431, No. 7006), pp. 350-355.

Ambs, S., Prueitt, R.L., Yi, M., Hudson, R.S., Howe, T.M., Petrocca, F., Wallace, T.A., Liu, C.G., Volinia, S., Calin, G.A., Yfantis, H.G., Stephens, R.M. & Croce, C.M. (2008). Genomic Profiling of microRNA and Messenger RNA Reveals Deregulated microRNA Expression in Prostate Cancer, *Cancer Research,* Vol. 68, No. 15, pp. 6162-6170.

American Cancer Society (2011) http://www.cancer.org.

Ascoli, M. & Puett, D. (2009). The Gonadotropins and Their Receptors, In *Yen and Jaffee`s Reproductive Endocrinology*. Strauss III, J.L. & Barbieri, R. (Editors). Philadelphia, Elsevier Publ. Co., pp. 35-55.

Asschert, J.G., Vellenga, E., Ruiters, M.H. & de Vries, E.G. (1999). Regulation of Spontaneous and TNF/IFN-Induced IL-6 Expression in Two Human Ovarian-carcinoma Cell Lines, *International Journal of Cancer,* Vol. 82, No. 2, pp. 244-249.

Bagnato, A. & Rosano, L. (2008). The Endothelin Axis in Cancer, Int*ernational Journal of Biochemistry and Cell Biology,* Vol. 40, No. 8, pp. 1443-1451.

Barlund, M., Monni, O., Kononen, J., Cornelison, R., Torhorst, J., Sauter, G., Kallioniemi, O.-P. & Kallioniemi, A. (2000). Multiple Genes at 17q23 Undergo Amplification and Overexpression in Breast Cancer, *Cancer Research,* Vol. 60, No. 19, pp. 5340-5344.

Bartel, D.P. (2004). MicroRNAs: Genomics, Biogenesis, Mechanism, and Function, *Cell,* Vol. 116, No. 2, pp. 281-297.

Bhalla, A., Haque, S., Taylor, I., Winslet, M. & Loizidou, M. (2009). Endothelin Receptor Antagonism and Cancer, *European Journal of Clinical Investigation,* Vol. 39, Suppl 2, pp. 74-77.

Bignell, G.R., Greenman, C.D., Davies, H., Butler, A.P., Edkins, S., Andrews, J.M., Buck, G., Chen, L., Beare, D., Latimer, C., Widaa, S., Hinton, J., Fahey, C., Fu, B., Swamy, S., Dalgliesh, G.L., Teh, B.T., Deloukas, P., Yang, F., Campbell, P.J., Futreal, P.A. & Stratton, M.R. (2010). Signatures of Mutation and Selection in the Cancer Genome, *Nature,* Vol. 463, No. 7283, pp. 893-898.

Bloomston, M., Frankel, W.L., Petrocca, F., Volinia, S., Alder, H., Hagan, J.P., Liu, C.G., Bhatt, D., Taccioli, C. & Croce, C.M. (2007). MicroRNA Expression Patterns to Differentiate Pancreatic Adenocarcinoma from Normal Pancreas and Chronic Pancreatitis. *Journal of the American Medical Association,* Vol. 297, No. 17, pp. 1901-1908.

Calin, G.A., Dumitru, C.D., Shimizu, M., Bichi, R., Zupo, S., Noch, E., Aldler, H., Rattan, S., Keating, M., Rai, K., Rassenti, L., Kipps, T., Negrini, M., Bullrich, F. & Croce, C.M.

(2002). Frequent Deletions and Down-Regulation of micro- RNA Genes miR15 and miR16 at 13q14 in Chronic Lymphocytic Leukemia. *Proceedings of the National Academy of Sciences USA*, Vol. 99, No. 24, pp. 15524-15529.

Calin, G.A., Sevignani, C., Dumitru, C.D., Hyslop, T., Noch, E., Yendamuri, S., Shimizu, M., Rattan, S., Bullrich, F., Negrini, M. & Croce, C.M. (2004). Human microRNA Genes are Frequently Located at Fragile Sites and Genomic Regions Involved in Cancers. *Proceedings of the National Academy of Sciences USA*, Vol. 101, No. 9, pp. 2999-3004.

Calin, G.A., Ferracin, M., Cimmino, A., Di Leva, G., Shimizu, M., Wojcik, S.E., Iorio, M.V., Visone, R., Sever, N.I., Fabbri, M., Iuliano, R., Palumbo, T., Pichiorri, F., Roldo, C., Garzon, R., Sevignani, C., Rassenti, L., Alder, H., Volinia, S., Liu, C.G., Kipps, T.J., Negrini, M. & Croce, C.M. (2005). A microRNA Signature Associated with Prognosis and Progression in Chronic Lymphocytic Leukemia. *New England Journal of Medicine*, Vol. 353, No. 17, pp. 1793-1801.

Choi, J.H., Wong, A.S., Huang, H.F. & Leung, P.C. (2007). Gonadotropins and Ovarian Cancer. *Endocrine Reviews*, Vol. 28, No. 4, pp. 440-461.

Chou, C.H., Wei, L.H., Kuo, M.L., Huang, Y.J., Lai, K.P., Chen, C.A. & Hsieh, C.Y. (2005). Up-Regulation of Interleukin-6 in Human Ovarian Cancer Cell via a Gi/PI3K-Akt/NF-kappaB Pathway by Lysophosphatidic Acid, an Ovarian Cancer-Activating Factor. *Carcinogenesis*, Vol. 26, No. 1, pp. 45-52.

Tatusov, R.L., Galperin, M.Y., Natale, D.A. & Koonin, E.V. (2000). The COG Database: A Tool for Genome-Scale Analysis of Protein Functions and Evolution. *Nucleic Acids Research,* Vol. 288, No. 1, pp. 33-36.

Croce, C.M. (2009). Causes and Consequences of microRNA Dysregulation in Cancer. *Nature Review of Genetics*, Vol. 10, No. 10, pp. 704-714.

Cui, J., Liu, Q., Puett, D. & Xu, Y. (2008). Computational Prediction of Human Proteins that can be Secreted into the Bloodstream. *Bioinformatics*, Vol. 24, No. 20, pp. 2370-2375.

Cui, J., Chen, Y., Chou, W.C., Sun, L., Chen, L., Suo, J., Ni, Z., Zhang, M., Kong, X., Hoffman, L.L., Kang, J., Su, Y., Olman, V., Johnson, D., Tench, D.W., Amster, I.J., Orlando, R., Puett, D., Li, F. & Xu, Y. (2011a). An Integrated Transcriptomic and Computational Analysis for Biomarker Identification in Gastric Cancer. *Nucleic Acids Research*, Vol. 39, No. 4, pp. 1197-1207.

Cui, J., Eldredge, J.B., Xu, Y. & Puett, D. (2011b). microRNA Expression and Regulation in Human Ovarian Carcinoma Cells by Luteinizing Hormone. *PLoS One* , Vol. 6, No. 7, e21730.

Cui, J., Miner, B., Eldredge, J.B., Warrenfeltz, S.W., Xu, Y. & Puett, D. (2011c). Gene Expression Profiling of Ovarian Cancer Cells: Alterations by Luteinizing Hormone Receptor Activation. *BMC Cancer*, Vol. 11: 280, pp. 1-16.

Dai, Y. & Zhou, X. (2010). Computational Methods for the Identificaiton of microRNA Targets. *Open Access Bioinformatics*, No. 2, pp. 29-39.

Garzon, R., Volinia, S., Liu, C.G., Fernandez-Cymering, C., Palumbo, T., Pichiorri, F., Fabbri, M., Coombes, K., Alder, H., Nakamura, T., Flomenberg, N., Marcucci, G., Calin, G.A., Kornblau, S.M., Kantarjian, H., Bloomfield, C.D., Andreeff, M. & Croce, C.M. (2008). MicroRNA Signatures Associated with Cytogenetics and Prognosis in Acute Myeloid Leukemia. *Blood*, Vol. 111, No. 6, pp. 3183-3189.

Gatcliffe, T.A., Monk, B.J., Planutis, K. & Holcombe, R.F. (2008). Wnt Signaling in Ovarian Tumorigenesis. *International Journal of Gynecological Cancer*, Vol. 18, No. 5, pp. 954-962.

GeneGo (2000). Ingenuity Pathways Analysis(IPA).

Hanahan, D. & Weinberg, R.A. (2011). The Hallmarks of Cancer: The Next Generation. *Cell*, Vol. 144, No. 5, pp. 646-674.

He, L., Thomson, J.M., Hemann, M.T., Hernando-Monge, E., Mu, D., Goodson, S., Powers, S., Cordon-Cardo, C., Lowe, S.W., Hannon, G.J. & Hammond, S.M. (2005). A microRNA Polycistron as a Potential Human Oncogene. *Nature*, Vol. 435, No. 7043, pp. 828-833.

Holder, J.W., Elmore, E. & Barrett, J.C. (1993). Gap Junction Function and Cancer. *Cancer Research*, Vol. 53, No. 15, pp. 3475-3485.

Hong, C.S., Cui, J., Ni, Z., Su, Y., Puett, D., Li, F. & Xu, Y. (2011). A Computational Method for Prediction of Excretory Proteins and Application to Identification of Gastric Cancer Markers in Urine. *PLoS One*, Vol. 6, No. 2, e16875.

Huhtaniemi, I. (2010). Are Gonadotrophins Tumorigenic--A Critical Review of Clinical and Experimental Data. *Molecular and Cellular Endocrinology*, Vol. 329, Nos. 1-2, pp. 56-61.

Jiang, Q., Wang, Y., Hao, Y., Juan, L., Teng, M., Zhang, X., Li, M., Wang, G. & Liu, Y. (2009). miR2Disease: A Manually Curated Database for microRNA Deregulation in Human Disease. *Nucleic Acids Research*, Vol. 37 (Database issue): D98-104.

Kang, H., Watkins, G., Parr, C., Douglas-Jones, A., Mansel, R.E. & Jiang, W.G. (2005). Stromal Cell Derived Factor-1: Its Influence on Invasiveness and Migration of Breast Cancer Cells in vitro, and Its Association with Prognosis and Survival in Human Breast Cancer. *Breast Cancer Research*, Vol. 7, No. 4, pp. R402-410.

Kohonen, T. (1982). Self-organized Formation of Topologically Correct Feature Maps. *Biological Cybernetics*, Vol. 43, pp. 59-69.

Lancaster, J.M., Dressman, H.K., Clarke, J.P., Sayer, R.A., Martino, M.A., Cragun, J.M., Henriott, A.H., Gray, J., Sutphen, R., Elahi, A., Whitaker, R.S., West,M., Marks, J.R., Nevins, J.R. & Berchuck, A. (2006). Identification of Genes Associated with Ovarian Cancer Metastasis Using Microarray Expression Analysis. *International Journal of Gynecological Cancer*, Vol. 16, No. 5, pp. 1733-1745.

Lau, M.T., Wong, A.S. & Leung, P.C. (2010). Gonadotropins Induce Tumor Cell Migration and Invasion by Increasing Cyclooxygenases Expression and Prostaglandin E(2) Production in Human Ovarian Cancer Cells. *Endocrinology*, Vol. 151, No. 7, pp. 2985-2993.

Leung, P.C. & Choi, J.H. (2007). Endocrine Signaling in Ovarian Surface Epithelium and Cancer. *Human Reproduction Update*, Vol. 13, No. 2, pp. 143-162.

Lewis, B.P., Burge, C.B. & Bartel, D.P. (2005). Conserved Seed Pairing, Often Flanked by Adenosines, Indicates that Thousands of Human Genes are microRNA Targets. *Cell*, Vol. 120, No. 1, pp. 15-20.

Mandai, M., Konishi, I., Kuroda, H. & Fujii, S. (2007). LH/hCG Action and Development of Ovarian Cancer--A Short Review on Biological and Clinical/Epidemiological Aspects. *Molecular and Cellular Endocrinology*, Vol. 269, Nos. 1-2, pp. 61-64.

Miranda, K.C., Huynh, T., Tay, Y., Ang, Y.S., Tam, W.L., Thomson, A.M., Lim, B. & Rigoutsos, I. (2006). A Pattern-Based Method for the Identification of microRNA

Binding Sites and Their Corresponding Heteroduplexes. *Cell*, Vol. 126, No. 6, pp. 1203-1217.

Mosgaard, B.J., Lidegaard, O., Kjaer, S.K., Schou, G. & Andersen, A.N. (1997). Infertility, Fertility Drugs, and Invasive Ovarian Cancer: A Case-control Study. *Fertility and Sterility*, Vol. 67, No. 6, pp. 1005-1012.

Pan, G., Ni, J., Wei, Y.F., Yu, G., Gentz, R. & Dixit, V.M. (1997). An Antagonist Decoy Receptor and a Death Domain-Containing Receptor for TRAIL. *Science*, Vol. 277, No. 5327, pp. 815-818.

Parrott, J.A., Doraiswamy, V., Kim, G., Mosher, R. & Skinner, M.K. (2001). Expression and Actions of Both the Follicle Stimulating Hormone Receptor and the Luteinizing Hormone Receptor in Normal Ovarian Surface Epithelium and Ovarian Cancer. *Molecular and Cellular Endocrinology*, Vol. 172, Nos. 1-2, pp. 213-222.

Peng, H., Xu, F., Pershad, R., Hunt, K.K., Frazier, M.L., Berchuck, A., Gray, J.W., Hogg, D., Bast, Jr., R.C. & Yu, Y. (2000). ARHI is the Center of Allelic Deletion on Chromosome 1p31 in Ovarian and Breast Cancers. *International Journal of Cancer*, Vol. 86, No. 5, pp. 690-694.

Puett, D., Angelova, K., da Costa, M.R., Warrenfeltz, S.W. & Fanelli, F. (2010). The Luteinizing Hormone Receptor: Insights into Structure-Function Relationships and Hormone-Receptor-Mediated Changes in Gene Expression in Ovarian Cancer Cells. *Molecular and Cellular Endocrinology*, Vol. 329, Nos. 1-2, pp. 47-55.

Rayhman, O., Klipper, E., Muller, L., Davidson, B., Reich, R. & Meidan, R. (2008). Small Interfering RNA Molecules Targeting Endothelin-Converting Enzyme-1 Inhibit Endothelin-1 Synthesis and the Invasive Phenotype of Ovarian Carcinoma Cells. *Cancer Research*, Vol. 68, No. 22, pp. 9265-9273.

Rosano, L., Spinella, F. & Bagnato, A. (2010). The Importance of Endothelin Axis in Initiation, Progression, and Therapy of Ovarian Cancer. *American Journal of Physiology: Regulatory, Integrative, and Comparative Physiology*, Vol. 299, No. 2, pp. R395-404.

Sabatier, R., Finetti, P., Cervera, N., Birnbaum, D. & Bertucci, F. (2009). Gene Expression Profiling and Prediction of Clinical Outcome in Ovarian Cancer. *Critical Reviews in Oncology and Hematology*, Vol. 72, No. 2, pp. 98-109.

Sanner, K., Conner, P., Bergfeldt, K., Dickman, P., Sundfeldt, K., Bergh, T., Hagenfeldt, K., Janson, P.O., Nilsson, S. & Persson, I. (2009). Ovarian Epithelial Neoplasia after Hormonal Infertility Treatment: Long-Term Follow-Up of a Historical Cohort in Sweden. *Fertility and Sterility*, Vol. 91, No. 4, pp. 1152-1158.

Schetter, A.J., Leung, S.Y., Sohn, J.J., Zanetti, K.A., Bowman, E.D., Yanaihara, N., Yuen, S.T., Chan, T.L., Kwong, D.L., Au, G.K., Liu, C.G., Calin, G.A., Croce, C.M. & Harris, C.C. (2008). microRNA Expression Profiles Associated with Prognosis and Therapeutic Outcome in Colon Adenocarcinoma. *Journal of the American Medical Association*, Vol. 299, No. 4, pp. 425-436.

Schwartz, B.M., Hong, G., Morrison, B.H., Wu, W., Baudhuin, L.M., Xiao, Y.J., Mok, S.C. & Xu, Y. (2001). Lysophospholipids Increase Interleukin-8 Expression in Ovarian Cancer Cells. *Gynecological Oncology*, Vol. 81, No. 2, pp. 291-300.

Sjolund, J., Manetopoulos, C., Stockhausen, M.T. & Axelson, H. (2005). The Notch Pathway in Cancer: Differentiation Gone Awry. *European Journal of Cancer*, Vol. 41, No. 17, pp. 2620-2629.

Wang, Y., Li, Y., Ma, Z., Yang, W. & Ai, C. (2010). Mechanism of microRNA-Target Interaction: Molecular Dynamics Simulations and Thermodynamics Analysis. *PLoS Computational Biology*, Vol. 6, No. 7: e1000866.

Warrenfeltz, S.W., Lott, S.A., Palmer, T.M., Gray, J.C. & Puett, D. (2008). Luteinizing Hormone-Induced Up-Regulation of ErbB-2 is Insufficient Stimulant of Growth and Invasion in Ovarian Cancer Cells. *Molecular Cancer Research*, Vol. 6, No. 11, pp. 1775-1785.

Wyman, S.K., Parkin, R.K., Mitchell, P.S., Fritz, B.R., O'Briant, K., Godwin, A.K., Urban, N., Drescher, C.W., Knudsen, B.S. & Tewari, M. (2009). Repertoire of microRNAs in Epithelial Ovarian Cancer as Determined by Next Generation Sequencing of Small RNA cDNA Libraries. *PLoS One*, Vol. 4, No. 4: e5311.

Xiao, F., Zuo, Z., Cai, G., Kang, S., Gao, X. & Li, T. (2009). miRecords: An Integrated Resource for microRNA-Target Interactions. *Nucleic Acids Research*, Vol. 37 (Database issue), pp. D105-110.

Yanaihara, N., Caplen, N., Bowman, E., Seike, M., Kumamoto, K., Yi, M., Stephens, R.M., Okamoto, A., Yokota, J., Tanaka, T., Calin, G.A., Liu, C.G., Croce, C.M. & Harris, C.C. (2006). Unique microRNA Molecular Profiles in Lung Cancer Diagnosis and Prognosis. *Cancer Cell*, Vol. 9, No. 3, pp. 189-198.

Zaina, S., Pettersson, L., Ahren, B., Branen, L., Hassan, A.B., Lindholm, M., Mattsson, R., Thyberg, J. & Nilsson, J. (2002). Insulin-Like Growth Factor II Plays a Central Role in Atherosclerosis in a Mouse Model. *Journal of Biological Chemistry*, Vol. 277, No. 6, pp. 4505-4511.

14

Ectoenzymes in Epithelial Ovarian Carcinoma: Potential Diagnostic Markers and Therapeutic Targets

Nicola Lo Buono, Simona Morone, Rossella Parrotta, Alice Giacomino, Erika Ortolan and Ada Funaro
Department of Genetics, Biology and Biochemistry, University of Torino Medical School, Torino Italy

1. Introduction

Ovarian cancer is one of the most lethal among the gynaecological malignancies, affecting 1-2% of women in developed countries (Cannistra, 2004). The lethality of ovarian cancer is primarily attributable to our current inability to detect the disease at an early stage, when it is still limited to the ovary. Therefore, the majority of patients are diagnosed when they have advanced-stage disease. Despite progresses in cytotoxic therapies, only 30% of patients with advanced-stage ovarian cancer survive 5 years after diagnosis. The insidious nature of ovarian cancer stems from its unique biological behaviour: ovarian carcinoma can spread by direct extension to adjacent organs, and exfoliated tumour cells can be transported in peritoneal fluid (Naora et al., 2005). Subsequent implants are characterised by their adhesion to mesothelial cells, migration throughout and invasion of the tumor cells into the omentum and peritoneum. This seeding of the peritoneal cavity is frequently associated with ascites formation. Only secondarily and rather late during the disease progression, are pelvic and para-aortic lymph nodes involved. However, the local peritoneal disease cannot be controlled and remains a factor leading to death (Feki et al., 2009). The cellular processes that lead to local and distant dissemination of ovarian cancer are not fully understood, and the mechanisms of interaction between cancer cells and mesothelium need to be further elucidated to achieve novel information on the biology of this highly aggressive form of cancer and possibly, to identify new potential targets for selective therapeutic strategies.
The combined effort of clinicians and researchers has led to the identification of a number of molecules that might facilitate screening, diagnosis, prognosis and monitoring response to treatment or relapse during follow-up. These new molecules might provide specific targets for anti-tumour therapy with antibody-directed treatments, gene therapy or specific inhibitory molecules. An unexpectedly high number of these newly identified molecules have turned out to be cell surface-expressed ectoenzymes. Ectoenzymes are a large, heterogeneous class of membrane proteins whose catalytically active sites face the extracellular environment. The products of their catalytic activities can influence the extracellular environment (for example, several of these products can function as second messengers or regulate the recruitment of cells). Moreover, many ectoenzymes can function

both as receptors and signalling molecules through mechanisms that are independent from their catalytic activity. The nomenclature of ectoenzymes is confusing: in addition to several original descriptive names, many of them also have a cluster designation (CD) given by immunologists and an EC number assigned by biochemists.
This chapter presents an overview of the ectoenzymes involved in ovarian cancer biology, development or progression (focusing on CD10, CD13, CD26, CD73, CD157, and Autotaxin/CD203c) and highlights the potential role of these molecules as markers for ovarian cancer outcome or as novel therapeutic targets.

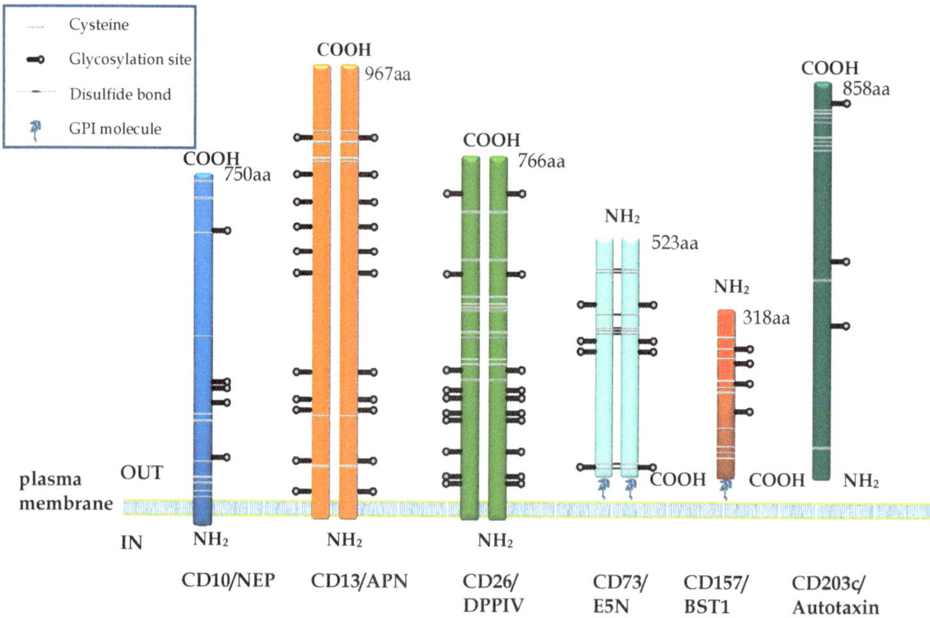

Fig. 1. Schematic representation of ectoenzymes involved in ovarian cancer progression.

2. CD10

2.1 Structure and expression

Human CD10 (also known as CALLA, NEP, Neprilysin, EC 3.4.24.11) is a 100 kDa cell surface aminopeptidase originally characterised as a T cell differentiation antigen (Common Acute Lymphoblastic Leukaemia Antigen, CALLA) identified for its expression in most acute lymphoblastic leukaemias (Shipp et al., 1989). Subsequently, its identity with neutral endopeptidase 24.11 (NEP) and KII-NA was unequivocally established and a wider distribution attributed to the protein (Shipp et al., 1993).
The CALLA/NEP gene spans more than 80 kilobases (kb) on chromosome 3q21-q27 and is composed of 24 exons (D'Adamio et al., 1989). CD10 is a 749-amino acid type II integral membrane glycoprotein with a single 24-amino acid hydrophobic segment that can function both as a transmembrane region and a signal peptide. The COOH-terminal is composed of 700-amino acids and forms the extracellular protein fragment, whereas the 25 amino-

terminal amino acids form the cytoplasmic tail (Ritz et al., 1980). CD10 is expressed by human lymphoblastic leukaemia cells, by early lymphoid progenitors (Greaves et al., 1983; Hoffmann-Fezer et al., 1982) and by other lymphoid malignancies (Greaves, et al., 1983). It is also expressed in terminally differentiated granulocytes and in non-lymphoid cells, including cultured fibroblasts and bone marrow stromal cells, implying that its biological function is not restricted to lymphoid development (Pesando et al., 1983). CD10 expression has been reported on epithelial cells of various tissues, such as bronchial epithelial cells, renal proximal tubular epithelial cells, small intestinal epithelium, biliary canaliculae (Loke et al., 1990), breast myoepithelium (O'Hare et al., 1991), prostate, endometrium (Suzuki et al., 2001) and placenta (Ino et al., 2000). Several reports have shown that CD10 is also expressed in selected solid tumours of the colon (Fujimoto et al., 2005), lung (Cohen et al., 1996), breast (Burns et al., 1999), prostate (Dai et al., 2001) and ovary (Khin et al., 2003).

2.2 Functions

CD10 is a cell membrane-associated zinc metalloproteinase that cleaves peptide bonds on the amino-terminal side of hydrophobic amino acids and inactivates a variety of peptides, cytokines and hormones (Shipp et al., 1988). CD10 plays an important role in the maintenance of homeostasis in normal tissues by degrading endothelin-1 (ET-1), enkephalin, oxytocin, neurotensin, bradykinin, bombesin-like peptides, and angiotensin I and II, among others (Erdos et al., 1989). In specific contexts, CD10 works in concert with CD13, BP-1 and CD26 to digest common substrates (Bowes et al., 1987). This enzyme network controls the local concentrations of these substrates, thus regulating their biological activities and the downstream signal transduction pathways (Shipp & Look, 1993).

CD10 has been implicated in a variety of processes including stromal cell-dependent B lymphopoiesis (Salles et al., 1992), chemotactic and inflammatory responses (Madara et al., 1993), and T cell activation (Massaia et al., 1988). Apart from the hematopoietic compartment, CD10 participates in the final stage of peptide hydrolysis in the renal proximal tubules and the small intestine.

Several reports showed that CD10 plays a role in neoplastic transformation and tumour progression in selected human malignancies by inactivating ET-1 or bombesin, both involved in autocrine/paracrine stimulation of tumour cell proliferation and migration in many epithelial cancers, including breast (Burns, et al., 1999), lung (Cohen, et al., 1996) and prostate cancers (Dai, et al., 2001).

CD10 is expressed in the stroma of malignant ovarian carcinomas, but not in benign adenomas or in normal ovaries, and its expression inversely correlates with histologic tumour grade (Khin, et al., 2003). In ovarian carcinoma, ET-1 promotes cell growth, invasion and angiogenesis by acting as an autocrine/paracrine growth factor (Bagnato et al., 1999; Salani et al., 2000). CD10 may directly influence the local concentration of ET-1 via its enzymatic activity thus contrasting the mitogenic effects of ET-1, suggesting that CD10 plays a role in the biology of neoplastic transformation or in the control of ovarian cancer progression (Kajiyama et al., 2005). It has been suggested that CD10 may function as a tumour suppressor factor in ovarian cancer progression, as well as in lung and prostate cancer (Papandreou et al., 1998).

In addition to its role in the control of ovarian carcinoma progression, Kajiyama et al. (Kajiyama, et al., 2005) demonstrated that CD10 enhances susceptibility to paclitaxel in the SKOV3 ovarian carcinoma cell line, resulting in increased apoptosis and reduced tumour formation and invasiveness in *in vivo* models. This evidence suggests that CD10 might serve as a potential target for gene therapy in metastatic ovarian carcinoma. However, no experimental data in this regard is so far available, and this aspect deserves further investigation.

3. CD13

3.1 Structure and expression

Human CD13 was isolated in 1963 from pig kidney (Pfleiderer et al., 1963) and is a transmembrane protein also known as aminopeptidase N (APN), alanine aminopeptidase, microsomal aminopeptidase, amino oligopeptidase, GP150. CD13 cleaves N-terminal neutral amino acids of a number of peptides and proteins. The CD13 gene is located on the long arm of chromosome 15 and the coding sequence spans 20 exons (Lerche et al., 1996). CD13 consists of 967 amino acids constituting a short N-terminal cytoplasmic domain, a single transmembrane fragment and a large ectodomain encompassing the active site (Olsen et al., 1988).

The CD13 protein is predominantly expressed in stem cells and cells of the granulocytic and monocytic lineages at discrete stages of differentiation (Razak et al., 1992). Non-hematopoietic cells, such as renal proximal tubular epithelial cells, small intestinal epithelium, biliary canaliculae, bone marrow stromal cells, fibroblasts and osteoclasts are also CD13-positive (Metzgar et al., 1981; Noren, 1986). Deregulated expression of membrane and/or soluble forms of CD13 has been observed in many diseases. For example, CD13 is overexpressed in acute and chronic myeloid leukaemias (Antczak et al., 2001) and in anaplastic large cell lymphomas (Dunphy et al., 2000). High expression of CD13 has been detected in various solid tumours such as melanoma (Fujii et al., 1995), renal (Kitamura et al., 1990), pancreas (Ikeda et al., 2003), colon (Hashida et al., 2002), prostate (Ishii et al., 2001a), gastric (Carl-McGrath et al., 2004), thyroid (Kehlen et al., 2003) and ovarian cancers (Yamashita et al., 2007). In ovarian cancer CD13 expression is associated with the histological subtype: over 80% of serous and mucinous carcinomas but only 20% of clear cell carcinomas are CD13-positive (van Hensbergen et al., 2004). Moreover, CD13 also exists as a soluble form, likely originating from shedding of the membrane protein, which has a potent enzymatic activity in the plasma and reactive effusions of cancer patients, such as ascites from ovarian cancer patients (van Hensbergen et al., 2002).

3.2 Functions

CD13 is a multifunctional protein acting as an enzyme, a receptor and a signalling molecule. As an enzyme, CD13 regulates the activity of numerous peptides involved in important biological processes by removing their N-terminal aminoacids, mainly neutral aminoacids (Noren, 1986). CD13 hydrolyses the N-terminal Arg of angiotensin III to generate angiotensin IV (Danziger, 2008) and participates in the metabolism of glutathione, somatostatin, thymopentin, neurokinin A, splenopentin, nociceptin FQ and peptides derived from the thrombin receptor (Noble et al., 1997). In the intestinal brush border, the CD13 enzymatic domain faces the lumen and has been supposed to play an important role in the final stages of the digestion of small peptides (Semenza, 1986). CD13 has been postulated to cooperate with CD10 in the hydrolysis of oligopeptides in the small intestine (Semenza, 1986), and to inactivate opioid peptides and enkephalins in the brain (Matsas et al., 1985) and the chemotactic peptide Met-Leu-Phe during neutrophil-mediated inflammatory responses (Connelly et al., 1985).

CD13 also acts as a receptor for coronaviruses, which exploit the endocytosis of the molecule to enter into respiratory and intestinal epithelial cells (Nomura et al., 2004). Moreover, CD13 is involved in transduction of intracellular signals, converging on mitogen-activated protein kinases, such as ERK1/2, JNK, and p38, in association with auxiliary proteins such as galectin-3 (Santos et al., 2000), galectin-4 (Danielsen et al., 1997), RECK (Miki et al., 2007) and the tumour-associated antigen L6 (Chang et al., 2005).

CD13 activates or inactivates bioactive peptides on the cell surface, thus regulating their activities on adjacent cells. CD13 has a wide range of functions, including a role in antigen presentation by processing antigenic peptides protruding from MHC class II molecules (Larsen et al., 1996), in phagocytosis (Mina-Osorio et al., 2005), in lymphocyte and monocyte adhesion and aggregation (Mina-Osorio et al., 2006) and intracellular signal transduction (Santos, et al., 2000), in stem cell differentiation (Chen et al., 2007), cholesterol uptake (Knopfel et al., 2007) and spermatozoid motility (Carlsson et al., 2006).

Several studies have confirmed a correlation between CD13 expression and increased malignant behaviour in melanoma (Carlsson, et al., 2006), prostate (Ishii, et al., 2001a), colon (Hashida, et al., 2002) and lung cancers (Chang, et al., 2005). In these tumours it is implicated in cell motility and in the degradation of and invasion through the extracellular matrix (ECM) (Saiki et al., 1993). By contrast, an inverse correlation has been reported between CD13 expression and tumour progression in renal cancer (Ishii et al., 2001b).

Several studies have demonstrated that CD13 expression is induced in tumour microvascular endothelial cell by angiogenic cytokines and hypoxia and that it regulates endothelial cell tube formation both in *in vitro* (Hashida, et al., 2002) and in *in vivo* models (Bhagwat et al., 2001).

Functional studies indicate that CD13 expression is associated with a long spindle fibroblast-like morphology and a migratory phenotype accompanied by enhanced secretion of MMP-2 in various ovarian cancer cell lines (Terauchi et al., 2007). Since CD13 is involved in cell motility, in the invasive potential of tumour cells and in the neoangiogenic processes, it holds promise as a therapeutic tumour target. In ovarian cancer it has been demonstrated that suppression of CD13 activity by specific inhibitors (including blocking antibodies, bestatin or actinonin) reduces the proliferative, migratory and angiogenic potential of tumour cells, as well as the peritoneal dissemination *in vivo* in mouse models, leading to prolonged survival (Terauchi, et al., 2007). It has also been determined that CD13 is involved in the chemosensivity and radiosensitivity of ovarian cancer cells. Indeed, combined treatment of tumour cells with bestatin and paclitaxel showed a significant increase in apoptosis and an improved outcome of ovarian cancer patients (Yamashita, et al., 2007).

Taken together, the results from these studies suggest that inhibition of CD13 enzymatic activity may provide a new approach for improving the efficacy of ovarian carcinoma therapy, leading to reduced cell proliferation, motility, invasiveness, angiogenesis and chemoresistance of ovarian cancer cells.

4. CD26

4.1 Structure and expression

CD26, also known as dipeptidyl peptidase IV (DPPIV), adenosine deaminase binding protein (ADAbp) or EC 3.4.14.5, is a multifunctional type II cell surface glycoprotein. CD26 is a 110 kDa aminopeptidase that is catalytically active only as a dimer. Each monomer consists of two domains, an α/β-hydrolase domain (residues 39–51 and 501–766) and an eight-blade β-propeller domain (residues 59–497), that enclose a large cavity of ~ 30–45A° in diameter. Access to this cavity is provided by a large side opening of ~15A°(Aertgeerts et al., 2004). However, only elongated peptides, or unfolded or partly unfolded protein fragments, can reach the small pocket within this cavity that contains the active site. The main enzymatic activity of CD26 is a serine protease activity with a post-proline dipeptidyl aminopeptidase activity, preferentially cleaving Xaa-Pro or Xaa-Ala dipeptides (where Xaa is any amino acid except Pro) from the N-terminus of polypeptides.

CD26 contains nine potential N-linked glycosylation sites that lie predominantly on the propeller domain, near the dimerization interface (Engel et al., 2003). The human CD26 gene consists of 26 exons and is located on the long arm of chromosome 2 (Tanaka et al., 1992).

4.2 Functions

CD26 exerts pivotal roles in nutrition, metabolism, immune and endocrine systems, bone marrow mobilization, cancer growth and cell adhesion. CD26 activates or deactivates various bioactive peptides on the cell surface or in the extracellular environment, by cleaving them enzymatically, therefore regulating their availability for adjacent cells. CD26 substrates include cytokines and several chemokines: substance P, chorionic gonadotropin, tumour necrosis factor α (TNF-α), interleukin-2, stromal cell-derived factor 1a, RANTES, neuropeptide Y, peptide YY, glucagon-like peptide (GLP)-1, GLP-2 and glucose-dependent insulinotropic peptide (Gorrell, 2005). Besides its enzymatic activity, CD26 shows a variety of functions, including regulation of inflammatory and immunological responses, signal transduction, interactions with extracellular matrix proteins and apoptosis.

CD26 ligands include adenosine deaminase (ADA) (Morrison et al., 1993), kidney Na^+/H^+ ion exchanger 3 (Girardi et al., 2001) and fibronectin (Cheng et al., 2003).

CD26 has been consistently associated with cancer since its identification (ten Kate et al., 1984). A number of recent studies have provided evidence that CD26 plays a role in discrete steps of tumour progression, such as cell adhesion, invasion and cell cycle arrest (Pethiyagoda et al., 2000). In selected carcinoma tissues, CD26 is misexpressed and it can function either as an oncogene or as a tumour suppressor gene. Its expression is upregulated and associated with tumour aggressiveness in T and B lymphomas and leukaemias (Bauvois et al., 1999; Carbone et al., 1995; Dang et al., 2003), thyroid follicular tumours (de Micco et al., 2008), papillary carcinomas, astrocytic tumours (Stremenova et al., 2007) and gastrointestinal stromal tumours (Yamaguchi et al., 2008). Conversely, loss of CD26 occurs during malignant transformation of melanocytes into melanoma (Wesley et al., 1999), indicating a possible role of the molecule in suppressing the malignant transformation of melanocytes.

The precise biological mechanism through which CD26 regulates tumour cell progression remains controversial. According to Wesley et al., high CD26 expression leads to a loss of tumorigenicity through its serine protease activity (Wesley, et al., 1999). On the other hand, the suppressive effect of CD26 on melanoma's malignant phenotype is related neither to the protease activity located at the extracellular domain nor to the signal transduction related to the cytoplasmic domain (Pethiyagoda et al., 2000).

In 2002 Kajiyama et al. first described the expression of CD26 in ovarian carcinoma cell lines and tissues. CD26 immunoreactivity was observed on surgically resected ovarian carcinoma of different histotypes, but was not found in stromal cells. CD26 expression in ovarian cancer cell lines is associated with an epithelioid morphology. Indeed, forced expression of

CD26 in an ovarian cancer cell line results in marked morphological changes from a fibroblastic/spindle-shaped appearance toward an epithelioid pattern, which is paralleled by the shift from mesenchymal to epithelial markers (Kajiyama et al., 2002).

Exogenous expression of CD26 leads to a significant reduction in the invasive potential in ovarian carcinoma cell lines *in vitro* and an increased E-cadherin expression. Indeed, CD26 expression in ovarian cancer cell lines positively correlates with E-cadherin expression and induces the upregulation of both E-cadherin and β-catenin, which play a key role in the suppression of invasive and metastatic phenotype of cancer cells (Kajiyama et al., 2003). Moreover, in ovarian carcinoma cell lines CD26 expression negatively correlates with MMP-2 expression, and the expression levels of both MMP-2 and MT1-MMP are significantly reduced in CD26-transfected cells. Overexpression of CD26 also increases expression levels of TIMP-1 and TIMP-2, known to be key inhibitors of tumour invasion, angiogenesis and metastasis (Kikkawa et al., 2005).

Overexpression of CD26 reduced intraperitoneal dissemination of carcinoma cells and prolonged survival time *in vivo* in a mouse orthotopic model. Ovarian carcinoma cell lines with higher CD26 expression has significantly less metastatic potential when injected into the abdominal cavity of nude mice than the CD26-negative control cells (Mizutani et al., 2003). Consistent with this, the intensity of CD26 immunohistochemical staining in tissues proved to be stronger in well-differentiated and non-infiltrating ovarian carcinomas, thus indicating that the decrease of CD26 is related to neoplastic transformation and tumour progression (Zhang et al., 2008).

A positive correlation between CD26 expression and sensitivity to paclitaxel has been described in several ovarian carcinoma cell lines. Forced expression of CD26 in a CD26-negative ovarian cancer cell line significantly enhanced sensitivity to paclitaxel by increasing the rate of apoptotic cells through the repression of the transcriptional factor Twist, a master regulator of epithelial-mesenchymal transition, linked to paclitaxel resistance. These data were corroborated by the observation that paclitaxel-resistant NOS-PR cells showed reduced expression of CD26. However, no significant alteration in paclitaxel sensitivity was observed in the presence of a specific inhibitor of DPPIV activity in CD26-transfected or natively CD26-overexpressing cells (Kajiyama et al., 2010).

Further understanding of the anti-invasive effect of CD26 may prove useful in devising new strategies in the control of ovarian cancer and other carcinomas. Like other membrane-bound peptidases, CD26 may soon be destined for use not only as a new diagnostic/prognostic marker, but also as a molecular target in novel therapeutic strategies.

5. CD73

5.1 Structure and expression

CD73, also known as ecto-5′-nucleotidase (ecto-5′-NT), is a glycosylphosphatidylinositol (GPI)-anchored ectoenzyme composed of two identical subunits of 70-74 kDa. The mature protein consists of 548 amino acids and corresponds to a molecular mass of ~63 kDa (Airas et al., 1993). The human CD73 gene has been mapped to region q14-q21 of chromosome 6. CD73 is abundantly expressed by vascular endothelial cells (Jalkanen et al., 2008) and by a subpopulation of peripheral blood lymphocytes represented by regulatory T cells and primed uncommitted CD4-positive T cells. Follicular dendritic cells (Airas, 1998), intestinal epithelial cells (Strohmeier et al., 1997), fibroblasts (Nemoto et al., 2004), cardiomyocytes

(Carneiro-Ramos et al., 2004), neurons, oligodendrocytes (Maienschein et al., 1996) and mesenchymal stem cells (Barry et al., 2001) have been reported to express CD73.

5.2 Functions

It has been proposed that CD73 behaves as an adhesion molecule modulating lymphocyte-endothelial cell interactions (Airas et al., 2000). Furthermore, CD73 is known to play a critical role *in vivo* in maintaining the integrity of the vascular endothelium during hypoxia (Colgan et al., 2006), in mediating efficient entry of lymphocytes into the central nervous system during experimental autoimmune encephalomyelitis and in regulating leukocyte-endothelium interaction during cardiac ischemia–reperfusion (Koszalka et al., 2004).

CD73 catalyzes the dephosphorylation of purine and pyrimidine ribo- and deoxyribonucleoside monophosphates to the corresponding nucleoside. This ectoenzymatic cascade operates in tandem with CD39 (ecto-ATPase) and catalyzes the conversion of AMP to bioactive adenosine from adenosine triphosphate (ATP) which is often released into the extracellular environment from damaged or inflamed target cells (Stagg et al., 2010b). Extracellular adenosine induces potent immunosuppressive effects, mainly mediated through four adenosine-binding G protein–coupled receptors. In addition to its enzymatic function, CD73 has been suggested to have a role in T cell signalling (Resta et al., 1998).

The resistance of many solid tumours to host immune responses has been largely attributed to a spectrum of tumour-associated immune-suppressive mechanisms. During tumour progression, tumour cells promote a tolerant microenvironment and activation of multiple immunosuppressive mechanisms, which may act in concert to attenuate an effective immune responses (Rabinovich et al., 2007). It is thought that tipping the balance from an immune-suppressive to an immune-active environment is necessary for effective cancer immunotherapy (Rabinovich et al., 2007). Adenosine is a purine nucleoside reaching high concentrations within solid tumours (Ohta et al., 2006) where it promotes tumour growth through the stimulation of tumour angiogenesis (Stagg & Smyth, 2010b) and inhibition of anti-tumour immune responses (Hoskin et al., 2008). However, the mechanisms whereby adenosine accumulates in solid tumours and the effects resulting from this accumulation are not completely understood.

CD73 expression has been reported in several tumour types (Stagg & Smyth, 2010b), including ovarian cancer (Jin et al., 2010) and its expression has been associated with a prometastatic phenotype in melanoma and breast cancer (Leth-Larsen et al., 2009). Although *in vitro* studies suggested that CD73 expression can enhance breast cancer cell migration and invasion, the underlying mechanisms remain elusive. In breast cancer cells, CD73 expression significantly inhibits endogenous adaptive anti-tumour immunosurveillance, in addition, CD73-derived adenosine enhances tumour cell migration *in vitro* and metastasis *in vivo* through the activation of A2B adenosine receptors (Stagg et al., 2010a). CD73 expression has been shown to be regulated by estrogen receptors, whereby loss of estrogen receptors significantly enhances CD73 expression (Spychala et al., 2004). CD73 is highly expressed in many human solid tumours (Salmi et al., 2011), and its high expression and activity are associated with tumour invasiveness and metastasis (Stagg et al., 2010a) and with shorter patient survival. Recently it has been demonstrated that exosomes released by cancer cells *in vitro* and in biological effusions are able to dephosphorylate exogenous ATP and 5'AMP to form adenosine. These hydrolytic activities have been in part attributed to expression of functional CD39 and CD73 by exosomes. This mechanism may contribute to augmenting

adenosine levels within the tumour microenvironment and hence participate to the negative regulation of T cell function (Clayton et al., 2011).
CD73 expressed in ovarian cancer negatively modulates tumour antigen-specific T cell immunity. Indeed, it has been demonstrated that knockdown of CD73 on tumour cells by siRNA improved anti-tumour T cell responses, completely restoring the efficacy of adoptive T cell therapy and leading to long-term tumour-free survival in tumour-bearing mice. Moreover, in a mouse model, host CD73 deficiency decreased the ovarian carcinoma burden and increased mouse survival in a T cell–dependent manner. Accordingly, reduction of both tumour and host CD73 resulted in an optimal anti-tumour effect (Jin et al., 2010).
Pharmacological blockade of CD73 using the specific inhibitor α,β-methylene adenosine 5'-diphosphate (APCP) or a blocking anti-CD73 monoclonal antibody inhibited tumour growth and promoted efficacy of adoptive T cell therapy (Zhang, 2010), suggesting that CD73-targeted therapy might be a promising and rational approach to cancer treatment (Häusler SF et al., 2011). In summary, detailed analysis of CD73 expression on tumour cells and/or host cells regulating anti-tumour immunity may have important consequences on our understanding of immunosuppressive mechanisms in the tumour microenvironment that support tumour evasion. Inhibition of CD73 could be a therapeutic adjuvant to improve cancer immunotherapy.

6. CD157

6.1 Structure and expression

CD157/BST-1 is a GPI-anchored glycoprotein encoded by a member of a gene family of NADase/ADP-ribosyl cyclase, which includes CD38. The CD38 and bone marrow stromal cell antigen 1 (BST-1) genes arose by gene duplication before the divergence of humans and rodents (Ferrero et al., 1997). The human CD157 gene is located on chromosome 4p15, it spans ~35 kb and consists of nine exons (Muraoka et al., 1996). Although CD157 was initially characterised as a stromal (Kaisho et al., 1994) and myeloid surface antigen (Goldstein et al., 1993), it is also expressed by certain other cell types that include vascular endothelial cells (Ortolan et al., 2002) and mesothelial cells (Ross et al., 1998).

6.2 Functions

CD157 is an ectoenzyme that cleave extracellular nicotinamide adenine dinucleotide (NAD) and NADP+, generating cyclic ADP ribose (cADPR), NAADP+, and ADPR. Beside their role as mediators of intracellular calcium release (Galione, 1994), the products of CD157-operated NAD cleavage can act as extracellular immunomodifiers (Haag et al., 2007). Emerging data indicated that these metabolites can act extracellularly as paracrine factors (Moreschi et al., 2008). Moreover, the catalytic reactions generate substrate for ADP-ribosyl transferases and polymerases involved in cell signalling, DNA repair and apoptosis (Haag et al., 2007). In addition, CD157 possesses receptor activity, indeed, it interacts with other surface molecules thus acquiring the ability to transduce signals (Malavasi et al., 2008). Accumulating evidence indicates that CD157 is a key molecule in the control of leukocyte adhesion, migration and diapedesis (Funaro, 2004; Ortolan, 2006). CD157 establishes a structural interaction with β1 and β2 integrins (Lavagno et al., 2007) and, following antibody-induced cross-linking, promotes their relocation into detergent-resistant membrane domains, thus driving the dynamic reorganization of signalling-competent membrane microdomains. Moreover, CD157 effectively contributes to the integrin-driven signalling network that is critical during leukocyte transmigration (Lo Buono et al., 2011).

Recently, we demonstrated that CD157 is expressed in epithelial ovarian cancer (EOC) primary cell cultures and tissues, and it is involved in interactions among EOC cells, extracellular matrix proteins, and mesothelial cells which ultimately control tumour cell migration and invasion. The results inferred *in vitro* were validated by clinical evidence: CD157 was expressed by 93% of EOC analysed and high CD157 expression was associated with rapid tumour relapse in patients. Moreover, CD157 appears to be a marker of poor prognosis in the serous subtype of ovarian cancer, which is the most frequent and aggressive type. Multivariate survival analysis showed that CD157 is an independent prognostic factor of tumour relapse shortly after surgical debulking of ovarian cancer (Ortolan et al., 2010). Several lines of evidence point to the fact that high levels of CD157 are associated with more aggressive ovarian cancer. First, forced expression of CD157 in CD157-negative NIH:OVCAR-3 cells substantially increased cell motility, a prerequisite for dissemination. Second, blockade of CD157 activity, either by a specific monoclonal antibody *in vitro* or by its weak expression in patients, was associated with reduced invasion and migration by tumour cells. Finally, clinical observations revealed that high CD157 correlated with rapid tumour relapse (Ortolan et al., 2010). However, how CD157 might contribute to a more aggressive ovarian cancer remains to be defined (Annunziata et al., 2010). Our results support the rationale for the future use of CD157 as a potential diagnostic target for EOC, providing the opportunity to develop new strategies using CD157 as a therapeutic target to prevent tumour dissemination in patients with serous ovarian cancer.

7. Autotaxin/CD203c

7.1 Structure and expression

Autotaxin (ATX) also known as CD203c or ENPP2 (ectonucleotide pyrophosphatase/phosphodiesterase 2), is a cell motility-stimulating factor originally isolated from human melanoma cells (Stracke et al., 1992). It is a member of the ENPP protein family, which includes membrane-associated or secreted ectoenzymes that hydrolyze pyrophosphate or phosphodiester bonds in various extracellular compounds, such as nucleotides and lysophospholipids (Tokumura et al., 2002). ATX/CD203c is a soluble 125 kDa glycoprotein encoded by a single gene located on human chromosome 8. Three alternatively spliced isoforms have been reported: α, β and γ. Isoform β, considered the canonical form, is the predominant one, and is expressed in peripheral tissues while isoform γ is more highly expressed in the central nervous system. Both β and γ variants are catalytically active, whereas the α isoform is rapidly degraded into smaller inactive forms (Giganti et al., 2008). Autotaxin contains a catalytic domain, which is responsible for enzymatic activity and two additional domains, a somatomedin-B-like domain and a nuclease-like domain, which are located at the N-terminus and C-terminus of the protein, respectively. The somatomedin-B-like domain is rich in cysteine residues and contains an RGD tripeptide motif that is possibly involved in cell-extracellular matrix interactions. The nuclease-like domain contains an EF hand-like motif, structurally similar to the DNA- or RNA-non-specific endonucleases but it is catalytically inactive. All three domains are required for the catalytic activity (Nishimasu et al., 2011).

ATX is predominantly expressed in brain, kidney, placenta, ovary, small intestine and in body fluids such as plasma (Tokumura et al., 2002), cerebral spinal fluid, saliva, and follicular and amniotic fluids (Giganti et al., 2008; Nishimasu et al., 2011).

7.2 Functions

Autotaxin is defined as a multi-functional protein producing *(i)* lysophosphatidic acid (LPA) by conversion of lysophosphatidylcholine (LPC), present in human serum or plasma, and *(ii)* cyclic phosphatidic acid (cPA), an LPA analogue with distinct physiological activities. ATX activity accounts for the majority of LPA production in blood (Nakanaga et al., 2010). The biological activity of LPA is largely mediated through the activation of five receptors, LPA1 to LPA5. All of these are type I, rhodopsin-like G protein-coupled receptors with seven-transmembrane alpha helices (Lin et al., 2010). LPA evokes a wide variety of cellular responses in different cell types including Ras-mediated cell proliferation and Rho/Rac-regulated cell migration (including vascular endothelial cells migration), neurite retraction, platelet aggregation, smooth muscle contraction, actin stress fibers formation and cytokine/chemokine secretion. LPA levels are increased during pathological conditions of the brain (neuropsychiatric disorders such as bipolar disorders, schizophrenia, etc.). Deregulation of LPA signalling is found in cardiovascular diseases: the formation of excess fibrous connective tissues is strongly influenced by receptor-mediated LPA signalling in different organs (for example, lung, kidney and liver) (Lin et al., 2010). Moreover, in both *in vivo* and *in vitro* systems, LPA has been shown to participate in critical events of cancer progression such as cell proliferation, growth, survival, migration, invasion, and promotion of angiogenesis (van Meeteren et al., 2007). Therefore, LPA signalling is worth considering for its involvement in disease processes as well as in normal physiological functions.

Autotaxin was originally identified as a tumour cell motility factor released in the spent medium of human melanoma cells. When overexpressed in Ras-NIH3T3 cells, ATX promotes tumour aggressiveness, metastasis and angiogenesis in nude mice (Nam et al., 2000). ATX is highly expressed in several human cancers, including glioblastoma, lung and breast cancer, renal cell carcinoma, neuroblastoma, thyroid carcinoma and Hodgkin's lymphoma (Mills et al., 2003). High ATX expression is detected in glioblastoma multiforme, a lethal cancer with a high infiltration rate (Hoelzinger et al., 2005). ATX has also been found upregulated in stromal cells from prostate carcinoma patients (Zhao et al., 2007) and its expression is strongly enhanced by v-Jun oncogene-induced transformation (Black et al., 2004) and by overexpression of cancer-associated $\alpha6\beta4$ integrin in breast cancer (Chen et al., 2005). In an *in vivo* angiogenesis model, ATX-transfected Ras-transformed NIH3T3 cells caused more prominent new blood vessel formation than control cells (Nam et al., 2000). In addition, ATX stimulates human vascular endothelial cells grown on Matrigel to form tubules, similarly to the effects induced by vascular endothelial growth factor (VEGF) (Nam et al., 2001).

Recent studies have demonstrated the molecular mechanisms underlying the ATX/LPA axis in cancer. ATX-induced motility of melanoma cells is mediated through the activation of focal adhesion kinase (FAK) (Jung et al., 2004) and, in the nucleus, by the DNA binding of necrosis factor kappa B (NF-kB) (Lee et al., 2006).

Another finding is that LPA strongly counteracts Taxol-induced death in the MCF-7 breast cancer cell line and in MDA-MB-435 melanoma cells, by activating phosphatidylinositol 3-kinase (PI3K), which antagonizes the Taxol-induced accumulation of cancer cells in the

G2/M phase of the cell cycle (Samadi et al., 2009). Recently it has been demonstrated that the ATX/LPA axis allows breast cancer cells to escape from mitotic arrest following the PI3K-dependent displacement of Taxol from polymerised tubulin (Samadi et al., 2011). Moreover, recent data from *in vivo* experiments indicate that increased expression of ATX, LPA1, LPA2 or LPA3 receptors in mice is associated with enhanced invasiveness of estrogen receptor-positive, metastatic breast cancers (Liu et al., 2009). Finally, the significance of the plasma or serum ATX levels in cancer patients has been reported in patients with follicular lymphoma, where serum ATX levels proved to be significantly higher than those in healthy subjects, to correlate with plasma LPA levels and to change according to patient clinical course (Masuda et al., 2008). Additional studies have reported an impressive and specific increase in serum ATX activity and plasma LPA in patients with chronic hepatitis C (Watanabe et al., 2007) and pancreatic cancer (Nakai et al., 2011).

In the last 20 years several studies have considered the potential role of the ATX/LPA axis in ovarian cancer. The high metastatic potential of ovarian carcinoma was suggested to be related to increased local production of LPA in the peritoneal cavity (Mills & Moolenaar, 2003). Levels of LPA are markedly elevated in the ascites of patients with EOC (Mills et al., 1988) and in the plasma of 90% of stage I ovarian cancer patients, compared with healthy women (Xu et al., 1998).

The outcomes of LPA-driven signalling are determined by the expression level of LPA receptors on the cell surfaces. Indeed, normal ovarian epithelial cells express low levels of mRNA for LPA2 and LPA3, whereas the mRNA levels for LPA2 and particularly LPA3, are elevated in EOC (Fang et al., 2002), suggesting a shift on ovarian cancer cells towards an LPA-dependent phenotype. Moreover >90% of LPA degradation by ovarian cancer cells is caused by the action of lipid phosphate phosphohydrolase-like (LPP-like) enzymes, whose expression differs between normal ovarian epithelium and epithelial ovarian cancer (Imai et al., 2000). This implies that LPA, its receptors and downstream metabolic cascade might be potential targets for the design of novel ovarian cancer therapies.

LPA has been found to induce VEGF expression (Hu et al., 2001) which in turn contributes to malignant ascites formation by increasing peritoneal microvessel permeability (Nagy et al., 1995). A feedback model between ATX, LPA and VEGF in ovarian cancer cells has been recently proposed (Ptaszynska et al., 2008). VEGF activates ATX transcription and subsequent protein secretion through VEGFR2. Increased secretion of ATX leads to an increased level of extracellular LPA. Completing the loop, LPA can stimulate VEGF and VEGFR2 expression through LPA receptor signalling thus enhancing tumour survival and growth. These data indicate that cross-talk between ATX and VEGF may be an important autocrine mechanism in the generation of an aggressive ovarian cancer phenotype. In addition, soluble ATX may be a beneficial target for cancer therapy because of its capacity to control both LPA production and signalling, and VEGF signalling.

The development of drug resistance to cytotoxic therapies such as carboplatin and paclitaxel as well as to newly emerging therapies (Agarwal et al., 2003), remains a high risk factor for ovarian cancer patients. Therefore, the identification of genes which confer drug resistance may offer novel therapeutic targets that can be exploited to develop drugs which re-sensitize tumour cells to chemotherapeutic agents (Richardson et al., 2005). ATX has been linked to chemoresistance due to its ability to inhibit apoptosis induced by paclitaxel in breast cancer cells (Samadi et al., 2009) and LPA can inhibit cell death induced by cisplatin (Frankel et al., 1996). It has been demonstrated that ATX may be a target for treating drug-resistant ovarian cancer. The ectopic expression of ATX leads to the activation of a PI3K/Akt-mediated survival pathway, suggesting that ATX can delay carboplatin-induced cell death through the generation of LPA and the subsequent activation of the PI3K/Akt pathway (Vidot et al., 2010). The inhibition of ATX in therapy has the advantage of providing a single extracellular drug target capable of blocking production of LPA. It has been observed that the primary effect of ATX is to delay apoptosis induced by carboplatin; since the exposure of tumour cells to carboplatin in patients is transient, accelerating the induction of apoptosis might be beneficial and may lead to improved tumour cell destruction.

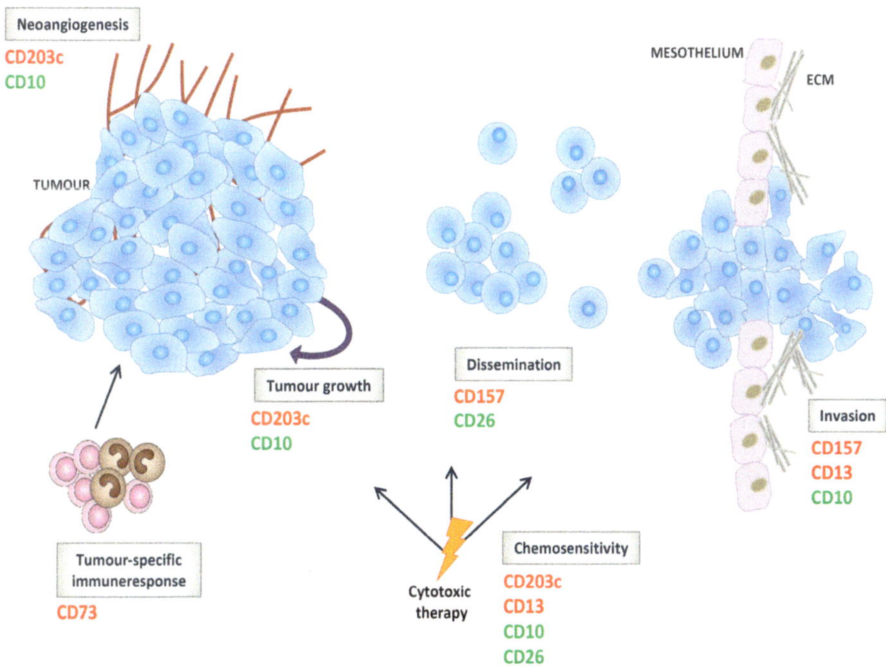

Fig. 2. Schematic representation of the role of ectoenzymes in the main steps of ovarian cancer progression. Ectoenzymes in red have stimulating effects, those in green have inhibitory effects on the indicated steps.

8. Conclusion

Improved understanding of the underlying biology of ovarian tumour progression and chemoresistance has led to the development of molecular targeted therapies. Ectoenzymes are attractive targets for designing new strategies to interfere with ovarian cancer progression and recurrence. This can be achieved by inhibiting the ectoenzymes that promote tumour migration and invasiveness (such as CD157 and CD13) or by inducing the activity of ectoenzymes that normally counteract tumour progression (such as CD26). In many cases, ectoenzymes can be inactivated either by specific monoclonal antibodies that block their function, or by small-molecule enzyme inhibitors. The dual nature of ectoenzymes warrants more detailed and vigorous investigation, because some of their functions seem to be independent of their enzymatic activities. It is conceivable that the large extracellular domains of ectoenzymes and their lateral interaction with other membrane proteins can mediate responses without involvement of their catalytic activity. However, many of the non-substrate ligands of ectoenzymes remain to be identified. Moreover, increasing evidence indicates that a number of ectoenzymes orchestrate the immune mechanisms underlying tumour progression and outcome and it is now evident that ovarian cancer features a number of different tumour evasion mechanisms. The future challenge will be to use a combinatorial approach to increase the existing anti-tumour response, dampen tumour evasion mechanisms and target crucial environmental players.

9. Acknowledgement

This work was supported by grants from the Italian Association for Cancer Research (MFAG 6312 to E.O.) and the Italian Ministry for University and Scientific Research (PRIN 2008 to A.F.). The Fondazione Internazionale Ricerche Medicina Sperimentale (FIRMS) provided financial and administrative assistance. N.LB. S.M. and A.G. are members of the Ph.D. program in "Complexity in Post-Genomic Biology" and R.P. is a member of the Ph.D. program in "Human Genetics", all at the University of Torino, Torino, Italy.

10. References

Aertgeerts, K., Ye, S., Shi, L., Prasad, S. G., Witmer, D., et al. (2004) N-linked glycosylation of dipeptidyl peptidase IV (CD26): effects on enzyme activity, homodimer formation, and adenosine deaminase binding, *Protein Science,* Vol. 13 N° 1 (Jan), pp. 145-154, ISSN 0961-8368

Agarwal, R., & Kaye, S. B. (2003) Ovarian cancer: strategies for overcoming resistance to chemotherapy, *Nature Reviews. Cancer,* Vol. 3 N° 7 (Jul), pp. 502-516, ISSN 1474-175X

Airas, L., Salmi, M., & Jalkanen, S. (1993) Lymphocyte-vascular adhesion protein-2 is a novel 70-kDa molecule involved in lymphocyte adhesion to vascular endothelium, *Journal of Immunology,* Vol. 151 N° 8 (Oct 15), pp. 4228-4238, ISSN 0022-1767

Airas, L. (1998) CD73 and adhesion of B-cells to follicular dendritic cells, *Leukemia and Lymphoma,* Vol. 29 N° 1-2 (Mar), pp. 37-47, ISSN 1042-8194

Airas, L., Niemela, J., & Jalkanen, S. (2000) CD73 engagement promotes lymphocyte binding to endothelial cells via a lymphocyte function-associated antigen-1-dependent mechanism, *Journal of Immunology,* Vol. 165 N° 10 (Nov 15), pp. 5411-5417, ISSN 0022-1767

Annunziata, C. M., & Birrer, M. J. (2010) CD157 in ovarian carcinoma: how does it help us?, *Journal of the National Cancer Institute,* Vol. 102 N° 15 (Aug 4), pp. 1104-1105, ISSN 1460-2105

Antczak, C., De Meester, I., & Bauvois, B. (2001) Ectopeptidases in pathophysiology, *Bioessays,* Vol. 23 N° 3 (Mar), pp. 251-260, ISSN 0265-9247

Bagnato, A., Salani, D., Di Castro, V., Wu-Wong, J. R., Tecce, R., et al. (1999) Expression of endothelin 1 and endothelin A receptor in ovarian carcinoma: evidence for an autocrine role in tumour growth, *Cancer Research,* Vol. 59 N° 3 (Feb 1), pp. 720-727, ISSN 0008-5472

Barry, F., Boynton, R., Murphy, M., Haynesworth, S., & Zaia, J. (2001) The SH-3 and SH-4 antibodies recognize distinct epitopes on CD73 from human mesenchymal stem cells, *Biochemical and Biophysical Research Communications*, Vol. 289 N° 2 (Nov 30), pp. 519-524, ISSN 0006-291X

Bauvois, B., De Meester, I., Dumont, J., Rouillard, D., Zhao, H. X., et al. (1999) Constitutive expression of CD26/dipeptidylpeptidase IV on peripheral blood B lymphocytes of patients with B chronic lymphocytic leukaemia, *British Journal of Cancer*, Vol. 79 N° 7-8 (Mar), pp. 1042-1048, ISSN 0007-0920

Bhagwat, S. V., Lahdenranta, J., Giordano, R., Arap, W., Pasqualini, R., et al. (2001) CD13/APN is activated by angiogenic signals and is essential for capillary tube formation, *Blood*, Vol. 97 N° 3 (Feb 1), pp. 652-659, ISSN 0006-4971

Black, E. J., Clair, T., Delrow, J., Neiman, P., & Gillespie, D. A. (2004) Microarray analysis identifies Autotaxin, a tumour cell motility and angiogenic factor with lysophospholipase D activity, as a specific target of cell transformation by v-Jun, *Oncogene*, Vol. 23 N° 13 (Mar 25), pp. 2357-2366, ISSN 0950-9232

Bowes, M. A., & Kenny, A. J. (1987) An immunohistochemical study of endopeptidase-24.11 and aminopeptidase N in lymphoid tissues, *Immunology*, Vol. 60 N° 2 (Feb), pp. 247-253, ISSN 0019-2805

Burns, D. M., Walker, B., Gray, J., & Nelson, J. (1999) Breast cancer cell-associated endopeptidase EC 24.11 modulates proliferative response to bombesin, *British Journal of Cancer*, Vol. 79 N° 2 (Jan), pp. 214-220, ISSN 0007-0920

Cannistra, S. A. (2004) Cancer of the ovary, *New England Journal of Medicine*, Vol. 351 N° 24 (Dec 9), pp. 2519-2529, ISSN 1533-4406

Carbone, A., Gloghini, A., Zagonel, V., Aldinucci, D., Gattei, V., et al. (1995) The expression of CD26 and CD40 ligand is mutually exclusive in human T-cell non-Hodgkin's lymphomas/leukemias, *Blood*, Vol. 86 N° 12 (Dec 15), pp. 4617-4626, ISSN 0006-4971

Carl-McGrath, S., Lendeckel, U., Ebert, M., Wolter, A. B., Roessner, A., et al. (2004) The ectopeptidases CD10, CD13, CD26, and CD143 are upregulated in gastric cancer, *International Journal of Oncology*, Vol. 25 N° 5 (Nov), pp. 1223-1232, ISSN 1019-6439

Carlsson, L., Ronquist, G., Eliasson, R., Egberg, N., & Larsson, A. (2006) Flow cytometric technique for determination of prostasomal quantity, size and expression of CD10, CD13, CD26 and CD59 in human seminal plasma, *International Journal of Andrology*, Vol. 29 N° 2 (Apr), pp. 331-338, ISSN 0105-6263

Carneiro-Ramos, M. S., da Silva, V. B., Coutinho, M. B., Jr., Battastini, A. M., Sarkis, J. J., et al. (2004) Thyroid hormone stimulates 5'-ecto-nucleotidase of neonatal rat ventricular myocytes, *Molecular and Cellular Biochemistry*, Vol. 265 N° 1-2 (Oct), pp. 195-201, ISSN 0300-8177

Chang, Y. W., Chen, S. C., Cheng, E. C., Ko, Y. P., Lin, Y. C., et al. (2005) CD13 (aminopeptidase N) can associate with tumour-associated antigen L6 and enhance the motility of human lung cancer cells, *International Journal of Cancer*, Vol. 116 N° 2 (Aug 20), pp. 243-252, ISSN 0020-7136

Chen, L., Gao, Z., Zhu, J., & Rodgers, G. P. (2007) Identification of CD13+CD36+ cells as a common progenitor for erythroid and myeloid lineages in human bone marrow, *Experimental Hematology*, Vol. 35 N° 7 (Jul), pp. 1047-1055, ISSN 0301-472X

Chen, M., & O'Connor, K. L. (2005) Integrin alpha6beta4 promotes expression of autotaxin/ENPP2 autocrine motility factor in breast carcinoma cells, *Oncogene,* Vol. 24 N° 32 (Jul 28), pp. 5125-5130, ISSN 0950-9232

Cheng, H. C., Abdel-Ghany, M., & Pauli, B. U. (2003) A novel consensus motif in fibronectin mediates dipeptidyl peptidase IV adhesion and metastasis, *Journal of Biological Chemistry,* Vol. 278 N° 27 (Jul 4), pp. 24600-24607, ISSN 0021-9258

Clayton A, Al-Taei S, Webber, D., M., Tabi, M., et al. (2011) Cancer Exosomes Express CD39 and CD73, Which Suppress T Cells through Adenosine Production, *Journal of Immunology,* Vol. 187 N° pp. 676-683

Cohen, A. J., Bunn, P. A., Franklin, W., Magill-Solc, C., Hartmann, C., et al. (1996) Neutral endopeptidase: variable expression in human lung, inactivation in lung cancer, and modulation of peptide-induced calcium flux, *Cancer Research,* Vol. 56 N° 4 (Feb 15), pp. 831-839, ISSN 0008-5472

Colgan, S. P., Eltzschig, H. K., Eckle, T., & Thompson, L. F. (2006) Physiological roles for ecto-5'-nucleotidase (CD73), *Purinergic Signal,* Vol. 2 N° 2 (Jun), pp. 351-360, ISSN 1573-9538

Connelly, J. C., Skidgel, R. A., Schulz, W. W., Johnson, A. R., & Erdos, E. G. (1985) Neutral endopeptidase 24.11 in human neutrophils: cleavage of chemotactic peptide, *Proceedings of the National Academy of Sciences of the United States of America,* Vol. 82 N° 24 (Dec), pp. 8737-8741, ISSN 0027-8424

D'Adamio, L., Shipp, M. A., Masteller, E. L., & Reinherz, E. L. (1989) Organization of the gene encoding common acute lymphoblastic leukemia antigen (neutral endopeptidase 24.11): multiple miniexons and separate 5' untranslated regions, *Proceedings of the National Academy of Sciences of the United States of America,* Vol. 86 N° 18 (Sep), pp. 7103-7107, ISSN 0027-8424

Dai, J., Shen, R., Sumitomo, M., Goldberg, J. S., Geng, Y., et al. (2001) Tumour-suppressive effects of neutral endopeptidase in androgen-independent prostate cancer cells, *Clinical Cancer Research,* Vol. 7 N° 5 (May), pp. 1370-1377, ISSN 1078-0432

Dang, N. H., Aytac, U., Sato, K., O'Brien, S., Melenhorst, J., et al. (2003) T-large granular lymphocyte lymphoproliferative disorder: expression of CD26 as a marker of clinically aggressive disease and characterization of marrow inhibition, *British Journal of Haematology,* Vol. 121 N° 6 (Jun), pp. 857-865, ISSN 0007-1048

Danielsen, E. M., & van Deurs, B. (1997) Galectin-4 and small intestinal brush border enzymes form clusters, *Molecular Biology of the Cell,* Vol. 8 N° 11 (Nov), pp. 2241-2251, ISSN 1059-1524

Danziger, R. S. (2008) Aminopeptidase N in arterial hypertension, *Heart Failure Reviews,* Vol. 13 N° 3 (Sep), pp. 293-298. ISSN 1382-4147

de Micco, C., Savchenko, V., Giorgi, R., Sebag, F., & Henry, J. F. (2008) Utility of malignancy markers in fine-needle aspiration cytology of thyroid nodules: comparison of Hector Battifora mesothelial antigen-1, thyroid peroxidase and dipeptidyl aminopeptidase IV, *British Journal of Cancer,* Vol. 98 N° 4 (Feb 26), pp. 818-823, ISSN 0007-0920

Dunphy, C. H., Gardner, L. J., Manes, J. L., Bee, C. S., & Taysi, K. (2000) CD30+ anaplastic large-cell lymphoma with aberrant expression of CD13: case report and review of the literature, *Journal of Clinical Laboratory Analysis,* Vol. 14 N° 6 pp. 299-304, ISSN 0887-8013

Engel, M., Hoffmann, T., Wagner, L., Wermann, M., Heiser, U., et al. (2003) The crystal structure of dipeptidyl peptidase IV (CD26) reveals its functional regulation and enzymatic mechanism, *Proceedings of the National Academy of Sciences of the United States of America,* Vol. 100 N° 9 (Apr 29), pp. 5063-5068, ISSN 0027-8424

Erdos, E. G., & Skidgel, R. A. (1989) Neutral endopeptidase 24.11 (enkephalinase) and related regulators of peptide hormones, *FASEB Journal,* Vol. 3 N° 2 (Feb), pp. 145-151, ISSN 0892-6638

Fang, X., Schummer, M., Mao, M., Yu, S., Tabassam, F. H., et al. (2002) Lysophosphatidic acid is a bioactive mediator in ovarian cancer, *Biochimica et Biophysica Acta,* Vol. 1582 N° 1-3 (May 23), pp. 257-264, ISSN 0006-3002

Feki, A., Berardi, P., Bellingan, G., Major, A., Krause, K. H., et al. (2009) Dissemination of intraperitoneal ovarian cancer: Discussion of mechanisms and demonstration of lymphatic spreading in ovarian cancer model, *Critical Reviews in Oncology/Hematology,* Vol. 72 N° 1 (Oct), pp. 1-9, ISSN 1879-0461

Ferrero, E., & Malavasi, F. (1997) Human CD38, a leukocyte receptor and ectoenzyme, is a member of a novel eukaryotic gene family of nicotinamide adenine dinucleotide+-converting enzymes: extensive structural homology with the genes for murine bone marrow stromal cell antigen 1 and aplysian ADP-ribosyl cyclase, *Journal of Immunology,* Vol. 159 N° 8 (Oct 15), pp. 3858-3865, ISSN 0022-1767

Frankel, A., & Mills, G. B. (1996) Peptide and lipid growth factors decrease cis-diamminedichloroplatinum-induced cell death in human ovarian cancer cells, *Clinical Cancer Research,* Vol. 2 N° 8 (Aug), pp. 1307-1313, 1078-0432

Fujii, H., Nakajima, M., Saiki, I., Yoneda, J., Azuma, I., et al. (1995) Human melanoma invasion and metastasis enhancement by high expression of aminopeptidase N/CD13, *Clinical and Experimental Metastasis,* Vol. 13 N° 5 (Sep), pp. 337-344, ISSN 0262-0898

Fujimoto, Y., Nakanishi, Y., Sekine, S., Yoshimura, K., Akasu, T., et al. (2005) CD10 expression in colorectal carcinoma correlates with liver metastasis, *Diseases of the Colon and Rectum,* Vol. 48 N° 10 (Oct), pp. 1883-1889, ISSN 0012-3706

Funaro, A., Ortolan, E., Ferranti, B., Gargiulo, L., Notaro, R., et al. (2004) CD157 is an important mediator of neutrophil adhesion and migration, *Blood,* Vol. 104 N° 13 (Dec 15), pp. 4269-4278, ISSN 0006-4971

Galione, A. (1994) Cyclic ADP-ribose, the ADP-ribosyl cyclase pathway and calcium signalling, *Molecular and Cellular Endocrinology,* Vol. 98 N° 2 (Jan), pp. 125-131, ISSN 0303-7207

Giganti, A., Rodriguez, M., Fould, B., Moulharat, N., Coge, F., et al. (2008) Murine and human autotaxin alpha, beta, and gamma isoforms: gene organization, tissue distribution, and biochemical characterization, *Journal of Biological Chemistry,* Vol. 283 N° 12 (Mar 21), pp. 7776-7789, ISSN 0021-9258

Girardi, A. C., Degray, B. C., Nagy, T., Biemesderfer, D., & Aronson, P. S. (2001) Association of Na(+)-H(+) exchanger isoform NHE3 and dipeptidyl peptidase IV in the renal proximal tubule, *Journal of Biological Chemistry,* Vol. 276 N° 49 (Dec 7), pp. 46671-46677, ISSN 0021-9258

Goldstein, S. C., & Todd, R. F., 3rd. (1993) Structural and biosynthetic features of the Mo5 human myeloid differentiation antigen, *Tissue Antigens,* Vol. 41 N° 4 (Apr), pp. 214-218, ISSN 0001-281

Gorrell, M. D. (2005) Dipeptidyl peptidase IV and related enzymes in cell biology and liver disorders, *Clinical Science,* Vol. 108 N° 4 (Apr), pp. 277-292, ISSN 0143-5221

Greaves, M. F., Hariri, G., Newman, R. A., Sutherland, D. R., Ritter, M. A., et al. (1983) Selective expression of the common acute lymphoblastic leukemia (gp 100) antigen on immature lymphoid cells and their malignant counterparts, *Blood,* Vol. 61 N° 4 (Apr), pp. 628-639, ISSN 0006-4971

Haag, F., Adriouch, S., Brass, A., Jung, C., Moller, S., et al. (2007) Extracellular NAD and ATP: Partners in immune cell modulation, *Purinergic Signal,* Vol. 3 N° 1-2 (Mar), pp. 71-81, ISSN 1573-9546

Hashida, H., Takabayashi, A., Kanai, M., Adachi, M., Kondo, K., et al. (2002) Aminopeptidase N is involved in cell motility and angiogenesis: its clinical significance in human colon cancer, *Gastroenterology,* Vol. 122 N° 2 (Feb), pp. 376-386, ISSN 0016-5085

Häusler SF, Montalbán Del Barrio I, Strohschein J, Anoop Chandran P, Engel JB, et al. (2011) Ectonucleotidases CD39 and CD73 on OvCA cells are potent adenosine-generating enzymes responsible for adenosine receptor 2A-dependent suppression of T cell function and NK cell cytotoxicity. *Cancer Immunology, Immunotherapy,* Vol.60 N°10 (Oct), pp. 1405-1418, ISSN 0340-7004

Hoelzinger, D. B., Mariani, L., Weis, J., Woyke, T., Berens, T. J., et al. (2005) Gene expression profile of glioblastoma multiforme invasive phenotype points to new therapeutic targets, *Neoplasia,* Vol. 7 N° 1 (Jan), pp. 7-16, ISSN 1522-8002

Hoffmann-Fezer, G., Knapp, W., & Thierfelder, S. (1982) Anatomical distribution of call antigen expressing cells in normal lymphatic tissue and in lymphomas, *Leukemia Research,* Vol. 6 N° 6 pp. 761-767, ISSN 0145-2126

Hoskin, D. W., Mader, J. S., Furlong, S. J., Conrad, D. M., & Blay, J. (2008) Inhibition of T cell and natural killer cell function by adenosine and its contribution to immune evasion by tumour cells (Review), *International Journal of Oncology,* Vol. 32 N° 3 (Mar), pp. 527-535, ISSN 1019-6439

Hu, Y. L., Tee, M. K., Goetzl, E. J., Auersperg, N., Mills, G. B., et al. (2001) Lysophosphatidic acid induction of vascular endothelial growth factor expression in human ovarian cancer cells, *Journal of the National Cancer Institute,* Vol. 93 N° 10 (May 16), pp. 762-768, ISSN 0027-8874

Ikeda, N., Nakajima, Y., Tokuhara, T., Hattori, N., Sho, M., et al. (2003) Clinical significance of aminopeptidase N/CD13 expression in human pancreatic carcinoma, *Clinical Cancer Research,* Vol. 9 N° 4 (Apr), pp. 1503-1508, ISSN 1078-0432

Imai, A., Furui, T., Tamaya, T., & Mills, G. B. (2000) A gonadotropin-releasing hormone-responsive phosphatase hydrolyses lysophosphatidic acid within the plasma membrane of ovarian cancer cells, *Journal of Clinical Endocrinology and Metabolism,* Vol. 85 N° 9 (Sep), pp. 3370-3375, ISSN 0021-972X

Ino, K., Suzuki, T., Uehara, C., Nagasaka, T., Okamoto, T., et al. (2000) The expression and localization of neutral endopeptidase 24.11/CD10 in human gestational trophoblastic diseases, *Laboratory Investigation,* Vol. 80 N° 11 (Nov), pp. 1729-1738, ISSN 0023-6837

Ishii, K., Usui, S., Sugimura, Y., Yamamoto, H., Yoshikawa, K., et al. (2001a) Inhibition of aminopeptidase N (AP-N) and urokinase-type plasminogen activator (uPA) by zinc suppresses the invasion activity in human urological cancer cells, *Biological and Pharmaceutical Bulletin,* Vol. 24 N° 3 (Mar), pp. 226-230, ISSN 0918-6158

Ishii, K., Usui, S., Yamamoto, H., Sugimura, Y., Tatematsu, M., et al. (2001b) Decreases of metallothionein and aminopeptidase N in renal cancer tissues, *Journal of Biochemistry,* Vol. 129 N° 2 (Feb), pp. 253-258, ISSN 0021-924X

Jalkanen, S., & Salmi, M. (2008) VAP-1 and CD73, endothelial cell surface enzymes in leukocyte extravasation, *Arteriosclerosis, Thrombosis, and Vascular Biology,* Vol. 28 N° 1 (Jan), pp. 18-26, ISSN 1524-4636

Jin, D., Fan, J., Wang, L., Thompson, L. F., Liu, A., et al. (2010) CD73 on tumour cells impairs antitumour T-cell responses: a novel mechanism of tumour-induced immune suppression, *Cancer Research,* Vol. 70 N° 6 (Mar 15), pp. 2245-2255, ISSN 1538-7445

Jung, I. D., Lee, J., Lee, K. B., Park, C. G., Kim, Y. K., et al. (2004) Activation of p21-activated kinase 1 is required for lysophosphatidic acid-induced focal adhesion kinase phosphorylation and cell motility in human melanoma A2058 cells, *European Journal of Biochemistry,* Vol. 271 N° 8 (Apr), pp. 1557-1565, ISSN 0014-2956

Kaisho, T., Ishikawa, J., Oritani, K., Inazawa, J., Tomizawa, H., et al. (1994) BST-1, a surface molecule of bone marrow stromal cell lines that facilitates pre-B-cell growth, *Proceedings of the National Academy of Sciences of the United States of America,* Vol. 91 N° 12 (Jun 7), pp. 5325-5329, ISSN 0027-8424

Kajiyama, H., Kikkawa, F., Suzuki, T., Shibata, K., Ino, K., et al. (2002) Prolonged survival and decreased invasive activity attributable to dipeptidyl peptidase IV overexpression in ovarian carcinoma, *Cancer Research,* Vol. 62 N° 10 (May 15), pp. 2753-2757, ISSN 0008-5472

Kajiyama, H., Kikkawa, F., Khin, E., Shibata, K., Ino, K., et al. (2003) Dipeptidyl peptidase IV overexpression induces up-regulation of E-cadherin and tissue inhibitors of matrix metalloproteinases, resulting in decreased invasive potential in ovarian carcinoma cells, *Cancer Research,* Vol. 63 N° 9 (May 1), pp. 2278-2283, ISSN 0008-5472

Kajiyama, H., Shibata, K., Terauchi, M., Morita, T., Ino, K., et al. (2005) Neutral endopeptidase 24.11/CD10 suppresses progressive potential in ovarian carcinoma in vitro and in vivo, *Clinical Cancer Research,* Vol. 11 N° 5 (Mar 1), pp. 1798-1808, ISSN 1078-0432

Kajiyama, H., Shibata, K., Ino, K., Mizutani, S., Nawa, A., et al. (2010) The expression of dipeptidyl peptidase IV (DPPIV/CD26) is associated with enhanced chemosensitivity to paclitaxel in epithelial ovarian carcinoma cells, *Cancer Science,* Vol. 101 N° 2 (Feb), pp. 347-354. ISSN 1349-7006

Kehlen, A., Lendeckel, U., Dralle, H., Langner, J., & Hoang-Vu, C. (2003) Biological significance of aminopeptidase N/CD13 in thyroid carcinomas, *Cancer Research,* Vol. 63 N° 23 (Dec 1), pp. 8500-8506. ISSN 0008-5472

Khin, E. E., Kikkawa, F., Ino, K., Suzuki, T., Shibata, K., et al. (2003) Neutral endopeptidase/CD10 expression in the stroma of epithelial ovarian carcinoma, *International Journal of Gynecological Pathology,* Vol. 22 N° 2 (Apr), pp. 175-180, ISSN 0277-1691

Kikkawa, F., Kajiyama, H., Shibata, K., Ino, K., Nomura, S., et al. (2005) Dipeptidyl peptidase IV in tumour progression, *Biochimica et Biophysica Acta,* Vol. 1751 N° 1 (Aug 1), pp. 45-51, ISSN 0006-3002

Kitamura, Y., Watanabe, M., Komatsubara, S., & Sakata, Y. (1990) [Urinary excretion of glycine.prolile dipeptidile aminopeptidase, N-acetyl-beta-D-glucosaminidase, alanine aminopeptidase and low molecular protein in patients with renal cell carcinoma], *Hinyokika Kiyo (Acta Urologica Japonica),* Vol. 36 N° 5 (May), pp. 535-539, ISSN 0018-1994

Knopfel, M., Davies, J. P., Duong, P. T., Kvaerno, L., Carreira, E. M., et al. (2007) Multiple plasma membrane receptors but not NPC1L1 mediate high-affinity, ezetimibe-sensitive cholesterol uptake into the intestinal brush border membrane, *Biochimica et Biophysica Acta,* Vol. 1771 N° 9 (Sep), pp. 1140-1147, ISSN 0006-3002

Koszalka, P., Ozuyaman, B., Huo, Y., Zernecke, A., Flogel, U., et al. (2004) Targeted disruption of cd73/ecto-5'-nucleotidase alters thromboregulation and augments vascular inflammatory response, *Circulation Research,* Vol. 95 N° 8 (Oct 15), pp. 814-821, ISSN 1524-4571

Larsen, S. L., Pedersen, L. O., Buus, S., & Stryhn, A. (1996) T cell responses affected by aminopeptidase N (CD13)-mediated trimming of major histocompatibility complex class II-bound peptides, *Journal of Experimental Medicine,* Vol. 184 N° 1 (Jul 1), pp. 183-189, ISSN 0022-1007

Lavagno, L., Ferrero, E., Ortolan, E., Malavasi, F., & Funaro, A. (2007) CD157 is part of a supramolecular complex with CD11b/CD18 on the human neutrophil cell surface, *Journal of Biological Regulators and Homeostatic Agents,* Vol. 21 N° 1-2 pp. 5-11.

Lee, J., Duk Jung, I., Gyo Park, C., Han, J. W., & Young Lee, H. (2006) Autotaxin stimulates urokinase-type plasminogen activator expression through phosphoinositide 3-kinase-Akt-nuclear [corrected] factor kappa B signaling cascade in human melanoma cells, *Melanoma Research,* Vol. 16 N° 5 (Oct), pp. 445-452, ISSN 0960-8931

Lerche, C., Vogel, L. K., Shapiro, L. H., Noren, O., & Sjostrom, H. (1996) Human aminopeptidase N is encoded by 20 exons, *Mammalian Genome,* Vol. 7 N° 9 (Sep), pp. 712-713, ISSN 0938-8990

Leth-Larsen, R., Lund, R., Hansen, H. V., Laenkholm, A. V., Tarin, D., et al. (2009) Metastasis-related plasma membrane proteins of human breast cancer cells identified by comparative quantitative mass spectrometry, *Molecular and Cellular Proteomics,* Vol. 8 N° 6 (Jun), pp. 1436-1449, ISSN 1535-9484

Lin, M. E., Herr, D. R., & Chun, J. (2010) Lysophosphatidic acid (LPA) receptors: signaling properties and disease relevance, *Prostaglandins and Other Lipid Mediators,* Vol. 91 N° 3-4 (Apr), pp. 130-138, ISSN 1098-8823

Liu, S., Umezu-Goto, M., Murph, M., Lu, Y., Liu, W., et al. (2009) Expression of autotaxin and lysophosphatidic acid receptors increases mammary tumourigenesis, invasion, and metastases, *Cancer Cell,* Vol. 15 N° 6 (Jun 2), pp. 539-550, ISSN 1878-3686

Lo Buono, N., Parrotta, R., Morone, S., Bovino, P., Nacci, G., et al. (2011) The CD157-integrin partnership controls transendothelial migration and adhesion of human monocytes *Journal of Biological Chemistry,* Vol. 286, N°21 (May) pp. 18681-18691, ISSN 0021-9258

Loke, S. L., Leung, C. Y., Chiu, K. Y., Yau, W. L., Cheung, K. N., et al. (1990) Localisation of CD10 to biliary canaliculi by immunoelectron microscopical examination, *Journal of Clinical Pathology,* Vol. 43 N° 8 (Aug), pp. 654-656, ISSN 0021-9746

Madara, J. L., Patapoff, T. W., Gillece-Castro, B., Colgan, S. P., Parkos, C. A., et al. (1993) 5'-adenosine monophosphate is the neutrophil-derived paracrine factor that elicits chloride secretion from T84 intestinal epithelial cell monolayers, *Journal of Clinical Investigation,* Vol. 91 N° 5 (May), pp. 2320-2325, ISSN 0021-9738

Maienschein, V., & Zimmermann, H. (1996) Immunocytochemical localization of ecto-5'-nucleotidase in cultures of cerebellar granule cells, *Neuroscience,* Vol. 70 N° 2 (Jan), pp. 429-438, ISSN 0306-4522

Malavasi, F., Deaglio, S., Funaro, A., Ferrero, E., Horenstein, A. L., et al. (2008) Evolution and function of the ADP ribosyl cyclase/CD38 gene family in physiology and pathology, *Physiological Reviews,* Vol. 88 N° 3 (Jul), pp. 841-886, ISSN 0031-9333

Massaia, M., Pileri, A., Boccadoro, M., Bianchi, A., Palumbo, A., et al. (1988) The generation of alloreactive cytotoxic T lymphocytes requires the expression of ecto-5'nucleotidase activity, *Journal of Immunology,* Vol. 141 N° 11 (Dec 1), pp. 3768-3775, ISSN 0022-1767

Masuda, A., Nakamura, K., Izutsu, K., Igarashi, K., Ohkawa, R., et al. (2008) Serum autotaxin measurement in haematological malignancies: a promising marker for follicular lymphoma, *British Journal of Haematology,* Vol. 143 N° 1 (Oct), pp. 60-70, ISSN 1365-2141

Matsas, R., Stephenson, S. L., Hryszko, J., Kenny, A. J., & Turner, A. J. (1985) The metabolism of neuropeptides. Phase separation of synaptic membrane preparations with Triton X-114 reveals the presence of aminopeptidase N, *Biochemical Journal,* Vol. 231 N° 2 (Oct 15), pp. 445-449, ISSN 0264-6021

Metzgar, R. S., Borowitz, M. J., Jones, N. H., & Dowell, B. L. (1981) Distribution of common acute lymphoblastic leukemia antigen in nonhematopoietic tissues, *Journal of Experimental Medicine,* Vol. 154 N° 4 (Oct 1), pp. 1249-1254, ISSN 0022-1007

Miki, T., Takegami, Y., Okawa, K., Muraguchi, T., Noda, M., et al. (2007) The reversion-inducing cysteine-rich protein with Kazal motifs (RECK) interacts with membrane type 1 matrix metalloproteinase and CD13/aminopeptidase N and modulates their endocytic pathways, *Journal of Biological Chemistry,* Vol. 282 N° 16 (Apr 20), pp. 12341-12352, ISSN 0021-9258

Mills, G. B., May, C., McGill, M., Roifman, C. M., & Mellors, A. (1988) A putative new growth factor in ascitic fluid from ovarian cancer patients: identification, characterization, and mechanism of action, *Cancer Research,* Vol. 48 N° 5 (Mar 1), pp. 1066-1071, ISSN 0008-5472

Mills, G. B., & Moolenaar, W. H. (2003) The emerging role of lysophosphatidic acid in cancer, *Nature Reviews. Cancer,* Vol. 3 N° 8 (Aug), pp. 582-591. 1474-175X

Mina-Osorio, P., & Ortega, E. (2005) Aminopeptidase N (CD13) functionally interacts with FcgammaRs in human monocytes, *Journal of Leukocyte Biology,* Vol. 77 N° 6 (Jun), pp. 1008-1017, ISSN 0741-5400

Mina-Osorio, P., Shapiro, L. H., & Ortega, E. (2006) CD13 in cell adhesion: aminopeptidase N (CD13) mediates homotypic aggregation of monocytic cells, *Journal of Leukocyte Biology,* Vol. 79 N° 4 (Apr), pp. 719-730, ISSN 0741-5400

Mizutani, S., Kajiyama, H., Suzuki, T., Shibata, K., Ino, K., et al. (2003) Survival time and invasive activity due to dipeptidyl peptidase IV overexpression in ovarian carcinoma, *Advances in Experimental Medicine and Biology,* Vol. 524 N° pp. 253-256, ISSN 0065-2598

Moreschi, I., Bruzzone, S., Bodrato, N., Usai, C., Guida, L., et al. (2008) NAADP+ is an agonist of the human P2Y11 purinergic receptor, *Cell Calcium,* Vol. 43 N° 4 (Apr), pp. 344-355, ISSN 0143-4160

Morrison, M. E., Vijayasaradhi, S., Engelstein, D., Albino, A. P., & Houghton, A. N. (1993) A marker for neoplastic progression of human melanocytes is a cell surface ectopeptidase, *Journal of Experimental Medicine,* Vol. 177 N° 4 (Apr 1), pp. 1135-1143, ISSN 0022-1007

Muraoka, O., Tanaka, H., Itoh, M., Ishihara, K., & Hirano, T. (1996) Genomic structure of human BST-1, *Immunology Letters,* Vol. 54 N° 1 (Dec 1), pp. 1-4, ISSN 0165-2478

Nagy, J. A., Masse, E. M., Herzberg, K. T., Meyers, M. S., Yeo, K. T., et al. (1995) Pathogenesis of ascites tumour growth: vascular permeability factor, vascular hyperpermeability, and ascites fluid accumulation, *Cancer Research,* Vol. 55 N° 2 (Jan 15), pp. 360-368, ISSN 0008-5472

Nakai, Y., Ikeda, H., Nakamura, K., Kume, Y., Fujishiro, M., et al. (2011) Specific increase in serum autotaxin activity in patients with pancreatic cancer, *Clinical Biochemistry,* Vol. 44 N° 8-9 (Jun), pp. 576-581, ISSN 1873-2933

Nakanaga, K., Hama, K., & Aoki, J. (2010) Autotaxin--an LPA producing enzyme with diverse functions, *J Biochem,* Vol. 148 N° 1 (Jul), pp. 13-24, ISSN 1756-2651

Nam, S. W., Clair, T., Campo, C. K., Lee, H. Y., Liotta, L. A., et al. (2000) Autotaxin (ATX), a potent tumour motogen, augments invasive and metastatic potential of ras-transformed cells, *Oncogene,* Vol. 19 N° 2 (Jan 13), pp. 241-247, ISSN 0950-9232

Nam, S. W., Clair, T., Kim, Y. S., McMarlin, A., Schiffmann, E., et al. (2001) Autotaxin (NPP-2), a metastasis-enhancing motogen, is an angiogenic factor, *Cancer Research,* Vol. 61 N° 18 (Sep 15), pp. 6938-6944, ISSN 0008-5472

Naora, H., & Montell, D. J. (2005) Ovarian cancer metastasis: integrating insights from disparate model organisms, *Nature Reviews. Cancer,* Vol. 5 N° 5 (May), pp. 355-366, ISSN 1474-175X

Nemoto, E., Kunii, R., Tada, H., Tsubahara, T., Ishihata, H., et al. (2004) Expression of CD73/ecto-5'-nucleotidase on human gingival fibroblasts and contribution to the inhibition of interleukin-1alpha-induced granulocyte-macrophage colony stimulating factor production, *Journal of Periodontal Research,* Vol. 39 N° 1 (Feb), pp. 10-19, ISSN 0022-3484

Nishimasu, H., Okudaira, S., Hama, K., Mihara, E., Dohmae, N., et al. (2011) Crystal structure of autotaxin and insight into GPCR activation by lipid mediators, *Nature Structural and Molecular Biology,* Vol. 18 N° 2 (Feb), pp. 205-212, ISSN 1545-9985

Noble, F., & Roques, B. P. (1997) Association of aminopeptidase N and endopeptidase 24.15 inhibitors potentiate behavioral effects mediated by nociceptin/orphanin FQ in mice, *FEBS Letters,* Vol. 401 N° 2-3 (Jan 20), pp. 227-229, ISSN 0014-5793

Nomura, R., Kiyota, A., Suzaki, E., Kataoka, K., Ohe, Y., et al. (2004) Human coronavirus 229E binds to CD13 in rafts and enters the cell through caveolae, *Journal of Virology,* Vol. 78 N° 16 (Aug), pp. 8701-8708, ISSN 0022-538X

Noren, O. (1986) The enzymes of the enterocyte plasma membrane, In: *Molecular and cellular basis of digestion,* Desnuelle P., 133-167, Elsevier, Amsterdam, Holland.

O'Hare, M. J., Ormerod, M. G., Monaghan, P., Lane, E. B., & Gusterson, B. A. (1991) Characterization in vitro of luminal and myoepithelial cells isolated from the human mammary gland by cell sorting, *Differentiation,* Vol. 46 N° 3 (Apr), pp. 209-221, ISSN 0301-4681

Ohta, A., Gorelik, E., Prasad, S. J., Ronchese, F., Lukashev, D., et al. (2006) A2A adenosine receptor protects tumours from antitumour T cells, *Proceedings of the National*

Academy of Sciences of the United States of America, Vol. 103 N° 35 (Aug 29), pp. 13132-13137, ISSN 0027-8424

Olsen, J., Cowell, G. M., Konigshofer, E., Danielsen, E. M., Moller, J., et al. (1988) Complete amino acid sequence of human intestinal aminopeptidase N as deduced from cloned cDNA, *FEBS Letters,* Vol. 238 N° 2 (Oct 10), pp. 307-314, ISSN 0014-5793

Ortolan, E., Vacca, P., Capobianco, A., Armando, E., Crivellin, F., et al. (2002) CD157, the Janus of CD38 but with a unique personality, *Cell Biochemistry and Function,* Vol. 20 N° 4 (Dec), pp. 309-322, ISSN 0263-6484

Ortolan, E., Tibaldi, E. V., Ferranti, B., Lavagno, L., Garbarino, G., et al. (2006) CD157 plays a pivotal role in neutrophil transendothelial migration, *Blood,* Vol. 108 N° 13 (Dec 15), pp. 4214-4222, ISSN 0006-4971

Ortolan, E., Arisio, R., Morone, S., Bovino, P., Lo-Buono, N., et al. (2010) Functional Role and Prognostic Significance of CD157 in Ovarian Carcinoma, *Journal of the National Cancer Institute,* Vol. 105 N° 16 (Jul 16), pp. 1160-1177, ISSN 1460-2105

Papandreou, C. N., Usmani, B., Geng, Y., Bogenrieder, T., Freeman, R., et al. (1998) Neutral endopeptidase 24.11 loss in metastatic human prostate cancer contributes to androgen-independent progression, *Nature Medicine,* Vol. 4 N° 1 (Jan), pp. 50-57, ISSN 1078-8956

Pesando, J. M., Tomaselli, K. J., Lazarus, H., & Schlossman, S. F. (1983) Distribution and modulation of a human leukemia-associated antigen (CALLA), *Journal of Immunology,* Vol. 131 N° 4 (Oct), pp. 2038-2045, ISSN 0022-1767

Pethiyagoda, C. L., Welch, D. R., & Fleming, T. P. (2000) Dipeptidyl peptidase IV (DPPIV) inhibits cellular invasion of melanoma cells, *Clinical and Experimental Metastasis,* Vol. 18 N° 5 pp. 391-400, ISSN 0262-0898

Pfleiderer, G., & Celliers, P. G. (1963) [Isolation of an Aminopeptidase from Kidney Particles], *Biochemische Zeitschrift,* Vol. 339 N° (Dec 3), pp. 186-189. ISSN 0366-0753

Ptaszynska, M. M., Pendrak, M. L., Bandle, R. W., Stracke, M. L., & Roberts, D. D. (2008) Positive feedback between vascular endothelial growth factor-A and autotaxin in ovarian cancer cells, *Molecular Cancer Research,* Vol. 6 N° 3 (Mar), pp. 352-363, ISSN 1541-7786

Rabinovich, G. A., Gabrilovich, D., & Sotomayor, E. M. (2007) Immunosuppressive strategies that are mediated by tumour cells, *Annual Review of Immunology,* Vol. 25 N° pp. 267-296, ISSN 0732-0582

Razak, K., & Newland, A. C. (1992) The significance of aminopeptidases and haematopoietic cell differentiation, *Blood Reviews,* Vol. 6 N° 4 (Dec), pp. 243-250, ISSN 0268-960X

Resta, R., Yamashita, Y., & Thompson, L. F. (1998) Ecto-enzyme and signaling functions of lymphocyte CD73, *Immunological Reviews,* Vol. 161 N° (Feb), pp. 95-109, ISSN 0105-2896

Richardson, A., & Kaye, S. B. (2005) Drug resistance in ovarian cancer: the emerging importance of gene transcription and spatio-temporal regulation of resistance, *Drug Resistance Updates,* Vol. 8 N° 5 (Oct), pp. 311-321, ISSN 1368-7646

Ritz, J., Pesando, J. M., Notis-McConarty, J., Lazarus, H., & Schlossman, S. F. (1980) A monoclonal antibody to human acute lymphoblastic leukaemia antigen, *Nature,* Vol. 283 N° 5747 (Feb 7), pp. 583-585, ISSN 0028-0836

Ross, J. A., Ansell, I., Hjelle, J. T., Anderson, J. D., Miller-Hjelle, M. A., et al. (1998) Phenotypic mapping of human mesothelial cells, *Advances in Peritoneal Dialysis,* Vol. 14 N° pp. 25-30. ISSN 1197-8554

Saiki, I., Fujii, H., Yoneda, J., Abe, F., Nakajima, M., et al. (1993) Role of aminopeptidase N (CD13) in tumour-cell invasion and extracellular matrix degradation, *International Journal of Cancer,* Vol. 54 N° 1 (Apr 22), pp. 137-143, ISSN 0020-7136

Salani, D., Di Castro, V., Nicotra, M. R., Rosano, L., Tecce, R., et al. (2000) Role of endothelin-1 in neovascularization of ovarian carcinoma, *American Journal of Pathology,* Vol. 157 N° 5 (Nov), pp. 1537-1547, ISSN 0002-9440

Salles, G., Chen, C. Y., Reinherz, E. L., & Shipp, M. A. (1992) CD10/NEP is expressed on Thy-1low B220+ murine B-cell progenitors and functions to regulate stromal cell-dependent lymphopoiesis, *Blood,* Vol. 80 N° 8 (Oct 15), pp. 2021-2029, ISSN 0006-4971

Salmi, M., & Jalkanen, S. (2011) Homing-associated molecules CD73 and VAP-1 as targets to prevent harmful inflammations and cancer spread, *FEBS Letters,* Vol. 585 N° 11 (Jun 6), pp. 1543-1550, ISSN 1873-3468

Samadi, N., Gaetano, C., Goping, I. S., & Brindley, D. N. (2009) Autotaxin protects MCF-7 breast cancer and MDA-MB-435 melanoma cells against Taxol-induced apoptosis, *Oncogene,* Vol. 28 N° 7 (Feb 19), pp. 1028-1039, ISSN 1476-5594

Samadi, N., Bekele, R. T., Goping, I. S., Schang, L. M., & Brindley, D. N. (2011) Lysophosphatidate induces chemo-resistance by releasing breast cancer cells from taxol-induced mitotic arrest, *PLoS ONE,* Vol. 6 N° 5 pp. e20608, ISSN 1932-6203

Santos, A. N., Langner, J., Herrmann, M., & Riemann, D. (2000) Aminopeptidase N/CD13 is directly linked to signal transduction pathways in monocytes, *Cellular Immunology,* Vol. 201 N° 1 (Apr 10), pp. 22-32, ISSN 0008-8749

Semenza, G. (1986) Anchoring and biosynthesis of stalked brush border membrane proteins: glycosidases and peptidases of enterocytes and renal tubuli, *Annual Review of Cell Biology,* Vol. 2 N° pp. 255-313, ISSN 0743-4634

Shipp, M. A., Richardson, N. E., Sayre, P. H., Brown, N. R., Masteller, E. L., et al. (1988) Molecular cloning of the common acute lymphoblastic leukemia antigen (CALLA) identifies a type II integral membrane protein, *Proceedings of the National Academy of Sciences of the United States of America,* Vol. 85 N° 13 (Jul), pp. 4819-4823, ISSN 0027-8424

Shipp, M. A., Vijayaraghavan, J., Schmidt, E. V., Masteller, E. L., D'Adamio, L., et al. (1989) Common acute lymphoblastic leukemia antigen (CALLA) is active neutral endopeptidase 24.11 ("enkephalinase"): direct evidence by cDNA transfection analysis, *Proceedings of the National Academy of Sciences of the United States of America,* Vol. 86 N° 1 (Jan), pp. 297-301, ISSN 0027-8424

Shipp, M. A., & Look, A. T. (1993) Hematopoietic differentiation antigens that are membrane-associated enzymes: cutting is the key!, *Blood,* Vol. 82 N° 4 (Aug 15), pp. 1052-1070, ISSN 0006-4971

Spychala, J., Lazarowski, E., Ostapkowicz, A., Ayscue, L. H., Jin, A., et al. (2004) Role of estrogen receptor in the regulation of ecto-5'-nucleotidase and adenosine in breast cancer, *Clinical Cancer Research,* Vol. 10 N° 2 (Jan 15), pp. 708-717, ISSN 1078-0432

Stagg, J., Divisekera, U., McLaughlin, N., Sharkey, J., Pommey, S., et al. (2010a) Anti-CD73 antibody therapy inhibits breast tumour growth and metastasis, *Proceedings of the*

National Academy of Sciences of the United States of America, Vol. 107 N° 4 (Jan 26), pp. 1547-1552, ISSN 1091-6490

Stagg, J., & Smyth, M. J. (2010b) Extracellular adenosine triphosphate and adenosine in cancer, *Oncogene,* Vol. 29 N° 39 (Sep 30), pp. 5346-5358, ISSN 1476-5594

Stracke, M. L., Krutzsch, H. C., Unsworth, E. J., Arestad, A., Cioce, V., et al. (1992) Identification, purification, and partial sequence analysis of autotaxin, a novel motility-stimulating protein, *Journal of Biological Chemistry,* Vol. 267 N° 4 (Feb 5), pp. 2524-2529, ISSN 0021-9258

Stremenova, J., Krepela, E., Mares, V., Trim, J., Dbaly, V., et al. (2007) Expression and enzymatic activity of dipeptidyl peptidase-IV in human astrocytic tumours are associated with tumour grade, *International Journal of Oncology,* Vol. 31 N° 4 (Oct), pp. 785-792, ISSN 1019-6439

Strohmeier, G. R., Lencer, W. I., Patapoff, T. W., Thompson, L. F., Carlson, S. L., et al. (1997) Surface expression, polarization, and functional significance of CD73 in human intestinal epithelia, *Journal of Clinical Investigation,* Vol. 99 N° 11 (Jun 1), pp. 2588-2601, ISSN 0021-9738

Suzuki, T., Kikkawa, F., Ino, K., Nagasaka, T., Tamakoshi, K., et al. (2001) Imbalance between neutral endopeptidase 24.11 and endothelin-1 expression in human endometrial carcinoma, *Oncology,* Vol. 60 N° 3 pp. 258-267, ISSN 0030-2414

Tanaka, T., Camerini, D., Seed, B., Torimoto, Y., Dang, N. H., et al. (1992) Cloning and functional expression of the T cell activation antigen CD26, *Journal of Immunology,* Vol. 149 N° 2 (Jul 15), pp. 481-486, ISSN 0022-1767

ten Kate, J., Wijnen, J. T., van der Goes, R. G., Quadt, R., Griffioen, G., et al. (1984) Quantitative changes in adenosine deaminase isoenzymes in human colorectal adenocarcinomas, *Cancer Research,* Vol. 44 N° 10 (Oct), pp. 4688-4692, ISSN 0008-5472

Terauchi, M., Kajiyama, H., Shibata, K., Ino, K., Nawa, A., et al. (2007) Inhibition of APN/CD13 leads to suppressed progressive potential in ovarian carcinoma cells, *BMC Cancer,* Vol. 7 N° pp. 140, ISSN 1471-2407

Tokumura, A., Majima, E., Kariya, Y., Tominaga, K., Kogure, K., et al. (2002) Identification of human plasma lysophospholipase D, a lysophosphatidic acid-producing enzyme, as autotaxin, a multifunctional phosphodiesterase, *Journal of Biological Chemistry,* Vol. 277 N° 42 (Oct 18), pp. 39436-39442, ISSN 0021-9258

van Hensbergen, Y., Broxterman, H. J., Hanemaaijer, R., Jorna, A. S., van Lent, N. A., et al. (2002) Soluble aminopeptidase N/CD13 in malignant and nonmalignant effusions and intratumoural fluid, *Clinical Cancer Research,* Vol. 8 N° 12 (Dec), pp. 3747-3754, ISSN 1078-0432

van Hensbergen, Y., Broxterman, H. J., Rana, S., van Diest, P. J., Duyndam, M. C., et al. (2004) Reduced growth, increased vascular area, and reduced response to cisplatin in CD13-overexpressing human ovarian cancer xenografts, *Clinical Cancer Research,* Vol. 10 N° 3 (Feb 1), pp. 1180-1191, ISSN 1078-0432

van Meeteren, L. A., & Moolenaar, W. H. (2007) Regulation and biological activities of the autotaxin-LPA axis, *Progress in Lipid Research,* Vol. 46 N° 2 (Mar), pp. 145-160, ISSN 0163-7827

Vidot, S., Witham, J., Agarwal, R., Greenhough, S., Bamrah, H. S., et al. (2010) Autotaxin delays apoptosis induced by carboplatin in ovarian cancer cells, *Cellular Signalling*, Vol. 22 N° 6 (Jun), pp. 926-935, ISSN 1873-3913

Watanabe, N., Ikeda, H., Nakamura, K., Ohkawa, R., Kume, Y., et al. (2007) Both plasma lysophosphatidic acid and serum autotaxin levels are increased in chronic hepatitis C, *Journal of Clinical Gastroenterology*, Vol. 41 N° 6 (Jul), pp. 616-623, ISSN 0192-0790

Wesley, U. V., Albino, A. P., Tiwari, S., & Houghton, A. N. (1999) A role for dipeptidyl peptidase IV in suppressing the malignant phenotype of melanocytic cells, *Journal of Experimental Medicine*, Vol. 190 N° 3 (Aug 2), pp. 311-322, ISSN 0022-1007

Xu, Y., Shen, Z., Wiper, D. W., Wu, M., Morton, R. E., et al. (1998) Lysophosphatidic acid as a potential biomarker for ovarian and other gynecologic cancers, *JAMA*, Vol. 280 N° 8 (Aug 26), pp. 719-723, ISSN 0098-7484

Yamaguchi, U., Nakayama, R., Honda, K., Ichikawa, H., Hasegawa, T., et al. (2008) Distinct gene expression-defined classes of gastrointestinal stromal tumour, *Journal of Clinical Oncology*, Vol. 26 N° 25 (Sep 1), pp. 4100-4108, ISSN 1527-7755

Yamashita, M., Kajiyama, H., Terauchi, M., Shibata, K., Ino, K., et al. (2007) Involvement of aminopeptidase N in enhanced chemosensitivity to paclitaxel in ovarian carcinoma in vitro and in vivo, *International Journal of Cancer*, Vol. 120 N° 10 (May 15), pp. 2243-2250, ISSN 0020-7136

Zhang, B. (2010) CD73: a novel target for cancer immunotherapy, *Cancer Research*, Vol. 70 N° 16 (Aug 15), pp. 6407-6411, ISSN 1538-7445

Zhang, M. Z., Qiao, Y. H., & Suo, Z. H. (2008) [Correlation of DPPIV expression with clinicopathological features and prognosis in epithelial ovarian carcinoma], *Zhonghua Zhong Liu Za Zhi (Chinese Journal of Oncology)*, Vol. 30 N° 11 (Nov), pp. 848-852, ISSN 0253-3766

Zhao, H., Ramos, C. F., Brooks, J. D., & Peehl, D. M. (2007) Distinctive gene expression of prostatic stromal cells cultured from diseased versus normal tissues, *Journal of Cellular Physiology*, Vol. 210 N° 1 (Jan), pp. 111-121, ISSN 0021-9541

15

VEGF Targeting Agents in Ovarian Cancer

Seiji Mabuchi, Atsuko Wakabayashi and Tadashi Kimura
Department of Obstetrics and Gynecology, Osaka University
Japan

1. Introduction

Angiogenesis, the formation of new blood vessels, is a critical component in the growth and metastasis of cancers and has been recognized as an attractive target for anticancer therapy (Ferrara, 2002). Among the pro-angiogenic factors, vascular endothelial growth factor (VEGF) is recognized as the predominant mediator of angiogenesis in tumor cells (Ferrara & Kerbel, 2005). As VEGF is overexpressed in most ovarian cancers, the VEGF pathway is a promising target for anti-angiogenic therapy against ovarian cancer (Burger, 2011).

Recent increases in our understanding of the molecular pathways that control tumor angiogenesis have led to the development of novel VEGF-targeting agents for the treatment of ovarian cancer (Burger, 2011). In addition to inhibiting neo-vascularization, anti-angiogenic agents are also believed to normalize intratumoral blood vessels. Intratumoral vessels are hyperpermeable, leading to interstitial hypertension and impaired perfusion in tumors. Normalization of the tumor vasculature results in a reduction in interstitial pressure and the improved delivery of oxygen, nutrients, and cytotoxic agents (Ferrara, 2002).

Many of these agents have been evaluated in clinical trials, and some of them have shown promising clinical activity against ovarian cancer (Burger, 2011). In this article, we review the emerging VEGF-targeting strategies for treating ovarian cancer and provide information about the latest clinical studies of VEGF-targeting agents that have been employed as treatments for ovarian cancer.

2. Angiogenesis overview

Angiogenesis is the process by which new blood vessels grow from the existing vasculature. A tumor is unable to grow beyond 2mm diameter without neoangiogenesis (Carmeliet, 2000), thus, angiogenesis plays an essential role in tumor growth, invasion, and metastasis (Carmeliet, 2000; Kerbel, 1991). Angiogenesis is tightly regulated by balancing pro- and anti-angiogenic factors. The transition of a tumor from "avascular phase" to "vascular phase" is termed "angiogenic switch". This switch is believed to be stimulated by an increase in expression of pro-angiogenic factors. A variety of pro-angiogenic factors have been identified and recognized as potential targets of antiangiogenic therapy (Ferrara & Kerbel, 2005). Vascular endothelial cell growth factor (VEGF), one of the key mediators of angiogenesis, promotes the proliferation, survival, and migration of endothelial cells and is essential for blood vessel formation (Ferrara & Kerbel, 2005). VEGF can also affect new vessel formation in tumors by acting as a chemoattractant for bone marrow-derived progenitor cells (Rafii et al., 2002). The major physiological stimulus for VEGF expression is hypoxia, which commonly develops within tumors when cancer cell proliferation exceeds the rate of blood vessel formation. Hypoxia inducible factor-1α (HIF-1α), a transcriptional activator that acts as a central regulator of oxygen homeostasis, regulates the expression of VEGF and promotes angiogenesis, which is essential for fulfilling the metabolic requirements of tumor growth (Forsythe et al., 1996).

3. Vascular endothelial growth factor (VEGF): Structure and function

VEGF (also referred to as VEGF-A) is a dimeric protein that has been shown to stimulate angiogenesis. As it also enhances vascular permeability, VEGF is also recognized as vascular permeability factor (VPF) (Ferrara & Kerbel, 2005).

VEGF is a member of the VEGF/PDGF gene family. Other members of this family include VEGF-B, VEGF-C, VEGF-D, PDGF, and PIGF (Ferrara & Kerbel, 2005). VEGF exerts its biological effects by interacting with the VEGF receptors (VEGFR) present on the cell surface (Figure 1). These transmembrane receptors include VEGFR-1 (also known as Flt-1) and VEGFR-2 (Flk-1), which are predominantly expressed on vascular endothelial cells. A third receptor, VEGFR-3 (Flt-4), is mainly involved in the regulation of lymphatic systems (Karkkainen et al., 2001). The binding of VEGF to its receptor causes the dimerization and phosphorylation of intracellular receptor kinases, which in turn activates a cascade of downstream signals responsible for tumor angiogenesis (Ferrara & Kerbel, 2005).

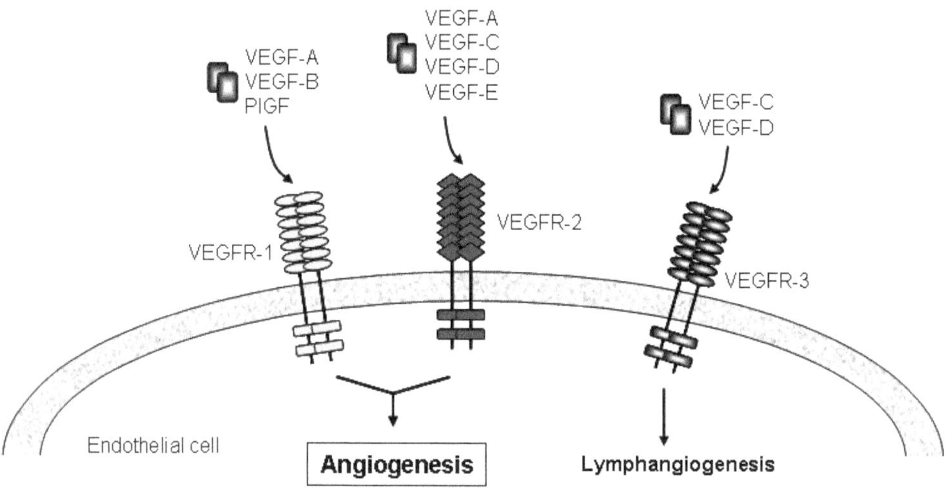

Fig. 1. VEGF signaling.

4. Role of VEGF in epithelial ovarian cancer: Preclinical findings

4.1 VEGF expression in epithelial ovarian cancer

VEGF expression in epithelial ovarian cancer has been intensively examined (Wong et al., 2003; Yamamoto et al., 1997; Brustmann, 2004; Mabuchi et al., 2010b). It has been generally accepted that VEGF expression is greater in ovarian cancers than in normal ovarian tissue or benign ovarian neoplasm. According to previous reports, in which common histological subtypes such as serous adenocarcinoma or endometrioid adenocarcinoma were investigated, the expression rate of VEGF was approximately 90% (Wong et al., 2003; Yamamoto et al., 1997; Brustmann, 2004). In a recent report about clear cell carcinoma of the ovary, strong VEGF expression was observed in 86% of cases (Mabuchi et al., 2010b). These results suggest that most epithelial ovarian cancers are dependent on VEGF for tumor progression, and hence, are candidates for VEGF targeting therapy.

4.2 VEGF expression and patient prognosis

In patients with ovarian cancer, high serum VEGF levels are an independent risk factor for advanced stage and decreased survival (Mabuchi et al., 2010b; Cooper et al., 2002; Li et al., 2004; Hefler et al., 2006). Moreover, previous immunohistochemical analyses have suggested that VEGF expression in ovarian cancer specimens is also associated with poor patient prognosis, advanced stage, and short survival (Mabuchi et al., 2010b; Cooper et al., 2002; Li et al., 2004; Hefler et al., 2006). For example, in a recent investigation of ovarian clear cell carcinomas (Mabuchi et al., 2010b), patients whose tumor showed strong immunoreactivity displayed significantly shorter survival than those with weak immunoreactivity for VEGF (mean: 60 months vs. 40 months, respectively). The association observed between VEGF expression and clinical outcome in ovarian cancer patients makes the VEGF pathway an attractive therapeutic target in this patient group.

4.3 VEGF expression and ascites formation

The effect of VEGF on vascular permeability is believed to be crucial for malignant ascites formation (Senger et al., 1983; Zhang et al., 2002). In patients with ovarian cancer, high serum VEGF levels was reported to be an independent risk factor for developing ascites formation (Cooper et al., 2002; Li et al., 2004; Hefler et al., 2006). In an in vivo investigation using an intraperitoneal ovarian cancer model, VEGF inhibition resulted in the complete inhibition of ascites formation (Mesiano et al., 1998; Mabuchi et al., 2008). Since patients with advanced or recurrent ovarian cancer frequently suffer from malignant ascites and require paracentesis for symptomatic relief, the ability of VEGF-targeting agents to inhibit ascites formation makes them attractive candidate treatments for ovarian cancer (Numnum et al., 2006).

4.4 VEGF expression and chemoresistance

It has been reported that chemoresistant tumors display greater VEGF expression than chemosensitive tumors (Mabuchi et al., 2010b; Schönau et al., 2007). For example, 5-fluorouracil-resistant colon adenocarcinoma subclones were found to display increased VEGF expression and enhanced pro-angiogenic activity compared to the corresponding primary adenocarcinoma cells (Schönau et al., 2007). Moreover, cisplatin-refractory ovarian cancer cell lines exhibit higher VEGF expression than their parental cisplatin-sensitive cell lines (Mabuchi et al., 2010b). As VEGF increases vascular permeability, which leads to interstitial hypertension and the impaired delivery of cytotoxic agents to tumors; theoretically, increased VEGF production in chemoresistant tumors might further limit the efficacy of chemotherapy (Gerber & Ferrara, 2005). Therefore, VEGF inhibition is a reasonable treatment strategy for overcoming chemoresistance or enhancing the sensitivity of ovarian cancer to chemotherapeutic agents.

4.5 VEGF receptor expression in epithelial ovarian cancer

VEGFR are predominantly expressed on vascular endothelial cells. However, recent reports have suggested that VEGFR are also expressed by some tumor cells including ovarian cancer cells (Sood et al., 2001; Spannuth et al., 2009). In a study by Spannuth et al, in situ hybridization revealed that VEGFR-1 and VEGFR-2 expression was observed in 85% and 15% of human ovarian cancer specimens, respectively. Moreover, using the ovarian cancer cell lines, the authors showed that functionally active VEGFR is present on most ovarian cancer cells (Spannuth et al., 2009). Although the biological role of the VEGFR expressed on tumor cells remains unclear, they might represent an additional target of ovarian cancer therapy.

5. VEGF targeting agents

It is generally accepted that, unlike normal vasculature, the intratumoral vessels produced by VEGF-mediated angiogenesis are hyperpermeable, leading to increased interstitial fluid pressure and the impaired perfusion of oxygen and cytotoxic agents into tumors. The resultant hypoxic conditions in tumor cells further increase the expression of VEGF and limit the efficacy of chemotherapy and radiotherapy (Gerber & Ferrara, 2005). Theoretically, the inhibition of VEGF by VEGF-targeting agents should inhibit neo-vascularization and "normalize" poorly formed, leaky intratumoral blood vessels. This could lead to the improved delivery of cytotoxic agents and oxygen to tumors (Gerber & Ferrara, 2005).

There are two major strategies used to inhibit the VEGF pathway in cancer therapy (Spannuth et al., 2008). One is the inhibition of the VEGF ligand with antibodies or soluble receptors, and the other is the inhibition of the VEGF receptor with tyrosine kinase inhibitors (TKI) or receptor antibodies (Figure 2). Various VEGF-targeting agents have been identified and are currently being evaluated clinically or preclinically. Of these, bevacizumab, aflibercept, and several TKI are currently being evaluated in phase III clinical trials for the treatment of epithelial ovarian cancer (Table 1-2).

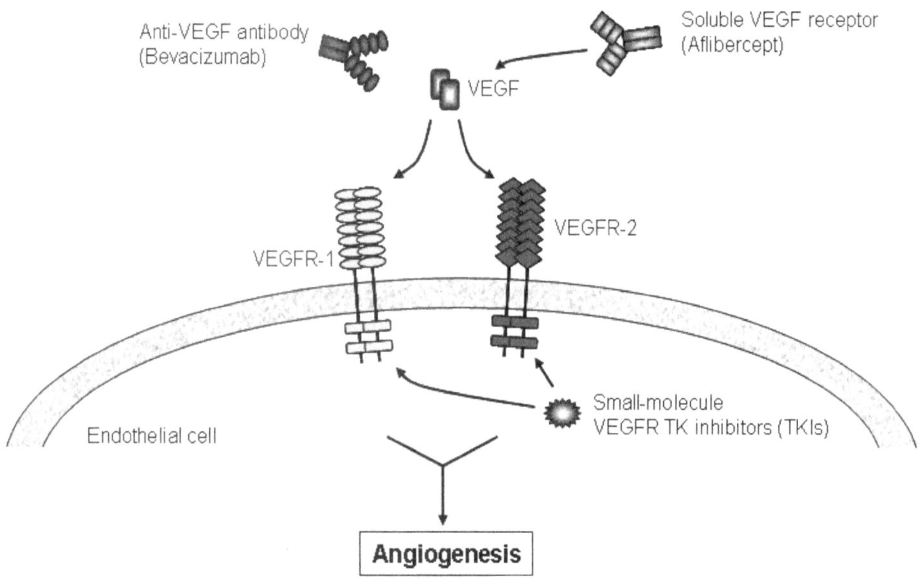

Fig. 2. Strategy to inhibit VEGF signaling

6. Therapeutic potential of VEGF targeted agents in ovarian cancer: Preclinical findings

Among the VEGF-targeting agents including bevacizumab, aflibercept, and TKI, bevacizumab has been used most commonly for the treatment of ovarian cancer in the clinical setting. Thus, we herein provide information regarding the preclinical activity of bevacizumab in ovarian cancer.

6.1 Monotherapy

Preclinical in vivo studies have demonstrated that inhibiting VEGF activity using a murine monoclonal antibody to human VEGF (A4.6.1) significantly inhibited the growth of subcutaneously inoculated ovarian tumors. Moreover, in mice carrying intraperitoneal tumors, treatment with A4.6.1 completely inhibited ascites production (Mesiano et al., 1998). Bevacizumab is the humanized form of A4.6.1, which was developed in 1997 (Presta et al., 1997). In a preclinical investigation, treatment with bevacizumab significantly inhibited the growth of intraperitoneally inoculated serous ovarian cancer. In addition, bevacizumab treatment significantly inhibited ascites production and prolonged survival of the mice (Mabuchi et al., 2008).

The single agent activity of bevacizumab on chemoresistant ovarian cancer has also been evaluated preclinically. According to a recent report, the growth inhibitory effect of bevaciumab on cisplatin-resistant ovarian cancer was similar to the effect of bevacizumab on cisplatin-sensitive ovarian cancer (Mabuchi et al., 2010b). Collectively, these results suggest that both platinum-sensitive and platinum-resistant ovarian cancer are the candidates for VEGF-targeting therapy.

6.2 Combination therapy

Not only to inhibit neo-vascularization, VEGF-targeted agents are believed to normalize intra-tumoral blood vessels and improved delivery of oxygen, nutrients, and cytotoxic agents (Gerber & Ferrara, 2005; Jain, 2005). Thus, theoretically, VEGF-targeting agents should be efficacious in combination with chemotherapy.

In a mouse model of ovarian cancer, treatment with bevacizumab in combination with paclitaxel significantly reduced tumor growth compared with paclitaxel alone (83.3% reduction in the combination arm versus 58.5% reduction in the paclitaxel alone arm) and resulted in the complete inhibition of ascites formation (Hu et al., 2002). Similarly, treatment with bevacizumab in combination with cisplatin significantly reduced tumor growth and ascites formation compared with cisplatin therapy alone (Mabuchi et al., 2008).

6.3 Maintenance therapy

There is a strong rationale for using angiogenesis targeted agents in the maintenance therapy setting. Since it has been reported that tumors require a vascular blood supply to grow beyond 2 mm (Gimbrone et al., 1972), any subclinical ovarian tumors that are present after a complete clinical response to first-line chemotherapy should require angiogenesis for their continued proliferation, invasion, and metastasis. Thus, VEGF-targeting maintenance therapy after standard primary treatment might be beneficial for patients with ovarian cancer.

The effect of VEGF-targeting agent as a maintenance therapy has been investigated in an *in vivo* ovarian cancer model (Mabuchi et al., 2008). In this investigation, athymic mice were intraperitoneally inoculated with serous ovarian cancer cells. When bevacizumab was used as a maintenance treatment after a complete clinical response to front-line chemotherapy had been obtained, bevacizumab significantly inhibited the recurrence of ovarian cancer and prolonged the survival of the mice (Mabuchi et al., 2008). This is the only preclinical report in which a survival benefit was derived from the use of a VEGF-targeting agent in the setting of maintenance therapy.

7. VEGF targeting agents in ovarian cancer: A clinical trial review

7.1 Bevacizumab

To date, bevacizumab, a recombinant human monoclonal antibody to the VEGF ligand, is the most studied VEGF-targeting agent in patients with ovarian cancer (Eskander & Randall, 2011).

7.1.1 Bevacizumab in the setting of front-line, maintenance, or salvage therapy

The clinical activity of bevacizumab as a single agent has been prospectively examined in two phase II trials involving patients with recurrent ovarian cancer (Cannistra et al., 2007; Burger et al., 2007). The gynecologic oncology group (GOG) evaluated the efficacy of bevacizumab in a phase II clinical trial involving 62 patients with recurrent ovarian cancer (GOG 170-D). Of the patients enrolled, 3 patients showed a complete response, and 4 patients demonstrated a partial response, giving an overall response rate of 18% and a median response duration of 10.25 months. Importantly, an additional 34 patients (55%) showed disease stabilization (Burger et al., 2007). Canninstra et al. also investigated the activity of single agent bevacizumab in 44 patients with platinum-resistant, heavily pretreated ovarian cancer. Of the 44 patients, according to the RECIST guidelines, there were no complete responders, but 7 partial responders were observed. The median duration of the response was 4.3 months (Cannistra et al., 2007).

The effect of bevacizumab has also been examined in the setting of combination therapy in two phase II studies. Garcia et al. evaluated the activity of a combination of bevacizumab and oral cyclophosphamide in patients with recurrent ovarian cancer. Of the 70 patients enrolled, 17 patients (24%) demonstrated a partial response, and 44 patients (63%) showed disease stabilization (Garcia et al., 2008). Penson et al. recently reported on the efficacy of bevacizumab in combination with carboplatin and paclitaxel as a first-line chemotherapy for patients with advanced Mullerian tumors, most of which (73%) were ovarian cancers. Of a total of 28 patients with measurable disease, 11 patients (39%) demonstrated a complete response, and 10 patients (36%) showed a partial response (Penson et al., 2010).

The evidence of clinical activity found in these phase II studies has led to the development of phase III trials examining the use of bevacizumab for the treatment of ovarian cancer (Teoh & Secord, 2011; Burger, 2011) (Table 1).

The efficacy of Bevacizumab in combination with carboplatin and paclitaxel as a primary treatment is being evaluated in three phase III trials. The first is a three-arm placebo-controlled trial, GOG 218 (NCT00262847): a 3-armed trial designed to investigate the clinical benefit of adding bevacizumab to front-line carboplatin-paclitaxel chemotherapy, as well as the benefit of bevacizumab maintenance therapy in patients with advanced stage epithelial ovarian, primary peritoneal, or fallopian tube cancer (Figure 3). After a median follow-up period of 17.4 months, the preliminary results from 1873 patients were presented at the 2010 meeting of the American Society of Clinical Oncology (ASCO) (Burger et al., 2010). The patients who were treated with concurrent or maintenance bevacizumab showed significantly longer PFS than the standard chemotherapy arm (14.1 months versus 10.3 months; hazard ratio, 0.717; 95% confidence interval, 0.625-0.824; p<0.0001). No significant difference in PFS was observed between the patients treated with concurrent bevacizumab and those treated with standard chemotherapy (11.2 months versus 10.3 months; HR, 0.908; 95% CI, 0.759-1.040; p=0.008). The OS data were not mature at the time of the presentation due to the cohort suffering a mortality rate of 24%.

Study	Setting	Trial design	Status	Outcome
GOG 218	First-line adjuvant	Arm 1: CT Arm 2: CT+Bev Arm 3: CT+Bev+maintenance Bev	Completed accrual	Favoring Arm 3; HR 0.717; p<0.0001.
ICON-7	First-line adjuvant	Arm 1: CT Arm 2: CT+Bev+maintenance Bev	Completed accrual	Favoring arm 2; HR 0.81; p<0.0041.
GOG 252	First-line adjuvant	Arm 1: PTX (iv,d1, 8, 15)+ CBDCA (iv,d1)+ Bev+ maintenance Bev Arm 2: PTX (iv, d1, 8, 15)+ CBDCA (ip, d1)+Bev+ maintenance Bev Arm 3: PTX (iv,d1)+ PTX (ip, d8)+ CDDP (ip, d2)+ Bev+maintenance Bev	Open to accrual	
GOG 213	Recurrent	Arm 1: CT Arm 2: CT+Bev+maintenance Bev	Open to accrual	
OCEANS	Recurrent	Arm 1: CG Arm 2: CG+Bev+maintenance Bev	Completed accrual	Results not yet available
AURELIA	Recurrent	Arm 1: PTX, Topo, or PLD Arm 2: PTX, Topo, or PLD+Bev	Open to accrual	

Table 1. Summary of randomized controlled trials evaluating bevacizumab in ovarian cancer. CT, carboplatin plus paclitaxel; CG, carboplatin plus gemcitabine, Bev, bevacizumab, PTX, paclitaxel; CBDCA, carboplatin; CDDP, cisplatin; Topo, topotecan; PLD, liposomal doxorubicin; HR, hazard ratio.

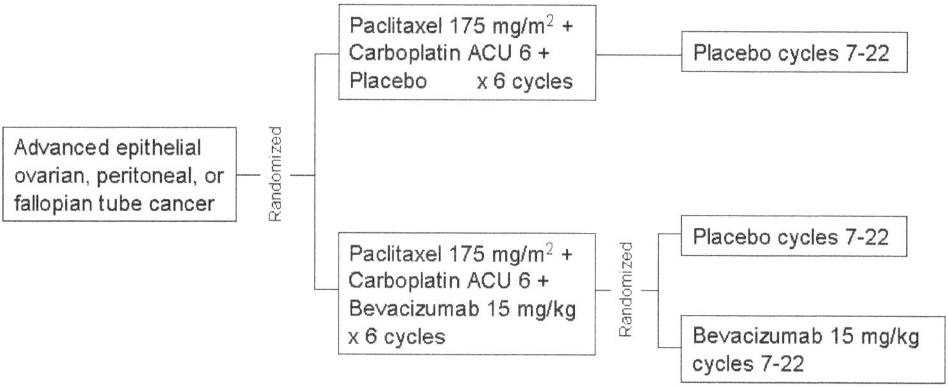

Fig. 3. GOG 218 schema.

The second study is a non-placebo-controlled trial organized by the International Collaborative Ovarian Neoplasm trial, ICON7 (NCT00483782). This study is 2-armed trial designed to compare carboplatin-paclitaxel with bevacizumab plus carboplatin-paclitaxel followed by maintenance bevacizumab therapy in patients with stage IIB-IV or early-stage high-risk ovarian (stage I-IIa with grade 3 or clear cell histology), primary peritoneal, or fallopian tube cancer (Figure 4). Data from the 1528 patients enrolled in this trial were presented at European Society of Medical Oncology meeting (ESMO) in 2010 (Perren et al 2010). The patients that were treated with concurrent and maintenance bevacizumab had a median PFS of 19 months, which was longer than the 17.3 months observed in the patients treated with chemotherapy alone (HR, 0.81; 95% CI, 0.70-0.94; p<0.0041). The result of interim analysis presented at the 2011 meeting of the ASCO also showed the superiority of the concurrent and maintenance bevacizumab compared to the standard chemotherapy (median PFS of 19.8 months versus 17.4 months; HR, 0.87; 95% CI, 0.77-0.99; p=0.039). Survival data will not be mature until 2013 (Kristensen et al., 2011).

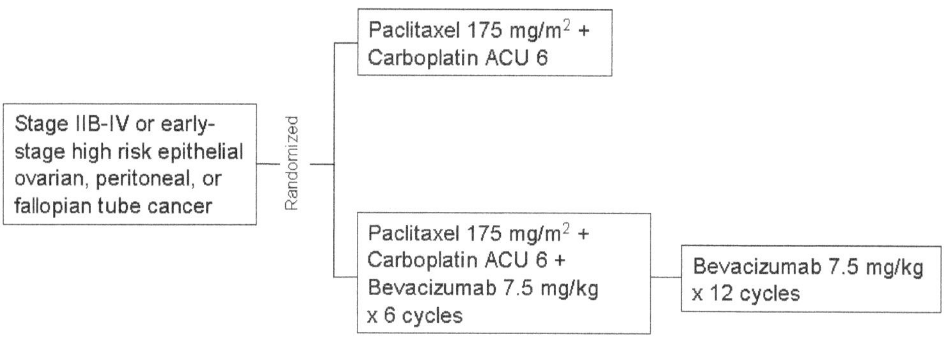

Fig. 4. ICON7 schema.

The last trial is GOG252 (NCT00951496), which will not determine the efficacy of additional bevacizumab, but rather is designed to compare intravenous versus intraperitoneal carboplatin, and intraperitoneal carboplatin versus intraperitoneal cisplatin plus paclitaxel in the setting of front-line therapy. All participants received bevacizumab in the front-line setting as well as bevacizumab consolidation chemotherapy (Figure 5).

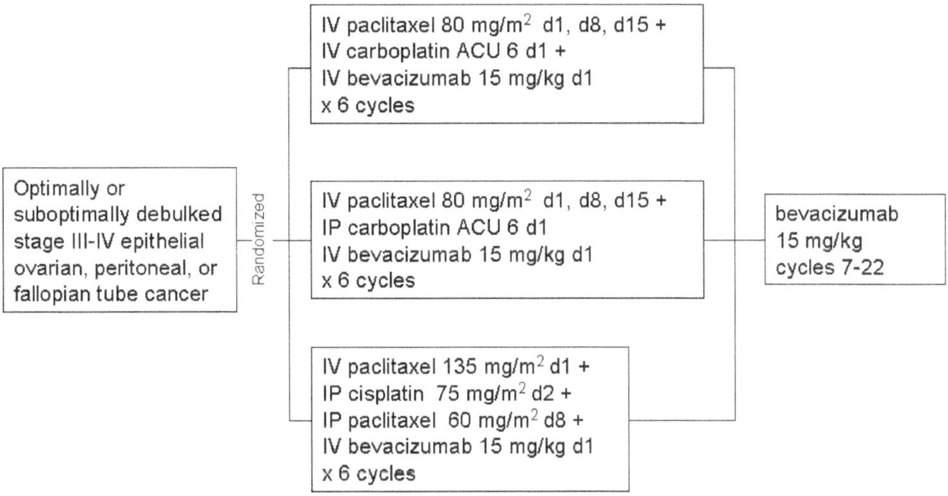

Fig. 5. GOG 252 schema.

The activity of bevacizumab in patients with recurrent ovarian cancer is currently being evaluated in several phase III trials. GOG 213 (NCT00565851) was designed to evaluate the roles of secondary cytoreductive surgery and bevacizumab in combination with carboplatin-paclitaxel in patients with platinum-sensitive recurrent ovarian cancer (Figure 6).

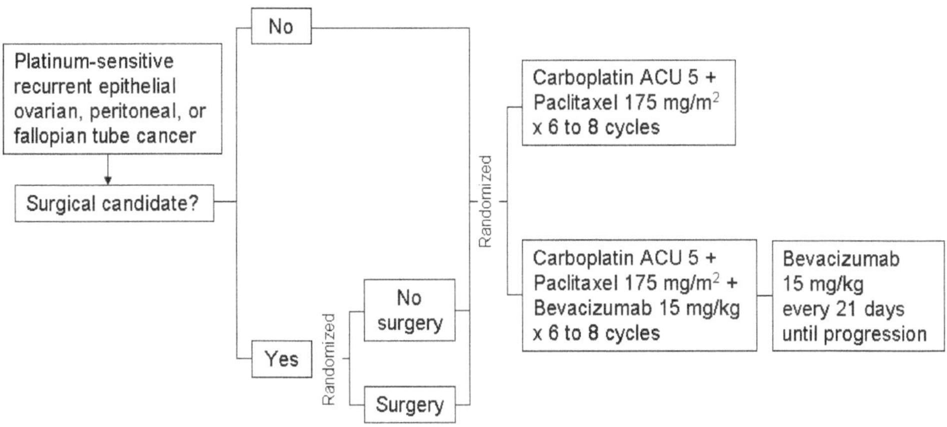

Fig. 6. GOG 213 schema.

The Ovarian Cancer Evaluation of Avastin and Safety-AVF4095g trial (OCEANS) is a phase III study designed to compare gemcitabine and carboplatin with or without bevacizumab in patients with platinum-sensitive recurrent ovarian, primary peritoneal, or fallopian tube cancer (NCT00434642). After 6 cycles of combination chemotherapy with carboplatin-gemcitabine, the patients will continue to receive bevacizumab or placebo consolidation therapy for up to 51 weeks (Figure 7). After a median follow-up period of 24 months, preliminary results from 484 patients were presented at the 2011 meeting of the ASCO

(Aghajanian et al., 2011). Patients treated with concurrent and maintenance bevacizumab showed significantly longer PFS compared to the standard chemotherapy arm (12.4 months versus 8.4 months; hazard ratio, 0.484; 95% Cl, 0.388-0.605; $p<0.0001$). The survival data are not mature.

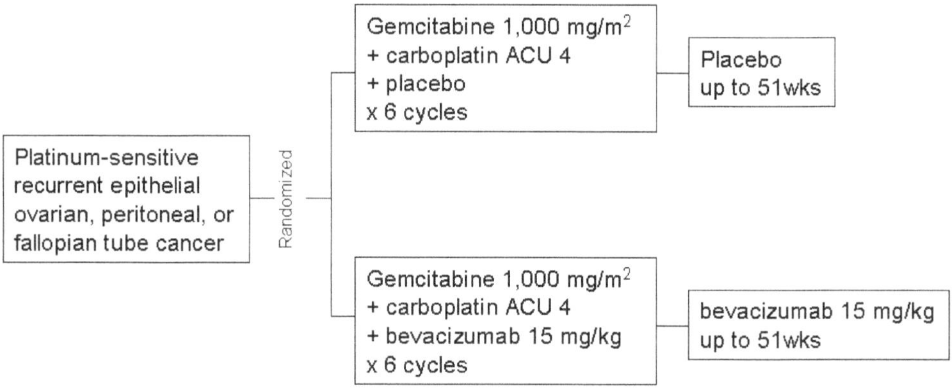

Fig. 7. OCEANS schema.

The AURELIA study (NCT00976911) is a phase III study designed to evaluate the benefit of adding bevacizumab to standard chemotherapy in patients with recurrent epithelial ovarian, fallopian tube, or primary peritoneal cancer who displayed disease progression within 6 months of platinum therapy. The patients will receive paclitaxel, topotecan, or liposomal doxorubicin with or without concomitant bevacizumab (Figure 8).

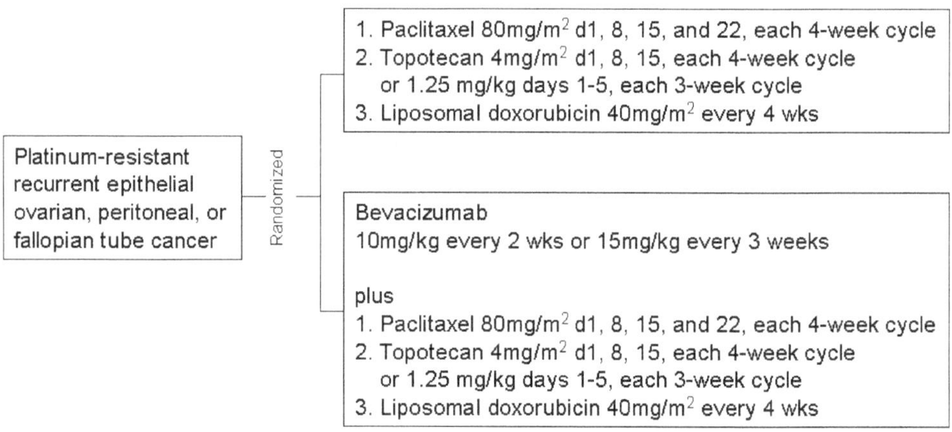

Fig. 8. AURELIA schema.

7.1.2 Bevacizumab for palliative treatment

The ability of bevacizumab as a palliative agent for symptomatic ascites has also been evaluated in several studies. In a report by Numnum et al, treatment with bevacizumab for patients with recurrent ovarian cancer with symptomatic ascites resulted in relief of symptoms associated with ascites formation. Moreover, objectively, no patient required a paracentesis after the initiation of bevacizumab therapy (Numnum et al., 2006). These results suggest that it is reasonable to consider the use of bevacizumab as a palliative agent in patients with end stage ovarian cancer with symptomatic ascites.

7.2 Aflibercept (AVE0005/VEGF trap)

Aflibercept (AVE0005/VEGF trap) is a fusion protein that inactivates VEGF by acting as a decoy receptor for VEGF, preventing VEGF binding to VEGFR. Preclinical in vivo studies have demonstrated that treatment with aflibercept resulted in a decreased tumor burden and reduced ascites formation as a result of tumor angiogenesis inhibition (Byrne et al., 2003).

The clinical activity of aflibercept in ovarian cancer has been evaluated in several phase I/II studies (Moroney et al., 2009). In a randomized, double-blind, phase II study of patients with recurrent ovarian cancer, aflibercept produced a significant tumor response (according to the RECIST criteria) or CA-125 response (defined as a 50% reduction in the CA-125 protein level) was observed in 18 (13.8%) out of 130 evaluable patients. In addition, of the 40 patients who had evaluable ascites at the baseline, 77.5% demonstrated the complete disappearance or stabilization of their ascites (Tew et al., 2007).

On the basis of the promising results from these preclinical and clinical investigations, aflibercept has been evaluated in a phase III trial (Table 2). In this trial, the effect of aflibercept on the necessity of repeated paracentesis for symptomatic ascites in patients with advanced ovarian cancer has been evaluated (NCT00327444) (Figure 9).

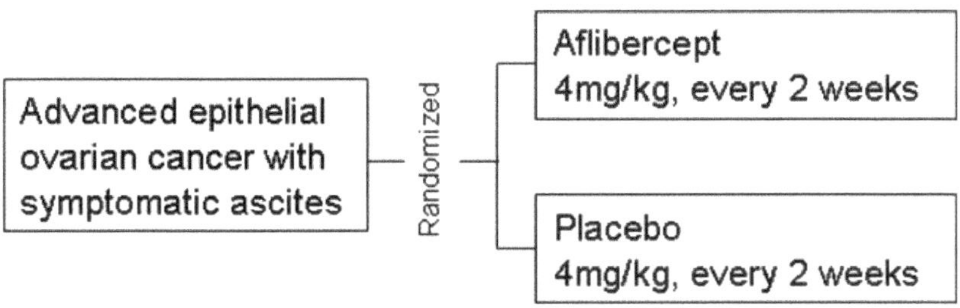

Fig. 9. NCT00327444 schema.

7.3 Tyrosine kinase inhibitors

Another strategy is the inhibition of the VEGF receptor using tyrosine kinase inhibitors (Teoh & Secord, 2011). In contrast to the specific inhibition of the VEGF pathway using bevacizumab or aflibercept, most TKI target multiple receptors responsible for tumor-angiogenesis. Theoretically, these multi-targeting anti-angiogenic agents inhibit tumor angiogenesis more completely than agents that specifically target VEGF, and thus, might have a greater therapeutic benefit. Several TKI have demonstrated clinical activity in phase I/II trials involving patients with ovarian cancer and are currently being evaluated in phase III trials (Table 2).

Compound	Target	Setting	Patients	Endopoint	Status
Aflibercept	VEGF	Recurrent	Arm 1: Placebo Arm 2: Aflibercept	Time to repeat para-centesis	Completed Results not yet available
Cediranib	VEGFR -1,2,3 PDGFR -β c-kit	Recurrent	Arm 1: CT Arm 2: CT+Ced Arm 3: CT+Ced+ maintenance Ced	PFS and OS	Open to accrual
Pazopanib	VEGFR -1,2,3 PDGFR -α, β c-kit	Maintenance*	Arm 1: Placebo Arm 2: Pazopanib	PFS	Completed accrual
BIBF 1120	VEGFR -1,2,3 PDGFR −α, β FGFR-1,2,3	Front-line adjuvant	Arm 1: CT Arm 2: CT+BIBF 1120	PFS	Open to accrual

Table 2. Summary of the randomized controlled trials evaluating the efficacy of tyrosine kinase inhibitors against ovarian cancer. Ced, Cediranib; PFS, progression free survival; OS, overall survival.

* Maintenance treatment for patients whose cancer had not progressed during first line chemotherapy.

7.3.1 Cediranib

Cediranib is an oral TKI that targets all three VEGFR, PDGFR, and c-kit. In the setting of a phase II study of patients with recurrent epithelial ovarian cancer or fallopian tube cancer, cediranib demonstrated significant clinical activity. In this trial, single agent cediranib showed a clinical benefit rate (complete response, partial response, stable disease, or CA125 non-progression) of 30% (Matulonis et al., 2009).

Cediranib is currently being evaluated in a phase III trial (ICON6), which was designed to investigate the clinical benefit of adding cediranib to carboplatin-paclitaxel, as well as the benefit of continuing cediranib as a maintenance therapy in patients with platinum-sensitive, recurrent ovarian cancer (NCT00532194) (Figure 10).

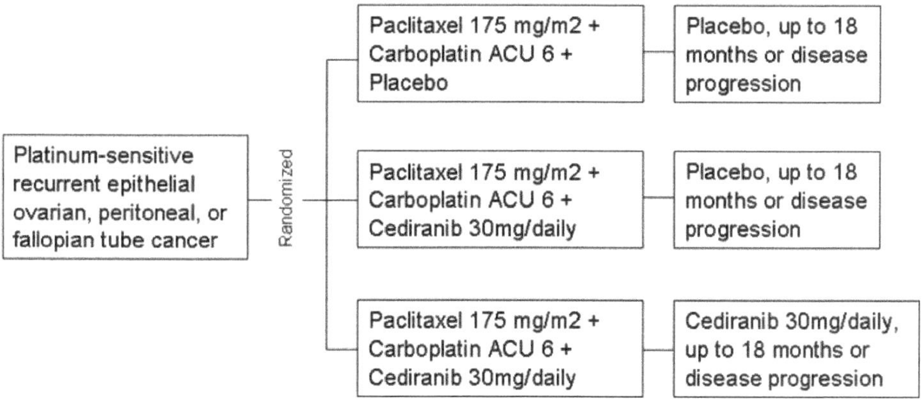

Fig. 10. NCT00532194 schema.

7.3.2 Pazopanib

Pazopanib, an oral TKI that targets all three VEGFR, PDGFR, and c-kit, was approved by the United States Food and Drug Administration in 2009 for the treatment of patients with advanced renal cell carcinoma. The clinical activity of pazopanib in ovarian cancer has been evaluated in several phase I/II trials (Monk et al., 2010; Friedlander et al., 2010). In a phase II trial in which the CA-125 response (≥50% decrease from baseline) was the primary endpoint, pazopanib demonstrated a CA-125 response rate of 31% (11 out of 36 patients). In 17 patients with measurable disease, the overall response rate (according to the RECIST criteria) was 18%.

On the basis of these results, the activity of pazopanib is currently being evaluated in a phase III study, which was designed to compare the efficacy of pazopanib versus placebo in women whose disease had not progressed after first-line chemotherapy for epithelial ovarian, fallopian tube, or primary peritoneal cancer (NCT00866697) (Figure 11).

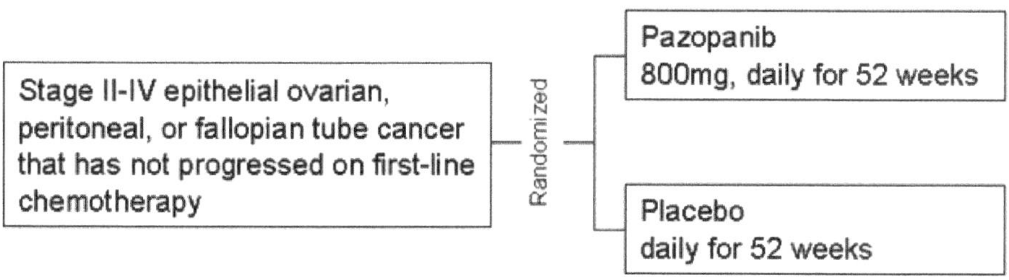

Fig. 11. NCT00866697 schema.

7.3.3 BIBF 1120

BIBF 1120 is an orally available TKI that binds and inhibits VEGFR, PDGFR, and FGFR tyrosine kinases. On the basis of a promising randomized controlled phase II trial highlighting the benefit of maintenance treatment with BIBF 1120 after salvage chemotherapy in patients with recurrent ovarian cancer (Ledermann et al., 2009), the

Arbeitsgemeinschaft Gynakologische Oncologie (AGO) is currently conducting a Phase III trial (AGO-OVAR-12). This trial was designed to evaluate the efficacy of BIBF 1120 in combination with carboplatin-paclitaxel in patients with advanced epithelial ovarian cancer in the setting of front-line treatment (NCT01015118) (Figure 12).

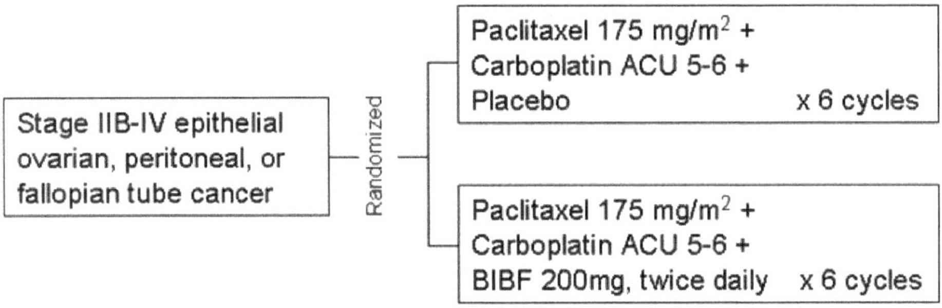

Fig. 12. NCT01015118 schema.

8. Toxic effects of VEGF-targeting agents

As VEGF mediates physiologically important processes in healthy tissues, VEGF-targeting agents are associated with unique and potentially problematic side effects (Stone et al., 2010).

Hypertension is the most common side effect of VEGF-targeting agents. It typically occurs within 3 weeks of the beginning of therapy. The pathogenesis of hypertension associated with VEGF-targeting agents is not fully understood. However, it is speculated that the suppression of nitric oxide production by VEGF antagonism leads to vasoconstriction and decreased sodium ion renal excretion, which results in elevated blood pressure (Izzedine et al., 2009). A recent review of the adverse effects of anti-angiogenic therapies suggested that the incidence of grade 3/4 hypertension in patients that had been treated with bevacizumab, aflibercept, or TKI was 8-26%, 9-32%, and 5-48%, respectively (Stone et al., 2010).

Proteinuria is another common side effect observed in patients treated with bevacizumab or aflibercept. In clinical trials of bevacizumab or aflibercept, grade 3/4 proteinuria occurred in approximately 1-4% of patients (Izzedine et al., 2010). Proteinuria is rare in patients treated with TKI. Such proteinuria is reported to occur as a result of the disruption of VEGF-dependent glomerular endothelial integrity (Ostendorf et al., 1999).

Wound healing complications is another serious side effect that is reported to occur in patients treated with VEGF-targeting agents. As the wound-healing process is dependent on angiogenesis, VEGF-targeting agents have the potential to delay the wound-healing process in patients who undergo surgery. On the basis of a previous report suggesting that patients who undergo surgery within 28-60 days of bevacizumab therapy are at an increased risk of wound-healing complications, physicians recommend avoiding major surgery at least 30 days after the completion of bevacizumab treatment (Shord et al., 2009).

The increased risk of atrial thromboembolic events (ATE), usually myocardial or cerebrovascular events, is another serious adverse effect associated with bevacizumab therapy. In a recent analysis of 1745 patients with colorectal, breast, or non-small-cell lung cancer from five randomized trials, the addition of bevacizumab to chemotherapy was associated with an increased risk of ATE (incidence of 3.8% in the combination therapy group vs 1.7% in the chemotherapy alone group) (Scappaticci et al., 2007). The precise incidence of ATE in patients with ovarian cancer who have been treated with VEGF-targeting agents is unknown; however, so far, 30 ATE events have been reported. ATE events are rarely reported in patients who have been treated with aflibercept or TKI (Stone et al., 2010).

The most serious complication of VEGF-targeting agents is bowel perforation. In a recent review of 9 clinical studies examining the use of bevacizumab in ovarian cancer patients, the overall frequency of bowel perforation was 5.4%, which was higher than the 2.4% observed in patients with colorectal cancer (Han & Monk, 2007). Bowel perforation was also observed in patients that had been treated with aflibercept (Colombo et al., 2008), however, there have been no reported cases of bowel perforation involving patients that were treated with TKI monotherapy (Stone et al., 2010). The management of bowel perforation is difficult because of the increased likelihood of surgical and postoperative complications, such as thrombosis or compromised wound healing caused by bevacizumab treatment, suggesting the importance of preventing this serious complication. The precise mechanisms of, and risk factors for, bowel perforation are largely unknown. However, Simpkins et al. suggested from their experience that bowel perforation can be avoided by carefully selecting patients without clinical symptoms of bowel obstruction, evidence of rectosigmoid involvement on a pelvic examination, or evidence of bowel involvement on a computed tomography (CT) scan (Simpkins et al., 2007).

At this point, no standard recommendations exist for the management of the adverse effects induced by VEGF-targeting agents. Further investigations are needed to solve this issue.

9. Conclusions and future directions

Recent increases in our understanding of cancer biology and the molecular pathways that control tumor angiogenesis have led to the identification of novel VEGF-targeting agents that can be used to treat ovarian cancer. Although VEGF-targeting agents have yielded promising results in ovarian cancer in the settings of front-line treatment and salvage treatment, several important clinical issues remain unanswered. The optimal methods for evaluating the efficacy of VEGF-targeting agents have yet to be clarified. As VEGF-targeting agents have cytostatic rather than cytotoxic effects, the traditional criteria applied to cytotoxic agents, such as the RECIST criteria, might be less applicable. The identification of surrogate biomarkers that can be used to guide drug choice or optimal dosing or to predict the tumor response or drug resistance is of paramount importance. In addition, increased understanding of the mechanisms underlying the unique toxic effects of VEFG-targeting agents, as well as the development of evidence-based management strategies for these adverse effects, are also necessary. Choosing the optimal VEGF-targeting agent for each patient will extend patient survival without reducing quality of life in the near future.

10. Acknowledgement

We thank Remina Emoto for providing secretarial assistance.

11. References

Aghajanian, C., Finkler, NJ., Rutherford, T. et al., OCEANS: A randomized, double-blinded, placebo-controlled phase III trial of chemotherapy with or without bevacizumab (BEV) in patients with platinum-sensitive recurrent epithelial ovarian (EOC), primary peritoneal (PPC), or fallopian tube cancer (FTC), Presented at: the 47th Annual Meeting of the American Society of Clinical Oncology; Chicago, IL, USA (June, 2011).

Brustmann, H. Vascular endothelial growth factor expression in serous ovarian carcinoma: relationship with topoisomerase II alpha and prognosis. Gynecol Oncol 2004;95:16-22.

Burger, RA., Sill, MW., Monk, BJ., Greer, BE., & Sorosk, JI. Phase II trial of bevacizumab in persistent or recurrent epithelial ovarian cancer or primary peritoneal cancer: a Gynecologic Oncology Group Study. J Clin Oncol 2007; 25:5165-5171.

Burger, RA., Brady, MF. Bookman, MA. et al., Phase III trial of bevacizumab (BEV) in the primary treatment of advanced epithelial ovarian cancer (EOC), primary peritoneal cancer (PPC), or fallopian tube cancer (FTC): a gynecologic oncology group study, Presented at: the 46th Annual Meeting of the American Society of Clinical Oncology; Chicago, IL, USA (June, 2010).

Burger, RA. Overview of anti-angiogenic agents in development for ovarian cancer. Gynecol Oncol. 2011;121:230-238.

Byrne, AT., Ross, L., Holash, J., Nakanishi, M., Hu, L., Hofmann, JI., Yancopoulos, GD., & Jaffe, RB. Vascular endothelial growth factor-trap decreases tumor burden, inhibits ascites, and causes dramatic vascular remodeling in an ovarian cancer model. Clin Cancer Res. 2003;9:5721-5728.

Cannistra, SA., Matulonis, UA., Penson, RT., Hambleton, J., Dupont, J., Mackey, H., Douglas, J., Burger, RA., Armstrong, D., Wenham, R., & McGuire, W. Phase II study of bevacizumab in patients with platinum-resistant ovarian cancer or peritoneal serous cancer. J Clin Oncol 2007;25:5180-5186.

Carmeliet, P. Mechanisms of angiogenesis and arteriogenesis. Nat Med. 2000;6:389-395.

Colombo, N., Mangili, G., Mammoliti, S. et al., Aflibercept (VEGF Trap) for advanced epithelial ovarian cancer (EOC) patients (pts) with symptomatic malignant ascites: Preliminary results of a pilot study, Presented at: the 44th Annual Meeting of the American Society of Clinical Oncology; Chicago, IL, USA (June, 2008).

Cooper, BC., Ritchie, JM., Broghammer, CL., Coffin, J., Sorosky, JI., Buller, RE., Hendrix, MJ., & Sood, AK.Preoperative serum vascular endothelial growth factor levels: significance in ovarian cancer. Clin Cancer Res. 2002;8:3193-3197.

Eskander, RN., & Randall, LM. Bevacizumab in the treatment of ovarian cancer. Biologics. 2011;5:1-5.

Ferrara, N. VEGF and the quest for tumour angiogenesis factors. Nat Rev Cancer 2002;2:795-803.

Ferrara, N., & Kerbel RS. Angiogenesis as a therapeutic target. Nature. 2005;438:967-974.

Forsythe, JA., Jiang, BH., Iyer, NV., Agani, F., Leung, SW., Koos, RD., & Semenza, GL. Activation of vascular endothelial growth factor gene transcription by hypoxia-inducible factor 1. Mol Cell Biol. 1996;16:4604-4613.

Friedlander, M., Hancock, KC., Rischin, D., Messing, MJ., Stringer, CA., Matthys, GM., Ma, B., Hodge, JP., & Lager, JJ. A Phase II, open-label study evaluating pazopanib in patients with recurrent ovarian cancer. Gynecol Oncol. 2010;119:32-37.

Garcia, AA., Hirte, H., Fleming, G., Yang, D., Tsao-Wei, DD., Roman, L., Groshen, S., Swenson, S., Markland, F., Gandara, D., Scudder, S., Morgan, R., Chen, H., Lenz, HJ., & Oza, AM. Phase II clinical trial of bevacizumab and low-dose metronomic oral cyclophosphamide in recurrent ovarian cancer: a trial of the California, Chicago, and Princess Margaret Hospital phase II consortia. J Clin Oncol 2008; 26:76-82.

Gerber, HP., & Ferrara, N. Pharmacology and pharmacodynamics of bevacizumab as monotherapy or in combination with cytotoxic therapy in preclinical studies. Cancer Res. 2005;65:671-680.

Gimbrone, MA. Jr., Leapman, SB., Cotran, RS., & Folkman, J. Tumor dormancy in vivo by prevention of neovascularization. J Exp Med 1972;136:261-276.

Han, ES., Monk, & BJ. What is the risk of bowel perforation associated with bevacizumab therapy in ovarian cancer? Gynecol Oncol. 2007;105:3-6.

Hefler, LA., Zeillinger, R., Grimm, C., Sood, AK., Cheng, WF., Gadducci, A., Tempfer, CB., & Reinthaller, A. Preoperative serum vascular endothelial growth factor as a prognostic parameter in ovarian cancer. Gynecol Oncol. 2006;103:512-517.

Hu, L., Hofmann, J., Zaloudek, C., Ferrara, N., Hamilton, T., & Jaffe, RB. Vascular endothelial growth factor immunoneutralization plus Paclitaxel markedly reduces tumor burden and ascites in athymic mouse model of ovarian cancer. Am J Pathol. 2002;161:1917-1924.

Izzedine, H., Ederhy, S., Goldwasser, F., Soria, JC., Milano, G., Cohen, A., Khayat, D., & Spano, JP. Management of hypertension in angiogenesis inhibitor-treated patients. Ann Oncol. 2009;20:807-815.

Izzedine, H., Massard, C., Spano, JP., Goldwasser, F., Khayat, D., & Soria, JC. VEGF signalling inhibition-induced proteinuria: Mechanisms, significance and management. Eur J Cancer. 2010;46:439-448.

Jain, RK. Normalization of tumor vasculature: an emerging concept in antiangiogenic therapy. Science 2005;307:58-62.

Karkkainen, MJ., Saaristo, A., Jussila, L., Karila, KA., Lawrence, EC., Pajusola, K., Bueler, H., Eichmann, A., Kauppinen, R., Kettunen, MI., Yla-Herttuala, S., Finegold, DN., Ferrell, RE., & Alitalo K. A model for gene therapy of human hereditary lymphedema. Proc Natl Acad Sci U S A. 2001;98:12677-12682.

Kerbel, RS. Inhibition of tumor angiogenesis as a strategy to circumvent acquired resistance to anti-cancer therapeutic agents. Bioessays. 1991;13:31-36.

Kristensen, G., Perren, T., Qian, W. et al., Result of interim analysis of overall survival in the GCIG ICON7 phase III randomized trial of bevacizumab in women with newly diagnosed ovarian cancer, Presented at: the 47th Annual Meeting of the American Society of Clinical Oncology; Chicago, IL, USA (June, 2011)

Ledermann, JA., Rustin, GJ., Hackshaw, A. et al., A randomised phase II placebo-controlled trial using maintenance therapy to evaluate the vascular targeting agent BIBF 1120 following treatment of relapsed ovarian cancer, Presented at: the 16th Biennial International Meeting of the European Society of Gynaecological Oncology; Belgrade, Serbia (October, 2009).

Li, L., Wang, L., Zhang, W., Tang, B., Zhang, J., Song, H., Yao, D., Tang, Y., Chen, X., Yang, Z., Wang, G., Li, X., Zhao, J., Ding, H., Reed, E., & Li, QQ. Correlation of serum VEGF levels with clinical stage, therapy efficacy, tumor metastasis and patient survival in ovarian cancer. Anticancer Res. 2004;24:1973-1979.

Mabuchi, S., Terai, Y., Morishige, K., Tanabe-Kimura, A., Sasaki, H., Kanemura, M., Tsunetoh, S., Tanaka, Y., Sakata, M., Burger, RA., Kimura, T., & Ohmichi, M. Maintenance treatment with bevacizumab prolongs survival in an in vivo ovarian cancer model. Clin Cancer Res 2008;14:7781-7789.

Mabuchi, S., Kawase, C., Altomare, DA., Morishige, K., Hayashi, M., Sawada, K., Ito, K., Terai, Y., Nishio, Y., Klein-Szanto, AJ., Burger, RA., Ohmichi, M., Testa, JR., & Kimura, T. Vascular endothelial growth factor is a promising therapeutic target for the treatment of clear cell carcinoma of the ovary. Mol Cancer Ther. 2010a;9:2411-2422.

Mabuchi, S., Morishige, K., & Kimura, T. Use of monoclonal antibodies in the treatment of ovarian cancer. Curr Opin Obstet Gynecol. 2010b;22:3-8.

Matulonis, UA., Berlin, S., Ivy, P., Tyburski, K., Krasner, C., Zarwan, C., Berkenblit, A., Campos, S., Horowitz, N., Cannistra, SA., Lee, H., Lee, J., Roche, M., Hill, M., Whalen, C., Sullivan, L., Tran, C., Humphreys, BD., & Penson, RT. Cediranib, an oral inhibitor of vascular endothelial growth factor receptor kinases, is an active drug in recurrent epithelial ovarian, fallopian tube, and peritoneal cancer. J Clin Oncol. 2009;27:5601-5606.

Mesiano, S., Ferrara, N., & Jaffe, RB. Role of vascular endothelial growth factor in ovarian cancer: inhibition of ascites formation by immunoneutralization. Am J Pathol. 1998;153:1249-1256.

Monk, BJ., Mas Lopez, L., Zarba, JJ., Oaknin, A., Tarpin, C., Termrungruanglert, W., Alber, JA., Ding, J., Stutts, MW., & Pandite, LN. Phase II, open-label study of pazopanib or lapatinib monotherapy compared with pazopanib plus lapatinib combination therapy in patients with advanced and recurrent cervical cancer. J Clin Oncol. 2010;28:3562-3569.

Moroney, JW., Sood, AK., & Coleman, RL. Aflibercept in epithelial ovarian carcinoma. Future Oncol. 2009;5:591-600.

Numnum, TM., Rocconi, RP., Whitworth, J., & Barnes, MN. The use of bevacizumab to palliate symptomatic ascites in patients with refractory ovarian carcinoma. Gynecol Oncol 2006;102:425-428.

Ostendorf, T., Kunter, U., Eitner, F., Loos, A., Regele, H., Kerjaschki, D., Henninger, DD., Janjic, N., & Floege, J. VEGF(165) mediates glomerular endothelial repair. J Clin Invest. 1999;104:913-923.

Penson, RT., Dizon, DS., Cannistra, SA., Roche, MR., Krasner, CN., Berlin, ST., Horowitz, NS., Disilvestro, PA., Matulonis, UA., Lee, H., King, MA., & Campos, SM. Phase II study of carboplatin, paclitaxel, and bevacizumab with maintenance bevacizumab as first-line chemotherapy for advanced mullerian tumors. J Clin Oncol 2010;28:154-159.

Perren, T. et al., ICON7: A phase III randomized gynecologic cancer intergroup trial of concurrent bevacizumab and chemotherapy followed by maintenance bevacizumab, versus chemotherapy alone in women with newly diagnosed epithelial ovarian (EOC), primary peritoneal (PPC), or fallopian tube cancer (FTC),

Presented at: the 35th European Society of Medical Oncology meeting; Milan, Italy (October, 2010).

Presta, LG., Chen, H., O'Connor, SJ., Chisholm, V., Meng, YG., Krummen, L., Winkler, M., & Ferrara, N. Humanization of an anti-vascular endothelial growth factor monoclonal antibody for the therapy of solid tumors and other disorders. Cancer Res. 1997;57:4593-4599.

Rafii, S., Lyden, D., Benezra, R., Hattori, K., & Heissig, B. Vascular and haematopoietic stem cells: novel targets for anti-angiogenesis therapy? Nat Rev Cancer. 2002;2:826-835.

Schönau, KK., Steger, GG., & Mader, RM. Angiogenic effect of naive and 5-fluorouracil resistant colon carcinoma on endothelial cells in vitro. Cancer Lett 2007;257:73-78.

Scappaticci, FA., Skillings, JR., Holden, SN., Gerber, HP., Miller, K., Kabbinavar, F., Bergsland, E., Ngai, J., Holmgren, E., Wang, J., & Hurwitz, H. Arterial thromboembolic events in patients with metastatic carcinoma treated with chemotherapy and bevacizumab. J Natl Cancer Inst. 2007;99:1232-1239.

Senger, DR., Galli, SJ., Dvorak, AM., Perruzzi, CA., Harvey, VS., & Dvorak, HF. Tumor cells secrete a vascular permeability factor that promotes accumulation of ascites fluid. Science 1983;219: 983-985.

Shord, SS., Bressler, LR., Tierney, LA., Cuellar, S., & George, A. Understanding and managing the possible adverse effects associated with bevacizumab. Am J Health Syst Pharm. 2009;66:999-1013.

Simpkins, F., Belinson, JL., Rose, & PG. Avoiding bevacizumab related gastrointestinal toxicity for recurrent ovarian cancer by careful patient screening. Gynecol Oncol. 2007;107:118-123.

Sood, AK., Seftor, EA., Fletcher, MS., Gardner, LM., Heidger, PM., Buller, RE., Seftor, RE., & Hendrix, MJ. Molecular determinants of ovarian cancer plasticity. Am J Pathol. 2001;158:1279-1288.

Spannuth, WA., Sood, AK., & Coleman, RL. Angiogenesis as a strategic target for ovarian cancer therapy. Nat Clin Pract Oncol. 2008;5:194-204.

Spannuth, WA., Nick, AM., Jennings, NB., Armaiz-Pena, GN., Mangala, LS., Danes, CG., Lin, YG., Merritt, WM., Thaker, PH., Kamat, AA., Han, LY., Tonra, JR., Coleman, RL., Ellis, LM., & Sood AK. Functional significance of VEGFR-2 on ovarian cancer cells. Int J Cancer. 2009;124:1045-1053.

Stone, RL., Sood, AK., & Coleman, RL. Collateral damage: toxic effects of targeted antiangiogenic therapies in ovarian cancer. Lancet Oncol. 2010;11:465-475.

Teoh, DG., & Secord, AA. Antiangiogenic therapies in epithelial ovarian cancer. Cancer Control. 2011;18:31-43.

Tew, WP., Colombo, N., Ray-Coquard, I. et al., VEGF-Trap for patients (pts) with recurrent platinum-resistant epithelial ovarian cancer (EOC): preliminary results of a randomized, multicenter phase II study, Presented at: the 43th Annual Meeting of the American Society of Clinical Oncology; Chicago, IL, USA (June, 2007).

Wong, C., Wellman, TL., & Lounsbury, KM. VEGF and HIF-1alpha expression are increased in advanced stages of epithelial ovarian cancer. Gynecol Oncol 2003;91: 513-517.

Yamamoto, S., Konishi, I., Mandai, M., Kuroda, H., Komatsu, T., Nanbu, K., Sakahara, H., & Mori, T. Expression of vascular endothelial growth factor (VEGF) in epithelial ovarian neoplasms: correlation with clinicopathology and patient survival, and analysis of serum VEGF levels. Br J Cancer 1997;76:1221-1227.

Zhang, L., Yang, N., Garcia, JR., Mohamed, A., Benencia, F., Rubin, SC., Allman, D., & Coukos, G. Generation of a syngeneic mouse model to study the effects of vascular endothelial growth factor in ovarian carcinoma. Am J Pathol 2002;161:2295-309.

16

Gene Amplification in Ovarian Carcinomas: Lessons from Selected Amplified Gene Families

Stéphanie Gaillard
Sidney Kimmel Comprehensive Cancer Center,
Johns Hopkins School of Medicine Baltimore
USA

1. Introduction

Ovarian cancer is the most malignant gynecologic cancer causing an estimated 140,000 deaths per year worldwide(Jemal et al 2011). In greater than 75% of incident cases, the disease is detected only after it has reached an advanced stage (stage III and IV) when standard therapy is unlikely to be curative. Even after maximal cytoreductive surgery followed by platinum-based chemotherapy, the survival rate at 5 years is only 15-30% (Kosary 1994). Epithelial ovarian cancer is a heterogeneous disease that can be subdivided into four histological categories: serous, clear cell, endometrial, and mucinous. The pathogenesis of the individual subtypes relies on different molecular and pathway aberrations and thus will likely respond with different sensitivities to systemic and targeted therapies(Kurman and Shih Ie 2008). The identification of critical molecular and pathway aberrations specific to each subtype could provide key insights into the mechanisms driving tumorigenesis and direct efforts in the development of targeted therapies.
Tumors characteristically display alterations in gene expression that lead to the acquisition of the hallmark features of cancer: uncontrolled proliferation, evasion of growth suppression and of the immune system, resistance to death signals, unlimited replicative potential, development of a supportive microenvironment (including angiogenesis), and ability to invade and metastasize(Hanahan and Weinberg 2011). Aberrant gene expression is manifest through a number of different mechanisms including DNA copy number alterations (amplifications, deletions, gains and losses of whole chromosomes resulting in aneuploidy), epigenetic regulation via methylation or histone acetylation, fusion proteins and individual gene mutations. Amplifications that are critical to tumorigenesis likely are essential because they result in the overexpression of gene products on which the tumor is dependent. These are often referred to as "driver" genes, as dysregulated expression leads to the activation of oncogenic pathways, while other genes in the amplified region may or may not be overexpressed and instead are "passenger" genes. Analysis of individual amplifications have elucidated driver pathways of cancer and revealed potential targets for drug development. For example, amplification of the Her-2/neu gene occurs in 25-30% of breast cancers and is associated with a more aggressive phenotype(Slamon et al 1989). However, treatment with HER-2 targeted therapy, in particular trastuzumab, has dramatically improved the natural history of HER2-positive breast cancer(Ferretti et al 2007). Similarly,

non-small cell lung cancers with mutations in or amplification of the EGFR gene benefit from EGFR inhibitors. Several amplified genes have been identified in epithelial ovarian cancers. The Cancer Genome Atlas (TCGA) project recently published their results from a multicenter comprehensive effort to characterize the molecular abnormalities in high-grade serous ovarian carcinomas. In this study 489 clinically annotated stage II-IV high-grade serous ovarian cancer samples were analyzed for changes in mRNA expression, microRNA expression, DNA copy number, and DNA promoter methylation. Interestingly, the TCGA found a relatively low rate of recurrent mutations while copy number changes were relatively abundant(Cancer Genome Atlas Research Network, 2011). In light of the recent results of the TCGA, this chapter will discuss the major pathways (Figure 1) frequently amplified in ovarian cancers and review the clinical efficacy of therapeutic agents targeting these genes.

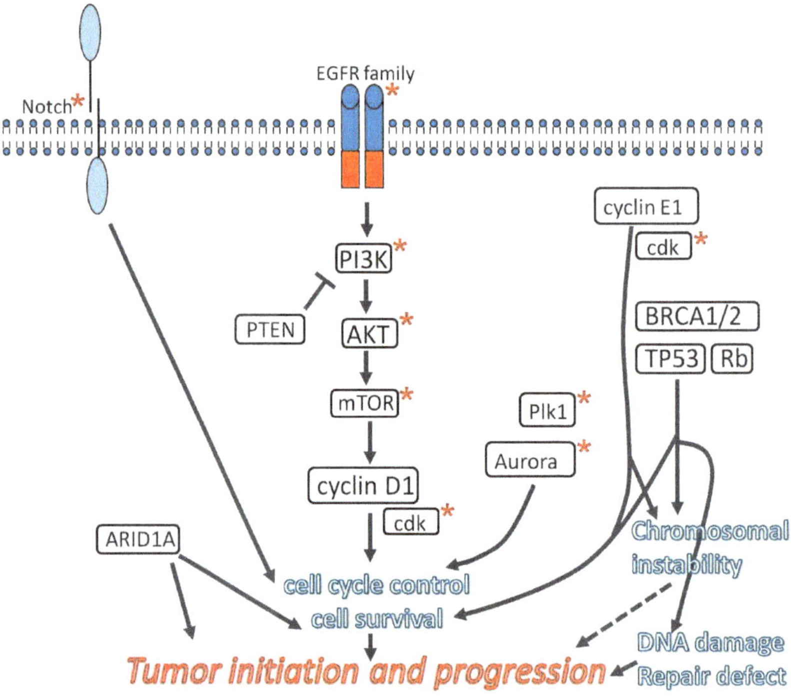

Fig. 1. Pathways amplified in epithelial ovarian cancer. *represents targetable pathways discussed in this chapter.

2. Global assessment of copy number variation in ovarian cancer

DNA copy number variations can be identified using several techniques including cytogenetics, fluorescence in situ hybridization (FISH), comparative genomic hybridization (CGH), and single nucleotide polymorphism (SNP) arrays. The latter two have the advantage of providing an unbiased genome wide assessment of copy number variation and have been widely used to characterize the complex genomic alterations attributable to ovarian cancer and reveal it to be a heterogeneous group of diseases(Gorringe et al 2010, Meinhold-Heerlein et al 2005, Nakayama et al 2007, Staebler et al 2002). Recent studies of the genomic alterations between invasive serous carcinomas and low grade or borderline serous tumors have identified dramatic differences in DNA copy number changes (Meinhold-Heerlein et al 2005, Nakayama et al 2007, Staebler et al 2002). High-grade serous carcinomas uniformly exhibited more extensive DNA copy number variations than borderline tumors or low-grade serous carcinomas (Figure 2). The frequency and amplitude of changes was higher in invasive serous carcinomas and involve the majority of chromosomes through gain or loss of discrete subchromosomal regions, chromosome arms, or whole chromosomes. By contrast, low-grade tumors exhibit significantly fewer copy number gains and few chromosomal losses. The pervasive changes seen within the chromosomes of high-grade serous ovarian carcinomas suggest that significant genomic instability is a critical feature of this disease.

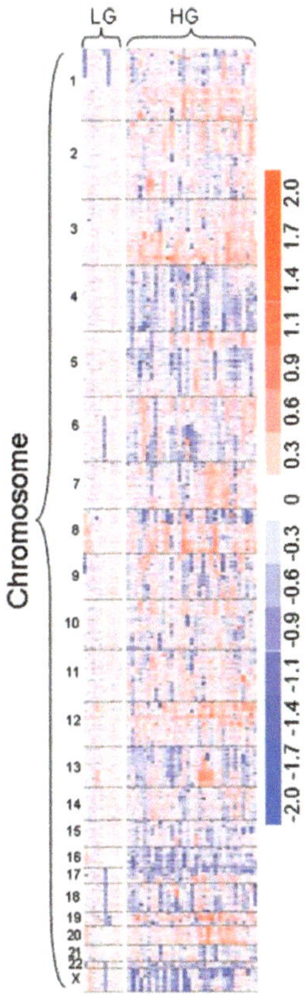

Fig. 2. Genome-wide distribution of DNA copy number changes in low-grade and high-grade ovarian serous carcinomas. Each column represents an individual tumor sample. DNA copy number changes are represented as pseudocolor gradients corresponding to the folds of increase (red boxes) and decrease (blue boxes), as compared to pooled normal samples. Reproduced with permission (Nakayama et al 2007).

Similar results were found in the TCGA analysis of the molecular aberrations in high-grade serous ovarian carcinomas. The project identified only 9 significant recurrently mutated genes, of which TP53, BRCA1, and BRCA2 were the most common(Cancer Genome Atlas Research Network, 2011). In contrast, copy number aberrations were abundant. One hundred and thirteen significant focal DNA copy number aberrations, including 8 regional recurrent gains, 22 regional recurrent losses, and 63 regions of focal amplification, were identified. Five of the regional gains were present in >50% of tumors. Analysis of the focal amplifications identified a number of genes that were highly amplified and potential therapeutic targets.

The results of these studies clearly highlight the complex molecular and genetic changes that are harbored by ovarian serous carcinomas. Copy number alteration alone, however, does not necessarily indicate that the region plays a causal role in tumorigenesis. One of the challenges with these studies is identifying the potential oncogenes or oncogenic pathways within the affected chromosomal regions that are likely to be responsible for the pathogenesis of ovarian cancer and/or should be a focus for drug development. In the following sections, we will discuss some of the candidate genes that have been identified and are being evaluated in clinical practice.

3. PIK3CA and AKT2

The phosphoinositide 3-kinase (PIK3)-AKT2 signaling pathway regulates diverse cellular functions including cellular proliferation, migration, metabolic homeostasis, apoptosis and survival, and the dysregulation of this pathway has been implicated in the tumorigenesis of a variety of cancers(Karakas et al 2006, Stokoe 2005). AKT2 is a serine/threonine protein kinase containing SH2-like (Src homology 2-like) domains and is a member of the AKT subfamily. It was originally identified as one of the putative human homologs of the v-akt oncogene of the retrovirus AKT8 (Staal 1987). AKT2 is activated by its upstream regulator PI3K. PIK3CA is the 110kD component of the catalytic subunit of PIK3 and aberrations in normal signaling of PIK3CA and AKT2 have been implicated in ovarian cancer pathogenesis making them potential targets for drug development(Cheng et al 1992, Dancey 2004, Hu et al 2005). Overexpression of activated PIK3CA results in phosphorylation of AKT and cellular transformation and inactivation of AKT by dominant negative mutants abrogates the survival advantage conferred by activated PI3K (Kang et al 2005, Link et al 2005). PTEN (phosphatase and tensin homologue deleted on chromosome 10) is a dual lipid and protein phosphatase that targets PIP3 (phosphatidylinositol-3,4,5- triphosphate), the target of PIK3. This pathway may be aberrantly activated by amplification or mutation of AKT2 or PIK3CA, or deletion, promoter methylation, or functional loss of PTEN which can lead to the excessive activation of downstream effectors, such as mTOR(Altomare et al 2004, Gao et al 2004, Mabuchi et al 2009).

AKT2 amplification has been reported in 5-29% of ovarian cancer cases(Bellacosa et al 1995, Cheng et al 1992, Courjal et al 1996, Nakayama et al 2006b, Park et al 2006). In comparison, AKT2 was not amplified in benign or borderline ovarian tumors(Bellacosa et al 1995, Nakayama et al 2006b). Similarly, low-level amplifications were present in PIK3CA in high-grade carcinomas but not in serous borderline tumors. Twenty seven percent of cases showed amplification in either gene emphasizing how frequently components of this pathway are amplified in ovarian cancer and coamplification of the two genes was seen in a small subset(Nakayama et al 2006b). The findings of this study also support the dualistic model of ovarian serous carcinogenesis in which high-grade and low-grade ovarian serous tumors develop along distinctly different molecular pathways(Kurman and Shih Ie 2008).

Pathway activation through PIK3CA can occur through either amplification or activating mutation of the catalytic subunit. Mutations of PIK3CA are typically associated with endometrioid and clear cell subtypes and are associated with lower tumor stage and grade(Campbell et al 2004, Kolasa et al 2009, Willner et al 2007). Amplifications, on the other hand, have been detected in all histological subtypes, though there was an association with poorer differentiation. PIK3CA amplification has been reported in 13-24% of ovarian carcinomas and is associated with increased expression of phosphorylated AKT indicating that amplification results in increased activation of the pathway(Campbell et al 2004, Kolasa et al 2009, Nakayama et al 2006b, Willner et al 2007, Woenckhaus et al 2007).

Clinical data is lacking in the majority of these studies and the prognostic role of AKT and mTOR in ovarian cancer is unclear. The median survival of patients with normal levels of AKT2 was longer than in patients whose tumors harbored AKT2 amplifications (45 versus 22 months, respectively), however the study was limited by the small number of patients for which survival data was available and did not reach statistical significance(Bellacosa et al 1995). The activation of AKT and increased downstream mTOR expression has been associated with more aggressive disease and shorter patient survival(Bunkholt Elstrand et al 2010). The effect of PIK3CA amplification on survival is also unclear with some studies showing no influence of amplification on overall survival while another showed that PIK3CA amplification was associated with shorter survival(Kolasa et al 2009, Willner et al 2007, Woenckhaus et al 2007).

PIK3-AKT2 pathway activation may affect response to therapy. PIK3CA amplification was identified more frequently in patients who were platinum resistant and in patients who did not achieve a complete remission to chemotherapy(Kolasa et al 2009). Disease recurrence was increased in the group with amplifications, however this study was limited by its small size and overall survival was not affected. Further studies in ovarian cancer cell lines with acquired cisplatin resistance shown that the cells harbor increased activation of the Akt/mTOR survival pathway and that inhibition of the pathway resensitizes the cells to cisplatin treatment(Lee et al 2005b, Peng et al 2010). However, whether they can be used as predictors of therapeutic response has not been established.

Given the relatively common activation of this pathway in tumorigenesis, there has been considerable interest in developing therapeutic drugs to target the PTEN/PIK3/AKT pathway for use in multiple cancers. The most successful approach thus far has been the development of mTOR inhibitors, which have been approved for use in renal cell carcinomas and pancreatic neuroendocrine tumors. Rapamycin, and its derivative inhibitors (temsirolimus, everolimus, and ridaforolimus) are currently in use in multiple clinical trials specifically evaluating their effectiveness for the treatment of advanced ovarian cancer. The current progress of the development of these drugs for ovarian cancer was the topic of a recent excellent review (Mabuchi et al 2011). Preclinical data suggest that these agents may be effective both as monotherapy as well as in combination with traditional cytotoxic chemotherapy and may even be effective as preventative agents. The majority of these studies are ongoing and have not completed recruitment, however the results of a few have been published (Table 1). In a phase I clinical trial designed to determine the recommended phase II dose of weekly temsirolimus and topotecan for the treatment of advanced and/or recurrent gynecologic malignancies, the toxicities of the combination were dose-limiting (Temkin et al 2010). Seven participants with ovarian cancer were enrolled in the study but the authors do not report the best response for these participants; nine of the 11 evaluable participants on the study had stable disease. In a Phase I study of temsirolimus, carboplatin, and paclitaxel in patients with endometrial and ovarian cancers, the combination was well tolerated and a recommended phase II dose was established(Oza et al 2009). In addition, 22 of the 26 participants with follow-up data showed either partial response (38.5%) or stable disease (46%) for a median duration of 7 months. In a phase II trial combining targeted therapies, temsirolimus and bevacizumab, a monoclonal antibody targeting VEGF-A, were given to patients with recurrent epithelial ovarian cancer who had received ≤2 chemotherapy regimens for recurrent disease. This study met its first stage goal of 14 participants remaining progression free at 6 months and has been reopened for second stage accrual(Morgan et al 2011). Rapamycin and its analogues predominantly inhibit mTOR complex 1 (mTORC1) without affecting the activity of mTORC2. A novel ATP-competitive inhibitor of mTOR kinase activity, AZD8055, inhibits both the mTORC1/mTORC2 and prevents the feedback activation of AKT that is observed with the rapalogues and has completed phase I clinical trial in advanced solid malignancies(Banerji et al 2011, Chresta et al 2010).

Therapy	Phase	# Pts	Selection Criteria	Outcome	Comments
Temsirolimus + Topotecan (Temkin et al 2010)	I	15 (7 ovarian cancer)	advanced or recurrent gynecologic malignancy refractory to curative therapy	9/11 SD	Toxicities of the combination were dose limiting, intolerable in pts previously treated with radiation
Temsirolimus + Carboplatin + Paclitaxel (Oza et al 2009)	I	31	advanced solid malignancies suitable for carboplatin and paclitaxel chemotherapy who had not received more than 2 prior lines of chemotherapy	10/26 PR 12/26 SD	Median duration of response 7 months
Temsirolimus + Bevacizumab (Morgan et al 2011)	II	31	recurrent epithelial OC who had received ≤ 2 chemotherapy regimens for recurrent disease	3/25 PR 9/25 SD	Met first stage goal, reopened for second stage accrual (NCT01010126)

Table 1. Selected Clinical Trials of mTOR inhibitors in Ovarian Cancer.

Several other PI3K-AKT pathway inhibitors (Table 2) are in early clinical development. Of these, GDC-0941, an inhibitor of PIK3CA, has shown early signs of possible clinical efficacy in an ovarian cancer patient with a PTEN negative tumor(Moreno Garcia et al 2011). MK-

2206, an allosteric AKT inhibitor, showed preclinical efficacy in ovarian cancer cell lines with synergistic responses when combined with other cytotoxic agents such as doxorubicin, docetaxel, and carboplatin. It is currently under investigation in a phase II trial evaluating its efficacy as monotherapy specifically in ovarian cancers exhibiting defects in the PI3K/AKT pathway while several other phase I trials are evaluating its safety in combination with other chemotherapeutic agents(Hirai et al 2010). The results of these and other ongoing studies of PI3K-AKT pathway inhibitors are eagerly awaited.

Drug	Target	Comments
Everolimus	mTOR inhibitor	Under evaluation in Phase I and II trials for ovarian cancer
OSI-027	ATP-competitive mTOR inhibitor	
AZD-8055	ATP-competitive mTOR inhibitor	Dual mTORC1/mTORC2 inhibitor, prevents feedback activation of AKT observed with rapalogues
CH5132799	Selective class I PI3K inhibitor	Anti-tumor activity in vitro and in animal models
GDC-0941	PIK3CA inhibitor	One ovarian cancer patient (PTEN negative) showed 30% response by PET & 80% by CA-125, stayed on study for ~5 months(Moreno Garcia et al 2011)
BEZ235	Dual PI3K/mTOR inhibitor	Anti-tumor activity in mouse model, undergoing evaluation as monotherapy and in combination with cytotoxic chemotherapy
MK-2206	Allosteric AKT inhibitor	Currently being evaluated in recurrent Grade 2 or 3 ovarian, fallopian tube, or primary peritoneal cancer with evidence of a defect in the PI3K/AKT pathway

Table 2. Other PI3K-AKT pathway inhibitors with pre-clinical efficacy in ovarian cancer.

4. Epidermal growth factor receptors

The epidermal growth factor receptor (EGFR) family of receptor tyrosine kinases has been implicated in the oncogenic transformation of a number of cancers. This family of genes encodes for four transmembrane tyrosine kinase receptors commonly referred to as EGFR (HER1/erbB1), HER2/neu (erbB2), HER3 (erbB2) and HER4 (erbB4). They each consist of a ligand-binding extracellular domain, an intracellular kinase domain, and a C-terminal signaling tail. The receptors are activated by binding to one of more than 30 ligands that then allow the formation of homodimers or heterodimers; except HER2 has no known ligand but is able to form heterodimers with other ligand-bound EGFR family members. Interestingly, HER3 lacks intrinsic kinase activity and therefore must form a heterodimer to be active and its preferred binding partner is HER2/neu. Activated dimers recruit signaling molecules through a phosphorylated cytoplasmic domain that initiates a signaling cascade leading to the activation of downstream pathways such as PI3K-AKT and MAPK that ultimately regulate cellular proliferation, migration, invasion, and apoptosis. Two recent excellent reviews have been published on the role of these receptors in ovarian cancer(Sheng and Liu 2011, Siwak et al 2010); herein we will focus on the clinical implications of EGFR, HER2/neu and HER3, the three receptors found to be amplified in ovarian cancers.

Amplification of the EGFR gene has been identified in 4-22% of ovarian cancers and, for the most part, amplification correlates with overexpression(Dimova et al 2006, Lassus et al 2006, Stadlmann et al 2006, Vermeij et al 2008). Some studies have delineated the level of amplification into high and low categories. While high level amplification occurs in a small percentage of tumors (4-12%), low level gain has been reported in as many as 43% of cases(Dimova et al 2006, Lassus et al 2006). High-level amplifications have been associated with malignant tumors and worse histologic grade. Results are mixed on the influence of EGFR overexpression on patient outcome. Several studies showed no association with survival, while EGFR overexpression was found to be a strong prognostic indicator in other studies(Baekelandt et al 1999, Elie et al 2004, Lassus et al 2006, Lee et al 2005a, Nicholson et al 2001). The discrepancy may be related to different methodologies used in staining and analysis.

Preclinical data suggests that targeting EGFR is an effective approach to treating ovarian cancer. Ovarian cancer cells treated with antisense RNA or dominant-negative approaches showed reduced proliferation, invasion, and tumorigenicity in a rat ovarian tumor model(Alper et al 2000, Alper et al 2001, Chan et al 2005). A human-mouse chimeric anti-EGFR monoclonal antibody (C225, cetuximab) resulted in decreased activity of cyclin dependent kinases and inhibition of ovarian cancer cellular proliferation by 40-50% and when combined with cytotoxic chemotherapy enhanced the efficacy of those agents(Ye et al 1999). However, the results have been inconsistent and targeting of EGFR with either gefitinib or cetuximab in several ovarian cancer cell lines showed minimal response(Bull Phelps et al 2008).

Two types of EGFR inhibitors are currently in clinical use: monoclonal antibodies (Table 3) and small molecule tyrosine kinase inhibitors (TKIs), and several have been evaluated for the treatment of ovarian cancer. The studies have taken different strategies, some requiring EGFR immunohistochemical positivity as an inclusion criterion, while others evaluated EGFR expression only after enrollment. Overall the results have been disappointing with some studies showing, at best, modest response. In the two studies using single agent EGFR monoclonal antibodies, cetuximab and matuzumab, overall response rates were 4% and 0%, respectively(Schilder et al 2009, Seiden et al 2007). There are five trials evaluating EGFR monoclonal antibodies in combination with cytotoxic chemotherapy, with three ongoing. Of the two involving cetuximab, a phase II trial of cetuximab in combination with carboplatin in recurrent, platinum-sensitive disease yielded an objective response rate of 34.6%, a rate that was too low to warrant further evaluation(Secord et al 2008). The other Phase II study that evaluated the combination of cetuximab, paclitaxel, and carboplatin in the initial treatment of advanced-stage ovarian, primary peritoneal, or fallopian tube cancers did not show an increase in progression free survival compared to historical controls(Konner et al 2008). Three separate phase II trials are evaluating panitumumab with cytotoxic chemotherapy; the results of these studies are not yet available but are eagerly awaited.

Small molecule tyrosine kinase inhibitors (TKI) targeting EGFR activity have been investigated in several trials specifically focused on ovarian cancer (Table 4). Single agent TKI did not show any substantial clinical benefit (0-9% for gefitinib(Posadas et al 2007,

Schilder et al 2005), 0% for CI-1033 an irreversible EGFR inhibitor(Campos et al 2005)). TKIs combined with cytotoxic chemotherapy, anti-angiogenic therapy, or hormonal therapy have also shown limited clinical efficacy and in some cases excessive toxicity(Campos et al 2010, Chambers et al 2010, Nimeiri et al 2008, Vasey et al 2008). The reason behind the relative failure of EGFR targeted therapies is not understood, but may be related to constitutive activation of downstream pathways, overexpression of ligands, or activation of alternative signaling pathways (reviewed in (Bianco et al 2007, Siwak et al 2010)). Despite the promising preclinical results based on the amplification data, these therapeutic agents cannot be recommended outside of a clinical trial setting for the treatment of ovarian cancer.

Therapy	Phase	# Pts	Selection Criteria	Outcome	Comments
Cetuximab (Schilder et al 2009)	II	25	Persistent/recurrent ovarian or primary peritoneal carcinoma	1/25 PR 9/25 SD	Median progression free survival 1.8 months
Matuzumab (Seiden et al 2007)	II	37	recurrent, EGFR-positive ovarian, or primary peritoneal cancer	6/37 SD	
Cetuximab + Carboplatin (Secord et al 2008)	II	28 (26 EGFR +)	relapsed platinum-sensitive ovarian or primary peritoneal carcinoma	3/28 CR 6/28 PR 8/28 SD	Did not meet criteria for a second stage of accrual
Cetuximab + Carboplatin + Paclitaxel (Konner et al 2008)	II	40	Initial treatment of stage III or IV, debulked tumor, EGFR positive by IHC	Median PFS 14.4 mths, PFS at 18 mths 38.8%	No prolongation of PFS when compared to historical data
Panitumumab + Gemcitabine	II		Persistent/recurrent platinum-resistant epithelial ovarian, primary peritoneal or fallopian tube cancer		Ongoing (NCT01296035)
Panitumumab + Pegylated Liposomal Doxorubicin	II		Platinum resistant epithelial primary ovarian, primary fallopian or primary peritoneal cancer		Ongoing (NCT00861120)
Panitumumab + Carboplatin + Pegylated Liposomal Doxorubicin	II		Platinum-sensitive recurrent epithelial ovarian cancer, primary peritoneal carcinomatosis or fallopian tube cancer, KRAS wild type		Opening soon (NCT01388621)

Table 3. Anti-EGFR monoclonal antibodies.

Therapy	Phase	# Pts	Selection Criteria	Outcome	Comments
CI-1033/ Canertinib (Campos et al 2005)	II	105	Persistent/recurrent epithelial ovarian cancer	18/52 SD at highest dose level	median PFS 2.2 mths, median OS 9.1 mths at highest dose level
Gefitinib (Posadas et al 2007)	II	24	Recurrent epithelial ovarian cancer	9/24 SD	EGFR and pEGFR levels decreased during therapy in >50%, however not associated with clinical benefit
Gefitinib (Schilder et al 2005)	II	27	Persistent/recurrent epithelial ovarian or primary peritoneal carcinoma	1/27 PR	4 pts with PFS ≥6 mths, trial did not continue to second stage, responder had activating EGFR mutation, trend towards response in EGFR positive pts
Gefitinib + Anastrazole (Krasner et al 2005)	II	35	Recurrent ovarian, peritoneal or tubal carcinoma, ER and/or PR positive by IHC	1/23 CR 14/23 SD	
Gefitinib + Tamoxifen (Wagner et al 2007)	II	56	Refractory, recurrent epithelial ovarian cancer	16/56 SD	Tumor did not need to be positive for ER or EGFR by IHC
Erlotinib (Gordon et al 2005)	II	34	Refractory, recurrent, ovarian cancer, EGFR positive by IHC	2/34 PR 15/34 SD	
Erlotinib + Carboplatin + Docetaxel (Vasey et al 2008)	Ib	45	Chemonaive	5/23 CR 7/23 PR	Objective response rate (52%) lower than in historical controls (59%), unselected for EGFR expression
Erlotinib + Bevacizumab (Chambers et al 2010)	II	40	Platinum resistant	1/39 CR 8/39 PR 10/39 SD	ORR not improved compared to historical controls of Bevacizumab alone
Erlotinib + Bevacizumab (Nimeiri et al 2008)	II	13	Recurrent ovarian, primary peritoneal or fallopian tube cancer	1/13 CR 1/13 PR 7/13 SD	Combination not superior to single-agent Bevacizumab, rate of GI perforation a concern

Table 4. Anti-EGFR small molecule inhibitors.

Expression and amplification levels of Her2/neu in ovarian cancer have been extensively evaluated, however the data is inconsistent and its significance is still controversial. Early studies showed amplification in 26% with corresponding overexpression and an analysis of the subset with available survival data showed a significantly longer median overall survival in women whose tumors did not exhibit Her2 amplification (1879, 959, and 243 days for women having one copy, 2-5 copies and >5 copies of Her2/neu gene, respectively, p <0.0001)(Slamon et al 1989). In subsequent studies, observed rates of Her2/neu amplification in ovarian cancer has been reported in up to 66% of epithelial ovarian cancers with overexpression reported in up to 76%(Camilleri-Broet et al 2004, Press et al 1990, Ross et al 1999, Serrano-Olvera et al 2006, Slamon et al 1989, Tuefferd et al 2007, Vermeij et al 2008). Levels of amplification differ with low copy number amplification (<2) observed in as many as 79%, 3-5 copies in 14%, >5 copies in 6.8%, and >10 copies in 1.8%(Lassus et al 2004). The level of amplification in general has correlated with level of overexpression by IHC, however this too has been called into question(Lassus et al 2004, Mano et al 2004, Pegram et al 1997, Wu et al 2004) and may be reflective of other mechanisms responsible for overexpression other than amplification.

Several studies have shown an association between Her2/neu overexpression/ amplification and poor response to therapy and prognosis, however more recent reports refute this association(Berchuck et al 1990, Bookman et al 2003, Farley et al 2009, Pegram et al 1997, Rubin et al 1994, Tuefferd et al 2007). In a recent Gynecologic Oncology Group study that evaluated Her2/neu amplification in 133 epithelial ovarian cancers, amplification (>2 copies) was only identified in 7% and was not an independent prognostic factor for progression free survival or overall survival(Farley et al 2009). A phase II trial evaluating the efficacy of trastuzumab, a monoclonal humanized anti-Her2 antibody, in patients with recurrent ovarian cancer showed that only 11% of tumor samples exhibited elevated expression of Her2 by immunohistochemistry. Of the participants treated with trastuzumab, the overall response rate was only 7% with a progression free interval of 2 months(Bookman et al 2003). Overall, it does not appear that Her2/neu amplification has predictive or prognostic value in epithelial ovarian cancer and the value of treatment with HER2 directed monotherapy is limited (Table 5). Despite, preclinical evidence of effectiveness(Gordon et al 2006), pertuzumab, a recombinant, humanized monoclonal antibody that binds the HER2 dimerization domain impeding dimerization of HER2 with other family members and thus prevents activation of downstream pathways, has shown similarly low response rates in clinical trials in the treatment of ovarian cancer. As a single agent, the response rate was only 4.3% and in a randomized phase II study the addition of pertuzumab to gemcitabine improved the objective response rate to 13.8% from 4.6%(Gordon et al 2006, Makhija et al 2010). Treatment response appeared to correlate with Her2 phosphorylation status in one study and low Her3 expression in another, however these markers have not yet been validated in further studies. Lapatinib, a dual EGFR/HER2 TKI, has also shown limited clinical response and excessive toxicity(Joly et al 2009, Kimball et al 2008). Preliminary results of a phase I/II trial combining lapatinib with carboplatin and paclitaxel showed promising preliminary results, but the final results of the trial have not been published(Rivkin et al 2008). Further studies will be necessary to determine whether lapatinib may be a useful agent in ovarian cancer.

Therapy	Phase	# Pts	Selection Criteria	Outcome	Comments
Trastuzumab (Bookman et al 2003)	II	41	persistent or recurrent epithelial ovarian cancer, 2/3+ HER2 by IHC	1/41 CR 2/41 PR 16/41 SD	serum HER2 was not associated with clinical outcome
Pertuzumab (Gordon et al 2006)	II	117	Recurrent epithelial ovarian cancer	5 PR 8 SD	Median PFS 6.6 wks, trend toward improved PFS for pts with pHER2+ disease
Pertuzumab + Gemcitabine vs Placebo + Gemcitabine (Makhija et al 2010)	II	65 (combo) 65 (placebo)	advanced, platinum-resistant epithelial ovarian, fallopian tube, or primary peritoneal cancer	9/65 PR (combo) 3/65 PR (placebo)	Low HER3 mRNA expression may predict pertuzumab clinical benefit
Lapatinib + Topotecan (Joly et al 2009)	II	39 (37 ovarian cancer)	Ovarian cancer relapsed w/in 12 months	0/2 PR 7/9 SD	Prematurely stopped for lack of efficacy
Lapatinib + Carboplatin (Kimball et al 2008)	I	12	Recurrent platinum sensitive epithelial ovarian carcinoma	3/11 PR 3/11 SD	unacceptable toxicities, excessive treatment delays and limited clinical responses
Lapatinib + Carboplatin + Paclitaxel (Rivkin et al 2008)	I/II	25	Recurrent ovarian cancer	CR 21% PR 29% SD 29%	final results not published

Table 5. Selected Clinical Trials of HER2/neu Targeted Agents in Ovarian Cancer.

The roles of HER3 and HER4 in ovarian cancer have been less extensively studied(Sheng and Liu 2011). HER3 amplification and overexpression in ovarian cancer has been described and in one study was significantly associated with poor survival (median survival time 3.3 years vs. 1.8 years for patients with low vs. high HER3 expression)(Sheng and Liu 2011, Tanner et al 2006, Tsuda et al 2004). Antibodies directed against the extracellular domain of HER3 diminished HER2 activity and attenuated the activation of downstream effectors(van der Horst et al 2005). Compensatory overexpression of HER3 has also been implicated as a mechanism of resistance to other EGFR inhibitors(Sheng and Liu 2011). These data suggest that targeting HER3 may be an effective treatment strategy and three monoclonal antibodies that target HER3 are being tested in early phase clinical trials for advanced solid tumors (U3-1287, MM-121, and MM-111 which targets both HER2 and HER3). The expression of

HER4 has been variably reported in ovarian cancer, ranging from nearly absent to almost ubiquitously expressed(Sheng and Liu 2011). Interestingly, overexpression of HER4 in ovarian cancer was associated with a trend toward improved progression free and overall survival, an effect that has also been seen in breast cancer possibly by promoting differentiation(Pejovic et al 2009, Rajkumar et al 1996). However, these results have not been confirmed and the role of HER4 in ovarian cancer is still undefined.

5. Notch signaling pathway

The Notch signaling pathway is an evolutionarily conserved pathway that regulates cellular differentiation, proliferation, and apoptosis. The family of Notch receptors (Notch 1-4) are large transmembrane proteins that consist of an extracellular ligand binding domain, a transmembrane domain, and an intracellular domain. Activation of the receptors is a multi-step process consisting of an initial cleavage event allowing the extracellular domain to heterodimerize with transmembrane ligands (Delta-like 1, 3, 4 and Jagged 1 and 2). Following ligand binding a second cleavage event releases the Notch extracellular domain (ECD) causing the ECD and the ligand to be endocytosed. Cleavage by gamma secretase following endocytosis releases the active Notch intracellular domain (NICD) allowing for translocation to the nucleus and heterodimerization to transcription factors and recruitment of coactivators to form a functionally active transcriptional complex(Rose 2009). Of the Notch receptors, Notch1 and Notch3 have been implicated in ovarian cancer. Reports of Notch1 expression in ovarian cancer are inconsistent with some showing increased expression in carcinomas compared to benign tumor or normal ovarian surface epithelium, while others showed decreased mRNA expression in carcinomas(Hopfer et al 2005, Rose et al 2010, Wang et al 2010).

The association between Notch3 and ovarian cancer has been more extensively studied. High level Notch3 amplification has been observed in 7.8% of high-grade serous carcinomas (Nakayama et al 2007), while high level protein overexpression was found in 63% of serous carcinomas and was significantly correlated with advanced stage, likelihood of metastasis, chemoresistance and poor overall survival(Jung et al 2010). Overexpression of the Notch ligands, Jagged-1 and Jagged-2, has also been identified in ovarian tumor cells lending support that activation of the Notch pathway promotes ovarian cancer proliferation and that inhibition of this pathway may be a viable therapeutic approach(Choi et al 2008, Hopfer et al 2005). Similarly, the TCGA identified alterations in the Notch pathway in 22% of high-grade serous ovarian carcinoma samples, which included amplification/mutation of Notch3, amplification of Jagged-1 and Jagged-2, and amplification/mutation of MAML1-3, a family of Notch transcriptional coactivators(Cancer Genome Atlas Research Network, 2011). Inactivation of Notch signaling through targeting Jagged-1 or direct inhibition of Notch by preventing cleavage with a gamma-secretase inhibitor decreases the proliferative potential of and increases apoptosis in ovarian cancer cell lines and xenograft models(Park et al 2006, Steg et al 2011). Targeting Jagged-1 also resulted in decreased microvessel density in xenografts suggesting Notch signaling may play a role in angiogenesis.

Notch pathway inhibitors have recently moved into clinical trials. Early reports of a phase I clinical trial of RO4929097, a selective oral gamma-secretase inhibitor, showed prolonged stable disease in 3 ovarian cancer patients (Table 6)(Tolcher et al 2010). Combination therapy is being evaluated in two ongoing early phase clinical trials in which RO4929097 is combined with either cediranib, a VEGF inhibitor, or GDC-0449, a hedgehog inhibitor. Whether this will be a useful agent in treating ovarian cancer remains to be seen.

Drug	Target	Comments
R04929097	Selective oral gamma-secretase inhibitor of Notch	Preliminary efficacy in 3 ovarian cancer patients(Tolcher et al 2010). Two early phase combination trials ongoing: NCT01131234 (+ cediranib), NCT01154452 (+ GDC-0449)
PD 0332991	CDK4/6 inhibitor	Current being tested in NCT01037790 which includes ovarian germ cell tumors
BMS-387032 (SNS-032)	CDK2 inhibitor	
Flavopiridol (Alvocidib)	Multi-CDK inhibitor	Ongoing phase II trial in combination with cisplatin in epithelial ovarian cancers (NCT00083122)
ON 01910.Na	Polo-Like Kinase 1 inhibitor	Durable response in a platinum-refractory ovarian cancer pt, maintained progression free for 24 months (Jimeno et al 2008)
MLN8237	Aurora A kinase inhibitor	Durable response (PR) in a pt with platinum-refractory ovarian cancer with continued treatment over 1.5 years(Dees et al 2010), ongoing phase II in combination with paclitaxel (NCT01091428)
ENMD-2076	Aurora kinase inhibitor	3/46 PR, 27/46 SD in preliminary report from phase II trial in platinum resistant ovarian cancer(Matulonis et al 2011)

Table 6. Other pathway inhibitors with pre-clinical efficacy in ovarian cancer.

6. Cell cycle regulatory proteins

Sustaining proliferative signaling through disruption of cell cycle regulatory checkpoints is one of the hallmarks of cancer(Hanahan and Weinberg 2011). Aberrant expression of cyclins, cyclin dependent kinases (Cdks), and cyclin-Cdk inhibitors has been linked to tumorigenesis in multiple cancer models(Deshpande et al 2005, Hwang and Clurman 2005). Studies in epithelial ovarian cancer have shown inconsistent associations between individual cell cycle regulatory protein expression and patient outcome (reviewed in Nam and Kim(Nam and Kim 2008)). Among the best studied in ovarian cancer is cyclin E. Amplification of the cyclin E gene occurs in 7-65% of ovarian cancers, typically resulting in overexpression of the cyclin E protein(Cancer Genome Atlas Research Network, 2011, Courjal et al 1996, Marone et al

1998, Mayr et al 2006, Nakayama et al 2007, Nakayama et al 2010, Park et al 2006, Schraml et al 2003a). Cyclin E expression has been found in as many as 97% of ovarian cancer/primary peritoneal cancer samples(Davidson et al 2006). In suboptimally debulked advanced epithelial ovarian cancers obtained from women enrolled in GOG111, the expression level of cyclin E correlated with a 6 month shorter median survival and worse overall survival(Farley et al 2003). Analysis of the subset of patients with serous carcinomas (72% of total study) showed an 11 month difference in median survival and suggested that the role of cyclin E was limited to the serous histology as nonserous tumors showed no statistically significant difference in survival based on cyclin E expression. The association between cyclin E amplification and poor outcome has also been identified in recent German and Japanese studies, although the correlation was not statistically significant in the latter(Mayr et al 2006, Nakayama et al 2010). Two independent labs have also suggested that amplification of the cyclin E gene was associated with primary treatment resistance and targeting cyclin E expression with siRNA reduced cell viability and increased apoptosis(Etemadmoghadam et al 2009, Etemadmoghadam et al 2010, Nakayama et al 2010). These studies suggest that cyclin E amplification/expression may serve as both a prognostic and predictive factor in ovarian cancer as well as a therapeutic target in the treatment of ovarian cancer.

Several studies have evaluated the expression levels of many other cell cycle regulatory proteins, however few appear to show gene amplification. Although overexpression of cyclin D has been reported, levels of expression did not correlate with clinical outcome and the mechanism of overexpression was not through amplification of the gene(Courjal et al 1996, Dhar et al 1999, Hung et al 1996, Masciullo et al 1997). High copy number amplification of cdk2 was found in only 4-6% of cases(Cancer Genome Atlas Research Network, 2011, Marone et al 1998). Genomic loss of the region containing the retinoblastoma (Rb) gene and loss of heterozygosity of Rb has been described, however loss of expression occurred in few cases leading the investigators to conclude that Rb did not play a significant role in high-grade ovarian carcinomas(Dodson et al 1994, Kim et al 1994, Li et al 1991). Recently, two families of mitotic kinases have been implicated in ovarian cancer: the Polo-like kinases and Aurora kinases. Overexpression of both has been associated with a shortened survival time in patients with ovarian cancer and these targets have been the focus of recent clinical trials, however only the Aurora A gene was found to be amplified (in 15-27% of ovarian carcinomas)(Chen et al 2009, Mendiola et al 2009, Tanner et al 2000, Weichert et al 2004). Level of amplification of the Aurora A gene has been inconsistent with regards to tumor characteristics (histology or grade), level of expression, or patient outcome, with reports of greater association with early stage and low grade ovarian cancers as well as an association with poor prognosis(Fu et al 2006).

Many cell cycle associated kinase inhibitors are in early phase development (reviewed in (De Falco and De Luca 2010)), but few have been tested in ovarian cancer (Table 6). Interestingly, a mitotic regulatory inhibitor that affects the polo-like kinases (among others), had clinical benefit for a chemorefractory ovarian cancer patient for 24 months(Jimeno et al 2008). Preliminary results with MLN8237, an Aurora A kinase inhibitor, in a phase I trial showed one long term response (>1.5 yrs) in a patient with platinum refractory ovarian cancer(Dees et al 2010). A phase II study of ENMD-2076, an oral small molecule kinase inhibitor with activity against aurora kinases among other kinases, showed modest activity in platinum-resistant ovarian cancer(Matulonis et al 2011). Inhibition of aurora kinase has been reported to sensitize cells to treatment with paclitaxel(Hata et al 2005, Scharer et al 2008) and the combination of paclitaxel and MLN8237 is being evaluated in a phase II randomized clinical trial. Results from these clinical trials are eagerly awaited.

7. Chromatin remodeling and transcription

Epigenetic modifications, such as DNA methylation and histone modifications, interact to remodel chromatin and result in the dysregulation of genes and pathways leading to uncontrolled cell growth. These mechanisms are primarily under the regulation of DNA methyltransferases (DNMTs) and histone decetylases (HDACs) and therapeutic agents inhibiting these epigenetic modifiers are currently in clinical use for the treatment of certain hematologic malignancies and are being evaluated in clinical trials for ovarian cancer (reviewed in Matei and Nephew(Matei and Nephew 2010)). Other chromatin remodeling proteins are emerging as potentially important in the pathogenesis of ovarian cancer and may be useful therapeutic targets. Amplification of the chromosome 11q13.5 locus is frequently detected in human cancers, including ovarian carcinomas. This region was amplified in 13-16% of high grade ovarian carcinomas but not in any of the normal ovarian tissues, benign ovarian tumors, or low grade ovarian carcinomas analyzed(Nakayama et al 2007, Shih Ie et al 2005). The only gene within the amplicon that showed consistent overexpression was the gene encoding HBXAP/Rsf-1, a subunit of the RSF chromatin assembly complex. Patients whose tumors harbored amplification of Rsf-1 had a shorter overall survival compared with those without amplification(Nakayama et al 2007, Sheu et al 2010, Shih Ie et al 2005). Rsf-1 amplification (and ensuing overexpression) was identified as an independent prognostic factor based on multivariate analysis and this may be secondary to its ability to confer resistance to treatment with paclitaxel(Choi et al 2009). Elevated levels of Rsf-1 was shown to induce chromosomal instability, and in non-transformed cells, induced growth arrest and activated DNA damage response pathways. However in the presence of an inactivated p53, long-term overexpression of Rsf-1 stimulated cellular proliferation. While Rsf-1 is only amplified in a subset of high-grade ovarian serous carcinomas, inactivation or disruption of the RSF complex may be a useful therapeutic approach for tumors that depend on this protein for a proliferative advantage.

Other genes, such as MYC, NACC1 (which encodes Nac1), EMSY, MECOM, and PAK1 involved in chromatin remodeling and transcription, have also been shown to be amplified in ovarian carcinomas(Dimova et al 2009, Schraml et al 2003b, Shih Ie et al 2011). The expression of some, such as Nac1, has been associated with poor progression-free survival and paclitaxel resistance(Davidson et al 2007, Jinawath et al 2009, Nakayama et al 2006a). For others, such as MYC and EMSY, the significance of the amplification in high grade serous carcinoma is unclear and they may not be the oncogenic driver within the amplicon(Shih Ie et al 2005). Others are likely only relevant for a subtype, as in ARID-1A in clear cell carcinomas. A number of amplified genes identified by the TCGA and others have potential drugs currently in preclinical development or early phase clinical trials. However further work is necessary to determine whether any of these are prognostic markers or predictive of response to therapy.

8. Conclusion

Despite the identification of several amplified pathways, the results of the clinical trials of therapeutic agents targeting these pathways in ovarian cancer have been disappointing. There are several potential reasons for the poor response rates. The majority of studies of new targeted agents enroll patients with advanced disease often after several lines of standard cytotoxic therapy have failed. Even when used in combination with cytotoxic chemotherapy, these agents may not be able to overcome the mechanisms of resistance that the tumor has developed. Of interest would be evaluating these drugs in low-volume or early (marker only) recurrent disease or in combination with initial chemotherapy. Another strategy would be to test these typically cytostatic agents as maintenance therapy in patients who are in a complete clinical remission.

Resistance to targeted agents is mediated through a variety of mechanisms including mutation of the target, constitutive activation of downstream effectors, or activation of compensatory pathways. Defining the mechanisms of constitutive or acquired resistance requires thorough investigation in cellular and animal models. Emphasis should be placed on characterizing resistance mechanisms and developing better predictive markers to identify subsets of patients who are more likely to respond to therapy.

Targeting codependent pathways, rather than the amplified genes directly, may be another approach to cancer treatment. Cancer cells typically co-opt metabolic and stress response pathways becoming functionally reliant on them for continued proliferation while normal cells are not dependent on their function. Raj et al. recently used this strategy to preferentially eliminate cancer cells by targeting the oxidative stress response pathway(Raj et al 2011). This approach is similar to the synthetic lethality seen with PARP inhibitors in tumors with BRCA mutations.

In summary, while at present there is not a clear role for targeting the amplified pathways in ovarian cancer outside of a clinical trial, elucidating strategies of tumor resistance and compensatory mechanisms may allow for the development of novel therapeutic agents or the rational combination of existing agents to improve the prognosis of patients with ovarian cancer.

9. Acknowledgement

Special thanks to Drs. Ie-Ming Shih and Tian-Li Wang for their help in the preparation of this manuscript.

10. References

(Cancer Genome Atlas Research Network, 2011). Integrated genomic analyses of ovarian carcinoma. *Nature* 474: 609-615.

Alper O, De Santis ML, Stromberg K, Hacker NF, Cho-Chung YS, Salomon DS (2000). Antisense suppression of epidermal growth factor receptor expression alters cellular proliferation, cell-adhesion and tumorigenicity in ovarian cancer cells. *Int J Cancer* 88: 566-574.

Alper O, Bergmann-Leitner ES, Bennett TA, Hacker NF, Stromberg K, Stetler-Stevenson WG (2001). Epidermal growth factor receptor signaling and the invasive phenotype of ovarian carcinoma cells. *J Natl Cancer Inst* 93: 1375-1384.

Altomare DA, Wang HQ, Skele KL, De Rienzo A, Klein-Szanto AJ, Godwin AK, Testa JR (2004). AKT and mTOR phosphorylation is frequently detected in ovarian cancer and can be targeted to disrupt ovarian tumor cell growth. *Oncogene* 23: 5853-5857.

Baekelandt M, Kristensen GB, Trope CG, Nesland JM, Holm R (1999). Epidermal growth factor receptor expression has no independent prognostic significance in advanced ovarian cancer. *Anticancer Res* 19: 4469-4474.

Banerji U, Aghajanian C, Raymond E, Kurzrock R, Blanco-Codesido M, Oelmann E, Grinsted L, Burke W, Kaye SB, Naing A (2011). First results from a phase I trial of AZD8055, a dual mTORC1 and mTORC2 inhibitor. *J Clin Oncol* 29: Abstr 3096.

Bellacosa A, de Feo D, Godwin AK, Bell DW, Cheng JQ, Altomare DA, Wan M, Dubeau L, Scambia G, Masciullo V, Ferrandina G, Benedetti Panici P, Mancuso S, Neri G, Testa JR (1995). Molecular alterations of the AKT2 oncogene in ovarian and breast carcinomas. *Int J Cancer* 64: 280-285.

Berchuck A, Kamel A, Whitaker R, Kerns B, Olt G, Kinney R, Soper JT, Dodge R, Clarke-Pearson DL, Marks P, et al. (1990). Overexpression of HER-2/neu is associated with poor survival in advanced epithelial ovarian cancer. *Cancer Res* 50: 4087-4091.

Bianco R, Damiano V, Gelardi T, Daniele G, Ciardiello F, Tortora G (2007). Rational combination of targeted therapies as a strategy to overcome the mechanisms of resistance to inhibitors of EGFR signaling. *Curr Pharm Des* 13: 3358-3367.

Bookman MA, Darcy KM, Clarke-Pearson D, Boothby RA, Horowitz IR (2003). Evaluation of monoclonal humanized anti-HER2 antibody, trastuzumab, in patients with recurrent or refractory ovarian or primary peritoneal carcinoma with overexpression of HER2: a phase II trial of the Gynecologic Oncology Group. *J Clin Oncol* 21: 283-290.

Bull Phelps SL, Schorge JO, Peyton MJ, Shigematsu H, Xiang LL, Miller DS, Lea JS (2008). Implications of EGFR inhibition in ovarian cancer cell proliferation. *Gynecol Oncol* 109: 411-417.

Bunkholt Elstrand M, Dong HP, Odegaard E, Holth A, Elloul S, Reich R, Trope CG, Davidson B (2010). Mammalian target of rapamycin is a biomarker of poor survival in metastatic serous ovarian carcinoma. *Hum Pathol* 41: 794-804.

Camilleri-Broet S, Hardy-Bessard AC, Le Tourneau A, Paraiso D, Levrel O, Leduc B, Bain S, Orfeuvre H, Audouin J, Pujade-Lauraine E (2004). HER-2 overexpression is an independent marker of poor prognosis of advanced primary ovarian carcinoma: a multicenter study of the GINECO group. *Ann Oncol* 15: 104-112.

Campbell IG, Russell SE, Choong DY, Montgomery KG, Ciavarella ML, Hooi CS, Cristiano BE, Pearson RB, Phillips WA (2004). Mutation of the PIK3CA gene in ovarian and breast cancer. *Cancer Res* 64: 7678-7681.

Campos S, Hamid O, Seiden MV, Oza A, Plante M, Potkul RK, Lenehan PF, Kaldjian EP, Varterasian ML, Jordan C, Charbonneau C, Hirte H (2005). Multicenter, randomized phase II trial of oral CI-1033 for previously treated advanced ovarian cancer. *J Clin Oncol* 23: 5597-5604.

Campos SM, Berlin ST, Parker LM, Chen WY, Bunnell CA, Atkinson T, Lee J, Matulonis U, Hirsch MS, Harris L, Krasner CN (2010). Phase I trial of liposomal doxorubicin and ZD1839 in patients with refractory gynecological malignancies or metastatic breast cancer. *Int J Clin Oncol* 15: 390-398.

Chambers SK, Clouser MC, Baker AF, Roe DJ, Cui H, Brewer MA, Hatch KD, Gordon MS, Janicek MF, Isaacs JD, Gordon AN, Nagle RB, Wright HM, Cohen JL, Alberts DS (2010). Overexpression of tumor vascular endothelial growth factor A may portend an increased likelihood of progression in a phase II trial of bevacizumab and erlotinib in resistant ovarian cancer. *Clin Cancer Res* 16: 5320-5328.

Chan JK, Pham H, You XJ, Cloven NG, Burger RA, Rose GS, Van Nostrand K, Korc M, Disaia PJ, Fan H (2005). Suppression of ovarian cancer cell tumorigenicity and evasion of Cisplatin resistance using a truncated epidermal growth factor receptor in a rat model. *Cancer Res* 65: 3243-3248.

Chen YJ, Chen CM, Twu NF, Yen MS, Lai CR, Wu HH, Wang PH, Yuan CC (2009). Overexpression of Aurora B is associated with poor prognosis in epithelial ovarian cancer patients. *Virchows Arch* 455: 431-440.

Cheng JQ, Godwin AK, Bellacosa A, Taguchi T, Franke TF, Hamilton TC, Tsichlis PN, Testa JR (1992). AKT2, a putative oncogene encoding a member of a subfamily of protein-serine/threonine kinases, is amplified in human ovarian carcinomas. *Proc Natl Acad Sci U S A* 89: 9267-9271.

Choi JH, Park JT, Davidson B, Morin PJ, Shih Ie M, Wang TL (2008). Jagged-1 and Notch3 juxtacrine loop regulates ovarian tumor growth and adhesion. *Cancer Res* 68: 5716-5723.

Choi JH, Sheu JJ, Guan B, Jinawath N, Markowski P, Wang TL, Shih Ie M (2009). Functional analysis of 11q13.5 amplicon identifies Rsf-1 (HBXAP) as a gene involved in paclitaxel resistance in ovarian cancer. *Cancer Res* 69: 1407-1415.

Chresta CM, Davies BR, Hickson I, Harding T, Cosulich S, Critchlow SE, Vincent JP, Ellston R, Jones D, Sini P, James D, Howard Z, Dudley P, Hughes G, Smith L *et al* (2010). AZD8055 is a potent, selective, and orally bioavailable ATP-competitive mammalian target of rapamycin kinase inhibitor with in vitro and in vivo antitumor activity. *Cancer Res* 70: 288-298.

Courjal F, Louason G, Speiser P, Katsaros D, Zeillinger R, Theillet C (1996). Cyclin gene amplification and overexpression in breast and ovarian cancers: evidence for the selection of cyclin D1 in breast and cyclin E in ovarian tumors. *Int J Cancer* 69: 247-253.

Dancey JE (2004). Molecular targeting: PI3 kinase pathway. *Ann Oncol* 15 Suppl 4: iv233-239.

Davidson B, Zhang Z, Kleinberg L, Li M, Florenes VA, Wang TL, Shih Ie M (2006). Gene expression signatures differentiate ovarian/peritoneal serous carcinoma from diffuse malignant peritoneal mesothelioma. *Clin Cancer Res* 12: 5944-5950.

Davidson B, Berner A, Trope CG, Wang TL, Shih Ie M (2007). Expression and clinical role of the bric-a-brac tramtrack broad complex/poxvirus and zinc protein NAC-1 in ovarian carcinoma effusions. *Hum Pathol* 38: 1030-1036.

De Falco M, De Luca A (2010). Cell cycle as a target of antineoplastic drugs. *Curr Pharm Des* 16: 1417-1426.

Dees EC, Infante JR, Burris HA, Astsaturov IA, Stinchcombe T, Liu H, Galvin K, Venkatakrishnan K, Fingert HJ, Cohen RB (2010). Phase I study of the investigational drug MLN8237, an Aurora A kinase (AAK) inhibitor, in patients (pts) with solid tumors. *J Clin Oncol* 28: Abstr 3010.

Deshpande A, Sicinski P, Hinds PW (2005). Cyclins and cdks in development and cancer: a perspective. *Oncogene* 24: 2909-2915.

Dhar KK, Branigan K, Parkes J, Howells RE, Hand P, Musgrove C, Strange RC, Fryer AA, Redman CW, Hoban PR (1999). Expression and subcellular localization of cyclin D1 protein in epithelial ovarian tumour cells. *Br J Cancer* 81: 1174-1181.

Dimova I, Zaharieva B, Raitcheva S, Dimitrov R, Doganov N, Toncheva D (2006). Tissue microarray analysis of EGFR and erbB2 copy number changes in ovarian tumors. *Int J Gynecol Cancer* 16: 145-151.

Dimova I, Raicheva S, Dimitrov R, Doganov N, Toncheva D (2009). Coexistence of copy number increases of c-Myc, ZNF217, CCND1, ErbB1 and ErbB2 in ovarian cancers. *Onkologie* 32: 405-410.

Dodson MK, Cliby WA, Xu HJ, DeLacey KA, Hu SX, Keeney GL, Li J, Podratz KC, Jenkins RB, Benedict WF (1994). Evidence of functional RB protein in epithelial ovarian carcinomas despite loss of heterozygosity at the RB locus. *Cancer Res* 54: 610-613.

Elie C, Geay JF, Morcos M, Le Tourneau A, Girre V, Broet P, Marmey B, Chauvenet L, Audouin J, Pujade-Lauraine E, Camilleri-Broet S (2004). Lack of relationship between EGFR-1 immunohistochemical expression and prognosis in a multicentre clinical trial of 93 patients with advanced primary ovarian epithelial cancer (GINECO group). *Br J Cancer* 91: 470-475.

Etemadmoghadam D, deFazio A, Beroukhim R, Mermel C, George J, Getz G, Tothill R, Okamoto A, Raeder MB, Harnett P, Lade S, Akslen LA, Tinker AV, Locandro B, Alsop K *et al* (2009). Integrated genome-wide DNA copy number and expression analysis identifies distinct mechanisms of primary chemoresistance in ovarian carcinomas. *Clin Cancer Res* 15: 1417-1427.

Etemadmoghadam D, George J, Cowin PA, Cullinane C, Kansara M, Gorringe KL, Smyth GK, Bowtell DD (2010). Amplicon-dependent CCNE1 expression is critical for clonogenic survival after cisplatin treatment and is correlated with 20q11 gain in ovarian cancer. *PLoS One* 5: e15498.

Farley J, Smith LM, Darcy KM, Sobel E, O'Connor D, Henderson B, Morrison LE, Birrer MJ (2003). Cyclin E expression is a significant predictor of survival in advanced, suboptimally debulked ovarian epithelial cancers: a Gynecologic Oncology Group study. *Cancer Res* 63: 1235-1241.

Farley J, Fuchiuji S, Darcy KM, Tian C, Hoskins WJ, McGuire WP, Hanjani P, Warshal D, Greer BE, Belinson J, Birrer MJ (2009). Associations between ERBB2 amplification and progression-free survival and overall survival in advanced stage, suboptimally-resected epithelial ovarian cancers: a Gynecologic Oncology Group Study. *Gynecol Oncol* 113: 341-347.

Ferretti G, Felici A, Papaldo P, Fabi A, Cognetti F (2007). HER2/neu role in breast cancer: from a prognostic foe to a predictive friend. *Curr Opin Obstet Gynecol* 19: 56-62.

Fu S, Hu W, Kavanagh JJ, Bast RC, Jr. (2006). Targeting Aurora kinases in ovarian cancer. *Expert Opin Ther Targets* 10: 77-85.

Gao N, Flynn DC, Zhang Z, Zhong XS, Walker V, Liu KJ, Shi X, Jiang BH (2004). G1 cell cycle progression and the expression of G1 cyclins are regulated by PI3K/AKT/mTOR/p70S6K1 signaling in human ovarian cancer cells. *Am J Physiol Cell Physiol* 287: C281-291.

Gordon AN, Finkler N, Edwards RP, Garcia AA, Crozier M, Irwin DH, Barrett E (2005). Efficacy and safety of erlotinib HCl, an epidermal growth factor receptor (HER1/EGFR) tyrosine kinase inhibitor, in patients with advanced ovarian carcinoma: results from a phase II multicenter study. *Int J Gynecol Cancer* 15: 785-792.

Gordon MS, Matei D, Aghajanian C, Matulonis UA, Brewer M, Fleming GF, Hainsworth JD, Garcia AA, Pegram MD, Schilder RJ, Cohn DE, Roman L, Derynck MK, Ng K, Lyons B *et al* (2006). Clinical activity of pertuzumab (rhuMAb 2C4), a HER dimerization inhibitor, in advanced ovarian cancer: potential predictive relationship with tumor HER2 activation status. *J Clin Oncol* 24: 4324-4332.

Gorringe KL, George J, Anglesio MS, Ramakrishna M, Etemadmoghadam D, Cowin P, Sridhar A, Williams LH, Boyle SE, Yanaihara N, Okamoto A, Urashima M, Smyth GK, Campbell IG, Bowtell DD (2010). Copy number analysis identifies novel interactions between genomic loci in ovarian cancer. *PLoS One* 5.

Hanahan D, Weinberg RA (2011). Hallmarks of cancer: the next generation. *Cell* 144: 646-674.

Hata T, Furukawa T, Sunamura M, Egawa S, Motoi F, Ohmura N, Marumoto T, Saya H, Horii A (2005). RNA interference targeting aurora kinase a suppresses tumor growth and enhances the taxane chemosensitivity in human pancreatic cancer cells. *Cancer Res* 65: 2899-2905.

Hirai H, Sootome H, Nakatsuru Y, Miyama K, Taguchi S, Tsujioka K, Ueno Y, Hatch H, Majumder PK, Pan BS, Kotani H (2010). MK-2206, an allosteric Akt inhibitor, enhances antitumor efficacy by standard chemotherapeutic agents or molecular targeted drugs in vitro and in vivo. *Mol Cancer Ther* 9: 1956-1967.

Hopfer O, Zwahlen D, Fey MF, Aebi S (2005). The Notch pathway in ovarian carcinomas and adenomas. *Br J Cancer* 93: 709-718.

Hu L, Hofmann J, Jaffe RB (2005). Phosphatidylinositol 3-kinase mediates angiogenesis and vascular permeability associated with ovarian carcinoma. *Clin Cancer Res* 11: 8208-8212.

Hung WC, Chai CY, Huang JS, Chuang LY (1996). Expression of cyclin D1 and c-Ki-ras gene product in human epithelial ovarian tumors. *Hum Pathol* 27: 1324-1328.

Hwang HC, Clurman BE (2005). Cyclin E in normal and neoplastic cell cycles. *Oncogene* 24: 2776-2786.

Jemal A, Bray F, Center MM, Ferlay J, Ward E, Forman D (2011). Global cancer statistics. *CA Cancer J Clin* 61: 69-90.

Jimeno A, Li J, Messersmith WA, Laheru D, Rudek MA, Maniar M, Hidalgo M, Baker SD, Donehower RC (2008). Phase I study of ON 01910.Na, a novel modulator of the Polo-like kinase 1 pathway, in adult patients with solid tumors. *J Clin Oncol* 26: 5504-5510.

Jinawath N, Vasoontara C, Yap KL, Thiaville MM, Nakayama K, Wang TL, Shih IM (2009). NAC-1, a potential stem cell pluripotency factor, contributes to paclitaxel resistance in ovarian cancer through inactivating Gadd45 pathway. *Oncogene* 28: 1941-1948.

Joly F, Weber B, Pautier P, Fabbro M, Selle F, Krieger S, Leconte A, Bourgeois H, Henry-Amar M (2009). Combined topotecan and lapatinib in patients with early recurrent ovarian or peritoneal cancer after first line of platinum-based chemotherapy: A French FEDEGYN-FNCLCC phase II trial. *J Clin Oncol* 27: Abstr 5555.

Jung SG, Kwon YD, Song JA, Back MJ, Lee SY, Lee C, Hwang YY, An HJ (2010). Prognostic significance of Notch 3 gene expression in ovarian serous carcinoma. *Cancer Sci* 101: 1977-1983.

Kang S, Bader AG, Vogt PK (2005). Phosphatidylinositol 3-kinase mutations identified in human cancer are oncogenic. *Proc Natl Acad Sci U S A* 102: 802-807.

Karakas B, Bachman KE, Park BH (2006). Mutation of the PIK3CA oncogene in human cancers. *Br J Cancer* 94: 455-459.

Kim TM, Benedict WF, Xu HJ, Hu SX, Gosewehr J, Velicescu M, Yin E, Zheng J, D'Ablaing G, Dubeau L (1994). Loss of heterozygosity on chromosome 13 is common only in the biologically more aggressive subtypes of ovarian epithelial tumors and is associated with normal retinoblastoma gene expression. *Cancer Res* 54: 605-609.

Kimball KJ, Numnum TM, Kirby TO, Zamboni WC, Estes JM, Barnes MN, Matei DE, Koch KM, Alvarez RD (2008). A phase I study of lapatinib in combination with carboplatin in women with platinum sensitive recurrent ovarian carcinoma. *Gynecol Oncol* 111: 95-101.

Kolasa IK, Rembiszewska A, Felisiak A, Ziolkowska-Seta I, Murawska M, Moes J, Timorek A, Dansonka-Mieszkowska A, Kupryjanczyk J (2009). PIK3CA amplification associates with resistance to chemotherapy in ovarian cancer patients. *Cancer Biol Ther* 8: 21-26.

Konner J, Schilder RJ, DeRosa FA, Gerst SR, Tew WP, Sabbatini PJ, Hensley ML, Spriggs DR, Aghajanian CA (2008). A phase II study of cetuximab/paclitaxel/carboplatin for the initial treatment of advanced-stage ovarian, primary peritoneal, or fallopian tube cancer. *Gynecol Oncol* 110: 140-145.

Kosary CL (1994). FIGO stage, histology, histologic grade, age and race as prognostic factors in determining survival for cancers of the female gynecological system: an analysis of 1973-87 SEER cases of cancers of the endometrium, cervix, ovary, vulva, and vagina. *Semin Surg Oncol* 10: 31-46.

Krasner CN, Debernardo RL, Findley M, Penson R, Matulonis U, Atkinson T, Roche M, Seiden MV (2005). Phase II Trial of Anastrazole in Combination with Gefitinib in Women with Asymptomatic Mullerian Cancer. *Journal of Clinical Oncology, 2005 ASCO Annual Meeting Proceedings* 23: Abstr 5063.

Kurman RJ, Shih Ie M (2008). Pathogenesis of ovarian cancer: lessons from morphology and molecular biology and their clinical implications. *Int J Gynecol Pathol* 27: 151-160.

Lassus H, Leminen A, Vayrynen A, Cheng G, Gustafsson JA, Isola J, Butzow R (2004). ERBB2 amplification is superior to protein expression status in predicting patient outcome in serous ovarian carcinoma. *Gynecol Oncol* 92: 31-39.

Lassus H, Sihto H, Leminen A, Joensuu H, Isola J, Nupponen NN, Butzow R (2006). Gene amplification, mutation, and protein expression of EGFR and mutations of ERBB2 in serous ovarian carcinoma. *J Mol Med (Berl)* 84: 671-681.

Lee CH, Huntsman DG, Cheang MC, Parker RL, Brown L, Hoskins P, Miller D, Gilks CB (2005a). Assessment of Her-1, Her-2, And Her-3 expression and Her-2 amplification in advanced stage ovarian carcinoma. *Int J Gynecol Pathol* 24: 147-152.

Lee S, Choi EJ, Jin C, Kim DH (2005b). Activation of PI3K/Akt pathway by PTEN reduction and PIK3CA mRNA amplification contributes to cisplatin resistance in an ovarian cancer cell line. *Gynecol Oncol* 97: 26-34.

Li SB, Schwartz PE, Lee WH, Yang-Feng TL (1991). Allele loss at the retinoblastoma locus in human ovarian cancer. *J Natl Cancer Inst* 83: 637-640.

Link W, Rosado A, Fominaya J, Thomas JE, Carnero A (2005). Membrane localization of all class I PI 3-kinase isoforms suppresses c-Myc-induced apoptosis in Rat1 fibroblasts via Akt. *J Cell Biochem* 95: 979-989.

Mabuchi S, Kawase C, Altomare DA, Morishige K, Sawada K, Hayashi M, Tsujimoto M, Yamoto M, Klein-Szanto AJ, Schilder RJ, Ohmichi M, Testa JR, Kimura T (2009). mTOR is a promising therapeutic target both in cisplatin-sensitive and cisplatin-resistant clear cell carcinoma of the ovary. *Clin Cancer Res* 15: 5404-5413.

Mabuchi S, Hisamatsu T, Kimura T (2011). Targeting mTOR Signaling Pathway in Ovarian Cancer. *Curr Med Chem* 18: 2960-2968.

Makhija S, Amler LC, Glenn D, Ueland FR, Gold MA, Dizon DS, Paton V, Lin CY, Januario T, Ng K, Strauss A, Kelsey S, Sliwkowski MX, Matulonis U (2010). Clinical activity of gemcitabine plus pertuzumab in platinum-resistant ovarian cancer, fallopian tube cancer, or primary peritoneal cancer. *J Clin Oncol* 28: 1215-1223.

Mano MS, Awada A, Di Leo A, Durbecq V, Paesmans M, Cardoso F, Larsimont D, Piccart M (2004). Rates of topoisomerase II-alpha and HER-2 gene amplification and expression in epithelial ovarian carcinoma. *Gynecol Oncol* 92: 887-895.

Marone M, Scambia G, Giannitelli C, Ferrandina G, Masciullo V, Bellacosa A, Benedetti-Panici P, Mancuso S (1998). Analysis of cyclin E and CDK2 in ovarian cancer: gene amplification and RNA overexpression. *Int J Cancer* 75: 34-39.

Masciullo V, Scambia G, Marone M, Giannitelli C, Ferrandina G, Bellacosa A, Benedetti Panici P, Mancuso S (1997). Altered expression of cyclin D1 and CDK4 genes in ovarian carcinomas. *Int J Cancer* 74: 390-395.

Matei DE, Nephew KP (2010). Epigenetic therapies for chemoresensitization of epithelial ovarian cancer. *Gynecol Oncol* 116: 195-201.

Matulonis U, Tew WP, Matei D, Behbakht K, Fleming GF, Oza AM (2011). A phase II study of ENMD-2076 in platinum-resistant ovarian cancer. *J Clin Oncol* 29: Abstr 5021.

Mayr D, Kanitz V, Anderegg B, Luthardt B, Engel J, Lohrs U, Amann G, Diebold J (2006). Analysis of gene amplification and prognostic markers in ovarian cancer using comparative genomic hybridization for microarrays and immunohistochemical analysis for tissue microarrays. *Am J Clin Pathol* 126: 101-109.

Meinhold-Heerlein I, Bauerschlag D, Hilpert F, Dimitrov P, Sapinoso LM, Orlowska-Volk M, Bauknecht T, Park TW, Jonat W, Jacobsen A, Sehouli J, Luttges J, Krajewski M, Krajewski S, Reed JC *et al* (2005). Molecular and prognostic distinction between serous ovarian carcinomas of varying grade and malignant potential. *Oncogene* 24: 1053-1065.

Mendiola M, Barriuso J, Marino-Enriquez A, Redondo A, Dominguez-Caceres A, Hernandez-Cortes G, Perez-Fernandez E, Sanchez-Navarro I, Vara JA, Suarez A, Espinosa E, Gonzalez-Baron M, Palacios J, Hardisson D (2009). Aurora kinases as prognostic biomarkers in ovarian carcinoma. *Hum Pathol* 40: 631-638.

Moreno Garcia V, Baird RD, Shah KJ, Basu B, Tunariu N, Blanco M, Cassier PA, Pedersen JV, Puglisi M, Sarker D, Papadatos-Pastos D, Omlin AG, Biondo A, Ware JA, Koeppen H *et al* (2011). A phase I study evaluating GDC-0941, an oral phosphoinositide-3 kinase (PI3K) inhibitor, in patients with advanced solid tumors or multiple myeloma. *J Clin Oncol* 29: Abstr 3021.

Morgan R, Oza AM, Qin R, Laumann KM, Mackay H, Strevel EL, Welch S, Sullivan D, Wenham RM, Chen HX, Doyle LA, Gandara DR, Erlichman C (2011). A phase II trial of temsirolimus and bevacizumab in patients with endometrial, ovarian, hepatocellular carcinoma, carcinoid, or islet cell cancer: Ovarian cancer (OC) subset—A study of the Princess Margaret, Mayo, Southeast phase II, and California Cancer (CCCP) N01 Consortia NCI#8233. *J Clin Oncol* 29: abstr 5015.

Nakayama K, Nakayama N, Davidson B, Sheu JJ, Jinawath N, Santillan A, Salani R, Bristow RE, Morin PJ, Kurman RJ, Wang TL, Shih Ie M (2006a). A BTB/POZ protein, NAC-1, is related to tumor recurrence and is essential for tumor growth and survival. *Proc Natl Acad Sci U S A* 103: 18739-18744.

Nakayama K, Nakayama N, Kurman RJ, Cope L, Pohl G, Samuels Y, Velculescu VE, Wang TL, Shih Ie M (2006b). Sequence mutations and amplification of PIK3CA and AKT2 genes in purified ovarian serous neoplasms. *Cancer Biol Ther* 5: 779-785.

Nakayama K, Nakayama N, Jinawath N, Salani R, Kurman RJ, Shih Ie M, Wang TL (2007). Amplicon profiles in ovarian serous carcinomas. *Int J Cancer* 120: 2613-2617.

Nakayama N, Nakayama K, Shamima Y, Ishikawa M, Katagiri A, Iida K, Miyazaki K (2010). Gene amplification CCNE1 is related to poor survival and potential therapeutic target in ovarian cancer. *Cancer* 116: 2621-2634.

Nam EJ, Kim YT (2008). Alteration of cell-cycle regulation in epithelial ovarian cancer. *Int J Gynecol Cancer* 18: 1169-1182.

Nicholson RI, Gee JM, Harper ME (2001). EGFR and cancer prognosis. *Eur J Cancer* 37 Suppl 4: S9-15.

Nimeiri HS, Oza AM, Morgan RJ, Friberg G, Kasza K, Faoro L, Salgia R, Stadler WM, Vokes EE, Fleming GF (2008). Efficacy and safety of bevacizumab plus erlotinib for patients with recurrent ovarian, primary peritoneal, and fallopian tube cancer: a trial of the Chicago, PMH, and California Phase II Consortia. *Gynecol Oncol* 110: 49-55.

Oza AM, Kollmannsberger C, Group NCT, Hirte H, Welch S, Siu L, Mazurka J, Sederias J, Doyle LA, Eisenhauer E (2009). Phase I study of temsirolimus (CCI-779), carboplatin, and paclitaxel in patients (pts) with advanced solid tumors: NCIC CTG IND 179. *J Clin Oncol* 27: abstr 3558.

Park JT, Li M, Nakayama K, Mao TL, Davidson B, Zhang Z, Kurman RJ, Eberhart CG, Shih Ie M, Wang TL (2006). Notch3 gene amplification in ovarian cancer. *Cancer Res* 66: 6312-6318.

Pegram MD, Finn RS, Arzoo K, Beryt M, Pietras RJ, Slamon DJ (1997). The effect of HER-2/neu overexpression on chemotherapeutic drug sensitivity in human breast and ovarian cancer cells. *Oncogene* 15: 537-547.

Pejovic T, Pande NT, Mori M, Mhawech-Fauceglia P, Harrington C, Mongoue-Tchokote S, Dim D, Andrews C, Beck A, Tarumi Y, Djilas J, Cappuccini F, Caballero O, Huang J, Levy S *et al* (2009). Expression profiling of the ovarian surface kinome reveals candidate genes for early neoplastic changes. *Transl Oncol* 2: 341-349.

Peng DJ, Wang J, Zhou JY, Wu GS (2010). Role of the Akt/mTOR survival pathway in cisplatin resistance in ovarian cancer cells. *Biochem Biophys Res Commun* 394: 600-605.

Posadas EM, Liel MS, Kwitkowski V, Minasian L, Godwin AK, Hussain MM, Espina V, Wood BJ, Steinberg SM, Kohn EC (2007). A phase II and pharmacodynamic study of gefitinib in patients with refractory or recurrent epithelial ovarian cancer. *Cancer* 109: 1323-1330.

Press MF, Jones LA, Godolphin W, Edwards CL, Slamon DJ (1990). HER-2/neu oncogene amplification and expression in breast and ovarian cancers. *Prog Clin Biol Res* 354A: 209-221.

Raj L, Ide T, Gurkar AU, Foley M, Schenone M, Li X, Tolliday NJ, Golub TR, Carr SA, Shamji AF, Stern AM, Mandinova A, Schreiber SL, Lee SW (2011). Selective killing of cancer cells by a small molecule targeting the stress response to ROS. *Nature* 475: 231-234.

Rajkumar T, Stamp GW, Hughes CM, Gullick WJ (1996). c-erbB3 protein expression in ovarian cancer. *Clin Mol Pathol* 49: M199-202.

Rivkin SE, Muller C, Iriarte D, Arthur J, Canoy A, Reid H (2008). Phase I/II lapatinib plus carboplatin and paclitaxel in stage III or IV relapsed ovarian cancer patients. *J Clin Oncol* 26: Abstr 5556.

Rose SL (2009). Notch signaling pathway in ovarian cancer. *Int J Gynecol Cancer* 19: 564-566.

Rose SL, Kunnimalaiyaan M, Drenzek J, Seiler N (2010). Notch 1 signaling is active in ovarian cancer. *Gynecol Oncol* 117: 130-133.

Ross JS, Yang F, Kallakury BV, Sheehan CE, Ambros RA, Muraca PJ (1999). HER-2/neu oncogene amplification by fluorescence in situ hybridization in epithelial tumors of the ovary. *Am J Clin Pathol* 111: 311-316.

Rubin SC, Finstad CL, Federici MG, Scheiner L, Lloyd KO, Hoskins WJ (1994). Prevalence and significance of HER-2/neu expression in early epithelial ovarian cancer. *Cancer* 73: 1456-1459.

Scharer CD, Laycock N, Osunkoya AO, Logani S, McDonald JF, Benigno BB, Moreno CS (2008). Aurora kinase inhibitors synergize with paclitaxel to induce apoptosis in ovarian cancer cells. *J Transl Med* 6: 79.

Schilder RJ, Sill MW, Chen X, Darcy KM, Decesare SL, Lewandowski G, Lee RB, Arciero CA, Wu H, Godwin AK (2005). Phase II study of gefitinib in patients with relapsed or persistent ovarian or primary peritoneal carcinoma and evaluation of epidermal growth factor receptor mutations and immunohistochemical expression: a Gynecologic Oncology Group Study. *Clin Cancer Res* 11: 5539-5548.

Schilder RJ, Pathak HB, Lokshin AE, Holloway RW, Alvarez RD, Aghajanian C, Min H, Devarajan K, Ross E, Drescher CW, Godwin AK (2009). Phase II trial of single agent cetuximab in patients with persistent or recurrent epithelial ovarian or primary peritoneal carcinoma with the potential for dose escalation to rash. *Gynecol Oncol* 113: 21-27.

Schraml P, Bucher C, Bissig H, Nocito A, Haas P, Wilber K, Seelig S, Kononen J, Mihatsch MJ, Dirnhofer S, Sauter G (2003a). Cyclin E overexpression and amplification in human tumours. *J Pathol* 200: 375-382.

Schraml P, Schwerdtfeger G, Burkhalter F, Raggi A, Schmidt D, Ruffalo T, King W, Wilber K, Mihatsch MJ, Moch H (2003b). Combined array comparative genomic hybridization and tissue microarray analysis suggest PAK1 at 11q13.5-q14 as a critical oncogene target in ovarian carcinoma. *Am J Pathol* 163: 985-992.

Secord AA, Blessing JA, Armstrong DK, Rodgers WH, Miner Z, Barnes MN, Lewandowski G, Mannel RS (2008). Phase II trial of cetuximab and carboplatin in relapsed platinum-sensitive ovarian cancer and evaluation of epidermal growth factor receptor expression: a Gynecologic Oncology Group study. *Gynecol Oncol* 108: 493-499.

Seiden MV, Burris HA, Matulonis U, Hall JB, Armstrong DK, Speyer J, Weber JD, Muggia F (2007). A phase II trial of EMD72000 (matuzumab), a humanized anti-EGFR monoclonal antibody, in patients with platinum-resistant ovarian and primary peritoneal malignancies. *Gynecol Oncol* 104: 727-731.

Serrano-Olvera A, Duenas-Gonzalez A, Gallardo-Rincon D, Candelaria M, De la Garza-Salazar J (2006). Prognostic, predictive and therapeutic implications of HER2 in invasive epithelial ovarian cancer. *Cancer Treat Rev* 32: 180-190.

Sheng Q, Liu J (2011). The therapeutic potential of targeting the EGFR family in epithelial ovarian cancer. *Br J Cancer* 104: 1241-1245.

Sheu JJ, Guan B, Choi JH, Lin A, Lee CH, Hsiao YT, Wang TL, Tsai FJ, Shih Ie M (2010). Rsf-1, a chromatin remodeling protein, induces DNA damage and promotes genomic instability. *J Biol Chem* 285: 38260-38269.

Shih Ie M, Sheu JJ, Santillan A, Nakayama K, Yen MJ, Bristow RE, Vang R, Parmigiani G, Kurman RJ, Trope CG, Davidson B, Wang TL (2005). Amplification of a chromatin remodeling gene, Rsf-1/HBXAP, in ovarian carcinoma. *Proc Natl Acad Sci U S A* 102: 14004-14009.

Shih Ie M, Nakayama K, Wu G, Nakayama N, Zhang J, Wang TL (2011). Amplification of the ch19p13.2 NACC1 locus in ovarian high-grade serous carcinoma. *Mod Pathol* 24: 638-645.

Siwak DR, Carey M, Hennessy BT, Nguyen CT, McGahren Murray MJ, Nolden L, Mills GB (2010). Targeting the epidermal growth factor receptor in epithelial ovarian cancer: current knowledge and future challenges. *J Oncol* 2010: 568938.

Slamon DJ, Godolphin W, Jones LA, Holt JA, Wong SG, Keith DE, Levin WJ, Stuart SG, Udove J, Ullrich A, et al. (1989). Studies of the HER-2/neu proto-oncogene in human breast and ovarian cancer. *Science* 244: 707-712.

Staal SP (1987). Molecular cloning of the akt oncogene and its human homologues AKT1 and AKT2: amplification of AKT1 in a primary human gastric adenocarcinoma. *Proc Natl Acad Sci U S A* 84: 5034-5037.

Stadlmann S, Gueth U, Reiser U, Diener PA, Zeimet AG, Wight E, Mirlacher M, Sauter G, Mihatsch MJ, Singer G (2006). Epithelial growth factor receptor status in primary and recurrent ovarian cancer. *Mod Pathol* 19: 607-610.

Staebler A, Heselmeyer-Haddad K, Bell K, Riopel M, Perlman E, Ried T, Kurman RJ (2002). Micropapillary serous carcinoma of the ovary has distinct patterns of chromosomal imbalances by comparative genomic hybridization compared with atypical proliferative serous tumors and serous carcinomas. *Hum Pathol* 33: 47-59.

Steg AD, Katre AA, Goodman BW, Han HD, Nick AM, Stone RL, Coleman RE, Alvarez RD, Lopez-Berestein G, Sood AK, Landen CN (2011). Targeting the Notch Ligand Jagged1 in Both Tumor Cells and Stroma in Ovarian Cancer. *Clin Cancer Res.*

Stokoe D (2005). The phosphoinositide 3-kinase pathway and cancer. *Expert Rev Mol Med* 7: 1-22.

Tanner B, Hasenclever D, Stern K, Schormann W, Bezler M, Hermes M, Brulport M, Bauer A, Schiffer IB, Gebhard S, Schmidt M, Steiner E, Sehouli J, Edelmann J, Lauter J *et al* (2006). ErbB-3 predicts survival in ovarian cancer. *J Clin Oncol* 24: 4317-4323.

Tanner MM, Grenman S, Koul A, Johannsson O, Meltzer P, Pejovic T, Borg A, Isola JJ (2000). Frequent amplification of chromosomal region 20q12-q13 in ovarian cancer. *Clin Cancer Res* 6: 1833-1839.

Temkin SM, Yamada SD, Fleming GF (2010). A phase I study of weekly temsirolimus and topotecan in the treatment of advanced and/or recurrent gynecologic malignancies. *Gynecol Oncol* 117: 473-476.

Tolcher AW, Mikulski SM, Messersmith WA, Kwak EL, Gibbon D, Boylan J, Xu ZX, DeMario M, Wheler JJ (2010). A phase I study of RO4929097, a novel gamma secretase inhibitor, in patients with advanced solid tumors. *J Clin Oncol* 28: Abstr 2502.

Tsuda H, Birrer MJ, Ito YM, Ohashi Y, Lin M, Lee C, Wong WH, Rao PH, Lau CC, Berkowitz RS, Wong KK, Mok SC (2004). Identification of DNA copy number changes in microdissected serous ovarian cancer tissue using a cDNA microarray platform. *Cancer Genet Cytogenet* 155: 97-107.

Tuefferd M, Couturier J, Penault-Llorca F, Vincent-Salomon A, Broet P, Guastalla JP, Allouache D, Combe M, Weber B, Pujade-Lauraine E, Camilleri-Broet S (2007). HER2 status in ovarian carcinomas: a multicenter GINECO study of 320 patients. *PLoS One* 2: e1138.

van der Horst EH, Murgia M, Treder M, Ullrich A (2005). Anti-HER-3 MAbs inhibit HER-3-mediated signaling in breast cancer cell lines resistant to anti-HER-2 antibodies. *Int J Cancer* 115: 519-527.

Vasey PA, Gore M, Wilson R, Rustin G, Gabra H, Guastalla JP, Lauraine EP, Paul J, Carty K, Kaye S (2008). A phase Ib trial of docetaxel, carboplatin and erlotinib in ovarian, fallopian tube and primary peritoneal cancers. *Br J Cancer* 98: 1774-1780.

Vermeij J, Teugels E, Bourgain C, Xiangming J, in 't Veld P, Ghislain V, Neyns B, De Greve J (2008). Genomic activation of the EGFR and HER2-neu genes in a significant proportion of invasive epithelial ovarian cancers. *BMC Cancer* 8: 3.

Wagner U, du Bois A, Pfisterer J, Huober J, Loibl S, Luck HJ, Sehouli J, Gropp M, Stahle A, Schmalfeldt B, Meier W, Jackisch C (2007). Gefitinib in combination with tamoxifen in patients with ovarian cancer refractory or resistant to platinum-taxane based therapy--a phase II trial of the AGO Ovarian Cancer Study Group (AGO-OVAR 2.6). *Gynecol Oncol* 105: 132-137.

Wang M, Wang J, Wang L, Wu L, Xin X (2010). Notch1 expression correlates with tumor differentiation status in ovarian carcinoma. *Med Oncol* 27: 1329-1335.

Weichert W, Denkert C, Schmidt M, Gekeler V, Wolf G, Kobel M, Dietel M, Hauptmann S (2004). Polo-like kinase isoform expression is a prognostic factor in ovarian carcinoma. *Br J Cancer* 90: 815-821.

Willner J, Wurz K, Allison KH, Galic V, Garcia RL, Goff BA, Swisher EM (2007). Alternate molecular genetic pathways in ovarian carcinomas of common histological types. *Hum Pathol* 38: 607-613.

Woenckhaus J, Steger K, Sturm K, Munstedt K, Franke FE, Fenic I (2007). Prognostic value of PIK3CA and phosphorylated AKT expression in ovarian cancer. *Virchows Arch* 450: 387-395.

Wu Y, Soslow RA, Marshall DS, Leitao M, Chen B (2004). Her-2/neu expression and amplification in early stage ovarian surface epithelial neoplasms. *Gynecol Oncol* 95: 570-575.

Ye D, Mendelsohn J, Fan Z (1999). Augmentation of a humanized anti-HER2 mAb 4D5 induced growth inhibition by a human-mouse chimeric anti-EGF receptor mAb C225. *Oncogene* 18: 731-738.

17

Nitric Oxide/Protein Kinase G-Iα Promotes c-Src Activation, Proliferation and Chemoresistance in Ovarian Cancer

Ronald R. Fiscus[1,2], Elaine L. Leung[1,2,3],
Janica C. Wong[1,2,4] and Mary G. Johlfs[1,2]
[1]Center for Diabetes and Obesity Prevention, Treatment, Research and Education, and the College of Pharmacy, Roseman University of Health Sciences (Formerly University of Southern Nevada), Henderson, Nevada,
[2]Cancer Molecular Biology Section, Nevada Cancer Institute, Las Vegas, Nevada,
[3]State Key Laboratory for Quality Research in Chinese Medicines, Macau University of Science and Technology, Taipa, Macau Special Administrative Region, and Shum Yiu Foon Shum Bik Chuen Memorial Centre for Cancer and Inflammation Research, School of Chinese Medicine, Hong Kong Baptist University, and Department of Pathology, Faculty of Medicine, The University of Hong Kong, Hong Kong Special Administrative Region,
[4]Department of Chemistry, University of Nevada Las Vegas, Las Vegas, Nevada,
[1,2,4]USA
[3]China

1. Introduction

Ovarian cancer is often associated with the development of resistance to chemotherapeutic agents (chemoresistance) and a recurrence of tumor growth, making this type of cancer especially difficult to treat by chemotherapy (Chien *et al*, 2007). The exaggerated cell growth and chemoresistance of ovarian cancer cells involve the dysregulation of multiple cell signaling (signal transduction) pathways that normally regulate cell proliferation and cell survival (Fraser *et al*, 2003). One particular cell signaling pathway that has recently become recognized as playing a central role in promoting cell proliferation and chemoresistance in human ovarian cancer cells is the nitric oxide (NO)/cyclic GMP (cGMP)/cGMP-dependent protein kinase [protein kinase G (PKG)] pathway (Fraser *et al*, 2006; Leung *et al*, 2008; Leung *et al*, 2010). Interestingly, two of the risk factors for developing ovarian cancer, i.e. advanced age and diabetes/obesity (Kulie *et al*, 2011), are known to cause dramatic dysregulations at multiple steps in the NO/cGMP/PKG signaling pathway in various organ systems, most notably the cardiovascular system (e.g. severe impairment of NO-mediated vasodilation and anti-hypertensive effects of the neuropeptide CGRP) (Chan & Fiscus, 2002; Fiscus *et al*, 2001; Fiscus & Ming, 2000; Fung *et al*, 2005) and the male reproductive system (e.g. diminished penile erection normally mediated by NO/cGMP/PKG signaling) (Fiscus, 2002; Fiscus *et al*, 2001; Fiscus & Ming, 2000; Fung *et al*, 2005). This dysregulation of the

NO/cGMP/PKG pathway contributes to the pathogenesis of various aging- and diabetes/ obesity-induced pathological complications, including hypertension, atherosclerosis and erectile dysfunction (Fiscus, 1988; Fiscus, 2002; Fiscus *et al*, 2001; Fiscus & Ming, 2000; Fung *et al*, 2005). However, until recently, the role of this signaling pathway in the pathogenesis of ovarian cancer had remained unrecognized. Recent data from our laboratory have now shown that the NO/cGMP/PKG signaling pathway, specifically involving the PKG type-Iα (PKG-Iα) isoform of PKG and its interaction with the c-Src tyrosine kinase pathway, plays a key role in promoting the exaggerated cell proliferation and chemoresistance in human ovarian cancer cells (Fraser *et al*, 2006; Leung *et al*, 2008; Leung *et al*, 2010).

Many of the early studies of NO in ovarian cancer had suggested that this small molecule mediates tumoricidal activity, including showing that NO donors added to ovarian cancer cells *in vitro* or the induction of high-level NO synthesis within the ovarian cancer cells by exposure to pro-inflammatory cytokines results in increased levels of apoptotic cell death (Cantuaria *et al*, 2000; Garban & Bonavida, 1999; Rieder *et al*, 2001). Furthermore, NO, released from activated macrophages, inhibits the growth of tumors in an animal model of ovarian cancer (Farias-Eisner *et al*, 1994). However, the molecular mechanisms mediating these tumoricidal actions of NO were not determined in the early studies. It is now recognized that NO has multiple actions in mammalian cells, including both toxic and cytoprotective effects, which greatly depend on the local concentration of NO and the micro-environmental conditions (e.g. whether there is a co-presence of elevated levels of superoxide, which can combine with high-level NO to form peroxynitrite, a toxic pro-oxidant mediating both oxidative and nitrosative stress) (Cheng Chew *et al*, 2003; Fiscus, 2002; Fiscus *et al*, 2002; Leung *et al*, 2008; Wong & Fiscus, 2010; Wong & Fiscus, 2011).

At lower physiological levels (0.01 - 1 nanomolar), NO selectively activates the PKG-Iα isoform (Batchelor *et al*, 2010; Nausch *et al*, 2008; Sato *et al*, 2006), which our laboratory has shown results in cytoprotection (i.e. inhibition of multiple steps in pro-apoptosis pathways, preventing both spontaneous and toxin-induced apoptosis) as well as stimulation of DNA synthesis and cell proliferation in many mammalian cells, including human ovarian cancer cells (Chan & Fiscus, 2003; Cheng Chew *et al*, 2003; Fiscus, 2002; Fiscus *et al*, 2002; Fraser *et al*, 2006; Fung *et al*, 2005; Leung *et al*, 2008; Leung *et al*, 2010; Wong & Fiscus, 2010; Wong & Fiscus, 2011). Although earlier studies had reported that "PKG expression is lost" when ovarian epithelial cells transform into cancer cells (Hou *et al*, 2006; Wong *et al*, 2001), our studies show that human ovarian cancer cells do indeed express PKG-Iα, which contributes to exaggerated cell proliferation and chemoresistance (Leung *et al*, 2008; Leung *et al*, 2010).

At higher concentrations (>100 nanomolar), as used in the earlier studies mentioned above, NO causes cytotoxic effects in many types of mammalian cells, both normal and cancer cells, which can involve both the direct S-nitrosylation of cysteine residues of proteins, altering their function (Nakamura & Lipton, 2010; Seth & Stamler, 2011), and the indirect nitration of tyrosine residues in proteins (via formation of peroxynitrite), further altering protein function (e.g. interferring with tyrosine phosphorylation) (Beckman & Koppenol, 1996; Fiscus, 2002; Fiscus *et al*, 2002; Ridnour *et al*, 2008; Thomas *et al*, 2008). Details of these cellular/molecular mechanisms mediating the concentration-dependent cytoprotective and cytotoxic actions of NO are discussed below and illustrated in the following figures.

2. Early studies identifying the important roles of NO, cGMP and PKG in controlling blood pressure and blood flow and mediating penile erection

Endogenous NO [originally referred to as EDRF (endothelium-derived relaxant factor)] in the cardiovascular system was first shown to play an important biological role in regulating arterial diameter [for reviews, see (Fiscus, 1988; Fiscus, 2002; Francis *et al*, 2010; Hofmann *et al*, 2006; Lincoln *et al*, 2001; Pilz & Casteel, 2003)]. In healthy arteries (i.e. arteries from individuals that are young and without diabetes, obesity or hypertension), endogenous NO is produced at physiological levels, now estimated to be in the range of 0.01 - 10 nanomolar (Batchelor *et al*, 2010; Sato *et al*, 2006), by the endothelial-form NO-synthase (eNOS) within the endothelial cells lining the arteries. Because of its high lipid solubility, NO readily diffuses into nearby cells, importantly vascular smooth muscle cells in blood vessels, where NO, via binding to the heme group of soluble guanylyl cyclase, enhances cGMP synthesis, resulting in elevation of intracellular levels of cGMP and activation of PKG.

Early studies throughout the 1970's and early 1980's, using purified PKG in *in vitro* experiments, had shown that the addition of cGMP to the purified PKG could enhance its kinase activity, suggesting that cGMP may be the intracellular chemical that serves as the allosteric activator of PKG within cells, similar to the role of cAMP in activating cAMP-dependent protein kinase (protein kinase A, PKA) [reviewed in (Fiscus, 1988; Fiscus, 2002; Francis *et al*, 1988; Hofmann *et al*, 2006; Lincoln *et al*, 2001; Pilz & Casteel, 2003)]. Thus, early on, it was suggested that NO, via its ability to elevate intracellular cGMP levels, may be causing vascular effects by activating PKG within the smooth muscle cells. However, the early attempts to prove this were found to be exceedingly difficult because of the uniquely unstable nature of the PKG activation that occurs within mammalian cells (Fiscus, 1988; Fiscus, 2002; Fiscus & Murad, 1988; Fiscus *et al*, 1983; Fiscus *et al*, 1984). It was not until 1983 and 1984 that NO was first shown to significantly stimulate the intracellular activation state of PKG in mammalian cells (Fiscus *et al*, 1983; Fiscus *et al*, 1984).

As a serine/threonine kinase, PKG phosphorylates numerous downstream target proteins in vascular smooth muscle cells, which ultimately results in the suppression of arterial vasoconstriction (i.e. vasodilation) (Fiscus, 1988; Fiscus, 2002; Fiscus & Murad, 1988; Francis *et al*, 1988; Hofmann *et al*, 2006; Lincoln *et al*, 2001; Pilz & Casteel, 2003). The NO/cGMP/PKG signaling pathway in vascular smooth muscle cells plays an essential role in preventing vasospasms and maintaining normal blood pressure and blood flow. Interestingly, even the basal release of NO from healthy endothelial cells, now estimated to generate a local concentration of NO of 0.01 - 0.1 nanomolar (Batchelor *et al*, 2010; Sato *et al*, 2006), was shown to cause significant increases in the intracellular PKG activation in vascular smooth muscle cells (Fiscus *et al*, 1983). This "basal activation" of PKG, induced by the basal, low-level (0.01 - 0.1 nanomolar) NO is now recognized to play a key role in protecting against the development of hypertension and other cardiovascular pathologies.

Advanced age (Chan & Fiscus, 2002; Fiscus, 1988; Fiscus, 2002; Fiscus & Ming, 2000; Fung *et al*, 2005) or diabetes and/or obesity in younger individuals (Fiscus, 2002; Fiscus *et al*, 2001; Fiscus & Ming, 2000) results in the dysregulation of NO production and NO's ability to activate PKG in both the cardiovascular system and the male reproductive system (Chang *et al*, 2004). This diminished capacity to generate the physiological levels of NO and for NO to activate PKG within cells is now recognized to play a key role in aging- and diabetes/obesity-induced pathological complications, including hypertension, athero-sclerosis (with increased risk of heart attack and stroke) and erectile dysfunction.

3. Anti-apoptotic effects mediated by the low-level-NO/cGMP/PKG-Iα signaling pathway in neural cells, uterine epithelial cells and human ovarian cancer cells

Further studies from our laboratory have shown that other types of mammalian cells, including uterine epithelial cells and many types of neural cells, possess all of the components of the NO/cGMP/PKG signaling pathway and that this pathway is biologically functional (Barger *et al*, 1995; Chan & Fiscus, 2003; Cheng Chew *et al*, 2003; Fiscus, 2002; Fiscus *et al*, 2002; Leung *et al*, 2010). However, in contrast to the contractile-regulatory role of the NO/cGMP/PKG pathway identified in vascular smooth muscle cells, these other mammalian cells utilize this pathway to regulate a very different biological function, i.e. cell survival. Activation of this signaling pathway by low, basal levels of endogenous NO (generated by either eNOS or neural-form NOS (nNOS) within these cells) results in the suppression of both spontaneous apoptosis and toxin-induced apoptosis in uterine epithelial cells and in the many different types of neural cells.

We had hypothesized that, if present in ovarian cancer cells, the NO/cGMP/PKG signaling pathway may also suppress the apoptosis of tumor cells, potentially contributing to the resistance to chemotherapeutic agents (i.e. chemoresistance). Our data have shown that human ovarian cancer cells do indeed express all of the key components of the NO/cGMP/PKG signaling pathway, including all three isoforms of NOS, i.e. eNOS (also called NOS3), nNOS (also called NOS1) and inducible NOS (iNOS, also called NOS2), thus providing an endogenous source of NO (Leung *et al*, 2008). Furthermore, ovarian cancer cells continuously produce NO at low physiological levels, which tonically activates the heme-dependent soluble guanylyl cyclase (Fraser *et al*, 2006), elevating cGMP levels sufficiently enough to cause continuous high-level activation of PKG (Leung *et al*, 2010). We have found that the type-Iα splice variant of PKG-I (i.e. PKG-Iα) appears to represent the predominant isoform of PKG expressed in two types of human ovarian cancer cells, OV2008 cells (possessing wild-type p53 and sensitivity to the toxic/pro-apoptotic effects of cisplatin) and A2780cp cells (possessing mutated p53 and resistance to the toxic/pro-apoptotic effects of cisplatin). The PKG-Iα isoform is the most sensitive of all of the three isoforms of PKG (PKG-Iα, PKG-Iβ and PKG -II) to stimulation by cGMP and thus is likely to be the only PKG isoform that is substantially activated by the presence of the lower physiological levels (0.01 - 1 nanomolar) of NO (see model in Figure 1).

4. Low-level-NO/cGMP/PKG-Iα pathway also promotes DNA synthesis and cell proliferation, which are biological responses opposite of those induced by high-level NO

Figure 1 illustrates the multiple (in some cases, opposite) biological effects of NO in human ovarian cancer cells, which greatly depend on the concentration [shown in nanomolar (nM)] of NO and the experimental conditions (e.g. whether there are elevated levels of superoxide, which is capable of reacting with high-level NO to form peroxynitrite). Most previous studies of NO's role in ovarian cancer have focused on the toxic effects of NO that occur at the higher concentrations (Cantuaria *et al*, 2000; Farias-Eisner *et al*, 1994; Garban & Bonavida, 1999; Rieder *et al*, 2001), which would lead to direct S-nitrosylation of cysteine residues of proteins (Nakamura & Lipton, 2010; Seth & Stamler, 2011) and indirect nitration (via production of peroxynitrite) of tyrosine residues of proteins (Beckman & Koppenol, 1996;

Fiscus, 2002; Fiscus *et al*, 2002) , as illustrated in Figure 1. In both cases, this can lead to cytotoxicity, with resulting inhibition of cell proliferation and induction of apoptosis.

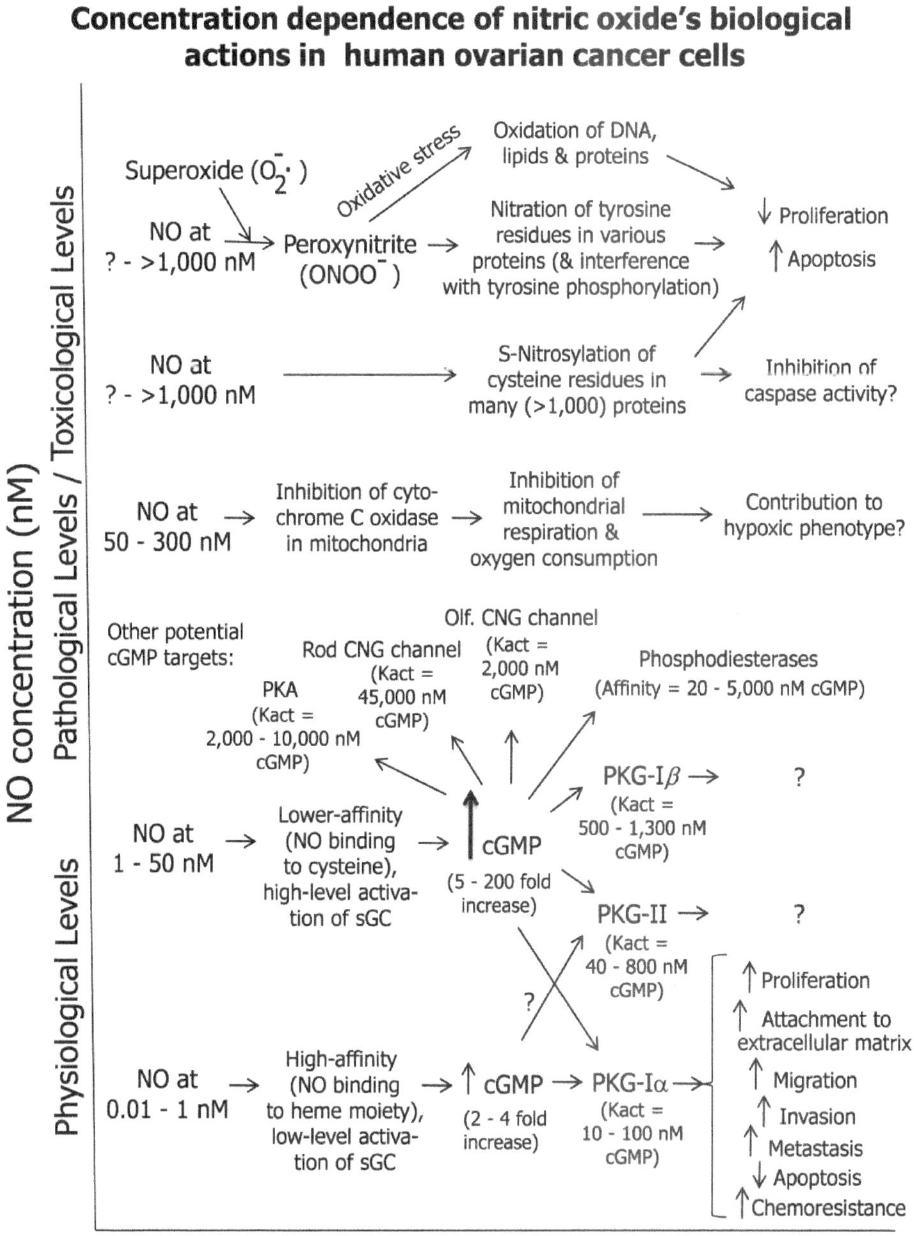

Fig. 1. Multiple cellular and molecular actions of NO in human ovarian cancer cells that occur at very different (local micro-environmental) NO concentrations [in nanomolar (nM)].

Figure 1 also illustrates how NO, at intermediate levels (i.e. 50 - 300 nanomolar), binds to the heme group of cytochrome C oxidase in the mitochondria, inhibiting the activity of this important metabolic enzyme (Bellamy *et al*, 2002). The biological role of this response to NO is currently unclear, but likely would result in decreased mitochondrial respiration and oxygen consumption and may possibly contribute to the hypoxic phenotype of cancer cells. At 1 - 50 nanomolar concentration, which is at the transition between the toxicological levels and the higher physiological levels, NO would cause high-level activation of soluble guanylyl cyclase, causing large increases in the intracellular levels of cGMP. Recently, this high-level activation was shown to be dependent not only on the binding of NO to the heme group of soluble guanylyl cyclase (which occurs at much lower concentrations, i.e. 0.01 - 1 nM, of NO) but also on the binding of higher-level NO to cysteine residues of soluble guanylyl cyclase (Fernhoff *et al*, 2009). It is not clear at present what effect this would have in human ovarian cancer cells. However, studies with other types of cells have shown that larger increases in cGMP levels would activate both the PKG-Iα and PKG-Iβ isoforms of PKG, and thus may result in biological responses that are very different from those mediated by the low-level-NO/cGMP/PKG-Iα pathway (for details, see Section 6. below). The large increases in cGMP caused by NO at 1 - 50 nanomolar may also regulate the activity of other potential cGMP-target proteins, including the olfactory- and rod-type CNG channels (cyclic nucleotide-gated cation channels), various phosphodiesterases and PKA (via "cross-activation" mediated by high-level cGMP binding to the cAMP-activation sites of PKA) [reviewed in (Fiscus, 2002; Francis *et al*, 2010; Hofmann *et al*, 2006; Lincoln *et al*, 2001; Pilz & Casteel, 2003)].

At the lower physiological levels (0.01 - 1 nanomolar) NO would selectively activate the PKG-Iα isoform of PKG in human ovarian cancer cells, which stimulates DNA synthesis/cell proliferation and suppresses apoptosis (promoting chemoresistance) (Leung *et al*, 2008; Leung *et al*, 2010), responses opposite to those of the high/toxic concentrations of NO. Studies in our laboratory, using both normal and malignant cells, including vascular smooth muscle cells, bone marrow-derived stromal cells and neuroblastoma cells, have suggested that a major role of the low-level-NO/cGMP/PKG-Iα signaling pathway is to protect these cells against the toxic/pro-apoptotic effects of high-level NO, as might occur during inflammation and exposure of cells to pro-inflammatory cytokines (Cheng Chew *et al*, 2003; Fiscus, 2002; Fiscus *et al*, 2002; Wong & Fiscus, 2010; Wong & Fiscus, 2011).

Recent evidence from our laboratory also suggests that the basal activation of PKG-Iα leads to increased attachment of cells to the extracellular matrix and increased cell migration, shown in bone marrow-derived stromal cells (Wong & Fiscus, 2011) as well as mesothelioma and non-small cell lung cancer cells (Fiscus & Johlfs, 2011). If similar attachment and migration responses occur in ovarian cancer cells, these PKG-Iα-mediated cellular effects could lead to increased invasion and metastasis. Further experiments are currently underway to test this possibility in models of ovarian cancer.

5. Interaction between c-Src and PKG-Iα in promoting DNA synthesis and cell proliferation

Studies from our laboratory suggest that the growth-promoting effect of PKG-Iα in ovarian cancer cells involves the enhancement of the tyrosine kinase activity of c-Src (Leung *et al*,

2010), an oncogenic protein often overexpressed and/or hyperactivated in many types of cancer cells, including ovarian cancer cells. The key role of PKG-Iα in activating c-Src and promoting cell proliferation was determined using siRNA gene knockdown techniques, which specifically silences the gene expression of PKG-Iα, and two types of pharmacological inhibitors, ODQ (1H-[1,2,4]oxadiazolo[4,3-a]quinozalin-1-one, an inhibitor of endogenous NO-induced, heme-dependent activation of soluble guanylyl cyclase) and DT-2 or DT-3 (two highly-specific inhibitors of the serine/threonine kinase activity of PKG-Iα) (Leung *et al*, 2010).

Epidermal growth factor (EGF)-induced activation of c-Src tyrosine kinase activity was found to cause tyrosine phosphorylation of PKG-Iα, increasing the serine/threonine kinase activity of PKG-Iα and its growth-promoting effects in ovarian cancer cells (Leung *et al*, 2010). Furthermore, we have found that PKG-Iα directly phosphorylates c-Src at serine-17, which enhances the tyrosine kinase activity of c-Src in both *in vitro* and intact-cell experiments (Fiscus & Johlfs, 2011). In human ovarian cancer cells, the c-Src-mediated tyrosine-phosphorylation of the EGF receptor was found to be highly dependent on PKG-Iα kinase activity (Leung *et al*, 2010). Thus, there appears to be a novel interaction between PKG-Iα and c-Src in human ovarian cancer cells. This interaction causes reciprocal phosphorylation, i.e. each protein kinase phosphorylating the other, potentially setting up an "oncogenic reinforcement" resulting in exaggerated DNA synthesis and cell proliferation.

6. Opposite effects of the two PKG-I splice variants, PKG-Iα and PKG-Iβ, on cell proliferation and apoptosis

Our studies of mammalian cells expressing both PKG-Iα and PKG-Iβ isoforms, such as vascular smooth muscle cells, show that exposure of these cells to NO in a wide concentration range results in biphasic responses of cell proliferation and apoptosis (Wong & Fiscus, 2010). For example, exposure to low physiological levels of NO tends to promote cell proliferation and suppress apoptosis (i.e. promote cytoprotection), whereas exposure to higher levels of NO has the opposite effects, suppressing cell proliferation and promoting apoptosis. Similar biphasic responses to different concentrations of NO have been reported in vascular endothelial cells (Isenberg *et al*, 2005). These opposite effects induced by the low and high levels of NO likely involve the many cellular and molecular mechanisms illustrated in the model of Figure 1. Of particular interest in our laboratory is the role played by the two splice variants of PKG-I, since both isozymes are expressed in vascular smooth muscle cells (Wong & Fiscus, 2010). At low levels, NO would selectively stimulate the kinase activity of PKG-Iα (but not PKG-Iβ), because the PKG-Iα isoform has a much higher sensitivity to NO and the cGMP-induced allosteric activation (illustrated in Figure 2). At higher levels, NO would activate both PKG-I isoforms. Importantly, PKG-Iβ requires at least 10-times higher levels of cGMP for activation (indicated by K_{act}), compared with PKG-Iα (Francis *et al*, 2010; Hofmann *et al*, 2006; Lincoln *et al*, 2001; Pilz & Casteel, 2003). Activation of PKG-Iβ by the high-level NO likely contributes to suppression of cell proliferation and induction of apoptosis [(Wong & Fiscus, 2010) and illustrated in Figure 2].

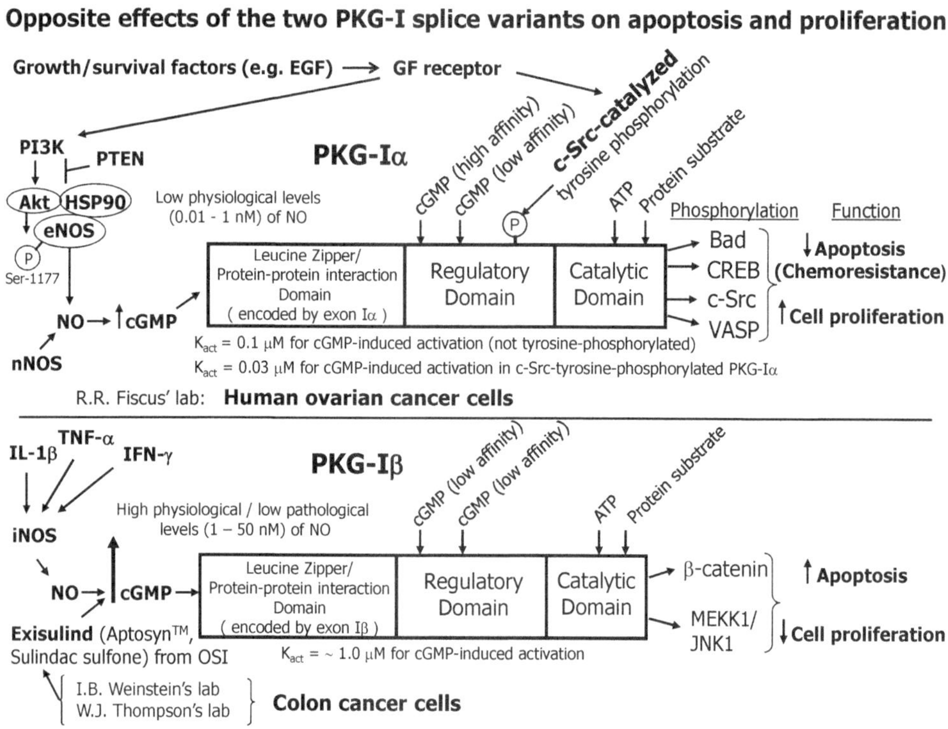

Fig. 2. Model of the two splice variants of PKG-I, illustrating their activation by different concentration ranges of NO and the downstream phosphorylation of different sets of target proteins. Also, the model for PKG-Iα illustrates the effects of growth factors (e.g. EGF), which stimulates both the PI3K/Akt pathway, enhancing eNOS activity and low-level NO generation, and c-Src activation, catalyzing downstream tyrosine-phosphorylation of PKG-Iα, enhancing its sensitivity to allosteric activation by cGMP (represented by the K_{act} values).

In human ovarian cancer cells, we found that endogenous PKG-Iα is tyrosine-phosphorylated, which depends on the high-level tyrosine kinase activity of c-Src (Leung *et al*, 2010). The tyrosine phosphorylation of PKG-Iα is known to cause a 3-fold decrease in the K_{act} for cGMP-induced activation, resulting in a substantial sensitization of the PKG-Iα to its activation by cGMP (illustrated in Figure 2). Earlier *in vitro* experiments, using purified PKG-Iα in a kinase reaction mixture with v-Src, the viral form of Src, had shown that tyrosine-phosphorylation of PKG-Iα results in a 3-fold shift downwards in the K_{act} (LaFevre-Bernt *et al*, 1998). The human form of c-Src, used in our studies, has the same catalytic domain as v-Src and thus catalyzes the same type of tyrosine-phosphorylation of PKG-Iα (Leung *et al*, 2010). Thus, in human ovarian cancer cells the tyrosine-phosphorylated PKG-Iα would be dramatically sensitized to the activation by basal intracellular cGMP levels, resulting in high-level activation (i.e. hyperactivation, estimated to be ~90% of maximal activity) of PKG-Iα within the ovarian cancer cells.

Our laboratory has shown that activation of PKG-Iα, which occurs tonically in cells that express either eNOS or nNOS, results in stimulation of DNA synthesis/cell proliferation and suppression of apoptosis in a variety of mammalian cells, notably human ovarian cancer cells (Fiscus, 2002; Fiscus *et al*, 2002; Fraser *et al*, 2006; Leung *et al*, 2008; Leung *et al*, 2010; Wong & Fiscus, 2010; Wong & Fiscus, 2011). In contrast, activation of both isoforms of PKG-I, following the exposure to higher-level NO in cells expressing both PKG-I isoforms, results in suppression of DNA synthesis/cell proliferation and induction of apoptosis (Wong & Fiscus, 2010). It appears that when PKG-Iβ is activated by the higher levels of NO, the growth-inhibitory and pro-apoptotic effects of PKG-Iβ predominate over the growth-stimulatory and anti-apoptotic effects mediated by PKG-Iα. Because of these differences in the biological responses mediated by the two isoforms of PKG-I and because most previous studies have used higher levels of NO, there has been confusion in the literature about the role of PKG in regulating cell proliferation and apoptosis.

Figure 2 illustrates the opposite biological effects of PKG-Iα and PKG-Iβ on cell proliferation and apoptosis, using, as examples, two types of cells that selectively express one isoform of PKG-I or the other. As stated above, our studies have shown that human ovarian cancer cells appear to express predominantly the PKG-Iα isoform, and that the activation of this kinase by endogenous low-level NO generated by eNOS and nNOS within ovarain cancer cells promotes DNA synthesis/cell proliferation and suppresses apoptosis, contributing to chemoresistance (i.e. interfering with the toxic/cancer-cell-killing effects of cisplatin) (Leung *et al*, 2008; Leung *et al*, 2010), shown in the upper model of Figure 2. The lower model in Figure 2 shows the regulation and downstream target proteins of PKG-Iβ, based in part on published data from the laboratories of I.B. Weinstein and W.J. Thompson. Their laboratories have shown that PKG-Iβ is the predominant isoform of PKG-I expressed in colon cancer cells and that, when activated [following the large increases in intracellular cGMP levels induced by Exisulind, a type-2/type-5 phosphodiesterase (PDE2/PDE5) inhibitor], PKG-Iβ phosphorylates two downstream target proteins, β-catenin and MEKK1, resulting in inhibition of cell proliferation and induction of apoptosis (Deguchi *et al*, 2004; Soh *et al*, 2000; Thompson *et al*, 2000). They also showed that the overexpression of PKG-Iβ in colon cancer cells causes a large suppression of cell proliferation and induction of apoptosis. Although their studies further showed that transfection of colon cancer cells with vectors causing overexpression of PKG-Iα also caused a small inhibition of cell proliferation, it appears likely that this forced overexpression of PKG-Iα may have resulted in the unnatural exposure of PKG-Iα to target proteins that normally would not be phosphorylated by naturally-expressed PKG-Iα (but rather by PKG-Iβ), leading to biological responses more like those of the PKG-Iβ isoform. Overall, the combined data from our laboratory using human ovarian cancer cells and the data from the laboratories of I.B. Weinstein and W.J. Thompson using colon cancer cells suggest that the two isoforms of PKG-I have opposite effects on cell proliferation and apoptosis. However, further studies will be needed to determine if cell-type differences may have also played a role in the opposite biological responses mediated by the two PKG-I isoforms.

In the model of PKG-Iβ shown in Figure 2, we have also included our current concept about the natural endogenous activator of PKG-Iβ within cancer cells, which we believe likely involves high-level NO generated by iNOS, either within the cancer cells themselves or within invading white blood cells (e.g. monocyte/macrophages), following their exposure to pro-inflammatory cytokines, such as interleukin-1β (IL-1β), tumor necrosis factor-α (TNF-α) and interferon-γ (IFN-γ). These pro-inflammatory cytokines are known to induce the gene expression of iNOS (Chan & Fiscus, 2004; Kleinert *et al*, 2003), which causes high-level production of NO and large increases in the intracellular levels of cGMP. Thus, the role of PKG-Iβ in regulating cell proliferation and apoptosis in cancer cells will depend on whether or not the cells actually express this isoform of PKG and whether or not there are concurrent inflammatory conditions in the tumor that would lead to the induction of iNOS and high levels of NO and cGMP, needed for activating PKG-Iβ.

Figure 2 further shows the difference between PKG-Iα and PKG-Iβ in terms of the immediate downstream target proteins that are being phosphorylated by the two protein kinases. Earlier studies had shown that PKG-Iα and PKG-Iβ have identical substrate specificities when tested in *in vitro* experiments (Francis *et al*, 2010; Hofmann *et al*, 2006; Lincoln *et al*, 2001), which used freely soluble kinases (either purified kinases or recombinant kinases) dissolved in an aqueous solution. The two isoforms of PKG-I have identical catalytic domains, which results in similar substrate specificity when tested *in vitro*. However, within intact cells, PKG-Iα and PKG-Iβ have very different subcellular localizations, because of their different localization domains (i.e. the leucine zipper/protein-protein-interaction domains), which represents the first 100 amino acids at the N-terminal encoded by the different first exons of the two splice variants of PKG-I. This difference in the subcellular localizations results in the exposure of the two PKG-I isoforms to very different sets of downstream target proteins, as illustrated in Figure 2.

Our studies have suggested that there is continuous high-level activation of PKG-Iα within cancer cells, which results in continuous downstream phosphorylation of four key regulatory proteins: 1) the apoptosis-regulating protein Bad (Johlfs & Fiscus, 2010), 2) the transcription factor CREB [(Fiscus, 2002), further supported by recent data from our laboratory using many types of cancer cells], 3) the oncogenic tyrosine kinase c-Src (Fiscus & Johlfs, 2011; Leung *et al*, 2010), and 4) the actin-filament- and focal-adhesion-associated protein VASP (vasodilator-stimulated phosphoprotein) (Leung *et al*, 2010; Wong & Fiscus, 2010; Wong & Fiscus, 2011). We have proposed that the PKG-Iα-mediated phosphorylations of Bad, CREB, c-Src and VASP play important roles in promoting chemoresistance, DNA synthesis/cell proliferation, cell attachment and cell migration. Others have shown that PKG-Iβ phosphorylates β-catenin and MEKK1 in colon cancer cells, which ultimately leads to increased levels of apoptosis and inhibition of cell proliferation in the colon cancer cells (Deguchi *et al*, 2004; Soh *et al*, 2000; Thompson *et al*, 2000).

7. Identification of PKG-Iα as the exclusive isoform of PKG-I expressed in A2780cp and OV2008 human ovarian cancer cells using the NanoPro100 system, a new ultrasensitive immuno-detection instrument based on capillary electrophoresis

Although our previous studies using Western blot analysis had suggested that PKG-Iα is the predominant isoform of PKG-I expressed in A2780cp and OV2008 human ovarian cancer cells (Leung *et al*, 2010), we had found it difficult to determine the PKG-I isozyme profile with certainty because of the relatively low abundance of the PKG-I isoforms in cancer cells and the difficulty in resolving and identifying the two isoforms of PKG-I using Western blot analysis. Other laboratories, also using Western blot analysis, were unable to detect PKG expression in ovarian cancer cells and various other types of cancer cells, which had lead them to conclude that "PKG expression is lost" in cancer cells (Hou *et al*, 2006; Wong *et al*, 2001). Our studies have now shown that all of the more than 25 different cancer cell lines tested in our laboratory, including breast cancer, colon cancer, lung cancer, melanoma, mesothelioma, ovarian cancer and prostate cancer cells, do indeed express PKG-I isoforms, with PKG-Iα expressed in all cell lines and PKG-Iβ co-expressed in about half of them. The misunderstanding about whether or not cancer cells actually express PKG-I isoforms had resulted from of the lack of sensitivity of conventional Western blot analysis (and the lack of sensitivity of conventional immunohistochemistry), resulting in the inability to detect the protein expression of the PKG-I isoforms. To avoid this technical problem caused by the inadequate sensitivity of conventional Western blot analysis, our laboratory has begun using a new, state-of-the-art methodology that utilizes the NanoPro100 system, a capillary-electrophoresis-based immuno-detection instrument, manufactured and marketed by ProteinSimple (previously named Cell Biosciences, Inc.), Santa Clara, CA, USA. The NanoPro100 system allows protein detection with a sensitivity that is >100-times better than conventional Western blot analysis, thus allowing clear identification of lower abundance proteins that have escaped detection by Western blot analysis. Furthermore, the NanoPro100 system is able to cleanly separate the two isoforms of PKG-I, thus making it much easier to identify which isoforms are expressed in cancer cells.

Figure 3 shows the dramatic improvement in sensitivity and resolving power of the NanoPro100 system for determining the PKG-I isoform expression profiles in human ovarian cancer cells, compared with conventional Western blot analysis (panel A). Recombinant PKG-Iα and PKG-Iβ were used as standards in the NanoPro100 system (panel B). The NCI-H2052 mesothelioma cell line, which expresses both isoforms of PKG-I, was used as a positive control, illustrating the correct positions for the two PKG-I isoforms in the NanoPro100 electropherograms following analysis of cell lysates (panel C). Both A2780cp and OV2008 human ovarian cancer cells were found to express exclusively the PKG-Iα isoform (panels D and E), thus confirming our earlier report using conventional Western blot analysis. Interestingly, because the NanoPro100 system separates proteins based on pI rather than molecular weight as in conventional Western blot analysis, this new state-of-the-art technology is able to separate and potentially identify the different phosphorylated forms (phospho-forms) of proteins, illustrated by the additional peaks to the left side of the main peak for PKG-Iα in panels D and E of Figure 3. The identification of these additional peaks as being phospho-forms of PKG-Iα is shown by their decrease after treatment of the cell lysates with lambda phosphatase, which removes the phosphate groups.

Based on the NanoPro100 data of Figure 3, the chemoresistant A2780cp cell line appears to have lower expression levels of PKG-Iα compared with the chemosensitive OV2008 cell line. On the surface, this seems to be opposite to what would be expected if PKG-Iα is contributing to chemoresistance in human ovarian cancer cells. However, it should be emphasized that protein expression levels do not indicate the functional activity of protein kinases. Much more important in determining the actual functional activity within cells are the levels of phosphorylation at regulatory sites (e.g. c-Src-mediate phosphorylation of tyrosine residues, in the case of PKG-Iα) and the intracellular concentrations of allosteric activators (e.g. cGMP, in the case of PKG-Iα). Another important determinant for functional kinase activity within cells is the subcellular localization, which determines the efficiency of phosphorylation and which of the potential downstream target proteins are actually phosphorylated (as illustrated in Figure 2 and discussed in Section 6.). Thus, the protein expression levels (of the total protein), as measured by Western blot analysis or NanoPro100 analysis, cannot directly predict the functional kinase activity of a protein kinase.

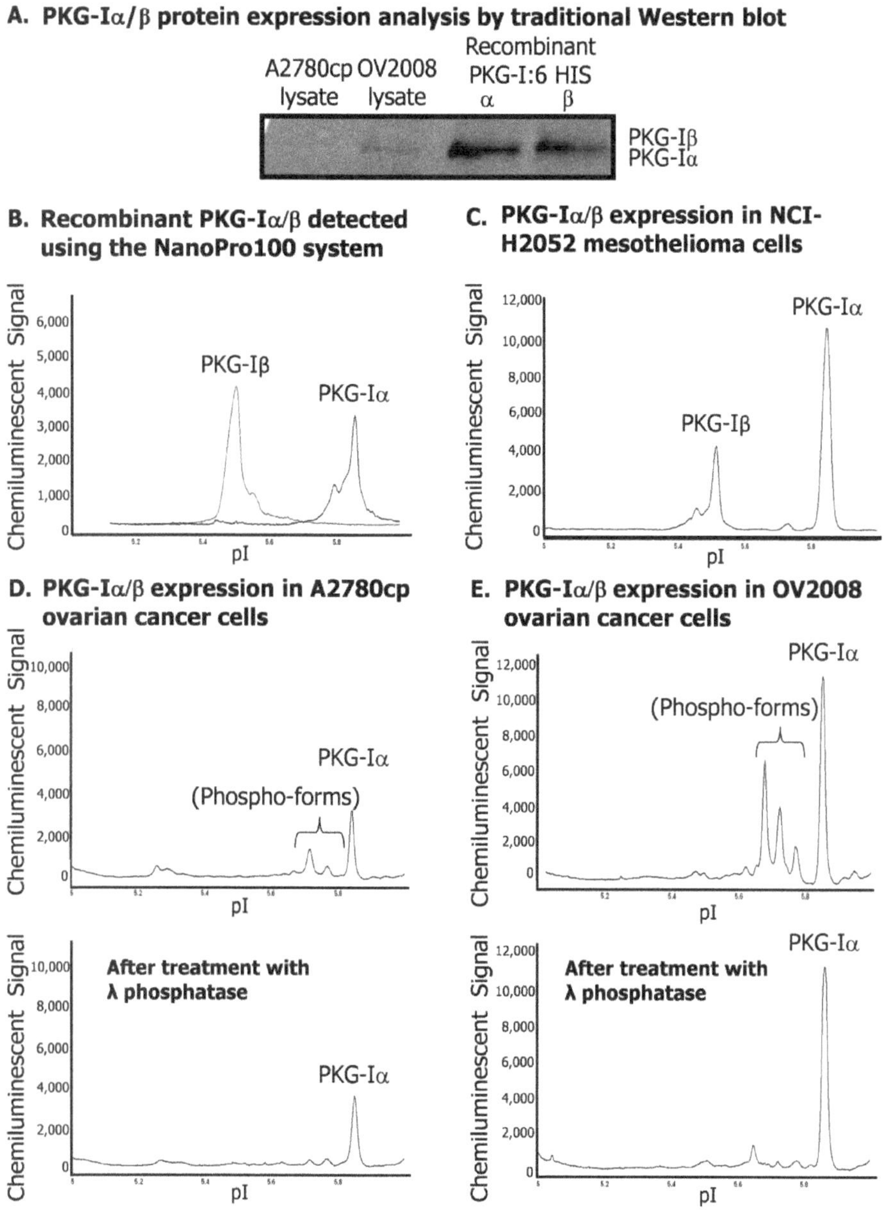

Fig. 3. Comparison between traditional Western blot analysis and the new ultrasensitive Nanopro100 system for identifying two PKG-I isoforms expressed in human ovarian cancer cell lysates. A. Western blot analysis of 1.56 μg total cellular protein in cell lysates of A2780cp and OV2008 cells. B – E. NanoPro100 analysis using 3.13 ng of total cellular protein in cell lysates. The lower electropherograms in D. & E. represent cell lysates treated for 30 minutes at 37° C with lambda phosphatase to remove phosphate groups from the proteins.

In many of our previous studies, there appears to be an inverse relationship between the protein expression levels and the kinase activity of PKG-Iα. For example, vascular smooth muscle cells have exceptionally high levels of PKG-Iα protein expression but relatively low levels of PKG-Iα kinase activation (e.g. 30% - 40% of maximal activity) (Fiscus, 1988; Fiscus & Murad, 1988; Fiscus *et al*, 1983). In contrast, many cancer cells, including human ovarian cancer cells, have relatively low levels of PKG-Iα protein expression but high levels of PKG-Iα kinase activation (i.e. hyperactivation, estimated to be ~90% of maximum activity) (Johlfs & Fiscus, 2010; Leung *et al*, 2010). We have proposed that the reason for this inverse relationship between protein expression levels and kinase activation levels is because of a negative-feedback mechanism, in which increases in PKG-Iα kinase activity (as, for example, resulting from c-Src-mediated tyrosine phosphorylation of PKG-Iα in cancer cells) would result in the negative modulation of PKG-Iα gene expression and protein expression, ultimately leading to the relatively low protein levels of PKG-Iα. However, in spite of lower protein levels (as measured in a Western blot analysis), the actual functional activity of PKG-Iα may remain quite high because of more-targeted subcellular localization, efficiently placing PKG-Iα in contact with its downstream target proteins. We have proposed that this may be the explanation for the low protein levels and high kinase activity of PKG-Iα in cancer cells, especially those overexpressing or having hyperactivated c-Src.

Negative feedback regulations of PKG-Iα expression at both the messenger RNA and protein levels have been shown in studies by Thomas Lincoln's laboratory at the University of South Alabama (Dey *et al*, 2009; Lincoln *et al*, 2001). Exposure of vascular smooth muscle cells to high levels of NO, causing large increases in intracellular cGMP levels, or to cell-permeable cGMP analogs that hyperactivate PKG-Iα, causes (negative-feedback) downregulation of PKG-Iα gene expression (Lincoln *et al*, 2001). Furthermore, high-level activation of PKG-Iα also results in the ubiquitination of PKG-Iα and its degradation by the proteasome (Dey *et al*, 2009). If such mechanisms are involved in regulating the protein expression levels of PKG-Iα in cancer cells, then the lower levels of protein expression of PKG-Iα, as was found in the chemoresistant A2780cp ovarian cancer cells (Figure 3), may actually reflect a higher level of functional PKG-Iα kinase activity. Future experiments will test this possibility.

8. Overall model of the involvement of the NO/cGMP/PKG-Iα signaling pathway in promoting tumor growth, chemoresistance and angiogenesis in ovarian cancer

Figure 4 illustrates our overall model showing the involvement of the NO/cGMP/PKG-Iα pathway in promoting cell proliferation and suppressing apoptosis in human ovarian cancer cells, which would contribute to enhanced tumor growth and chemoresistance. Also shown in the model is the potential role of nearby endothelial cells, which would provide an additional source of endogenous NO within the growing tumor, potentially contributing to the "angiogenic switch", i.e. the increased tumor growth that occurs after the invasion of endothelial cells into the tumor. Many factors are released from the endothelial cells that can stimulate the growth and chemoresistance of the tumor. Because low physiological levels (0.01 - 1 nM) of NO are now recognized to play a key role in promoting cancer cell proliferation and the development of chemoresistance, the NO released from nearby endothelial cells may have an important role in the tumor growth and chemoresistance commonly found in ovarian cancer. Endothelial cells also play another important role in tumor growth by providing new blood vessels (i.e. angiogenesis) needed for the vascularization and blood perfusion of the growing tumor.

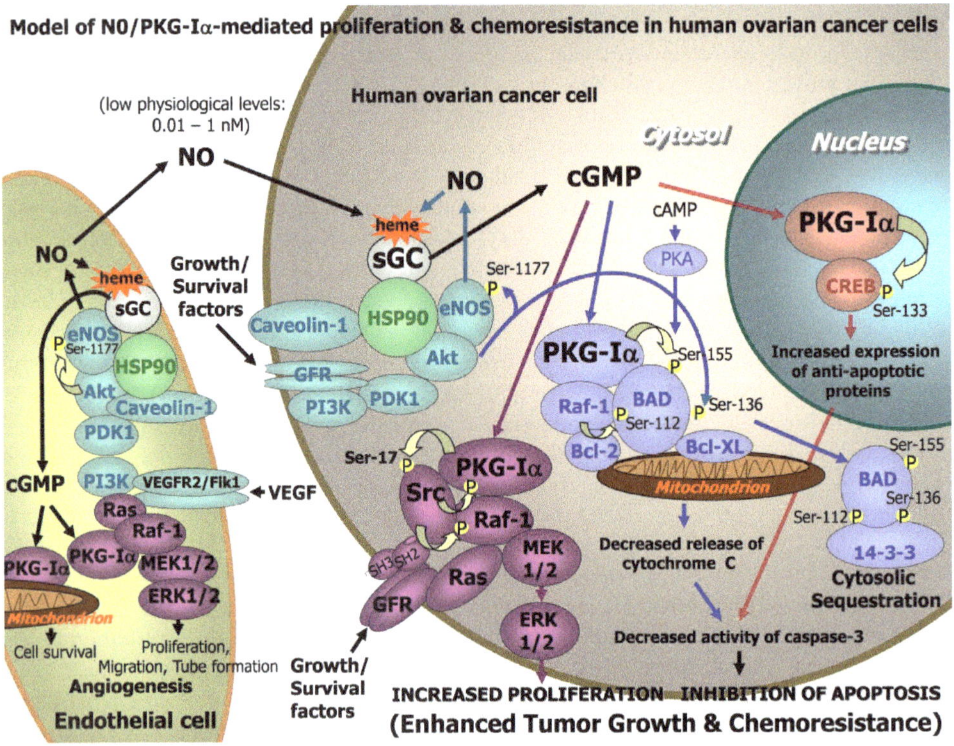

Fig. 4. Cellular model of the involvement of the NO/cGMP/PKG-Iα signaling pathway in promoting chemoresistance, tumor growth and angiogenesis in ovarian cancer.

Angiogenesis, especially that stimulated by VEGF (vascular endothelial growth factor), is now recognized to involve the stimulation of NO synthesis by eNOS within endothelial cells, which results in PKG activation and PKG-mediated downstream stimulation of MEK and ERK [reviewed in (Pilz & Casteel, 2003)]. This activation of the ERK signaling pathway is thought to result in enhanced proliferation, migration and tube formation of endothelial cells, key components of angiogenesis, all dependent on the NO/cGMP/PKG pathway. Although it has not yet been reported which isoform of PKG is involved in the multiple pro-angiogenesis responses of endothelial cells, our recent studies suggest that endothelial cells express predominantly the PKG-I**α** isoform (unpublished observations by J.C. Wong and R.R. Fiscus), which likely mediates the stimulation of downstream growth-promoting and pro-angiogenesis pathways in endothelial cells.

Figure 4 illustrates the interaction between PKG-Iα and c-Src, which results in the reciprocal phosphorylation, i.e. each kinase phosphorylating the other. Our studies have shown that activation of EGF receptors in human ovarian cancer cells causes downstream activation of c-Src, which is completely dependent on the kinase activity of PKG-Iα (Leung et al., 2010).

At the time, it was not completely clear how PKG-Iα was able to promote the activation of c-Src by EGF, but we had hypothesized that PKG-Iα may be able to catalyze the phosphorylation of a serine or threonine residence of c-Src that was important for enhancing c-Src's tyrosine kinase activity. Upon reviewing the amino acid sequence of c-Src, we recognized that serine-17 could possibly serve as a phosphorylation site for PKG-Iα, based on the surrounding amino acids that provided a good consensus sequence for PKG-Iα-catalyzed phosphorylation. To test this idea, we have worked with Cell Signaling Technologies (Danvers, MA, USA) over the last three years to develop an antibody that specifically recognizes the phosphorylated-form of serine-17 in c-Src. Using this antibody, we have shown that recombinant human-form PKG-Iα directly phosphorylates the serine-17 site in recombinant human-form c-Src, resulting in enhanced tyrosine kinase activity of c-Src (Fiscus & Johlfs, 2011). Using intact-cell experiments, involving two mesothelioma cell lines and a non-small cell lung cancer (NSCLC) cell line, we have further shown that gene knockdown of PKG-Iα expression (using siRNA and shRNA) or pharmacological inhibition of PKG-Iα activation resulted in dramatically suppressed levels of c-Src phosphorylation at serine-17, which corresponded to the inhibition of cell proliferation, increased levels of apoptosis and decreased attachment of the cells to the extracellular matrix (Fiscus & Johlfs, 2011). These recent studies have shown a clear role of the PKG-Iα-mediated phosphorylation of c-Src at serine-17 in preventing apoptosis and promoting proliferation, attachment and migration in the mesothelioma and NSCLC cells. It is very likely that a similar PKG-Iα-catalyzed phosphorylation of c-Src at serine-17 occurs in human ovarian cancer cells, which can explain the dependence of the c-Src activation by EGF on the presence of PKG-Iα, contributing to the stimulation of ovarian cancer cell proliferation, as reported in our earlier study (Leung *et al*, 2010).

Also shown in the model of Figure 4 is the interaction of PKG-Iα with two other downstream target proteins, Bad (shown in the model as BAD) and CREB. Previous studies from our laboratory and other laboratories have shown that the nuclear transcription factor CREB can be directly phosphorylated at its serine-133 site by PKG, which results in increased transcriptional activity and downstream regulation of gene expression [reviewed in (Fiscus, 2002; Pilz & Casteel, 2003)]. Also, we have recently shown that PKG-Iα directly phosphorylates BAD at serine-155, using *in vitro* experiments, and have further shown that a large part of the serine-155 phosphorylation of BAD within neuroblastoma cells is dependent on endogenous PKG-Iα kinase activity (Johlfs & Fiscus, 2010). Thus, BAD and CREB may be important downstream target proteins mediating the anti-apoptotic and pro-chemoresistant effects of the NO/cGMP/PKG-Iα pathway in human ovarian cancer cells.

9. Future research

Future studies will need to determine: 1) if PKG-Iα is the only isoform of PKG expressed in other human ovarian cancer cell lines as well as in tumor samples of patients with ovarian cancer, as we have shown for the A2780cp and OV2008 cell lines described herein and shown in Figure 3, or if there is a co-expression of the PKG-Iβ isoform in some ovarian cancer cells, like in the NCI-H2052 mesothelioma cell line (Figure 3), 2) what is the subcellular localization (e.g. plasma membrane, mitochondrial, nuclear, and/or cytosolic localization) of PKG-Iα (and possibly PKG-Iβ in some ovarian cancer cells) and how this determines which downstream target proteins are phosphorylated by the different PKG isoforms, 3) if the NO/cGMP/PKG-Iα signaling pathway is involved in promoting cell invasion and metastasis of ovarian cancer cells, 4) if there are other downstream target proteins that contribute to mediating the stimulation of DNA synthesis/cell proliferation, chemoresistance and metastasis of ovarian cancer cells, and 5) if the low-level-NO/cGMP/PKG-Iα and the higher-level-NO/cGMP/PKG-Iβ signaling pathways are involved in regulating apoptosis, proliferation and differentiation in the subset of ovarian cancer cells known as the ovarian tumor-initiating cells (or ovarian cancer stem cells) that may contribute to the tumorigenesis in ovarian cancer.

Our future studies will utilize the new ultrasensitive NanoPro100 system to determine the expression levels of PKG isoforms in human ovarian cancer cells. Because the NanoPro100 system separates proteins based on pI, rather than molecular weight as in conventional Western blot analysis, the new instrument can cleanly resolve the different phosphorylated forms of proteins, as shown in Figure 3. We will use this capability to identify the different phosphorylated forms of the PKG-I isoforms as well as the downstream phosphorylation of the different target proteins of the PKG isoforms.

10. Conclusions

Our studies suggest that the NO/cGMP/PKG-Iα signaling pathway and its interaction with the c-Src tyrosine kinase pathway play an essential role in promoting cell proliferation and chemoresistance in human ovarian cancer cells. The interaction with c-Src involves a novel reciprocal phosphorylation mechanism, which includes c-Src mediating the tyrosine-phosphorylation of PKG-Iα, enhancing PKG-Iα's serine/threonine kinase activity, and PKG-Iα mediating the serine-phosphorylation of c-Src (at serine-17), enhancing c-Src's tyrosine kinase activity. We propose that this novel interaction results in an "oncogenic reinforcement" in human ovarian cancer cells, leading to the exaggerated cell proliferation and chemoresistance, illustrated in the model in Figure 4.

This new understanding of the NO/cGMP/PKG-Iα pathway and its interaction with c-Src in human ovarian cancer cells provides new molecular targets that can be used for developing novel anti-cancer therapeutic agents. However, because NO has multiple cellular and molecular actions, illustrated in Figure 1, and the two PKG-I isoforms mediate very different biological effects, illustrated in Figure 2, future studies will need to recognize these complexities and their importance in development of new therapies for ovarian cancer.

New state-of-the-art instruments, like the NanoPro100 system, which provides >100-times higher sensitivity and much better specificity in identifying and quantifying protein expression and site-specific protein phosphorylation, compared with conventional Western blot analysis, will greatly facilitate our future studies. It is anticipated that the new information that will be learned about the low-level-NO/cGMP/PKG-Iα signaling pathway and its interaction with the c-Src tyrosine kinase pathway in human ovarian cancer cells will ultimately lead to new therapies that can successfully treat ovarian cancer.

11. Acknowledgements

Financial support for the research involving the NanoPro100 instrument and the preparation of this book chapter was provided by Start-up Funding from Roseman University of Health Sciences (formerly named University of Southern Nevada), Henderson,

Nevada, USA. Other parts of our research reported herein were conducted at the Nevada Cancer Institute, Las Vegas, Nevada, USA, and were supported by a grant from the U.S. Department of Defense (Grant # W81XWH-07-1-0543) and Start-up Funding from the Nevada Cancer Institute, Las Vegas, Nevada, USA, awarded to Dr. Fiscus.

12. References

Barger SW, Fiscus RR, Ruth P, Hofmann F, Mattson MP (1995) Role of cyclic GMP in the regulation of neuronal calcium and survival by secreted forms of beta-amyloid precursor. *J Neurochem* 64(5): 2087-96.

Batchelor AM, Bartus K, Reynell C, Constantinou S, Halvey EJ, Held KF, Dostmann WR, Vernon J, Garthwaite J (2010) Exquisite sensitivity to subsecond, picomolar nitric oxide transients conferred on cells by guanylyl cyclase-coupled receptors. *Proc Natl Acad Sci U S A* 107(51): 22060-5.

Beckman JS, Koppenol WH (1996) Nitric oxide, superoxide, and peroxynitrite: the good, the bad, and the ugly. *Am J Physiol* 271(5 Pt 1): C1424-37.

Bellamy TC, Griffiths C, Garthwaite J (2002) Differential sensitivity of guanylyl cyclase and mitochondrial respiration to nitric oxide measured using clamped concentrations. *J Biol Chem* 277(35): 31801-7.

Cantuaria G, Magalhaes A, Angioli R, Mendez L, Mirhashemi R, Wang J, Wang P, Penalver M, Averette H, Braunschweiger P (2000) Antitumor activity of a novel glyco-nitric oxide conjugate in ovarian carcinoma. *Cancer* 88(2): 381-8.

Chan GH, Fiscus RR (2002) Severe impairment of CGRP-induced hypotension in vivo and vasorelaxation in vitro in elderly rats. *Eur J Pharmacol* 434(3): 133-9.

Chan GH, Fiscus RR (2004) Exaggerated production of nitric oxide (NO) and increases in inducible NO-synthase mRNA levels induced by the pro-inflammatory cytokine interleukin-1beta in vascular smooth muscle cells of elderly rats. *Exp Gerontol* 39(3): 387-94.

Chan SL, Fiscus RR (2003) Guanylyl cyclase inhibitors NS2028 and ODQ and protein kinase G (PKG) inhibitor KT5823 trigger apoptotic DNA fragmentation in immortalized uterine epithelial cells: anti-apoptotic effects of basal cGMP/PKG. *Mol Hum Reprod* 9(12): 775-83.

Chang S, Hypolite JA, Velez M, Changolkar A, Wein AJ, Chacko S, DiSanto ME (2004) Downregulation of cGMP-dependent protein kinase-1 activity in the corpus cavernosum smooth muscle of diabetic rabbits. *Am J Physiol Regul Integr Comp Physiol* 287(4): R950-60.

Cheng Chew SB, Leung PY, Fiscus RR (2003) Preincubation with atrial natriuretic peptide protects NG108-15 cells against the toxic/proapoptotic effects of the nitric oxide donor S-nitroso- N-acetylpenicillamine. *Histochem Cell Biol* 120(3): 163-71.

Chien JR, Aletti G, Bell DA, Keeney GL, Shridhar V, Hartmann LC (2007) Molecular pathogenesis and therapeutic targets in epithelial ovarian cancer. *J Cell Biochem* 102(5): 1117-29.

Deguchi A, Thompson WJ, Weinstein IB (2004) Activation of protein kinase G is sufficient to induce apoptosis and inhibit cell migration in colon cancer cells. *Cancer Res* 64(11): 3966-73.

Dey NB, Busch JL, Francis SH, Corbin JD, Lincoln TM (2009) Cyclic GMP specifically suppresses Type-Ialpha cGMP-dependent protein kinase expression by ubiquitination. *Cell Signal* 21(6): 859-66.

Farias-Eisner R, Sherman MP, Aeberhard E, Chaudhuri G (1994) Nitric oxide is an important mediator for tumoricidal activity in vivo. *Proc Natl Acad Sci U S A* 91(20): 9407-11.

Fernhoff NB, Derbyshire ER, Marletta MA (2009) A nitric oxide/cysteine interaction mediates the activation of soluble guanylate cyclase. *Proc Natl Acad Sci U S A* 106(51): 21602-7.

Fiscus RR (1988) Molecular mechanisms of endothelium-mediated vasodilation. *Semin Thromb Hemost* 14 Suppl: 12-22.

Fiscus RR (2002) Involvement of cyclic GMP and protein kinase G in the regulation of apoptosis and survival in neural cells. *Neurosignals* 11(4): 175-90.

Fiscus RR, Chan GHH, Ma ACY (2001) Diabetes mellitus (DM) causes severe impairment of hypotensive response in vivo and vasorelaxant response in vitro to the neuropeptide CGRP. In *Peptides: The Wave of the Future*, Lebl M, Houghten RA (eds), pp 973-974. San Diego, California, U.S.A.: American Peptide Society.

Fiscus RR, Johlfs MG (2011) Protein kinase G type-I phosphorylates c-Src at serine-17 and promotes cell survival, proliferation and attachment in human mesothelioma and non-small cell lung cancer cells. *BMC Pharmacology* 11(Suppl. 1): 031.

Fiscus RR, Ming SK (2000) Biology of ageing. In *Medicine and Surgery in the Older Person*, Pang WS, Teoh MK, Ming SK (eds), pp 29-42. Singapore: Armour Publishing Pte Ltd.

Fiscus RR, Murad F (1988) cGMP-dependent protein kinase activation in intact tissues. *Methods Enzymol* 159: 150-9.

Fiscus RR, Rapoport RM, Murad F (1983) Endothelium-dependent and nitrovasodilator-induced activation of cyclic GMP-dependent protein kinase in rat aorta. *J Cyclic Nucleotide Protein Phosphor Res* 9(6): 415-25.

Fiscus RR, Torphy TJ, Mayer SE (1984) Cyclic GMP-dependent protein kinase activation in canine tracheal smooth muscle by methacholine and sodium nitroprusside. *Biochim Biophys Acta* 805(4): 382-92.

Fiscus RR, Yuen JP, Chan SL, Kwong JH, Chew SB (2002) Nitric oxide and cyclic GMP as pro- and anti-apoptotic agents. *J Card Surg* 17(4): 336-9.

Francis SH, Busch JL, Corbin JD, Sibley D (2010) cGMP-dependent protein kinases and cGMP phosphodiesterases in nitric oxide and cGMP action. *Pharmacol Rev* 62(3): 525-63.

Francis SH, Woodford TA, Wolfe L, Corbin JD (1988) Types I alpha and I beta isozymes of cGMP-dependent protein kinase: alternative mRNA splicing may produce different inhibitory domains. *Second Messengers Phosphoproteins* 12(5-6): 301-10.

Fraser M, Chan SL, Chan SS, Fiscus RR, Tsang BK (2006) Regulation of p53 and suppression of apoptosis by the soluble guanylyl cyclase/cGMP pathway in human ovarian cancer cells. *Oncogene* 25(15): 2203-12.

Fraser M, Leung B, Jahani-Asl A, Yan X, Thompson WE, Tsang BK (2003) Chemoresistance in human ovarian cancer: the role of apoptotic regulators. *Reprod Biol Endocrinol* 1: 66.

Fung E, Fiscus RR, Yim AP, Angelini GD, Arifi AA (2005) The potential use of type-5 phosphodiesterase inhibitors in coronary artery bypass graft surgery. *Chest* 128(4): 3065-73.

Garban HJ, Bonavida B (1999) Nitric oxide sensitizes ovarian tumor cells to Fas-induced apoptosis. *Gynecol Oncol* 73(2): 257-64.

Hofmann F, Feil R, Kleppisch T, Schlossmann J (2006) Function of cGMP-dependent protein kinases as revealed by gene deletion. *Physiol Rev* 86(1): 1-23.

Hou Y, Gupta N, Schoenlein P, Wong E, Martindale R, Ganapathy V, Browning D (2006) An anti-tumor role for cGMP-dependent protein kinase. *Cancer Lett* 240(1): 60-8.

Isenberg JS, Ridnour LA, Perruccio EM, Espey MG, Wink DA, Roberts DD (2005) Thrombospondin-1 inhibits endothelial cell responses to nitric oxide in a cGMP-dependent manner. *Proc Natl Acad Sci U S A* 102(37): 13141-6.

Johlfs MG, Fiscus RR (2010) Protein kinase G type-Ialpha phosphorylates the apoptosis-regulating protein Bad at serine 155 and protects against apoptosis in N1E-115 cells. *Neurochem Int* 56(4): 546-53.

Kleinert H, Schwarz PM, Forstermann U (2003) Regulation of the expression of inducible nitric oxide synthase. *Biol Chem* 384(10-11): 1343-64.

Kulie T, Slattengren A, Redmer J, Counts H, Eglash A, Schrager S (2011) Obesity and women's health: an evidence-based review. *J Am Board Fam Med* 24(1): 75-85.

LaFevre-Bernt M, Corbin JD, Francis SH, Miller WT (1998) Phosphorylation and activation of cGMP-dependent protein kinase by Src. *Biochimica et biophysica acta* 1386(1): 97-105.

Leung EL, Fraser M, Fiscus RR, Tsang BK (2008) Cisplatin alters nitric oxide synthase levels in human ovarian cancer cells: involvement in p53 regulation and cisplatin resistance. *Br J Cancer* 98(11): 1803-9.

Leung EL, Wong JC, Johlfs MG, Tsang BK, Fiscus RR (2010) Protein kinase G type Ialpha activity in human ovarian cancer cells significantly contributes to enhanced Src activation and DNA synthesis/cell proliferation. *Mol Cancer Res* 8(4): 578-91.

Lincoln TM, Dey N, Sellak H (2001) Invited review: cGMP-dependent protein kinase signaling mechanisms in smooth muscle: from the regulation of tone to gene expression. *J Appl Physiol* 91(3): 1421-30.

Nakamura T, Lipton SA (2010) Redox regulation of mitochondrial fission, protein misfolding, synaptic damage, and neuronal cell death: potential implications for Alzheimer's and Parkinson's diseases. *Apoptosis* 15(11): 1354-63.

Nausch LW, Ledoux J, Bonev AD, Nelson MT, Dostmann WR (2008) Differential patterning of cGMP in vascular smooth muscle cells revealed by single GFP-linked biosensors. *Proc Natl Acad Sci U S A* 105(1): 365-70.

Pilz RB, Casteel DE (2003) Regulation of gene expression by cyclic GMP. *Circ Res* 93(11): 1034-46.

Ridnour LA, Thomas DD, Switzer C, Flores-Santana W, Isenberg JS, Ambs S, Roberts DD, Wink DA (2008) Molecular mechanisms for discrete nitric oxide levels in cancer. *Nitric Oxide* 19(2): 73-6.

Rieder J, Jahnke R, Schloesser M, Seibel M, Czechowski M, Marth C, Hoffmann G (2001) Nitric oxide-dependent apoptosis in ovarian carcinoma cell lines. *Gynecol Oncol* 82(1): 172-6.

Sato M, Nakajima T, Goto M, Umezawa Y (2006) Cell-based indicator to visualize picomolar dynamics of nitric oxide release from living cells. *Anal Chem* 78(24): 8175-82.

Seth D, Stamler JS (2011) The SNO-proteome: causation and classifications. *Curr Opin Chem Biol* 15(1): 129-36.

Soh JW, Mao Y, Kim MG, Pamukcu R, Li H, Piazza GA, Thompson WJ, Weinstein IB (2000) Cyclic GMP mediates apoptosis induced by sulindac derivatives via activation of c-Jun NH2-terminal kinase 1. *Clin Cancer Res* 6(10): 4136-41.

Thomas DD, Ridnour LA, Isenberg JS, Flores-Santana W, Switzer CH, Donzelli S, Hussain P, Vecoli C, Paolocci N, Ambs S, Colton CA, Harris CC, Roberts DD, Wink DA (2008) The chemical biology of nitric oxide: implications in cellular signaling. *Free Radic Biol Med* 45(1): 18-31.

Thompson WJ, Piazza GA, Li H, Liu L, Fetter J, Zhu B, Sperl G, Ahnen D, Pamukcu R (2000) Exisulind induction of apoptosis involves guanosine 3',5'-cyclic monophosphate phosphodiesterase inhibition, protein kinase G activation, and attenuated beta-catenin. *Cancer Res* 60(13): 3338-42.

Wong AS, Kim SO, Leung PC, Auersperg N, Pelech SL (2001) Profiling of protein kinases in the neoplastic transformation of human ovarian surface epithelium. *Gynecol Oncol* 82(2): 305-11.

Wong JC, Fiscus RR (2010) Protein kinase G activity prevents pathological-level nitric oxide-induced apoptosis and promotes DNA synthesis/cell proliferation in vascular smooth muscle cells. *Cardiovasc Pathol* 19(6): e221-31.

Wong JC, Fiscus RR (2011) Essential roles of the nitric oxide (NO)/cGMP/protein kinase G type-Ialpha (PKG-Ialpha) signaling pathway and the atrial natriuretic peptide (ANP)/cGMP/PKG-Ialpha autocrine loop in promoting proliferation and cell survival of OP9 bone marrow stromal cells. *J Cell Biochem* 112(3): 829-39.

18

Autotaxin – A Target for the Treatment of Drug-Resistant Ovarian Cancer?

John King-Underwood[1], Steven M. Allin[2],
Charles W. Redman[3] and Alan Richardson[2]
[1]*CompchemRes*
[2]*Keele University*
[3]*University Hospital of North Staffordshire*
UK

1. Introduction

It has been known for a number of years that many patients with ovarian cancer suffer an accumulation of ascites fluid that contains a factor which supports the intraperitoneal growth of ovarian cancer cells (Mills et al. 1990). Following from the identification of lysophosphatidic acid (LPA) as a major growth factor in serum (van Corven et al. 1989), LPA was identified as the major "ovarian cancer activating factor" in ascites fluid (Xu et al. 1995). LPA was shown to accumulate to high concentrations (up to 80 μM) in ascites fluid. Since then, numerous publications have demonstrated the role of LPA in several biological processes relevant to cancer including cell migration and invasion, inhibition of apoptosis and senescence, angiogenesis and chemoresistance. Increases in plasma LPA are also being considered as a diagnostic biomarker of ovarian cancer (e.g. (Bese et al. 2010)). It is perhaps surprising then, that compounds interfering with this pathway have made slow progress to the clinic. Part of the reason for this likely reflects the complexity of the LPA signalling pathway. However, recent work has delineated many of the enzymes and receptors involved in regulating the LPA signalling pathways, revealing complexity in different LPA species, in the pathways involved in the metabolism of LPA, in LPA receptors and finally in the (patho)physiological responses to LPA. An understanding of how these pathways are deregulated in ovarian cancer has begun to suggest potential targets for the development of therapeutic drugs. One such target is autotaxin, an enzyme involved in the synthesis of LPA. Recently, several crystal structures of autotaxin have been solved, and these provide powerful tools to aid the development of autotaxin inhibitors. However, to fully appreciate the potential of autotaxin as a drug target, we first review LPA signalling pathways.

2. The LPA signalling pathway

2.1 Complexity in LPA

LPA (Fig. 1) itself provides a first example of complexity in this pathway, as it comprises a family of molecules. In general, LPA consists of a glycerol moiety linked as an ester to phosphate and fatty acid moieties. However, LPA molecules may differ in the length and the degree of unsaturation of the fatty acid, and the fatty acid may be attached to the *sn*1 or *sn*2 positions on the glycerol. In some cases, the fatty acid is replaced by an alkyl chain attached via an ether linkage. The phosphate may be attached to both the second and third glycerol hydroxyl groups, forming a cyclophosphate.

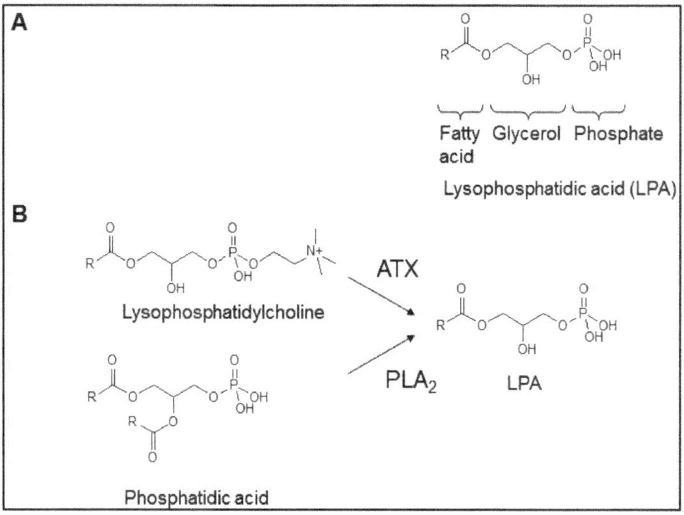

Fig. 1. **A** Lysophosphatidic acid is comprised of fatty acid, glycerol and phosphate moieties. **B**. Principle routes to the biosynthesis of LPA. ATX, autotaxin; PLA_2, phospholipase A_2. Note that autotaxin behaves as a phosopholipase D that uses *lyso* substrates, i.e. those lacking one fatty acid attached to the glycerol.

2.2 Complexity in the synthesis of LPA

There are a number of enzymes which can catalyze the synthesis of LPA in ovarian cancer and it is becoming more clear which of these contribute to the accumulation of LPA in ovarian cancer. LPA is synthesized both intracellularly and extracellularly, by ovarian cancer cells as well as mesothelial cells. Autotaxin is a secreted phospholipase that catalyses the hydrolysis of lysophosphatidyl choline to produce LPA and choline (fig. 2). Increased expression of autotaxin is observed in several cancers including renal (Stassar et al. 2001), thyroid (Kehlen et al. 2004), glioblastoma (Hoelzinger et al. 2005; Kishi et al. 2006), follicular lymphoma (Masuda et al. 2008), hepatic (Wu et al. 2010), prostate (Nouh et al. 2009) and pancreatic cancer (Nakai et al. 2011). Autotaxin expression is also increased in chemoresistant ovarian cancer compared to chemosensitive disease (Jazaeri et al. 2005). Ectopic expression of autotaxin in mammary epithelium is sufficient to cause high frequency breast cancer (Liu et al. 2009). Together these observations point to role for autotaxin in several cancer types. The elevated levels of LPA observed in ascites obtained from patients with ovarian cancer suggests a role in ovarian cancer. The increase in LPA levels are accompanied by elevated LPC, the substrate of autotaxin (Liu et al. 2009). Autotaxin itself is also present in ascites fluid (Tokumura et al. 2007). Although transgenic mice lacking autotaxin die as embryos, heterozygotes with one functional allele encoding autotaxin show a 50% reduction in plasma LPA (Tanaka et al. 2006), suggesting that autotaxin is the enzyme primarily responsible for the synthesis of LPA in plasma. However, it remains a possibility that autotaxin is not the enzyme responsible for the accumulation of LPA observed in ovarian cancer. In addition to autotaxin, extracellular LPA could potentially also be derived from the hydrolysis of phosphatidic acid by secreted phospholipase A_2 ($sPLA_2$).

A number of intracellular enzymes including glycerol 3-phosphate fatty acid transferase (GPFAT) and phospholipase D (PLD) and phospholipase A_2 may also contribute to the production of LPA at the cell membrane. It is possible that intracellular enzymes contribute to the accumulation of extracellular LPA. Although GPFAT has not received much attention in ovarian cancer, PLD_2 has recently been shown to contribute to EGF-induced LPA production (Snider et al. 2010). Other potential sources of LPA include intracellular isoforms of phospholipase A_2 which use phosphatidic acid as a substrate (Fig. 1). $cPLA_2$ is a calcium-dependant phospholipase implicated in cell migration whereas $iPLA_2$ is a calcium-independent phospholipase. Which cells are the potential sources of LPA? Platelets have previously been shown to be an important source of LPA in serum (Boucharaba et al. 2004), and Xu and co-workers have clearly shown in a murine model of ovarian cancer that both host and tumor cells contribute to the formation of LPA in ascites and this is catalysed by $iPLA_2$ (Li et al. 2010). Peritoneal mesothelial cells are one potential source of extracellular LPA produced by PLA_2 (Ren et al. 2006).

If both host and tumor cells contribute to the accumulation of peritoneal LPA, and there are several pathways capable of contributing to the formation of LPA, it seems reasonable to ask whether animal models accurately reflect clinical reality. In xenograft studies it is common to implant a human tumor cell into a murine host. Is the relative contribution of different LPA biosynthetic pathways in xenograft studies quantitatively similar to that observed in ovarian cancer? This is important because the relative contribution of, e.g., autotaxin and iPLA2 to the generation of LPA will likely influence the success of inhibitors of these individual enzymes when used in patients. Thus, we consider that although preclincial experiments may continue to shed light on validity of the different LPA biosynthetic pathways as drug targets, a definitive answer will only be provided by clinical studies.

The concentration of LPA in ascites fluid is controlled by its rate of elimination as well as its rate of synthesis. It is important, therefore, to consider also pathways of LPA catabolism. Two lipid phosphatases, LPP1 and LPP3, have been implicated in the hydrolysis of LPA. Importantly, LPP1 shows reduced expression in ovarian cancer cells, suggesting that this might contribute to increased levels of LPA (Tanyi et al. 2003; Tanyi et al. 2003). Correspondingly, expression of these genes has been shown to inhibit several of the responses ascribed to LPA, for example colony formation and cell migration. Understanding the pathways that regulate the expression of these phosphatases is important, as it might provide targets which can be used to increase the expression of LPP1 or LPP3 and so develop drugs to increase LPA catabolism.

It is also worth considering how the expression of LPA anabolic and catabolic enzymes might vary between patients as this may influence the design of clinical trials. Although we await further data to address this, it is worth considering the potential impact on the clinical use of drugs regulating the LPA pathway. It seems that it will be appropriate to select patients most likely to benefit from a particular enzyme inhibitor taking into account which biosynthetic pathways are deregulated. For example, PLD_2 has been implicated in EGF-driven LPA production (Snider et al. 2010), so patients whose tumors are driven by the EGF pathway may be more dependent on PLD_2 than other LPA producing enzymes. Similarly, VEGF regulates autotaxin production (see below), so tumors in which VEGF production is substantially elevated may be more dependent on autotaxin for LPA production. The expression level of LPP1 or LPP3 may also influence the response to drugs inhibiting the production of LPA. We speculate that inter-patient variability in the enzymes catalysing LPA catabolism may lead to different response to drugs which inhibit LPA synthesis and evaluating the extent of any clinical variation may prove to be important.

2.3 Complexity in LPA receptors

Two classes of cell surface receptors for LPA have been described, all of which are G-protein coupled receptors (Tigyi 2010). The first of these classes comprise the receptors LPA_1, LPA_2 and LPA_3. These are closely related and form part of the EDG (endothelial differentiation gene) family of receptors which also includes receptors for the bioactive lipid sphingosine 1-phosphate (S1P). At high (μM) concentrations, LPA may also bind to S1P receptors. A second set of LPA receptors are more closely related to purinergic receptors including LPA_4 (also known as P2Y9), LPA_5 (GPR95). There are several additional receptors that are also reported to respond to LPA including GPR35, GPR87, P2Y5 and P2Y10 and further characterization of these is on-going. Clearly, it is important to consider which of these receptors should be exploited as drug targets in ovarian cancer.

LPA_2 and LPA_3 appear to promote ovarian tumorigenesis. The expression of LPA_2 and LPA_3 is increased in ovarian cancer, (Fang et al. 2002; Wang et al. 2007; Murph et al. 2008) and over- expression of these receptors in Sk-Ov-3 cells promotes growth of primary tumors and metastasis (Yu et al. 2008). In clinical samples, expression of LPA_2 and LPA_3 correlates with tumor stage (Wang et al. 2007). In contrast, the expression of LPA_1 is decreased in ovarian cancer and expression of LPA_1 promotes apoptosis (Furui et al. 1999). These observations are important from a therapeutic perspective, because it suggest that ovarian cancer patients might benefit from a drug which is an LPA_2, LPA_3 antagonist but it may be preferable that such a drug does not bind with high affinity to LPA_1. However, it should be noted that the growth inhibitory properties of LPA_1 were found to be independent of LPA (Furui et al. 1999) and encouraging results have already been obtained with a pan-LPA receptor antagonist in xenograft studies (Zhang et al. 2009). We already have substantial experience developing (non-oncological) drugs using G-protein coupled receptors as drug targets, suggesting this may be a fruitful avenue for therapeutic research.

As well as binding to cell surface receptors, LPA has been proposed to activate the nuclear hormone receptor PPARγ. These intracellular receptors function as transcription factors and drive the expression of genes involved in diverse physiological responses including glucose and lipid metabolism, inflammatory response and apoptosis. PPARγ is over-expressed in ovarian cancer (Zhang et al. 2005) and its expression is associated with a poor response to chemotherapy and shortened survival (Davidson et al. 2009). Although this might lead to the hypothesis that activation of PPARγ by LPA is tumorigenic, confusingly synthetic PPAR agonists (the "glitazones") inhibit the proliferation of ovarian cancer cells and induce apoptosis (Yang et al. 2007). Glitazones also display synergistic activity with platinum chemotherapy through down-regulation of metallothionines involved in the detoxification of platinum (Girnun et al. 2007). Thus, the contribution of the activation of PPARγ by LPA to ovarian tumorigenesis remains to be further clarified.

Finally, it has also been pointed out that LPA binds to a number of intracellular cytoskeletal proteins (Tigyi 2010) possibly reflecting an intracellular role for LPA in regulating cell migration.

3. Physiological and pathophysiological functions of LPA

3.1 LPA/autotaxin and migration and invasion

LPA has several well characterized effects upon ovarian cancer cell migration and invasion. Firstly, activation of Src kinase by LPA leads to the breakdown of cell-cell junctions, promoting cell scattering (Huang et al. 2008). The breakdown of cell junctions is facilitated by activation uPA (urokinase plasminogen activator) by LPA, which leads to proteolysis of E-cadherin. Secondly, LPA triggers cytoskeletal reorganization (Do et al. 2007; Kim et al. 2011) and reorganization of cell contacts with the extracellular matrix which promotes cell motility (Sawada et al. 2002; Bian et al. 2004; Bian et al. 2006). Thirdly, LPA induces the expression of several proteases including uPA (Pustilnik et al. 1999; Li et al. 2005), MMP1 (Wang et al. 2011), MMP2 (Fishman et al. 2001) MMP7 and MMP9 (Park et al. 2011) which contribute to the breakdown of extracellular matrix allowing invasion through basement membrane. In addition, LPA decreases expression of TIMP metalloprotease inhibitors (Sengupta et al. 2007), thereby potentiating the effect of activation of proteases.

Although the role of autotaxin in migration and invasion has not yet been studied in ovarian cancer to the same level of detail as in other cancers, the role of autotaxin in these processes is well founded. Indeed, autotaxin was first identified through its activity as an autocrine motility factor (Stracke et al. 1992) and integrin $\alpha_6\beta_4$, which is associated with and invasive phenotype, can increase the expression of autotaxin (Chen and O'Connor 2005). Autotaxin and LPA promote the expression of the extracellular matrix protein osteopontin which promotes migration (Zhang et al. 2011). Autotaxin activates the small G-proteins cdc42 and Rac (Jung et al. 2002; Hoelzinger et al. 2008; Harper et al. 2010) and focal adhesion kinase (Jung et al. 2002), proteins which are key regulators of cell motility. More direct evidence comes from the observation that knockdown of autotaxin inhibits cell migration in several cancer types (Kishi et al. 2006; Gaetano et al. 2009; Harper et al. 2010) and over-expression of autotaxin increases motility (Kishi et al. 2006; Harper et al. 2010). Autotaxin regulates the formation of invadopodia (Harper et al. 2010) and induces the expression of uPA (Lee et al. 2006) and MMP3 (Haga et al. 2009). Correspondingly, knockdown of autotaxin inhibits invasion (Hoelzinger et al. 2008) while over-expression promotes invasion (Nam et al. 2000; Yang et al. 2002). Finally, autotaxin promotes osteolytic bone metastases derived from breast cancer cells (David et al. 2010). Taken together, these observations suggest that LPA and autotaxin are likely to promote an invasive phenotype in ovarian cancer cells. We discuss below the therapeutic implications of these observations.

3.2 LPA/autotaxin and a supportive microenvironment

LPA contributes to providing a microenvironment that is conducive to tumor growth. It does this in part by supressing apoptosis and senescence. LPA is itself a growth factor (van Corven et al. 1989) for several cell types. It stimulates the growth of cultures of ovarian cancer cells (Xu et al. 1995; Hu et al. 2003) by several pathways (Hurst and Hooks 2009). It also induces the expression of the growth factor Groα (Lee et al. 2006). Finally, iPLA2, one of the enzymes involved in the synthesis of LPA, can promote cell cycle progression in the absence of exogenous growth factors (Song et al. 2007).

LPA induces the production of the major angiogenic factor VEGF by ovarian cancer cells (Hu et al. 2001) and mesenchymal stem cells (Jeon et al. 2010). LPA also increases VEGF receptor expression on endothelial cells. The effect of LPA is apparently amplified by VEGF-induced expression of autotaxin by ovarian cancer cells (Ptaszynska et al. 2008) and endothelial cells (Ptaszynska et al. 2010) thereby potentiating LPA production. LPA also promotes the expression of other pro-angiogenic factors including IL-8 by tumor cells and SDF-1 by mesenchymal stem cells (Jeon et al. 2010). These observations suggest a key role for autotaxin and LPA in ovarian cancer driven angiogenesis and have led to the suggestion that autotaxin may also be a therapeutic target for inhibiting angiogenesis (Ptaszynska et al. 2010). In addition to its role in angiogenesis VEGF has also been implicated in LPA induced invasion (So et al. 2005; Wang et al. 2009; Wang et al. 2011).

3.3 LPA/autotaxin and inhibition of apoptosis and chemoresistance

The potential contribution of LPA to resistance to chemotherapy is of considerable therapeutic significance. Patients with ovarian cancer often receive chemotherapy comprising a taxane and a platinum-based compound, often paclitaxel and carboplatin. Although these drugs are initially effective, many patients eventually relapse with a disease that has become resistant to chemotherapy. Thus, a key reason that approximately 30% of patients diagnosed with ovarian cancer survive only 5-years post-diagnosis is the development of drug resistance. Understanding the molecular basis of drug resistance and developing drugs which restore drug sensitivity is one strategy to improve the treatment of ovarian cancer.

LPA causes the translocation of the pro-apoptotic receptor Fas from the cell surface, making tumor cells less responsive to stimuli that activate the extrinsic apoptosis pathway (Meng et al. 2005). Fas activates an intracellular caspase protease cascade to drive apoptosis. cFLIP is an inhibitor of caspase-8 activation, and the increased expression of cFLIP that is induced by LPA further contributes to suppression of apoptosis by LPA (Kang et al. 2004). At the same time, LPA induces the expression of Fas ligand (FasL) on tumor cells, and this promotes apoptosis of lymphocytes (Meng et al. 2004; Meng et al. 2005) presumably allowing tumor cells to avoid immune surveillance. LPA also increases the expression of the survival factor GEP (Kamrava et al. 2005). LPA inhibits the intrinsic apoptosis pathway by promoting phosphorylation of the pro-apoptotic protein BAD (Kang et al. 2004), which prevents BAD from promoting apoptosis through activation of Bak and Bax and permeabilization of the mitochondrial outer membrane. These observations suggest that LPA can regulate both the intrinsic and extrinsic apoptosis pathways, underlining the importance of this pathway as a therapeutic target.

In addition to LPA, there is evidence directly linking autotaxin to cell survival. Expression of autotaxin suppresses apoptosis in response to serum starvation (Song et al. 2005). LPA has been shown to activate the PI 3-kinase/Akt pathway in several cell types, including in ovarian cancer cells (Baudhuin et al. 2002). This pathway is a well described cell survival pathway and contributes to LPA suppressing both the extrinsic and the intrinsic apoptosis pathways (Kang et al. 2004). Similarly, inhibition of apoptosis by autotaxin is dependent on the PI 3-kinase pathway (Song et al. 2005).

As well as inhibition of apoptosis, one of the hallmarks of cancer is the avoidance of senescence. LPA suppresses p53-dependant replicative senescence (Kortlever et al. 2008), at least in part through induction of telomerase (Bermudez et al. 2007; Yang et al. 2008).

Along with many other chemotherapeutic agents, carboplatin and paclitaxel induce apoptosis. It seems reasonable to presume that the ability of autotaxin and LPA to suppress apoptosis contributes to resistance to paclitaxel and carboplatin. As these drugs are the cornerstone of ovarian cancer chemotherapy, the potential of the LPA pathway as a therapeutic target is again underlined. Early work demonstrated that LPA confers resistance to cisplatin (Frankel and Mills 1996) and this has also been observed in colon cancer cells (Sun et al. 2009). We conducted a screen to identify genes that confer resistance to carboplatin, and one of the hits identified in that screen was autotaxin. Expression of autotaxin delayed apoptosis induced by carboplatin, while apoptosis was accelerated after inhibition of autotaxin by either siRNA or with a small molecule inhibitor (Vidot et al. 2010). More recently, LPA and autotaxin have been shown to confer resistance of breast and melanoma cancer cells to paclitaxel (Samadi et al. 2009). Resistance to paclitaxel depends on PI 3-kinase, presumably reflecting the role of PI 3-kinase downstream of LPA in survival signalling that was noted above. Remarkably, resistance to paclitaxel conferred by LPA by restores normal spindle function in cells exposed to paclitaxel and the cells escape M-phase arrest (Samadi et al. 2011). The LPA_2 receptor is one candidate for mediating chemoresistance, because $LPA_2^{-/-}$ mice exhibit increased radiation-induced apoptosis (Deng et al. 2007). Thus, there is direct evidence linking autotaxin to resistance to both chemotherapeutic agents used to treat ovarian cancer.

Other proteins in the LPA pathway may also contribute to chemoresistance. RGS proteins (Regulator of G-protein signalling) attenuate signalling by LPA receptors by increasing the GTPase activity of G-proteins that are activated by LPA receptors (Hurst et al. 2008). Expression of several RGS proteins is decreased in ovarian cancer cell lines that are resistant to cisplatin (Hooks et al. 2010). Knockdown of expression of two RGS protein, RGS10 and RGS17, causes a 2-3 fold reduction in the potency but a striking 6-fold reduction in cisplatin potency is observed when the expression of both RGS proteins is inhibited. This suggests that loss of expression of RGS proteins, leading to increased activity of LPA receptor signalling through G-proteins, may contribute to resistance to chemotherapy.

In addition to inhibiting apoptosis through G-protein signalling, the LPA_2 receptor also regulates the pro-apoptotic protein Siva-1. Activation of p53 following DNA damage increases the expression of pro-apoptotic Siva-1 and this contributes to cisplatin-induced apoptosis (Barkinge et al. 2009), as well apoptosis induced by uvltraviolet light (Chu et al. 2004). LPA causes ubiquitination and turnover of Siva-1 and this contributes to suppression of apoptosis by LPA (Lin et al. 2007). This may be mediated by the LPA_2 receptor. LPA_2 is distinct from other LPA receptors in containing zinc finger and a C-terminal PDZ binding motifs. These motifs serve to recruit NHERF2 and TRIP6, which form a ternary complex with Siva-1. Both NHERF2 and TRIP6 are required for LPA to confer resistance to cisplatin (E et al. 2009). But how does Siva-1 induce apoptosis? In part, this probably reflects inhibition of the cell survival driven by the transcription factor NFκB. Intriguingly, Siva-1 can also inhibit Bcl-X_L, a member of the anti-apoptotic Bcl-2 family proteins that suppress activation of Bak and Bax in the intrinsic apoptosis pathway (Xue et al. 2002). We have shown previously that inhibition of Bcl-X_L increases sensitivity to carboplatin (Witham et al. 2007). Together with our observation that autotaxin confers resistance to carboplatin (Vidot et al. 2010), these data suggest that autotaxin may confer resistance to carboplatin by suppressing the intrinsic apoptosis pathway (fig. 2). As we discuss below, this predicts that autotaxin inhibitors may be useful in the treatment of drug-resistant ovarian cancer.

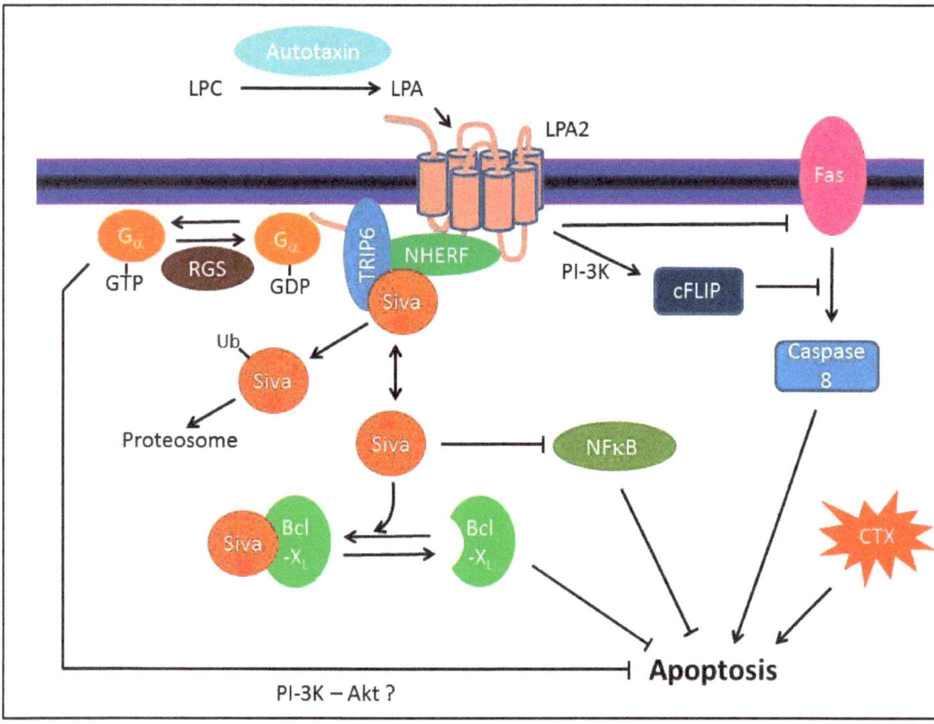

Fig. 2. Regulation of chemoresistance by LPA and autotaxin. CTX denotes chemotherapy, PI-3K, PI 3-kinse.

The observation that RGS and Siva pathways both contribute to chemoresistance in different cell lines highlights the point that there are multiple mechanisms that can cause drug resistance. Thus, if the signalling pathways that are activated by LPA receptors are used as therapeutic targets to restore chemosensitivity, it may be necessary to develop several different therapeutic agents and use them in accordance with the particular pathway that is driving chemoresistance in a individual patient's tumor. If multiple pathways promote resistance, several drugs may be necessary. Alternatively, it may be more straight forwards to develop drugs which either inhibit the LPA receptor(s) or prevent the production of LPA itself.

As well as contributing to resistance to chemotherapy, autotaxin also confer resistance to histone deacetylase inhibitors. HDAC3 and HDAC7 repress the expression of autotaxin. Consequently, exposure to the HDAC inhibitor trichostatin (TSA) increases the expression of autotaxin and the subsequent production of LPA inhibits apoptosis induced by TSA. This suggests that autotaxin confers resistance to HDAC inhibitors (Li et al. 2011). One clinical use of autotaxin inhibitors may be in combination with HDAC inhibitors.

4. Is autotaxin a valid target in ovarian cancer?

A starting point for drug discovery is "target validation" - a process in which data is amassed to give confidence that inhibiting a particular drug target will afford the desired therapeutic outcome. The foregoing discussion highlights several points in the LPA signalling pathway which might provide drug targets to treat ovarian cancer. Drugs could be developed which: inhibit the synthesis of LPA; increase the catabolism of LPA; up-regulate LPA binding proteins to sequester LPA; inhibit LPA binding to its receptors or inhibit LPA receptor expression; inhibit downstream signalling. (Note that strategies to modulate the tumor environment are already being explored as inhibitors of the VEGF pathway, e.g. bevacizumab, are currently in clinical trials in ovarian cancer and encouraging results have been obtained.)

Although several of these approaches are feasible, in several cases we consider that there is currently insufficient data to identify a drug target as well validated in ovarian cancer. For example, there are multiple signalling pathways activated by LPA receptors. Although experimental data is accumulating, several potential drug targets in these signalling pathways activated by LPA receptors require validation in additional cell lines and evaluation in clinical samples. Until such data is forthcoming, we consider that developing drugs which inhibit the synthesis of LPA or which inhibit LPA receptors are currently the most promising avenues. As we have discussed, there are difficulties with these approaches too. The complexity of the LPA pathway suggests to us that it may be difficult to gather robust target validation data with preclinical studies alone, and that well designed clinical research with inhibitors of autotaxin, iPLA2 or LPA receptors will be necessary to confirm the best approach(s). Thus, for the remainder of this review we will focus on autotaxin as one potential target to inhibiting the LPA pathway.

5. Current status of autotaxin inhibitors

To date a number of metal chelators, lipid analogues and non-lipid small molecules have been discovered to be inhibitors of autotaxin. In this section we have concentrated on recent reports of small molecule inhibitors of autotaxin.

Cui and Macdonald have developed a series of tyrosine-derived β-hydroxyphosphonates as analogues of LPA that display activity as inhibitors of autotaxin (Cui et al. 2007; Cui et al. 2008). The synthesis of this series of compounds is highlighted in Figure 3. The sodium borohydride reduction step gave rise to a mixture of two diasteroisomeric products that were separated and isolated by column chromatography. In the initial publications (Cui et al. 2007; Cui et al. 2008) the relative stereochemistry at the new chiral centre had not been determined, but later work from this group on a more advanced series of inhibitors gave insight to the relationship between stereochemistry and activity in the lead compounds (East et al. 2010). From an initial series of targets prepared ($R^1 = C_{15}H_{31}$, variation of R^2), the most active compound to be identified was compound **1a**, derived from *S*-tyrosine and later confirmed to have the relative stereochemistry shown (Fig. 3), which was able to inhibit 73% of autotaxin activity when tested at a concentration of 1 μM. The *syn* isomer, **1b**, was less active achieving 37% inhibition at the same concentration. Interestingly, the corresponding isomers of compound **1** prepared from the enantiomer *R*-tyrosine did *not* show potent inhibition of autotaxin even though they contained the same pyridyl subunit. Structural modification based around varying the length of, or incorporation of unsaturation into, the lipophilic side chains (R^1, Fig. 3) of compounds **1a** and **1b** did not result in an increase in activity from that originally seen with **1a**.

In a follow-up study (East et al. 2010) the SAR of the pyridyl region was further explored and important structural features were determined to be: the nitrogen heteroatom, the presence of the methoxy substituent, the presence of methyl groups. Extending the alkyl

chain of the alkyloxy substituent to ethyl or propyl led to a fall in activity. Activity was retained on removing the heteroatom as long as the methoxy group and methyl substitution were also retained. In all cases the *anti*-isomer was more active than the *syn* isomer.
Docking studies were carried out on compound **1a** and suggested the proximity of the phosphonate to the two zinc centres at the active site and that the lipophilic side chain was able to fill a large lipophilic pocket, thought to bind the lipid tail of LPC. An aromatic-guanidine binding interaction was also suggested between the benzyl substituent and Arg^{456} and a weak H-bonding interaction between the methoxy substituent and Lys^{209} within the hydrophilic leaving group pocket of autotaxin. The degree of interaction was dependent upon the electron density of the aryl ring, with more electron rich substituents on the pyridyl ring favouring the interaction. Interestingly the aromatic ring of the tyrosine unit appeared to act solely as an appropriate spacer unit between the more important pharmacophore groups.

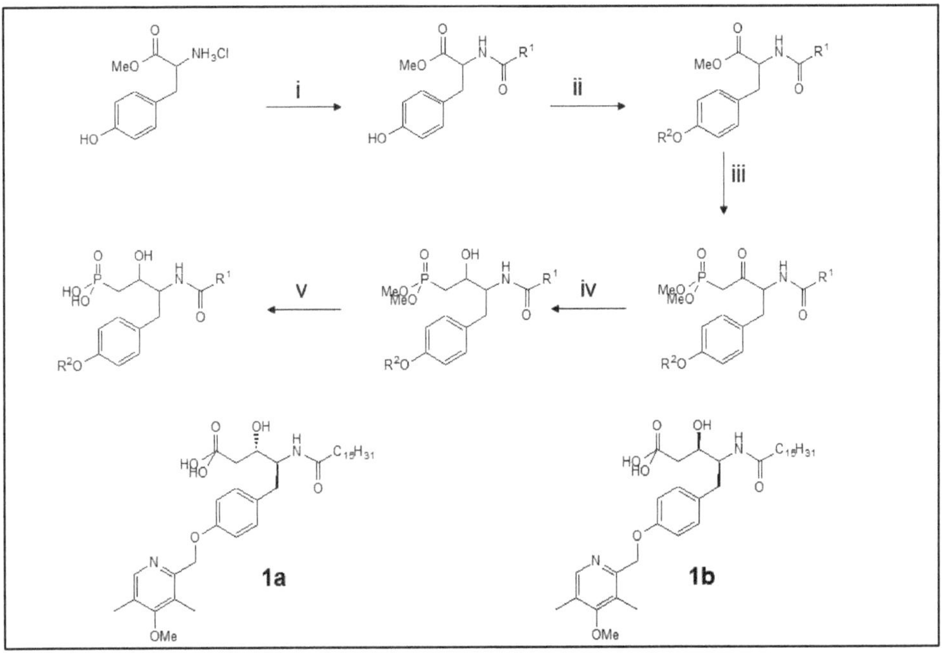

Fig. 3. Tyrosine based inhibitors of autotaxin. (i) Acid chloride, Et_3N, DCM, 0 °C, 3 h; (ii) Appropriate mesylate, K_2CO_3, 18-crown-6, acetone, reflux, overnight; (iii) *n*-BuLi, dimethyl methylphosphonate, -78 °C, 3 h; (iv) $NaBH_4$, THF, EtOH, 0 °C, 2 h; (v) TMSBr, pyridine, DCM, rt, 4 h, then H_2O/MeOH overnight.

A study by Ovaa and co-workers (Albers et al. 2010; Albers et al. 2010) on a collection of *ca.* 40,000 compounds has allowed the identification of a group of thiazolidinediones as autotaxin inhibitors. The general class of compound was prepared as outlined in Figure 4. From the initial screen, compound **2** was found to be the most active (IC_{50} = 56nM) and was selected for further optimization. Although structural variation at the benzylidene and benzyl groups did not lead to an increase in activity, the opportunity was taken to investigate pharmacophoric variation of the carboxylic acid substituent.

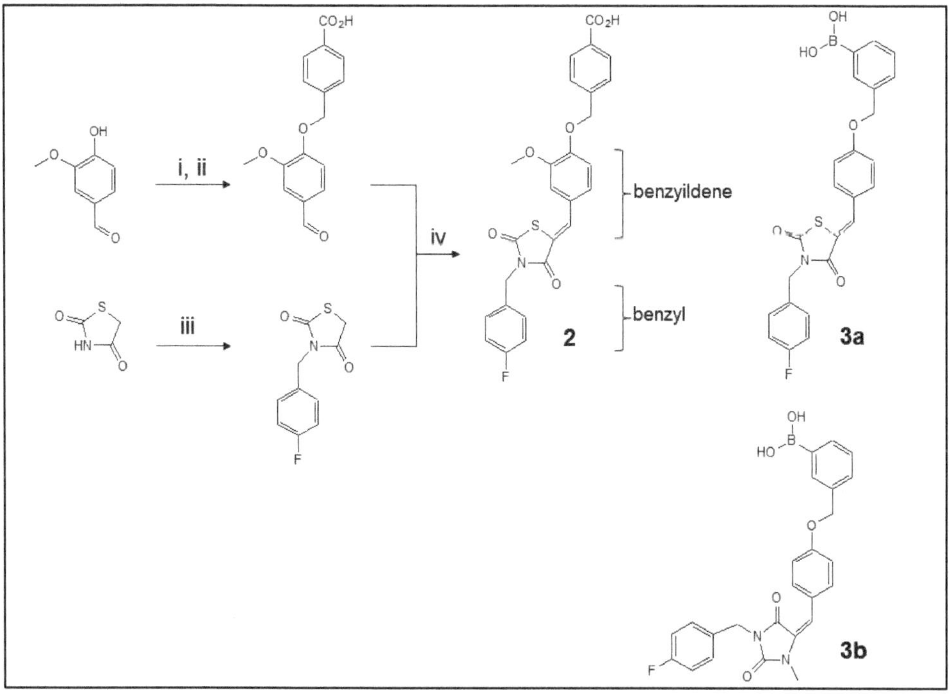

Fig. 4. (i) KOH, DMSO, appropriate benzyl bromide (as methyl ester), rt, 30 min; (ii) NaOH, DMSO/H_2O, reflux, 4 h, 91% yield; (iii) NaH, DMF, rt, appropriate benzyl chloride, 22 h, 74% yield; (iv) piperidine, EtOH, reflux, 20 h, 63% yield.

Replacing this group with a boronic acid moiety gave compound **3** that was found to be a potent inhibitor of autotaxin both *in vitro* and *in vivo* (IC_{50} = 6 nM). These results were rationalized on the basis that since the carboxylic acid group in **2** was expected to bind close to the active site threonine (Thr^{210}) in autotaxin, a boronic acid moiety might be expected to do the same. There was a precedent for this since the proteasome inhibitor bortezomib binds to a threonine oxygen nucleophile at the active site through a boronic acid group (Groll et al. 2006). The boronic acid-based thiazolidinediones showed greater affinity for autotaxin and are expected to show improved selectivity over other hydrolytic enzymes. The boronic acids such as **3** are expected to have the same binding site as the original lead **2**, but they show mixed-type inhibition rather than the competitive inhibition displayed by **2**. Ovaa has recently extended this work and has reported that the imidazolidine analogues such as **3b** show a similar level of activity to **3a** (Albers et al. 2011).

Virtual screening techniques have been used by Parrill, Baker and co-workers (Parrill et al. 2008; Hoeglund et al. 2010; Hoeglund et al. 2010; North et al. 2010). This has led to series of autotaxin inhibitors with pipemidic acid or pthalimide cores and related compounds (fig. 5). Of the pipemidic acid-based inhibitors (eg **4**, **5**, fig. 5), compound **4** (IC_{50} = 1.6 μM) was used as a lead to investigate the activity of a range of analogues with varying substitution on the pendent benzene ring. The synthetic approach was straightforward (fig. 6), starting with commercially available pipemidic acid and a range of substituted phenyl isothiocyanates to produce 30 compounds for evaluation. Themes to emerge were that *meta* substitution is preferred regardless of substituent, suggesting steric or conformational preferences rather than electronic effects are playing a role here. Within the *meta* class of compounds, inhibition was improved in the order: $\mathrm{OMe<F<Cl<I,<CF_3}$, reflecting neither size nor electronic trends. A single *meta*-trifluoromethyl group was preferred over two, and the singly substituted compound showed three times greater affinity for the enzyme than the original lead compound **4**. Of the compounds screened, compound **7** emerged as the most potent analogue in this study (IC_{50} = 0.9 μM; K_i = 0.7 μM), and showed competitive inhibition.

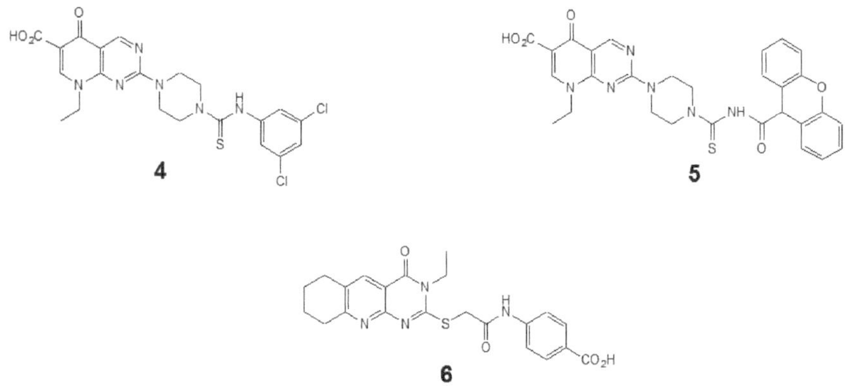

Fig. 5. Hits identified by virtual screening by Parrill and co-workers all of which inhibited autotaxin with IC_{50} ~ 2μM. Compounds **4** and **5** are pipemidic acid derivatives.

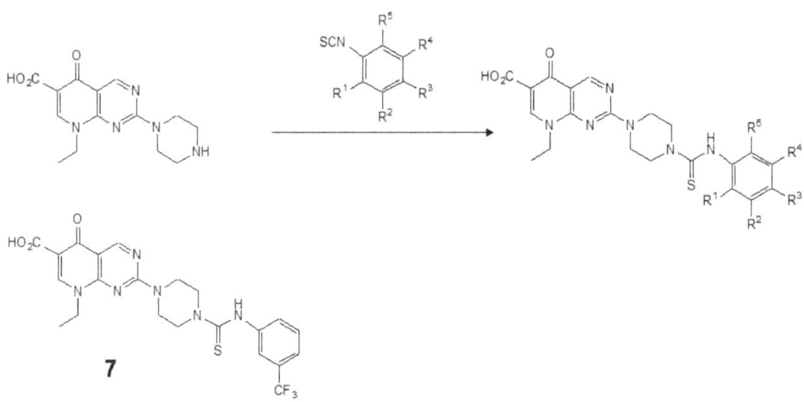

Fig. 6. Synthesis of autotaxin inhibitors basded on pipemidic acid. Compound 7 was the most potent analog reported (IC_{50} ~ 1 μM).

The phthalimide-derived small molecule lead inhibitors that were identified in the virtual screen by the Parrill and co-workers were also further evaluated including some dimeric examples, (Fig. 7) (Hoeglund et al. 2010). It is noticeable that these compounds contain terminal functionality that would be expected to contribute towards binding to zinc at the active site. Compounds **8** and **10** showed mixed-mode inhibition, whereas compound **9** showed competitive inhibition of autotaxin.

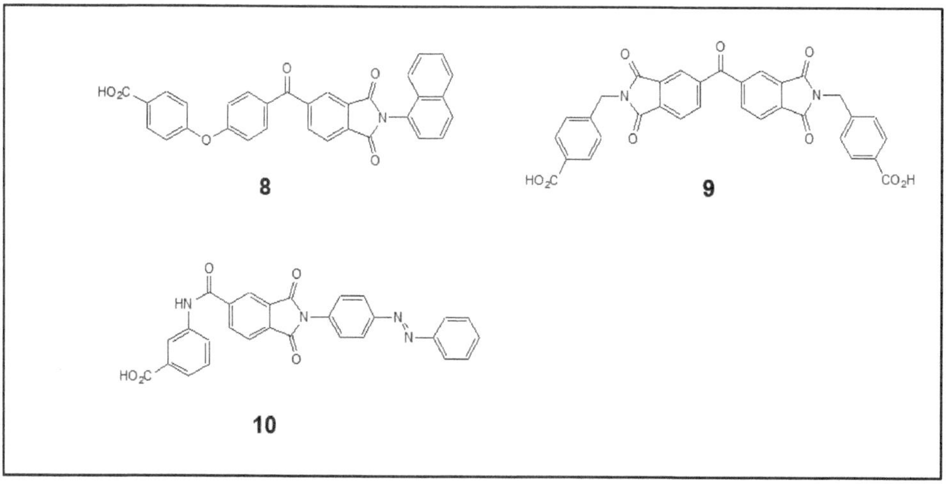

Fig. 7. Phthalimide-derived autotaxin inhibitors, all of which showed moderate potency (IC_{50} = 5 - 10μM) against autotaxin.

A recent report by Miller and Tigyi (Gupte et al. 2011) has built upon work carried out by Ferry and co-workers reporting that compound **11** (known as S32826, fig. 8; (Ferry et al. 2008)) possessed nanomolar activity as an autotaxin inhibitor. S32826 was inactive when evaluated using *in vivo* systems, and it has been presumed by Miller and Tigyi (Gupte et al. 2011) that this is due to the propensity for hydrolysis of the amide bond, making S32826 relatively unstable. In their own work Miller and Tigyi report a series of benzyl and naphthalene methyl phosphonic acid-derived compounds, of which **12** and **13** are most active, as inhibitors of autotaxin and that possess anti-invasive and anti-metastatic activity (Gupte et al. 2011). The synthetic approach to compound **12** (fig. 8) begins with a Heck coupling of the benzoic acid derivative to introduce the long alkyl side chain.

Compound **12** shows 94.8% inhibition of autotaxin and has an IC_{50} of 0.17 μM, with a K_i of 0.27 μM and displays a mixed mode of inhibition. In addition to inhibiting the invasion of MM1 hepatoma cells *in vitro* in a dose-dependent fashion, compound **13** significantly decreases lung metastasis of B16-F10 syngeneic mouse melanoma. Compound **12** has an average terminal half-life of 10 ± 5 hours and causes a long-lasting decrease in plasma LPA levels.

Prestwich has recently reported the synthesis of a hydroxylated S32826 analogue, (fig. 8, **14**), that retains acceptable levels of solubility (4mg/ml) whilst maintaining its potency as an inhibitor of autotaxin (K_i = 24.2 nM) and has potential for *in vivo* utility (Jiang et al. 2011). Compound **14** is currently undergoing further preclinical study.

Metabolically stable analogues of LPA, **15** and **16**, were designed by Prestwich and co-workers (Jiang et al. 2007). Compound **15** showed selective agonist activity for LPA_2, whereas **16** is a selective antagonist of LPA_4 and indeed is the first antagonist of this receptor to be reported. Compound **15** was found to be as effective as natural LPA as an inhibitor of autotaxin. Arguably the most interesting compound though, **16**, showed pan-antagonism of LPA GPCR's and was also active as an autotaxin inhibitor, thus having potential in anticancer and anti-metastasis models in cancer therapy (Zhang et al. 2009).

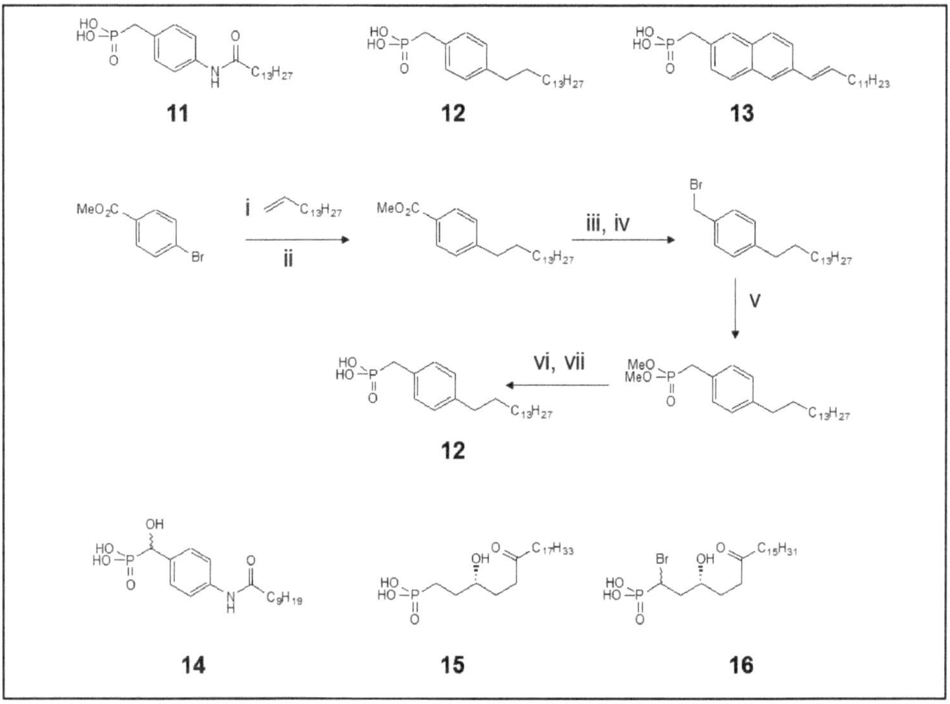

Fig. 8. (i) $Pd(OAc)_2$, Et_3N, DMF, reflux, 16 h; (ii) LAH, THF, 0 °C-rt, 4 h; (iii) H_2, Pd/C, MeOH, rt, 2 h; (iv) PBr_3, Et_2O, rt, 30 min; (v) $P(OMe)_3$, reflux, 18 h; (vi) TMSBr, CH_3CN, reflux, 1 h; (vii) MeOH, rt, 30 min.

6. Structure of autotaxin and molecular modelling to aid drug design

6.1 Autotaxin structure

The availability of data describing the structure of autotaxin is a superb tool to support drug discovery. Of the 8 protein crystal structures of autotaxin (*ENPP2*) that have thus far been described (Hausmann et al. 2011; Nishimasu et al. 2011) only one (2XRG.pdb; Table 1) has a small drug-like molecule bound in the active site. There are two unliganded structures. The others contain a range of phospholipids and LPA analogues with a variety of fatty chains and LPA analogues. The overall architecture of autotaxin is shown in figure 9. The N-terminus begins with a pair of somatomedin-B like (SMB) domains (residues 56-96 and 96-140) which lead into a phosphodiesterase domain (160-539) which contains a catalytic zinc binding site, a lasso loop (residues 539-590) and finally a nuclease domain (residues 539-862). It has also been suggested that a glycan chain located between the phosphodiesterase and nuclease domains is essential for correct folding of the protein. Strong bonding and electrostatic interactions are observed between the phosphodiesterase and the C-terminal region of the NUC domains including a disulphide cysteine bridge between residues 413 and 805 along with seven hydrogen bonds and nine salt bridges. This, combined with the extension of the Lasso loop from the PDE domain around the NUC domain, makes for a tight and well-ordered protein.

PDB CODE	Description	Reference
2XRG.pdb	Rat ATX with ligand	Hausmann et al
2XRN.pdb	Rat ATX no ligand	Hausmann et al
3NKM.pdb	Mouse ATX	Nishimasu et al
3NKN.pdb	Mouse ATX 14:0 LPA	Nishimasu et al
3NKO.pdb	Mouse ATX 16:0 LPA	Nishimasu et al
3NKP.pdb	Mouse ATX 18:1 LPA	Nishimasu et al
3NKQ.pdb	Mouse ATX 18:3 LPA	Nishimasu et al
3NKR.pdb	Mouse ATX 22:6 LPA	Nishimasu et al

Table 1. Structures of human autotaxin available in the Protein database. (www.pdb.org)

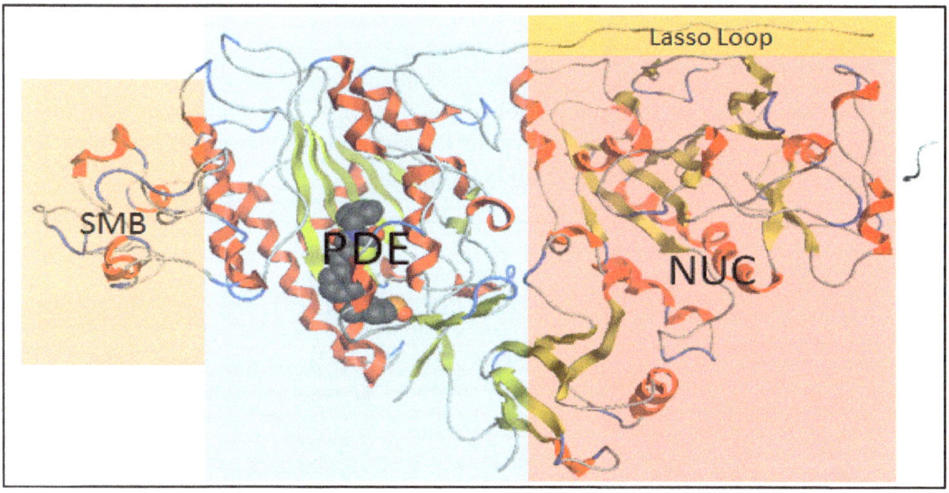

Fig. 9. The domain structure of autotaxin. The figure shows the location of the somatomedin domain (SMB), the phosphodiesterase domain (PDE) containing the catalytic site, the lasso loop and the nuclease domain (NUC).

The SMB domains are required for integrin binding and so may play a role in recruiting autotaxin to the cell surface where LPA receptors are located. A tunnel between one of the SMB domains and the ligand binding pocket has been suggested to facilitate delivery of LPA to cell surface receptors (Tabchy et al. 2011). The location of the tunnel compared to the catalytic site is shown in figure 10. Many lipophilic molecules are transported bound to protein carrier, such as albumin, so it seems reasonable that the tunnel fulfils a carrier role.

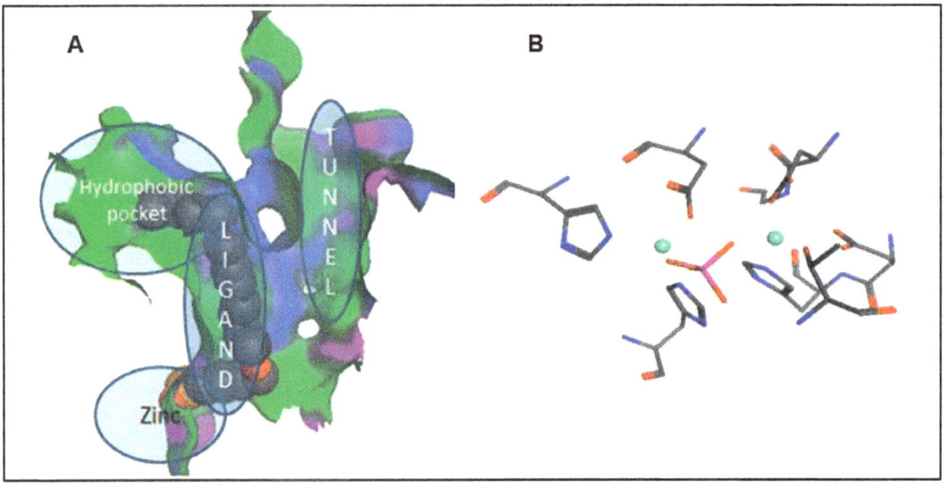

Fig. 10. **A**. A cut away diagram of the hydrophobic channel (right) adjacent to the ligand binding pocket. The main features of the binding site are highlighted with ovals. **B.** A close-up view of the local environment of catalytic zincs. The residues are coloured: grey, carbon; blue, nitrogen; red oxygen, light blue, zinc.

6.2 Ligand binding site

The overlay of several published X-ray structures of autotaxin shows a high conservation of ligand binding sites with only a few mobile residues. It is important to consider these as they may change the shape of the pocket or the electronic environment presented to the ligand and consequently affect ligand binding (fig 11).

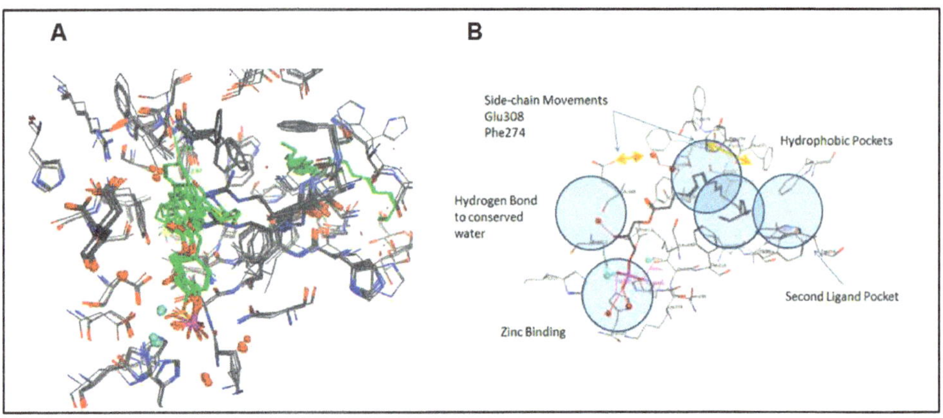

Fig. 11. **A**. The overlay of the active sites of 8 published protein structures of autotaxin. Residues whose positions have moved significantly between the structures are shown emboldened. Carbon atoms in LPA are shown in green whereas autotaxin carbon atoms are coloured grey; other atoms are coloured purple (phosphate), blue (nitrogen), red (oxygen) and light blue (zinc). **B.** An annotated view of the main features of the ligand binding site

The main features of the catalytic site are shown in figure 11. There are two di-cationic zinc atoms (fig 10 and fig. 11). The first is fully co-ordinated with a histidine, and threonine and two aspartate residues. The second zinc ion is co-ordinated by an aspartate and two histidine residues, leaving it available for co-ordination by a further negatively charged species such as phosphate or carboxylate.

Asn^{231} and Thr^{210} have been shown to be crucial for catalysis. These are located close to one zinc ions and provide a hydrogen bonding environment. Asn^{231} gives a preference for hydrogen bond acceptors while Thr^{210} provides an opportunity for irreversible (covalently bonded) ligands such as boronic acids to react. The conserved water that is held by hydrogen bonds between Asp^{311} and Glu^{308} can also play a role in control of ligand orientation and enantio-selectivity of ligand recognition.

The remainder of the site consists of a large hydrophobic pocket which has recognition features for the lipophilic chain of LPA. Within this pocket most of the side chains appear to be less mobile, although there are however three notable exceptions, Glu^{308}, Phe^{274} and Arg^{244}, some of which may help determine the potency with which ligands bind to autotaxin. Movement of Glu^{308} seems to displace a water molecule. Phe^{274} is mobile and unresolved in some structures but is shown to occupy various positions (fig. 12) in the hydrophobic pocket in others crystal structures in some cases moving to accommodate the ligand. We speculate that movement of this residue allows LPA to move from the active site into the hydrophobic tunnel. Arg^{244} is also mobile but its location adjacent to the solvent suggests that it may not be as important for ligand recognition.

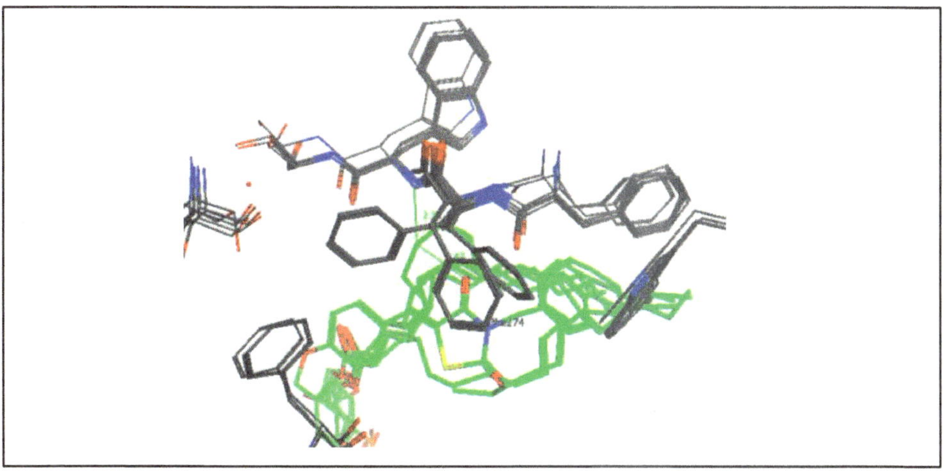

Fig. 12. This diagram shows the movement of side-chain Phe^{274} (grey, in centre of diagram) within the ligand binding site. The green shows the bound boronic acid inhibitor.

6.3 Docking methods

We have used the published crystal structures in an effort to understand the activity of several of the compounds described in section 5. In particular we evaluated whether the reported ligands were involved in zinc binding or whether they could occupy the hydrophobic pocket. Pharmacophoric overlay of autotaxin ligands has previously been reported to give a reasonable explanation of their relative binding modes by assuming that the ligands all make the same interactions within the autotaxin pocket (North et al. 2010). Here, however, we have used docking models of the catalytic zinc pocket to identify and compare the interactions of reported inhibitors. Ligands were placed within the binding pocket by aligning them with the pharmacophore map that had been overlaid onto the inhibitor bound in structure 2XRG. The steric requirements of the pocket were then used to refine our understanding of the activities of the ligands.

The pharmacophore map of the active site was constructed based on the binding of the boronic acid inhibitor HA155 (fig. 13). Docking to this map was performed using MOE software from the Chemical Computing Group. The placements of ligands were constrained to pharmacophoric points within the active site and refinement was performed with the MMFF94x force field (Halgren 1996).

The docking model faithfully reproduced the position of the ligand from 2xrg.pdb and its close analogues. This gives us confidence in the docking models used. While the pharmacophore map suggests a rich hydrogen bonding network around the ligand, most of the "linker" region of the ligands fail to interact with the pocket other than with a few hydrophobic contacts. The conserved nature of the ligands' hydrogen bonding motif, as can be seen from previous pharmacophore modelling efforts (North et al. 2010), suggests that there may be unresolved water atoms which are located in the site (large blue spheres in fig. 13).

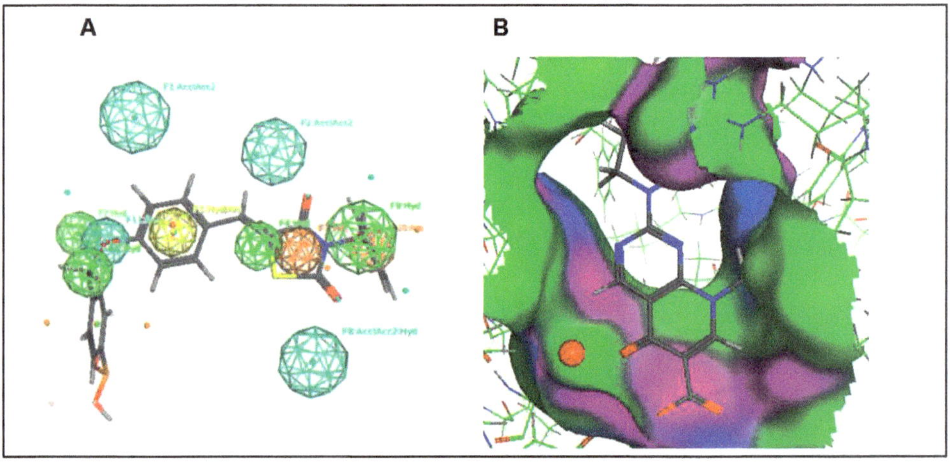

Fig. 13. **A** Pharmacophoric map and shape of ligand from 2XRG.pdb which takes into account the steric and electronic requirements of the pocket when placing the ligand. (Blue Mesh= hydrogen bond acceptor projected points, Green Mesh=Hydrophobic areas, Brown/yellow Mesh=Aromatic centers) B. The zinc binding portion of molecule **5** after docking to the pharmacophore map in the binding site.

The best fit to the zinc pocket was obtained for the carboxylic acid group from molecules **4** and **5** which appear to satisfy all the steric and electronic requirements of the local pocket (Fig below) When the hydrophobic tail of the docked molecules is prevented from occupying the ligand binding pocket because of a lack of ligand flexibility, it is often placed by the docking software in the tunnel region of the protein. This may be influenced by Phe^{274} which may act as a switch closing one or the other of these sites. Stabilization of this residue may contribute to ligand affinity.

Ligands which bind with high affinity interacted with both the zinc ion and also occupied the hydrophobic pocket e.g. with a benzyl group. In contrast, ligands which bind with low affinity failed to bridge the zinc ion and the hydrophobic portion of the ligand binding site. This leads us to conclude that for ligands to bind with high affinity, they should preferably bind both these sites. Docking studies also suggest that the hydrophobic tunnel provides an alternative location for ligands but these ligands identified so far fail to achieve better than micromolar activities. These observations may be used to design improved autotaxin inhibitors.

7. Potential clinical uses of autotaxin inhibitors

Once inhibitors of autotaxin complete preclinical evaluation, how could these be evaluated in clinical trials? As we have discussed above, autotaxin may not be the only enzyme that contributes to the formation of LPA in ovarian cancer and so it is possible that inhibition of autotaxin may not elicit the desired therapeutic effect. It will be important, therefore, to include in early clinical trials a measurement of the change in LPA in ascites following treatment with an autotaxin inhibitor and to establish biomarkers (e.g. measurement of autotaxin in ascites fluid) to stratify the patients which are likely to respond.

The data we have reviewed also suggests a number of different settings in which autotaxin inhibitors could be used. Autotaxin inhibitors may be useful to inhibit the growth of primary tumors or to inhibit tumor cell migration, invasion and metastases. Clinical trials to evaluate these may differ somewhat, for example using different surrogate endpoints (tumor shrinkage versus decreased metastasis). Different schedules of drug administration may also be appropriate. To cause tumor cell death, relatively short term treatment with the drug may suffice, but suppression of metastasis may require prolonged treatment. This highlights the importance of considering the therapeutic goal that is being evaluated with an autotaxin inhibitor at the outset.

As we have discussed, there is a large body of evidence indicating a role for LPA in cancer cell migration and invasion. In addition, several studies demonstrate in animal models of metastasis that inhibitors of autotaxin reduce colonization of the lung by tumors cells (Baker et al. 2006; Gupte et al. 2010; Gupte et al. 2011). Thus, one potential clinical use of autotaxin inhibitors is to inhibit metastasis. Unfortunately, many ovarian cancer patients present with advanced disease, and significant dissemination of the tumor within the peritoneal cavity has already taken place by the time of diagnosis. Although it may be beneficial to prevent further metastasis and progression to later stage disease, there may also be micro-metastases that are not evident on examination. It is not clear, then, whether inhibiting further metastasis would be helpful. Evaluation of autotaxin inhibitors as anti-metastatic agents in patients with early stage disease will also be challenging. Relatively few patients are diagnosed with early stage disease and these patients generally have a good prognosis, with 90% of patients surviving more than 5 years. A large cohort of patients may also be required to ensure sufficient patients are evaluated who lack pre-existing micro-metastases but who will progress to more advanced disease. The cost of such a large and long trial may be prohibitive unless an alternative is found.

We have also reviewed the substantial evidence linking LPA and autotaxin to cell survival. Autotaxin inhibitors may have an indirect cytotoxic effect or inhibit the growth of primary (and secondary) tumors. This might reflect deprivation of LPA directly causing apoptosis of the tumor cells, or it might reflect a less supportive microenvironment. In support of this approach, BrP-LPA (Bromophosfono-lysophosphatidic acid; **16**, fig. 8) causes regression of breast tumor cells both in 3D *in vitro* models (Xu and Prestwich 2010) and as a xenograft (Zhang et al. 2009), although as the authors clearly state, this drug is also a pan LPA receptor antagonist and its activity cannot be ascribed to inhibition of autotaxin alone. Also, over-expression of autotaxin is sufficient to induce breast cancer, suggesting that selective inhibition of autotaxin may be sufficient to cause regression of comparable tumor types. An alternative to using an autotaxin inhibitor as a single agent is to use it in combination with chemotherapy and this is supported by the data implicating autotaxin and LPA in chemoresistance that we have discussed. Clearly this strategy has potential in patients who have developed chemoresistant disease, but it may also be useful to increase the response in patients whose tumors are sensitive to chemotherapy.

A pragmatic solution may be to evaluate autotaxin inhibitors first for their ability to inhibit tumor growth (either as a single agent or in combination with chemotherapy) and if this is successful evaluate their use as anti-metastatic agents after drug receives marketing approval. This may mitigate some of the risk associated with following a purely anti-metastatic approach to drug development.

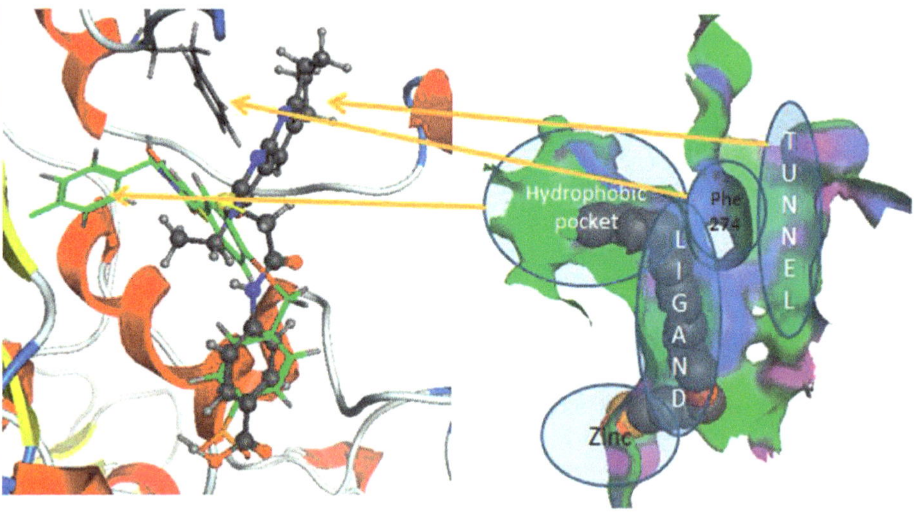

Fig. 14. The hydrophobic "tail" in ligands may occupy the hydrophobic pocket or the hydrophobic tunnel and Phe^{274} divides the two hydrophobic ligand binding sites.

8. Conclusion

Our understanding of autotaxin, in terms of it biological function, its structure and its potential as a drug target in ovarian cancer is rapidly evolving. Several compounds are currently undergoing preclinical discovery, and it cannot be long before the first of these enter clinic trials. In this review, we have focused on the role of autotaxin in ovarian cancer, but it also plays a role in other cancer types as well as other pathophysiological conditions such as neuropathic pain. It seems plausible that autotaxin inhibitors will serve as new medicines and perhaps none of these applications is as exciting as the potential to treat drug-resistant ovarian cancer, a disease for which therapeutic options are currently limited.

9. References

Albers, H. M., A. Dong, L. A. van Meeteren, D. A. Egan, M. Sunkara, E. W. van Tilburg, K. Schuurman, O. van Tellingen, A. J. Morris, S. S. Smyth, W. H. Moolenaar & H. Ovaa (2010). Boronic acid-based inhibitor of autotaxin reveals rapid turnover of LPA in the circulation. *Proc Natl Acad Sci U S A* vol. 107(16) pp. 7257-7262

Albers, H. M., L. J. Hendrickx, R. J. van Tol, J. Hausmann, A. Perrakis & H. Ovaa (2011). Structure-based design of novel boronic Acid-based inhibitors of autotaxin. *J Med Chem* vol. 54(13) pp. 4619-4626

Albers, H. M., L. A. van Meeteren, D. A. Egan, E. W. van Tilburg, W. H. Moolenaar & H. Ovaa (2010). Discovery and optimization of boronic acid based inhibitors of autotaxin. *J Med Chem* vol. 53(13) pp. 4958-4967

Baker, D. L., Y. Fujiwara, K. R. Pigg, R. Tsukahara, S. Kobayashi, H. Murofushi, A. Uchiyama, K. Murakami-Murofushi, E. Koh, R. W. Bandle, H. S. Byun, R. Bittman, D. Fan, M. Murph, G. B. Mills & G. Tigyi (2006). Carba analogs of cyclic phosphatidic acid are selective inhibitors of autotaxin and cancer cell invasion and metastasis. *J Biol Chem* vol. 281(32) pp. 22786-22793

Barkinge, J. L., R. Gudi, H. Sarah, F. Chu, A. Borthakur, B. S. Prabhakar & K. V. Prasad (2009). The p53-induced Siva-1 plays a significant role in cisplatin-mediated apoptosis. *J Carcinog* vol. 8 pp. 2

Baudhuin, L. M., K. L. Cristina, J. Lu & Y. Xu (2002). Akt activation induced by lysophosphatidic acid and sphingosine-1-phosphate requires both mitogen-activated protein kinase kinase and p38 mitogen-activated protein kinase and is cell-line specific. *Mol Pharmacol* vol. 62(3) pp. 660-671

Bermudez, Y., H. Yang, B. O. Saunders, J. Q. Cheng, S. V. Nicosia & P. A. Kruk (2007). VEGF- and LPA-induced telomerase in human ovarian cancer cells is Sp1-dependent. *Gynecol Oncol* vol. 106(3) pp. 526-537

Bese, T., M. Barbaros, E. Baykara, O. Guralp, S. Cengiz, F. Demirkiran, C. Sanioglu & M. Arvas (2010). Comparison of total plasma lysophosphatidic acid and serum CA-125 as a tumor marker in the diagnosis and follow-up of patients with epithelial ovarian cancer. *J Gynecol Oncol* vol. 21(4) pp. 248-254

Bian, D., C. Mahanivong, J. Yu, S. M. Frisch, Z. K. Pan, R. D. Ye & S. Huang (2006). The G12/13-RhoA signaling pathway contributes to efficient lysophosphatidic acid-stimulated cell migration. *Oncogene* vol. 25(15) pp. 2234-2244

Bian, D., S. Su, C. Mahanivong, R. K. Cheng, Q. Han, Z. K. Pan, P. Sun & S. Huang (2004). Lysophosphatidic Acid Stimulates Ovarian Cancer Cell Migration via a Ras-MEK Kinase 1 Pathway. *Cancer Res* vol. 64(12) pp. 4209-4217

Boucharaba, A., C. M. Serre, S. Gres, J. S. Saulnier-Blache, J. C. Bordet, J. Guglielmi, P. Clezardin & O. Peyruchaud (2004). Platelet-derived lysophosphatidic acid supports the progression of osteolytic bone metastases in breast cancer. *J Clin Invest* vol. 114(12) pp. 1714-1725

Chen, M. & K. L. O'Connor (2005). Integrin alpha6beta4 promotes expression of autotaxin/ENPP2 autocrine motility factor in breast carcinoma cells. *Oncogene* vol. 24(32) pp. 5125-5130

Chu, F., A. Borthakur, X. Sun, J. Barkinge, R. Gudi, S. Hawkins & K. V. Prasad (2004). The Siva-1 putative amphipathic helical region (SAH) is sufficient to bind to BCL-XL and sensitize cells to UV radiation induced apoptosis. *Apoptosis* vol. 9(1) pp. 83-95

Cui, P., W. F. McCalmont, J. L. Tomsig, K. R. Lynch & T. L. Macdonald (2008). alpha- and beta-substituted phosphonate analogs of LPA as autotaxin inhibitors. *Bioorg Med Chem* vol. 16(5) pp. 2212-2225

Cui, P., J. L. Tomsig, W. F. McCalmont, S. Lee, C. J. Becker, K. R. Lynch & T. L. Macdonald (2007). Synthesis and biological evaluation of phosphonate derivatives as autotaxin (ATX) inhibitors. *Bioorg Med Chem Lett* vol. 17(6) pp. 1634-1640

David, M., E. Wannecq, F. Descotes, S. Jansen, B. Deux, J. Ribeiro, C. M. Serre, S. Gres, N. Bendriss-Vermare, M. Bollen, S. Saez, J. Aoki, J. S. Saulnier-Blache, P. Clezardin & O. Peyruchaud (2010). Cancer cell expression of autotaxin controls bone metastasis formation in mouse through lysophosphatidic acid-dependent activation of osteoclasts. *PLoS One* vol. 5(3) pp. e9741

Davidson, B., R. Hadar, H. T. Stavnes, C. G. Trope & R. Reich (2009). Expression of the peroxisome proliferator-activated receptors-alpha, -beta, and -gamma in ovarian carcinoma effusions is associated with poor chemoresponse and shorter survival. *Hum Pathol* vol. 40(5) pp. 705-713

Deng, W., E. Shuyu, R. Tsukahara, W. J. Valentine, G. Durgam, V. Gududuru, L. Balazs, V. Manickam, M. Arsura, L. VanMiddlesworth, L. R. Johnson, A. L. Parrill, D. D. Miller & G. Tigyi (2007). The lysophosphatidic acid type 2 receptor is required for protection against radiation-induced intestinal injury. *Gastroenterology* vol. 132(5) pp. 1834-1851

Do, T. V., J. C. Symowicz, D. M. Berman, L. A. Liotta, E. F. Petricoin, 3rd, M. S. Stack & D. A. Fishman (2007). Lysophosphatidic acid down-regulates stress fibers and up-regulates pro-matrix metalloproteinase-2 activation in ovarian cancer cells. *Mol Cancer Res* vol. 5(2) pp. 121-131

E, S., Y. J. Lai, R. Tsukahara, C. S. Chen, Y. Fujiwara, J. Yue, J. H. Yu, H. Guo, A. Kihara, G. Tigyi & F. T. Lin (2009). Lysophosphatidic acid 2 receptor-mediated supramolecular complex formation regulates its antiapoptotic effect. *J Biol Chem* vol. 284(21) pp. 14558-14571

East, J. E., A. J. Kennedy, J. L. Tomsig, A. R. De Leon, K. R. Lynch & T. L. Macdonald (2010). Synthesis and structure-activity relationships of tyrosine-based inhibitors of autotaxin (ATX). *Bioorg Med Chem Lett* vol. 20(23) pp. 7132-7136

Fang, X., M. Schummer, M. Mao, S. Yu, F. H. Tabassam, R. Swaby, Y. Hasegawa, J. L. Tanyi, R. LaPushin, A. Eder, R. Jaffe, J. Erickson & G. B. Mills (2002). Lysophosphatidic acid is a bioactive mediator in ovarian cancer. *Biochim Biophys Acta* vol. 1582(1-3) pp. 257-264

Ferry, G., N. Moulharat, J. P. Pradere, P. Desos, A. Try, A. Genton, A. Giganti, M. Beucher-Gaudin, M. Lonchampt, M. Bertrand, J. S. Saulnier-Blache, G. C. Tucker, A. Cordi & J. A. Boutin (2008). S32826, a nanomolar inhibitor of autotaxin: discovery, synthesis and applications as a pharmacological tool. *J Pharmacol Exp Ther* vol. 327(3) pp. 809-819

Fishman, D. A., Y. Liu, S. M. Ellerbroek & M. S. Stack (2001). Lysophosphatidic acid promotes matrix metalloproteinase (MMP) activation and MMP-dependent invasion in ovarian cancer cells. *Cancer Res* vol. 61(7) pp. 3194 3199

Frankel, A. & G. B. Mills (1996). Peptide and lipid growth factors decrease cis-diamminedichloroplatinum-induced cell death in human ovarian cancer cells. *Clin Cancer Res* vol. 2(8) pp. 1307-1313

Furui, T., R. LaPushin, M. Mao, H. Khan, S. R. Watt, M. A. Watt, Y. Lu, X. Fang, S. Tsutsui, Z. H. Siddik, R. C. Bast & G. B. Mills (1999). Overexpression of edg-2/vzg-1 induces apoptosis and anoikis in ovarian cancer cells in a lysophosphatidic acid-independent manner. *Clin Cancer Res* vol. 5(12) pp. 4308-4318

Gaetano, C. G., N. Samadi, J. L. Tomsig, T. L. Macdonald, K. R. Lynch & D. N. Brindley (2009). Inhibition of autotaxin production or activity blocks lysophosphatidylcholine-induced migration of human breast cancer and melanoma cells. *Mol Carcinog* vol. 48(9) pp. 801-809

Girnun, G. D., E. Naseri, S. B. Vafai, L. Qu, J. D. Szwaya, R. Bronson, J. A. Alberta & B. M. Spiegelman (2007). Synergy between PPARgamma ligands and platinum-based drugs in cancer. *Cancer Cell* vol. 11(5) pp. 395-406

Groll, M., C. R. Berkers, H. L. Ploegh & H. Ovaa (2006). Crystal structure of the boronic acid-based proteasome inhibitor bortezomib in complex with the yeast 20S proteasome. *Structure* vol. 14(3) pp. 451-456

Gupte, R., R. Patil, J. Liu, Y. Wang, S. C. Lee, Y. Fujiwara, J. Fells, A. L. Bolen, K. Emmons-Thompson, C. R. Yates, A. Siddam, N. Panupinthu, T. C. Pham, D. L. Baker, A. L. Parrill, G. B. Mills, G. Tigyi & D. D. Miller (2011). Benzyl and naphthalene methylphosphonic acid inhibitors of autotaxin with anti-invasive and anti-metastatic activity. *ChemMedChem* vol. 6(5) pp. 922-935

Gupte, R., A. Siddam, Y. Lu, W. Li, Y. Fujiwara, N. Panupinthu, T. C. Pham, D. L. Baker, A. L. Parrill, M. Gotoh, K. Murakami-Murofushi, S. Kobayashi, G. B. Mills, G. Tigyi & D. D. Miller (2010). Synthesis and pharmacological evaluation of the stereoisomers of 3-carba cyclic-phosphatidic acid. *Bioorg Med Chem Lett* vol. 20(24) pp. 7525-7528

Haga, A., H. Nagai & Y. Deyashiki (2009). Autotaxin promotes the expression of matrix metalloproteinase-3 via activation of the MAPK cascade in human fibrosarcoma HT-1080 cells. *Cancer Invest* vol. 27(4) pp. 384-390

Halgren, T. A. (1996). Merck molecular force field .1. Basis, form, scope, parameterization, and performance of MMFF94. *Journal of Computational Chemistry* vol. 17(5-6) pp. 490-519

Harper, K., D. Arsenault, S. Boulay-Jean, A. Lauzier, F. Lucien & C. M. Dubois (2010). Autotaxin promotes cancer invasion via the lysophosphatidic acid receptor 4: participation of the cyclic AMP/EPAC/Rac1 signaling pathway in invadopodia formation. *Cancer Res* vol. 70(11) pp. 4634-4643

Hausmann, J., S. Kamtekar, E. Christodoulou, J. E. Day, T. Wu, Z. Fulkerson, H. M. Albers, L. A. van Meeteren, A. J. Houben, L. van Zeijl, S. Jansen, M. Andries, T. Hall, L. E. Pegg, T. E. Benson, M. Kasiem, K. Harlos, C. W. Kooi, S. S. Smyth, H. Ovaa, M. Bollen, A. J. Morris, W. H. Moolenaar & A. Perrakis (2011). Structural basis of substrate discrimination and integrin binding by autotaxin. *Nat Struct Mol Biol* vol. 18(2) pp. 198-204

Hoeglund, A. B., H. E. Bostic, A. L. Howard, I. W. Wanjala, M. D. Best, D. L. Baker & A. L. Parrill (2010). Optimization of a pipemidic acid autotaxin inhibitor. *J Med Chem* vol. 53(3) pp. 1056-1066

Hoeglund, A. B., A. L. Howard, I. W. Wanjala, T. C. Pham, A. L. Parrill & D. L. Baker (2010). Characterization of non-lipid autotaxin inhibitors. *Bioorg Med Chem* vol. 18(2) pp. 769-776

Hoelzinger, D. B., L. Mariani, J. Weis, T. Woyke, T. J. Berens, W. S. McDonough, A. Sloan, S. W. Coons & M. E. Berens (2005). Gene expression profile of glioblastoma multiforme invasive phenotype points to new therapeutic targets. *Neoplasia* vol. 7(1) pp. 7-16

Hoelzinger, D. B., M. Nakada, T. Demuth, T. Rosensteel, L. B. Reavie & M. E. Berens (2008). Autotaxin: a secreted autocrine/paracrine factor that promotes glioma invasion. *J Neurooncol* vol. 86(3) pp. 297-309

Hooks, S. B., P. Callihan, M. K. Altman, J. H. Hurst, M. W. Ali & M. M. Murph (2010). Regulators of G-Protein signaling RGS10 and RGS17 regulate chemoresistance in ovarian cancer cells. *Mol Cancer* vol. 9 pp. 289

Hu, Y. L., C. Albanese, R. G. Pestell & R. B. Jaffe (2003). Dual mechanisms for lysophosphatidic acid stimulation of human ovarian carcinoma cells. *J Natl Cancer Inst* vol. 95(10) pp. 733-740

Hu, Y. L., M. K. Tee, E. J. Goetzl, N. Auersperg, G. B. Mills, N. Ferrara & R. B. Jaffe (2001). Lysophosphatidic acid induction of vascular endothelial growth factor expression in human ovarian cancer cells. *J Natl Cancer Inst* vol. 93(10) pp. 762-768

Huang, R. Y., S. M. Wang, C. Y. Hsieh & J. C. Wu (2008). Lysophosphatidic acid induces ovarian cancer cell dispersal by activating Fyn kinase associated with p120-catenin. *Int J Cancer* vol. 123(4) pp. 801-809

Hurst, J. H., P. A. Henkel, A. L. Brown & S. B. Hooks (2008). Endogenous RGS proteins attenuate Galpha(i)-mediated lysophosphatidic acid signaling pathways in ovarian cancer cells. *Cell Signal* vol. 20(2) pp. 381-389

Hurst, J. H. & S. B. Hooks (2009). Lysophosphatidic acid stimulates cell growth by different mechanisms in SKOV-3 and Caov-3 ovarian cancer cells: distinct roles for Gi- and Rho-dependent pathways. *Pharmacology* vol. 83(6) pp. 333-347

Jazaeri, A. A., C. S. Awtrey, G. V. Chandramouli, Y. E. Chuang, J. Khan, C. Sotiriou, O. Aprelikova, C. J. Yee, K. K. Zorn, M. J. Birrer, J. C. Barrett & J. Boyd (2005). Gene expression profiles associated with response to chemotherapy in epithelial ovarian cancers. *Clin Cancer Res* vol. 11(17) pp. 6300-6310

Jeon, E. S., S. C. Heo, I. H. Lee, Y. J. Choi, J. H. Park, K. U. Choi, Y. Park do, D. S. Suh, M. S. Yoon & J. H. Kim (2010). Ovarian cancer-derived lysophosphatidic acid stimulates secretion of VEGF and stromal cell-derived factor-1 alpha from human mesenchymal stem cells. *Exp Mol Med* vol. 42(4) pp. 280-293

Jiang, G., D. Madan & G. D. Prestwich (2011). Aromatic phosphonates inhibit the lysophospholipase D activity of autotaxin. *Bioorg Med Chem Lett*

Jiang, G., Y. Xu, Y. Fujiwara, T. Tsukahara, R. Tsukahara, J. Gajewiak, G. Tigyi & G. D. Prestwich (2007). Alpha-substituted phosphonate analogues of lysophosphatidic acid (LPA) selectively inhibit production and action of LPA. *ChemMedChem* vol. 2(5) pp. 679-690

Jung, I. D., J. Lee, S. Y. Yun, C. G. Park, W. S. Choi, H. W. Lee, O. H. Choi, J. W. Han & H. Y. Lee (2002). Cdc42 and Rac1 are necessary for autotaxin-induced tumor cell motility in A2058 melanoma cells. *FEBS Lett* vol. 532(3) pp. 351-356

Kamrava, M., F. Simpkins, E. Alejandro, C. Michener, E. Meltzer & E. C. Kohn (2005). Lysophosphatidic acid and endothelin-induced proliferation of ovarian cancer cell lines is mitigated by neutralization of granulin-epithelin precursor (GEP), a prosurvival factor for ovarian cancer. *Oncogene* vol. 24(47) pp. 7084-7093

Kang, Y. C., K. M. Kim, K. S. Lee, S. Namkoong, S. J. Lee, J. A. Han, D. Jeoung, K. S. Ha, Y. G. Kwon & Y. M. Kim (2004). Serum bioactive lysophospholipids prevent TRAIL-induced apoptosis via PI3K/Akt-dependent cFLIP expression and Bad phosphorylation. *Cell Death Differ* vol. 11(12) pp. 1287-1298

Kehlen, A., N. Englert, A. Seifert, T. Klonisch, H. Dralle, J. Langner & C. Hoang-Vu (2004). Expression, regulation and function of autotaxin in thyroid carcinomas. *Int J Cancer* vol. 109(6) pp. 833-838

Kim, E. K., J. M. Park, S. Lim, J. W. Choi, H. S. Kim, H. Seok, J. K. Seo, K. Oh, D. S. Lee, K. T. Kim, S. H. Ryu & P. G. Suh (2011). Activation of AMP-activated Protein Kinase Is Essential for Lysophosphatidic Acid-induced Cell Migration in Ovarian Cancer Cells. *J Biol Chem* vol. 286(27) pp. 24036-24045

Kishi, Y., S. Okudaira, M. Tanaka, K. Hama, D. Shida, J. Kitayama, T. Yamori, J. Aoki, T. Fujimaki & H. Arai (2006). Autotaxin is overexpressed in glioblastoma multiforme and contributes to cell motility of glioblastoma by converting lysophosphatidylcholine to lysophosphatidic acid. *J Biol Chem* vol. 281(25) pp. 17492-17500

Kortlever, R. M., T. R. Brummelkamp, L. A. van Meeteren, W. H. Moolenaar & R. Bernards (2008). Suppression of the p53-dependent replicative senescence response by lysophosphatidic acid signaling. *Mol Cancer Res* vol. 6(9) pp. 1452-1460

Lee, J., I. Duk Jung, C. Gyo Park, J. W. Han & H. Young Lee (2006). Autotaxin stimulates urokinase-type plasminogen activator expression through phosphoinositide 3-kinase-Akt-nuclear [corrected] factor kappa B signaling cascade in human melanoma cells. *Melanoma Res* vol. 16(5) pp. 445-452

Lee, Z., R. F. Swaby, Y. Liang, S. Yu, S. Liu, K. H. Lu, R. C. Bast, Jr., G. B. Mills & X. Fang (2006). Lysophosphatidic acid is a major regulator of growth-regulated oncogene alpha in ovarian cancer. *Cancer Res* vol. 66(5) pp. 2740-2748

Li, H., X. Ye, C. Mahanivong, D. Bian, J. Chun & S. Huang (2005). Signaling mechanisms responsible for lysophosphatidic acid-induced urokinase plasminogen activator expression in ovarian cancer cells. *J Biol Chem* vol. 280(11) pp. 10564-10571

Li, H., Z. Zhao, G. Wei, L. Yan, D. Wang, H. Zhang, G. E. Sandusky, J. Turk & Y. Xu (2010). Group VIA phospholipase A2 in both host and tumor cells is involved in ovarian cancer development. *FASEB J* vol. 24(10) pp. 4103-4116

Li, S., B. Wang, Y. Xu & J. Zhang (2011). Autotaxin is induced by TSA through HDAC3 and HDAC7 inhibition and antagonizes the TSA-induced cell apoptosis. *Mol Cancer* vol. 10 pp. 18

Lin, F. T., Y. J. Lai, N. Makarova, G. Tigyi & W. C. Lin (2007). The lysophosphatidic acid 2 receptor mediates down-regulation of Siva-1 to promote cell survival. *J Biol Chem* vol. 282(52) pp. 37759-37769

Liu, S., M. Umezu-Goto, M. Murph, Y. Lu, W. Liu, F. Zhang, S. Yu, L. C. Stephens, X. Cui, G. Murrow, K. Coombes, W. Muller, M. C. Hung, C. M. Perou, A. V. Lee, X. Fang & G. B. Mills (2009). Expression of autotaxin and lysophosphatidic acid receptors increases mammary tumorigenesis, invasion, and metastases. *Cancer Cell* vol. 15(6) pp. 539-550

Masuda, A., K. Nakamura, K. Izutsu, K. Igarashi, R. Ohkawa, M. Jona, K. Higashi, H. Yokota, S. Okudaira, T. Kishimoto, T. Watanabe, Y. Koike, H. Ikeda, Y. Kozai, M. Kurokawa, J. Aoki & Y. Yatomi (2008). Serum autotaxin measurement in haematological malignancies: a promising marker for follicular lymphoma. *Br J Haematol* vol. 143(1) pp. 60-70

Meng, Y., L. Graves, T. V. Do, J. So & D. A. Fishman (2004). Upregulation of FasL by LPA on ovarian cancer cell surface leads to apoptosis of activated lymphocytes. *Gynecol Oncol* vol. 95(3) pp. 488-495

Meng, Y., S. Kang & D. A. Fishman (2005). Lysophosphatidic acid stimulates fas ligand microvesicle release from ovarian cancer cells. *Cancer Immunol Immunother* vol. 54(8) pp. 807-814

Meng, Y., S. Kang, J. So, S. Reierstad & D. A. Fishman (2005). Translocation of Fas by LPA prevents ovarian cancer cells from anti-Fas-induced apoptosis. *Gynecol Oncol* vol. 96(2) pp. 462-469

Mills, G. B., C. May, M. Hill, S. Campbell, P. Shaw & A. Marks (1990). Ascitic fluid from human ovarian cancer patients contains growth factors necessary for intraperitoneal growth of human ovarian adenocarcinoma cells. *J Clin Invest* vol. 86(3) pp. 851-855

Murph, M. M., G. H. Nguyen, H. Radhakrishna & G. B. Mills (2008). Sharpening the edges of understanding the structure/function of the LPA1 receptor: expression in cancer and mechanisms of regulation. *Biochim Biophys Acta* vol. 1781(9) pp. 547-557

Nakai, Y., H. Ikeda, K. Nakamura, Y. Kume, M. Fujishiro, N. Sasahira, K. Hirano, H. Isayama, M. Tada, T. Kawabe, Y. Komatsu, M. Omata, J. Aoki, K. Koike & Y. Yatomi (2011). Specific increase in serum autotaxin activity in patients with pancreatic cancer. *Clin Biochem* vol. 44(8-9) pp. 576-581

Nam, S. W., T. Clair, C. K. Campo, H. Y. Lee, L. A. Liotta & M. L. Stracke (2000). Autotaxin (ATX), a potent tumor motogen, augments invasive and metastatic potential of ras-transformed cells. *Oncogene* vol. 19(2) pp. 241-247

Nishimasu, H., S. Okudaira, K. Hama, E. Mihara, N. Dohmae, A. Inoue, R. Ishitani, J. Takagi, J. Aoki & O. Nureki (2011). Crystal structure of autotaxin and insight into GPCR activation by lipid mediators. *Nat Struct Mol Biol* vol. 18(2) pp. 205-212

North, E. J., A. L. Howard, I. W. Wanjala, T. C. Pham, D. L. Baker & A. L. Parrill (2010). Pharmacophore development and application toward the identification of novel, small-molecule autotaxin inhibitors. *J Med Chem* vol. 53(8) pp. 3095-3105

Nouh, M. A., X. X. Wu, H. Okazoe, H. Tsunemori, R. Haba, A. M. Abou-Zeid, M. D. Saleem, M. Inui, M. Sugimoto, J. Aoki & Y. Kakehi (2009). Expression of autotaxin and acylglycerol kinase in prostate cancer: association with cancer development and progression. *Cancer Sci* vol. 100(9) pp. 1631-1638

Park, S. Y., K. J. Jeong, N. Panupinthu, S. Yu, J. Lee, J. W. Han, J. M. Kim, J. S. Lee, J. Kang, C. G. Park, G. B. Mills & H. Y. Lee (2011). Lysophosphatidic acid augments human hepatocellular carcinoma cell invasion through LPA1 receptor and MMP-9 expression. *Oncogene* vol. 30(11) pp. 1351-1359

Parrill, A. L., U. Echols, T. Nguyen, T. C. Pham, A. Hoeglund & D. L. Baker (2008). Virtual screening approaches for the identification of non-lipid autotaxin inhibitors. *Bioorg Med Chem* vol. 16(4) pp. 1784-1795

Ptaszynska, M. M., M. L. Pendrak, R. W. Bandle, M. L. Stracke & D. D. Roberts (2008). Positive feedback between vascular endothelial growth factor-A and autotaxin in ovarian cancer cells. *Mol Cancer Res* vol. 6(3) pp. 352-363

Ptaszynska, M. M., M. L. Pendrak, M. L. Stracke & D. D. Roberts (2010). Autotaxin signaling via lysophosphatidic acid receptors contributes to vascular endothelial growth factor-induced endothelial cell migration. *Mol Cancer Res* vol. 8(3) pp. 309-321

Pustilnik, T. B., V. Estrella, J. R. Wiener, M. Mao, A. Eder, M. A. Watt, R. C. Bast, Jr. & G. B. Mills (1999). Lysophosphatidic acid induces urokinase secretion by ovarian cancer cells. *Clin Cancer Res* vol. 5(11) pp. 3704-3710

Ren, J., Y. J. Xiao, L. S. Singh, X. Zhao, Z. Zhao, L. Feng, T. M. Rose, G. D. Prestwich & Y. Xu (2006). Lysophosphatidic acid is constitutively produced by human peritoneal mesothelial cells and enhances adhesion, migration, and invasion of ovarian cancer cells. *Cancer Res* vol. 66(6) pp. 3006-3014

Samadi, N., R. T. Bekele, I. S. Goping, L. M. Schang & D. N. Brindley (2011). Lysophosphatidate induces chemo-resistance by releasing breast cancer cells from taxol-induced mitotic arrest. *PLoS One* vol. 6(5) pp. e20608

Samadi, N., C. Gaetano, I. S. Goping & D. N. Brindley (2009). Autotaxin protects MCF-7 breast cancer and MDA-MB-435 melanoma cells against Taxol-induced apoptosis. *Oncogene* vol. 28(7) pp. 1028-1039

Sawada, K., K. Morishige, M. Tahara, R. Kawagishi, Y. Ikebuchi, K. Tasaka & Y. Murata (2002). Alendronate inhibits lysophosphatidic acid-induced migration of human ovarian cancer cells by attenuating the activation of rho. *Cancer Res* vol. 62(21) pp. 6015-6020

Sengupta, S., K. S. Kim, M. P. Berk, R. Oates, P. Escobar, J. Belinson, W. Li, D. J. Lindner, B. Williams & Y. Xu (2007). Lysophosphatidic acid downregulates tissue inhibitor of metalloproteinases, which are negatively involved in lysophosphatidic acid-induced cell invasion. *Oncogene* vol. 26(20) pp. 2894-2901

Snider, A. J., Z. Zhang, Y. Xie & K. E. Meier (2010). Epidermal growth factor increases lysophosphatidic acid production in human ovarian cancer cells: roles for phospholipase D2 and receptor transactivation. *Am J Physiol Cell Physiol* vol. 298(1) pp. C163-170

So, J., F. Q. Wang, J. Navari, J. Schreher & D. A. Fishman (2005). LPA-induced epithelial ovarian cancer (EOC) in vitro invasion and migration are mediated by VEGF receptor-2 (VEGF-R2). *Gynecol Oncol* vol. 97(3) pp. 870-878

Song, J., T. Clair, J. H. Noh, J. W. Eun, S. Y. Ryu, S. N. Lee, Y. M. Ahn, S. Y. Kim, S. H. Lee, W. S. Park, N. J. Yoo, J. Y. Lee & S. W. Nam (2005). Autotaxin (lysoPLD/NPP2) protects fibroblasts from apoptosis through its enzymatic product, lysophosphatidic acid, utilizing albumin-bound substrate. *Biochem Biophys Res Commun* vol. 337(3) pp. 967-975

Song, Y., P. Wilkins, W. Hu, K. S. Murthy, J. Chen, Z. Lee, R. Oyesanya, J. Wu, S. E. Barbour & X. Fang (2007). Inhibition of calcium-independent phospholipase A2 suppresses proliferation and tumorigenicity of ovarian carcinoma cells. *Biochem J* vol. 406(3) pp. 427-436

Stassar, M. J., G. Devitt, M. Brosius, L. Rinnab, J. Prang, T. Schradin, J. Simon, S. Petersen, A. Kopp-Schneider & M. Zoller (2001). Identification of human renal cell carcinoma associated genes by suppression subtractive hybridization. *Br J Cancer* vol. 85(9) pp. 1372-1382

Stracke, M. L., H. C. Krutzsch, E. J. Unsworth, A. Arestad, V. Cioce, E. Schiffmann & L. A. Liotta (1992). Identification, purification, and partial sequence analysis of autotaxin, a novel motility-stimulating protein. *J Biol Chem* vol. 267(4) pp. 2524-2529

Sun, H., J. Ren, Q. Zhu, F. Z. Kong, L. Wu & B. R. Pan (2009). Effects of lysophosphatidic acid on human colon cancer cells and its mechanisms of action. *World J Gastroenterol* vol. 15(36) pp. 4547-4555

Tabchy, A., G. Tigyi & G. B. Mills (2011). Location, location, location: a crystal-clear view of autotaxin saturating LPA receptors. *Nat Struct Mol Biol* vol. 18(2) pp. 117-118

Tanaka, M., S. Okudaira, Y. Kishi, R. Ohkawa, S. Iseki, M. Ota, S. Noji, Y. Yatomi, J. Aoki & H. Arai (2006). Autotaxin stabilizes blood vessels and is required for embryonic vasculature by producing lysophosphatidic acid. *J Biol Chem* vol. 281(35) pp. 25822-25830

Tanyi, J. L., Y. Hasegawa, R. Lapushin, A. J. Morris, J. K. Wolf, A. Berchuck, K. Lu, D. I. Smith, K. Kalli, L. C. Hartmann, K. McCune, D. Fishman, R. Broaddus, K. W. Cheng, E. N. Atkinson, J. M. Yamal, R. C. Bast, E. A. Felix, R. A. Newman & G. B. Mills (2003). Role of decreased levels of lipid phosphate phosphatase-1 in accumulation of lysophosphatidic acid in ovarian cancer. *Clin Cancer Res* vol. 9(10 Pt 1) pp. 3534-3545

Tanyi, J. L., A. J. Morris, J. K. Wolf, X. Fang, Y. Hasegawa, R. Lapushin, N. Auersperg, Y. J. Sigal, R. A. Newman, E. A. Felix, E. N. Atkinson & G. B. Mills (2003). The human lipid phosphate phosphatase-3 decreases the growth, survival, and tumorigenesis of ovarian cancer cells: validation of the lysophosphatidic acid signaling cascade as a target for therapy in ovarian cancer. *Cancer Res* vol. 63(5) pp. 1073-1082

Tigyi, G. (2010). Aiming drug discovery at lysophosphatidic acid targets. *Br J Pharmacol* vol. 161(2) pp. 241-270

Tokumura, A., T. Kume, K. Fukuzawa, M. Tahara, K. Tasaka, J. Aoki, H. Arai, K. Yasuda & H. Kanzaki (2007). Peritoneal fluids from patients with certain gynecologic tumor contain elevated levels of bioactive lysophospholipase D activity. *Life Sci* vol. 80(18) pp. 1641-1649

van Corven, E. J., A. Groenink, K. Jalink, T. Eichholtz & W. H. Moolenaar (1989). Lysophosphatidate-induced cell proliferation: identification and dissection of signaling pathways mediated by G proteins. *Cell* vol. 59(1) pp. 45-54

Vidot, S., J. Witham, R. Agarwal, S. Greenhough, H. S. Bamrah, G. J. Tigyi, S. B. Kaye & A. Richardson (2010). Autotaxin delays apoptosis induced by carboplatin in ovarian cancer cells. *Cell Signal* vol. 22(6) pp. 926-935

Wang, F. Q., E. Barfield, S. Dutta, T. Pua & D. A. Fishman (2009). VEGFR-2 silencing by small interference RNA (siRNA) suppresses LPA-induced epithelial ovarian cancer (EOC) invasion. *Gynecol Oncol* vol. 115(3) pp. 414-423

Wang, F. Q., J. Fisher & D. A. Fishman (2011). MMP-1-PAR1 axis mediates LPA-induced epithelial ovarian cancer (EOC) invasion. *Gynecol Oncol* vol. 120(2) pp. 247-255

Wang, P., X. Wu, W. Chen, J. Liu & X. Wang (2007). The lysophosphatidic acid (LPA) receptors their expression and significance in epithelial ovarian neoplasms. *Gynecol Oncol* vol. 104(3) pp. 714-720

Witham, J., M. R. Valenti, A. K. De-Haven-Brandon, S. Vidot, S. A. Eccles, S. B. Kaye & A. Richardson (2007). The Bcl-2/Bcl-XL family inhibitor ABT-737 sensitizes ovarian cancer cells to carboplatin. *Clin Cancer Res* vol. 13(23) pp. 7191-7198

Wu, J. M., Y. Xu, N. J. Skill, H. Sheng, Z. Zhao, M. Yu, R. Saxena & M. A. Maluccio (2010). Autotaxin expression and its connection with the TNF-alpha-NF-kappaB axis in human hepatocellular carcinoma. *Mol Cancer* vol. 9 pp. 71

Xu, X. & G. D. Prestwich (2010). Inhibition of tumor growth and angiogenesis by a lysophosphatidic acid antagonist in an engineered three-dimensional lung cancer xenograft model. *Cancer* vol. 116(7) pp. 1739-1750

Xu, Y., D. C. Gaudette, J. D. Boynton, A. Frankel, X. J. Fang, A. Sharma, J. Hurteau, G. Casey, A. Goodbody, A. Mellors & et al. (1995). Characterization of an ovarian cancer activating factor in ascites from ovarian cancer patients. *Clin Cancer Res* vol. 1(10) pp. 1223-1232

Xue, L., F. Chu, Y. Cheng, X. Sun, A. Borthakur, M. Ramarao, P. Pandey, M. Wu, S. F. Schlossman & K. V. Prasad (2002). Siva-1 binds to and inhibits BCL-X(L)-mediated protection against UV radiation-induced apoptosis. *Proc Natl Acad Sci U S A* vol. 99(10) pp. 6925-6930

Yang, K., D. Zheng, X. Deng, L. Bai, Y. Xu & Y. S. Cong (2008). Lysophosphatidic acid activates telomerase in ovarian cancer cells through hypoxia-inducible factor-1alpha and the PI3K pathway. *J Cell Biochem* vol. 105(5) pp. 1194-1201

Yang, S. Y., J. Lee, C. G. Park, S. Kim, S. Hong, H. C. Chung, S. K. Min, J. W. Han, H. W. Lee & H. Y. Lee (2002). Expression of autotaxin (NPP-2) is closely linked to invasiveness of breast cancer cells. *Clin Exp Metastasis* vol. 19(7) pp. 603-608

Yang, Y. C., Y. P. Tsao, T. C. Ho & I. P. Choung (2007). Peroxisome proliferator-activated receptor-gamma agonists cause growth arrest and apoptosis in human ovarian carcinoma cell lines. *Int J Gynecol Cancer* vol. 17(2) pp. 418-425

Yu, S., M. M. Murph, Y. Lu, S. Liu, H. S. Hall, J. Liu, C. Stephens, X. Fang & G. B. Mills (2008). Lysophosphatidic acid receptors determine tumorigenicity and aggressiveness of ovarian cancer cells. *J Natl Cancer Inst* vol. 100(22) pp. 1630-1642

Zhang, G. Y., N. Ahmed, C. Riley, K. Oliva, G. Barker, M. A. Quinn & G. E. Rice (2005). Enhanced expression of peroxisome proliferator-activated receptor gamma in epithelial ovarian carcinoma. *Br J Cancer* vol. 92(1) pp. 113-119

Zhang, H., X. Xu, J. Gajewiak, R. Tsukahara, Y. Fujiwara, J. Liu, J. I. Fells, D. Perygin, A. L. Parrill, G. Tigyi & G. D. Prestwich (2009). Dual activity lysophosphatidic acid receptor pan-antagonist/autotaxin inhibitor reduces breast cancer cell migration in vitro and causes tumor regression in vivo. *Cancer Res* vol. 69(13) pp. 5441-5449

Zhang, R., J. Wang, S. Ma, Z. Huang & G. Zhang (2011). Requirement of Osteopontin in the migration and protection against Taxol-induced apoptosis via the ATX-LPA axis in SGC7901 cells. *BMC Cell Biol* vol. 12 pp. 11

19

Potential Monoclonal Antibody Therapy for the Treatment of Ovarian Cancer

Gregory Lee, Mingang Zhu and Bixia Ge
UBC Center for Reproductive Health,
The University of British Columbia Vancouver
Canada

1. Introduction

Although ovarian cancer is the fifth most common cancer among women, it causes more death than any other type of female reproductive cancer (Mørch et al., 2009). Besides difficulties in early detection, limited options for the treatment of ovarian cancer at late stages have been the major cause of high mortality rate (Jemal et al., 2003). About 76% of women with ovarian cancer survive 1 year after diagnosis, but only about 45% will live 5 years after diagnosis (Choi et al., 2008). Therefore, it may be desirable to look for alternative means of treating this type of cancer rather than the conventional ones including chemo- or radiotherapy.

During the last two decades, target-oriented antibody-based anti-cancer drugs have become the main stream choices for cancer treatments in humans. Although the efficacy of cancer treatments varies greatly with individual cases, overall improvements of patients' care and survival are significant, when compared to those of the conventional ones. Besides those approved by the FDA of the United States of America for the clinical treatments of cancer, numerous antibody-drug candidates are still at various stages of clinical trials and pending for the final approval by the FDA (Waldmann, 2003).

Generally speaking, the majority of antibody-based anti-cancer drugs are target-oriented and the adverse side effects upon infusion of the antibody drugs are relatively mild as compared to those of the traditional ones. Therefore, selections of suitable targets against the tumor cells have become an essential step for the long term antibody drug development. In general, the ideal tumor target for the antibody drugs can be selected based on its accessibility, high abundance and surface homogeneity. Moreover, it should not be highly expressed on normal cells or tissues, especially the vital organs in humans (McGuire et al., 1996).

Recently, two monoclonal antibodies were identified and selected based on these criteria for ovarian cancer. One is RP215 which recognizes a carbohydrate-associated epitope found preferentially in cancer cell-expressed immunoglobulin superfamily proteins, designated in general as CA215. The other is GHR106 which was shown to react with the extracellular domain of human GnRH receptor. Both CA215 and GnRH receptor are widely expressed among cancer cells of different tissue origins, especially those of the human ovary with positive rates ranging from 60-80% (Lee et al., 2008, 2009; Lee & Ge,

2010a). The binding of either of these two monoclonal antibodies was found to inhibit the growth of ovarian cancer cells *in vitro* and *in vivo* through studies of induced apoptosis and complement-dependent cytotoxicity. Therefore, additional preclinical studies were performed to elucidate the mechanisms of action of these monoclonal antibodies as anti-cancer drugs for the treatment of ovarian cancer. These studies should represent our efforts to demonstrate the potential use of these monoclonal antibodies as the anti-ovarian cancer drugs in the future.

2. Results and discussion

In this study, two monoclonal antibodies, RP215 and GHR106, were evaluated to see if they are suitable drug candidates for the potential treatment of ovarian cancer. Several *in vitro* and *in vivo* experiments were performed including (1) immunohistochemical staining and Western blot assay to reveal the relative abundance of target antigens, CA215 and GnRH receptor, respectively, each of which appears on the surface of cancer cells of the ovary, (2) apoptosis and complement-dependent cytotoxicity assays to demonstrate the respective anti-cancer efficacy of these two monoclonal antibodies, (3) elucidation of respective molecular mechanisms of action of RP215 and GHR106 as anti-cancer drugs through gene expression/regulation studies, (4) nude mouse experiments to reveal the dose-dependent inhibition of the growth of tumor cells and (5) construction of chimeric forms of RP215 and GHR106 monoclonal antibodies for future preclinical and clinical studies, (6) clinical evaluations of CA215 levels from serum specimens of cancer patients by using the established enzyme immunoassay kits, and (7) glycoanalysis to elucidate the proposed structure of carbohydrate-associated epitope(s) recognized by RP215 in CA215.

2.1 Immunohistochemical studies and Western blot assay

RP215 and GHR106 monoclonal antibodies were found to react with antigens localized on the surface of a variety of cancer cells including that of the ovary. By indirect immunohistochemical studies, it can be shown that three of the selected ovarian cancer cell lines, including OC-3-VGH, OVCAR-3, and SKOV-3, were strongly stained with RP215 and GHR106, respectively, whereas normal mouse IgG as the negative control gave little or no colour staining. The results of such an analysis are presented in Figure 1A (Lee et al., 1992, 2008, 2009; Lee & Ge, 2010a). The immunohistochemical studies of selected cancerous tissue sections of the human ovary were also performed with RP215 as the primary antibody probe. The results are presented in Figure 1B for comparisons. In a separate study, GHR106 was used as a probe to carry out immunohistochemical staining of cancerous tissue sections of the ovary from patients at four various stages of ovarian cancer (Chien et al., 2004). From the results of this analysis, it was generally concluded that the positive staining rates of ovarian cancer tissue sections increase with the stages of this disease (37.5% at stage I to 100% at stage IV) (Chien et al., 2004). In contrast, the immunohistochemical staining of tissue sections of the normal ovary showed negative staining results. The results of such analysis are summarized in Figure 1C.

The antigens recognized by RP215 and GHR106 in the cell extract of ovarian cancer cells were also determined by Western blot assay (Lee et al., 2008, 2009; Lee & Ge, 2010a). In the case of RP215, the corresponding antigen, CA215, was found to have a molecular size ranging from 50 to 75 kDa for the cell extract from either of the three ovarian cancer cell lines (OC-3-VGH, OVCAR-3 and SKOV-3). When GHR106 was used as the probe for the same assay, the molecular weight of GnRH receptor of these cancer cells was found to be 60 kDa. The results were consistent with those reported previously for human GnRH receptor (Lee & Ge, 2010a). The results of such analysis are presented in Figure 2.

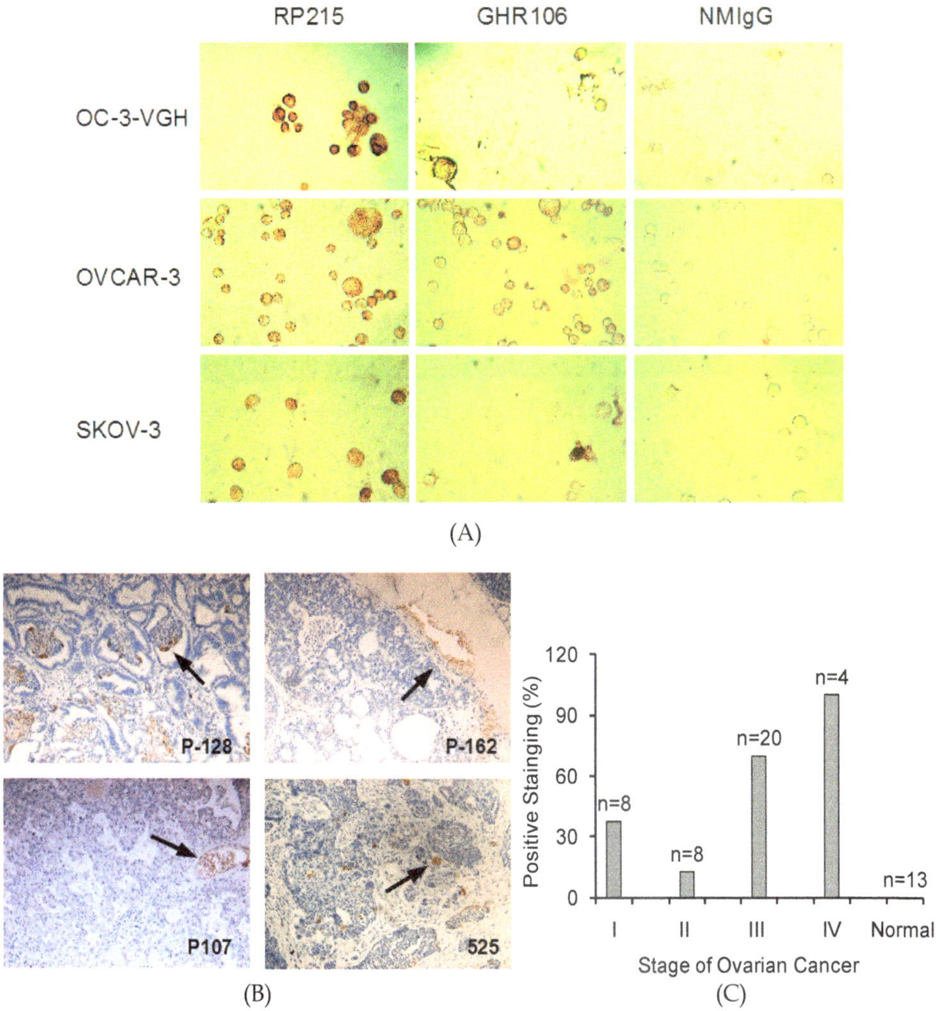

Fig. 1. (A) Immunohistochemical study to reveal staining of three different ovarian cancer cell lines, OC-3-VGH, OVCAR-3 and SKOV-3 with RP215, GHR106 and normal mouse IgG (NMIgG, negative control); (B) Immunohistochemical study to reveal staining of selected ovarian cancer tissue sections (P-128, P-162, P107 and 525) with RP215. The areas of staining are highlighted with the arrows; (C) Results of immunohistochemical staining of GnRH receptor of ovarian tissue sections at different stages (I to IV) of ovarian cancer. n = total number of specimens.

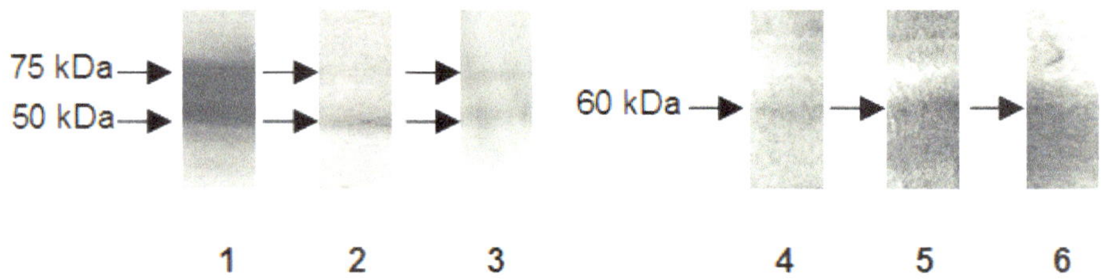

Fig. 2. Western blot assay to reveal protein bands from the extract of three ovarian cancer cell lines, OC-3-VGH (1 and 4), SKOV-3 (2 and 5) and OVCAR-3 (3 and 6), respectively, when probed with RP215 (lanes 1, 2 and 3) as well as GHR106 (lanes 4, 5 and 6). The molecular weight markers of 50 kDa, 60 kDa and 75 kDa are indicated by arrows.

2.2 Effects of RP215 and GHR106 monoclonal antibodies on the induction of apoptosis to ovarian cancer cells

By using terminal deoxynucleotidyl transferase dUTP nick end labelling (TUNEL) assay, the induced apoptosis of cancer cells upon incubation with RP215 and GHR106 could be clearly demonstrated. As shown in Figure 3A, all of the three ovarian cancer cell lines were found to undergo significant cellular apoptosis, when incubated with 10 μg/mL of either RP215 or GHR106 (24 - 48 h). A significant apoptosis of cancer cells was also induced upon treatments with 0.1 μg/mL of a GnRH antagonist, Antide or GnRH. Under the same assay conditions, the chimeric form of RP215, ChRP215, was found to induce apoptosis of the OC-3-VGH cancer cell line, similar to that observed for murine RP215. The results of such a comparative analysis are also summarized in Figure 3B. Similarly, chimeric form of GHR106, ChGHR106, was found to have the same effects as that of GHR106 in inducing apoptosis of the ovarian cancer cells (Figure 3B).

In addition to RP215, the induction of apoptosis to OC-3-VGH ovarian cancer cell has also been confirmed with other RP215-related monoclonal antibodies (RCA10, RCA100, RCA104, RCA110 and RCA111, see section 2.11), as demonstrated in Figure 3C.

2.3 Effects of RP215 and GHR106 monoclonal antibodies on complement-dependent cytotoxicity of ovarian cancer cells

The complement-dependent cytotoxicity assay was also employed to study the induction of complement-dependent cell lysis to OC-3-VGH ovarian cancer cells in the presence of complement and RP215 or GHR106 (10 μg/mL for 2 h incubation). The chimeric forms of monoclonal antibodies, ChRP215 or ChGHR106, also demonstrated a similar degree of complement-dependent cytotoxicity reaction to cultured ovarian cancer cells under the same conditions of incubation. In contrast, complement alone or complement with GnRH antagonist, Antide (0.1 μg/mL), revealed no effect on complement-dependent cytotoxicity to ovarian cancer cells (data not shown). Results of this complement-dependent cytotoxicity assay with different monoclonal antibodies plus complement are summarized in Figure 4 for comparisons.

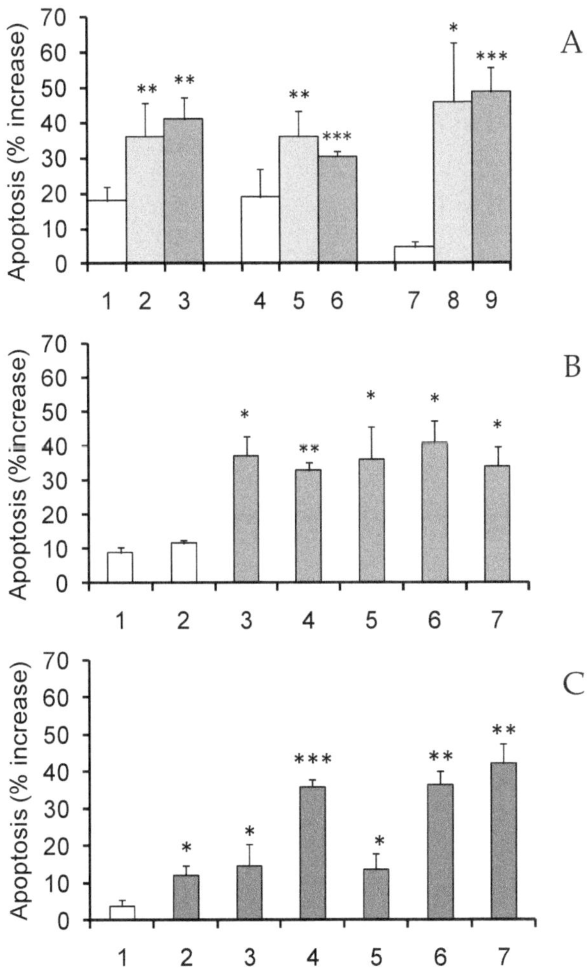

Fig. 3. (A) The TUNEL assay to demonstrate the increase in apoptosis of cancer cells in response to the treatment of cultured OC-3-VGH (Lanes 1-3), OVCAR-3 (Lanes 4-6) and SKOV-3 (Lanes 7-9) cells for 48 h with either of the following monoclonal antibodies (dose: 10 μg/mL each): normal mouse IgG (Lanes 1, 4, 7), RP215 (Lanes 2, 5, 8) and GHR106 (Lanes 3, 6,9), respectively; (B) The TUNEL assay to demonstrate the increase in apoptosis of OC-3-VGH cells in response to the treatment by chimeric as well as murine monoclonal antibodies (dose: 10 μg/mL each) for 48 h: Lane 1: non treatment; Lane 2: normal mouse IgG; Lane 3: ChRP215; Lane 4: ChGHR106; Lane 5: RP215; Lane 6: GHR106; and Lane 7: 0.1 μg/mL Antide; (C) The TUNEL assay to demonstrate the increase in apoptosis of cancer cells in response to the incubation of OC-3-VGH cancer cells for 48 h with the following antibodies (1 μg/mL each): Lanes 1-7 correspond to that of normal mouse IgG, RCA10, RCA100, RCA104, RCA110, RCA111, and RP215, respectively (to be described in section 2.11). All data presented are statistically significant at * $P < 0.05$, ** $P < 0.01$, and *** $P<0.001$.

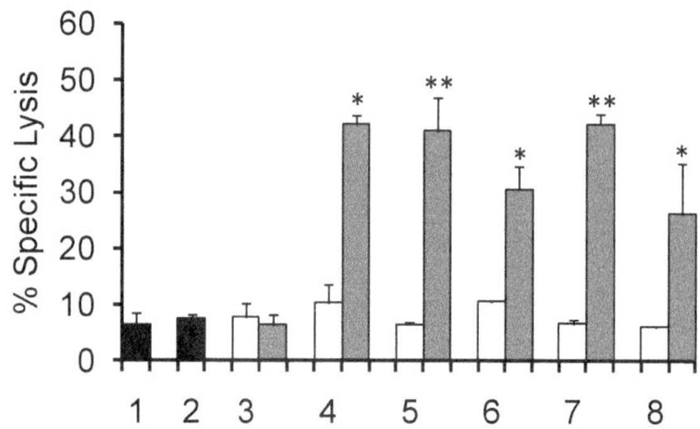

Fig. 4. Complement-dependent cytotoxicity assay to demonstrate the respective effects of normal mouse IgG (Lane 3), ChRP215 (Lane 4), ChGHR106 (Lane 5), RP215 (Lane 6), GHR106 (Lane 7), and goat anti-human IgG (Lane 8) on the complement-dependent lysis of OC-3-VGH ovarian cells. White, monoclonal antibody (10 µg/mL) alone; Grey, monoclonal antibody (10 µg/ml) plus complement; Black, non-treatment (Lane 1) or 3 µL freshly prepared rabbit baby complement (Lane 2) as control. * and ** indicate statistical significance of $P<0.05$ and $P<0.01$, respectively.

2.4 Effects of RP215 or GHR106 monoclonal antibodies on the expression of selected genes in ovarian cancer cells

Molecular mechanisms of action by which RP215 or GHR106 inhibit the growth of OC-3-VGH ovarian cancer cells were elucidated through the studies of gene regulation by qualitative and semi-quantitative RT-PCR (Lee & Ge, 2010a; Kang et al., 2003; Leung et al., 2003; Gründker et.al., 2000). A number of genes related to the growth of cancer cells were examined for their expressions in response to the treatment of cultured ovarian cancer cells with either of these two monoclonal antibodies for 48 h. The results of this qualitative analysis with a number of selected genes are summarized in Table 1.

Parallel to this gene expression study, the effects of GnRH antagonist, Antide, on the expression of selected genes in ovarian cancer cells are also presented for comparisons with those of GHR106. Based on the results of this comparative analysis, it was clearly demonstrated that both GHR106 and Antide induce the same patterns of gene regulations to ovarian cancer cells upon their respective ligand binding.

Generally speaking, the incubation of RP215 with OC-3-VGH ovarian cancer cells was found to increase the gene expression of IgG and NFKB1 (Li & Verma, 2002), but genes of ribosomal proteins, P0, P1 and P2 were significantly down-regulated (Lee & Ge, 2010b). RP215 incubation to cultured cancer cells were found to have no effect on EGF (epidermal growth factor) (Gründker et al., 2000), but caused a significant decrease in the gene expression of *c-fos* (Dragunow & Faull, 1989). On the other hand, under the same incubation conditions, both GHR106 monoclonal antibody and GnRH antagonist, Antide, were shown to up-regulate the expression of GnRH gene, but not that of GnRH receptor (Lee & Ge, 2010b). Gene regulations of ribosomal proteins by GHR106 or Antide were also different from those by RP215. While P0 gene was found to be down-regulated, P1 gene was up-regulated instead (Lee & Ge, 2010b). Although no changes in *c-fos* gene regulation were observed, EGF was found to be down-regulated significantly with the treatment of GHR106 or Antide. The results of such a comprehensive analysis with OC-3-VGH ovarian cancer cells are presented in Table 1. From this gene regulation analysis, it can be shown that the molecular mechanisms of action by which the apoptosis of cancer cells is induced with RP215 are quite different from those of GHR106 or GnRH antagonists, Antide.

Gene	RP215 (10 μg/ml)	GHR106 (10 μg/ml)	Antide (0.1 μg/ml)
GnRH	N.T[a]	↑	↑
GnRH receptor	N.T	N.C	N.C
IgG	↑[c]	N.T	N.T
NFKB1[b]	↑	N.T	N.T
P0	↓[c]	↓	↓
P1	↓	↑	↑
P2	↓	N.C	N.C
EGF	N.C[a]	↓	↓
c-fos	↓	N.C	N.C

[a]N.T: not tested; N.C: not changed

[b]Abbrevations used: NFKB1: nuclear factor of kappa light polypeptide gene enhancer in B cells 1; P0, P1 and P2 are genes expressed by selected ribosomal proteins; c-fos: cellular oncogene proteins; EGF: epidermal growth factor.

[c]↑ and ↓ indicate significant up and down gene regulations, respectively when compared to that of GAPDH (Glyceraldehyde 3-phosphate dehydrogenase).

Table 1. Gene regulation studies in cultured OC-3-VGH ovarian cancer cells using RP215, GHR106 and Antide.

2.5 Expressions of immunoglobulins of different classes from ovarian cancer cells derived from a single clone

OC-3-VGH ovarian cancer cells which were derived from a single clone were found to express IgG, IgA and IgM, simultaneously. This is in contrast with those of B cells, each of which expresses only a single class of immunoglobulins. (Qiu et.al., 2003; Huang et al.,2008; Zhang et al., 2010). This observation strongly suggests that immunoglobulins may be expressed by cancer cells through different mechanisms as compared to those of normal human B cells (Zheng et al., 2009).

2.6 Nude mouse experiments

Our previous studies have demonstrated that CA215 and GHR106 receptor are expressed on the surface of many human cancer cells including those of the ovary. Through *in vitro* studies with induced apoptosis and complement-dependent cytotoxicity reactions, it was clearly demonstrated that CA215 and GnRH receptor on the surface of cancer cells may be suitable targets by the respective monoclonal antibodies (Lee et al., 2009; Lee & Ge, 2010a). Therefore, nude mouse experiments were performed with OC-3-VGH ovarian cancer cell line as the model to evaluate the anti-tumor efficacy of RP215 monoclonal antibody.

Following a single injection of three different doses of RP215 (1-10 mg/kg doses) at the time of tumor implantation, a significant inhibition of tumor growth was observed in a dose dependent manner. Fifteen days after the tumor implant and antibody treatments, the tumor volumes were compared. As shown in the histogram of Figure 5, the dose-dependent inhibition of tumor growth by RP215 was statistically significant as compared to that of the

negative control. In addition, I^{131}-labelled RP215 (12 μCi/mg) was found to be more effective in the suppression of tumor growth than the unlabelled antibody.
Several nude mouse experiments were also performed with models of several other cancer cell lines. These included: C33A (cervix) and SK-MES-1 (lung) for RP215 as well as Hep2G (liver) for GHR106. In each case, significant tumor reduction or inhibition of tumor growth was observed 14-17 days after tumor implantation and subsequent injection of antibody drugs (RP215 or GHR106: dose 10 mg/kg) according to similar protocols for nude mouse experiments as described above (data not presented).

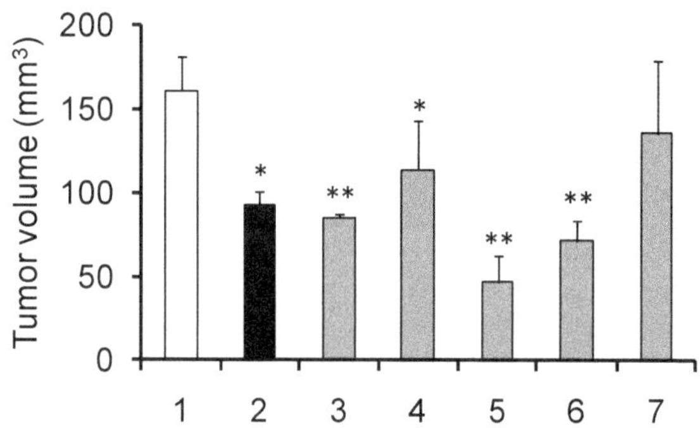

Fig. 5. Tumor volumes at Day 15 were compared for nude mice treated by RP215 in unlabelled and I^{131}-labelled form (specific activity 12 μCi/mg): Lane 1: negative control (no treatment, open column); Lane 2: positive control (black column, 60 mg/kg cyclophosphamide); Lane 3: AH (antibody high dose: 10 mg/kg); Lane 4: AM (antibody medium dose: 5 mg/kg); Lane 5: I-AH (I^{131}-labeled antibody high dose: 10 mg/kg); Lane 6: I-AM (I^{131}-labeled antibody median dose: 5 mg/kg); Lane 7: I-AL (I^{131}-labeled antibody low dose: 2 mg/kg). Data are statistically significant at $*P<0.05$, $**P<0.01$.

2.7 Anti-idiotypic monoclonal antibodies as anti-cancer vaccines

RP215 monoclonal antibody was shown to recognize carbohydrate-associated epitope which is preferentially expressed in a mixture of different glycoproteins designated as CA215 identified in many cancer cells in humans. Polyclonal and rat monoclonal antibodies against the Fab-idiotypic domains of RP215 were generated and characterized (Lee et al., 2010a and 2010b; Lee & Ge, 2010a and 2010b). The anti-idiotypic (aid) antibodies were found to bear the internal images of the RP215-specific carbohydrate-associated epitope. Following immunizations in mice with rat anti-idiotypic monoclonal antibody, the resulting anti-aid or Ab3 sera were found to behave like RP215 in biochemical and immunological properties (Lee et al., 2010a and 2010b; Lee & Ge, 2010a and 2010b).
By Western blot assay, Ab3 antisera were found to react with protein bands identical to those recognized by RP215. By immunohistochemical staining study, the majority of cancer cells from different tissue origins were positively stained by both Ab3 antisera and RP215. Ab3 antisera were shown to induce apoptosis, similar to that observed for RP215. Based on these experimental observations, it was therefore hypothesized that rat anti-idiotypic monoclonal antibodies or its Fab fragments bear the internal images of RP215-specific epitope (Lee et al., 2010a and 2010b; Lee & Ge, 2010a and 2010b) and may be suitable as anti-cancer vaccines to induce Ab3 responses in humans for cancer treatments or preventions (Lee et al., 2010b).

2.8 Molecular identity of CA215 and expression of immunoglobulin superfamily proteins by cancer cells

RP215 monoclonal antibody was shown to react with carbohydrate-associated epitope preferentially expressed by cancer cells in a mixture of glycoproteins designated as CA215. To reveal the molecular identity of CA215, MALDI-TOF MS (matrix assisted laser desorption ionization time-of-flight mass spectrometry) analysis was performed for more than one hundred tryptic peptides of CA215 affinity-purified from the shed medium of cultured OC-3-VGH ovarian cancer cells. It was generally concluded that CA215 consists mainly of immunoglobulin superfamily proteins (61%) including immunoglobulins (42%), T cell receptors (6%) and cell adhesion molecules (8%) as well as mucins (7%) and other unrelated ones. Results of this analysis are summarized in Table 2.

Molecular Function/Category	Number of Peptides Matched Total = 124 (Percentage)
I. Antigen receptors	
Antibodies and immunoglobulins	52 (42.0%)
T cell receptor chains	7 (5.7%)
II. Antigen presenting molecules	
MHC I and MHC II	6 (4.9%)
III. Adhesion molecules	10 (8.1%)
IV.Cytokine and growth factors	8 (6.5%)
V. Receptor tyrosine kinase/phosphatise	7 (5.7%)
VI. Others	
Immunoglobulin superfamily related (e.g. titin)	12 (9.7%)
	Total with homology[a]: 75/124 (60.5%)
Immunoglobulin superfamily unrelated (e.g. mucin)	9 (7.3%)

[a] Excluding overlapping matched peptides

Table 2. MALDI-TOF MS analysis of tryptic peptides derived from affinity-purified CA215.

By using semi-quantitative RT-PCR of the cell extract of over 20 cancer cell lines, it was observed that as many as 80% of these cancer cells express T cell receptors (α and β chains) at significantly high levels including OC-3-VGH, OVCAR-3 and SKOV-3 cell lines. Results of such an analysis are summarized in Table 3. In contrast with the exception of Raji (lymphoma) and Jurkat (T cell leukemia) cell lines, none of these cancer cell lines express CD3, CD4 and CD8 co-receptors and/or co-stimulator genes, indicating the non-functional nature of most of the cancer cell-expressed T cell receptors. In addition, numerous immunoglobulin superfamily protein-like cell adhesion molecules such as CD47, CD54, CD58 and CD147 are also highly expressed among all the cancer cell lines. Widespread T cell receptor expressions among cancer cells may have implications on cancer immunotherapy via T cell activation as well as the induced tolerance of T cells caused by tumor-associated antigens in humans (Lee et al., 2011a).

Origin	Human Ovarian			Lymphoma	T-cell leukemia
Designation cell line	SKOV-3	OVCAR-3	OC-3-VGH	Raji	Jurkat
ATCC NO.	HTB-77			CCL-86	TIB-152
TCR (α)[a]	+++[b]	+	++	+++	+++
TCR (β)	+	±	+	+++	+++
IgG (Fc)	+	++	+	++	+
CD3	-	-	-	+	+
CD4	-	-	-	-	-
CD8	-	-	-	-	-
CD47	++	++	++	++	++
CD54	++	++	+	+	++
CD58	++	++	++	++	++
CD147	++	++	++	++	++

[a] Abbreviations used: TCR, T cell receptor (α chain or β chain)
[b] Signal intensities follow the order of +++ (strongest), ++, +, ±, - (neg), GAPDH was used as the internal standards.

Table 3. Gene expressions of immunoglobulin superfamily proteins by RT-PCR.

2.9 Structural elucidations of carbohydrate-associated epitope recognized by RP215 monoclonal antibody

In collaboration with Complex Carbohydrate Research Center at University of Georgia, efforts have been made to elucidate the carbohydrate-associated epitope(s) recognized by RP215 in CA215. (Lee & Ge, 2009). By using CA215 affinity-purified from OC-3-VGH ovarian and C33A cervical cancer cell lines, profiles of N-linked and O-linked glycans were analyzed and compared with those of other known glycoproteins from normal and cancerous tissues. In the case of N-linked glycans, high mannose and complex bisecting structures with terminal N-glycolylneuraminic acid were detected in CA215. In the case of O-linked glycans, several oligosaccharides were detected in CA215 with structures similar to those of mucins, but with terminal N-glycolylneuraminic acid. N-linked and O-linked glycosylation site mappings of CA215 were performed. A total of two N-linked and eight O-linked glycopeptides were detected. Protein BLAST search of peptide sequence homology revealed that two N-linked and six O-linked glycopeptides were almost 100% matched to human immunoglobulin heavy chains. One of the remaining O-linked ones was matched to immunoglobulin superfamily proteins such as titin and hemicentin. Results of N-linked and O-linked glycosylation site mappings are summarized in Table 4. Based on the results of this extensive glyconanalysis, it can be suggested that both N-linked and O-linked glycans with unique terminal N-glycolylneuraminic acid in CA215 are structurally related to those of mucins. However, N-glycolylneuraminic acid might not to be directly involved in the RP215 epitope recognition as no loss of CA215 activity was found when OC-3-VGH cells were cultured in medium containing human serum instead of fetal calf serum as culture medium supplement (Lee & Azadi, 2011).

Accession Number	Peptide Detected[a]	Peptide Sequence Homology of Proteins (%)
CAC12842.1	EEQF**N**STFR[a]	Immunoglobulin heavy chain (Fc) (100%)[b]
CAA04843.1	EEQF**N**STYR	Immunoglobulin heavy chain (Fc) (100%)
AAB60643.2	L**S**VP**TS**EWQR	Cathepsin S (100%
AAK68690.1	F**T**CLA**T**NDAGD**S**SK	Hemicentin (100%) Titin (100%) Palladin isoform 4 (92%) LRN4 (78%) Immunoglobulin superfamily proteins
AAD38158.1	D**T**LMI**S**R	Immunoglobulin heavy chain (Fc) (100%)
AAC39746.2	GYLPEPV**T**V**T**WN**S**G**T**L**T**NGVR	Immunoglobulin heavy chain (Fab) (90%)[c]
AAN76042.1	**S**V**S**L**T**CMINGFYP**S**DI**S**VEWEK	Immunoglobulin heavy chain (Fc) (90%)
CAJ75462.1	Q**SS**GLY**S**L**SS**VVSVT**SSS**QPVTCNV	Immunoglobulin heavy chain (Fab and Fc) (100%)
ABY48864.2	VY**T**MGPPREEL**SS**R	Immunoglobulin heavy chain (Fc) (98%) IgA variable region (89%) IgM (98%)
NP_001139647.1	**T**FP**S**VR	Zinc finger protein 414 isoform I (100%) Forkhead box protein C2 (100%) Immunoglobulin heavy chain variable region (83%)

[a]Bold letters indicate glycosylation sites
[b]Fc: constant region of immunoglobulins
[c]Fab: variable region of immunoglobulins

Table 4. Results of N-linked and O-linked glycosylation site mappings of CA215.

2.10 Clinical diagnostic applications of RP215-based immunoassays

RP215 was found to recognize carbohydrate-associated epitope(s) detected preferentially in the cancer cell-expressed CA215, but rarely found in normal cells. This monoclonal antibody alone can be used in sandwich immunoassays for the determination of soluble CA215, if multi-RP215-specific epitope exists in a given CA215 glycoprotein molecule. Therefore, serum levels of CA215 can be determined quantitatively by using RP215 for both capturing and signal detection in a typical sandwich enzyme immunoassay. This enzyme immunoassay has been used in the diagnostics and monitoring of ovarian cancer and cervical cancers (Lee, 2009). CA215 levels in serum specimens of cancer patients at different disease stages can be determined by this enzyme immunoassay kit. Typical results of this analysis from a group of ovarian cancer patients at different stages are presented in Figure 6.

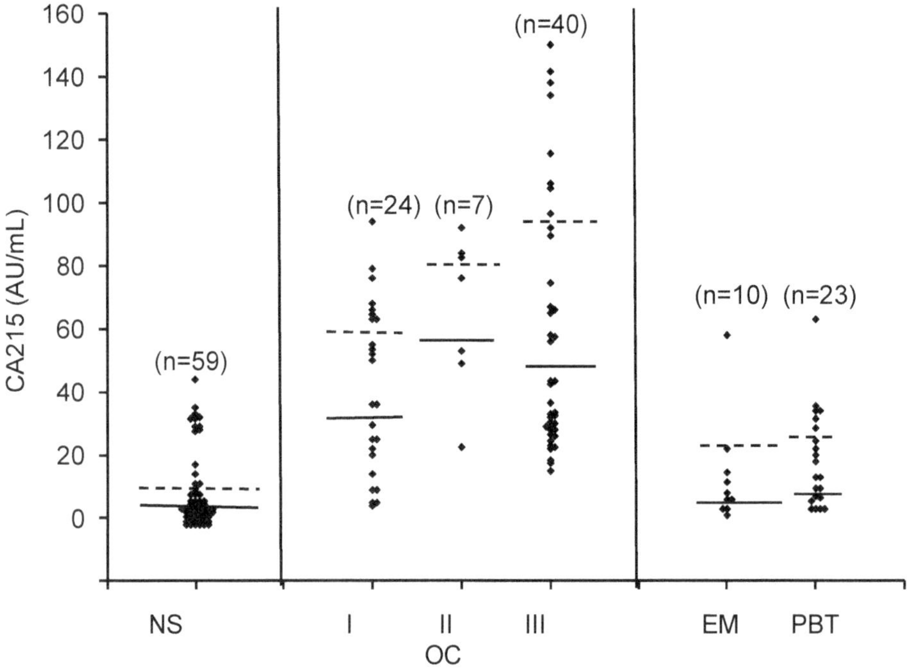

Fig. 6. Serum levels of CA215 pan cancer marker (expressed in AU/mL) for normal healthy individuals (NS) and for patients with ovarian cancer (OC) defined by respective stages (I, II, and III) of disease conditions and those with endometriosis (EM) and pelvic benign tumor (PET). Solid lines indicate the mean (M) serum CA215 levels in each category and dotted lines represent the mean values plus one standard deviation (SD). The number of cases in each category is indicated on the top of the scattered gram.

Statistics:

1. Normal control vs. ovarian carcinoma stage I ($P < 0.001$); stage II ($P < 0.001$); stage III ($P < 0.001$); stage I vs. stage III ($P < 0.05$); stage II vs. stage III ($P > 0.05$).
2. Normal control vs. endometriosis ($P > 0.05$).
3. Normal control vs. pelvic benign tumors ($P = 0.05$).

Compared to the known biomarker for ovarian cancer, such as CA125, enzyme immunoassay for CA215 revealed a similar degree of sensitivity and specificity to those of the known biomarker, CA125. When both biomarkers are combined for clinical diagnosis, the detection sensitivity was found to increase significantly (from 68% to 87%, n=31) (Lee, 2009).

Serum CA215 levels were also found to be correlated with the conditions of clinical treatments. It is interesting to note that the mean serum CA215 levels remained at relatively high levels including those at pre-operative stages and within 7 days following surgical operations. In contrast, serum CA215 levels decreased significantly when determined 7 days after the surgical operations. (Lee, 2009).

By employing the same enzyme immunoassay kit, the clinical utility of CA215 as a pan cancer biomarker was evaluated with clinically defined serum specimens from over 500 cancer patients and compared with results obtained by nine other established cancer biomarkers including AFP, CEA, CA215, CA19-9, CA15-3, Cyfra21, etc. (Lee et al., 2010b). A combination of CA215 with other tissue-associated cancer markers generally resulted in much higher cancer detection rates. By Western blot assay with RP215, it was revealed that cancer cell-expressed IgG's with RP215-specific epitope were detected in patients' serum specimens which were shown to have high levels of CA215 by enzyme immunoassay. In contrast, normal human serum specimens revealed the absence of cancer cell-expressed CA215 as determined by the same enzyme immunoassay (Lee et al., 2010b).

In conclusion, RP215-based immunoassay kit may be suitable for the monitoring of cancer in patients including that of the ovary in terms of disease conditions as well as clinical treatments.

2.11 Immunodominance of carbohydrate-associated epitope(s) recognized by RP215 in CA215

During our investigation of the carbohydrate-associated epitope(s) recognized by RP215, it was observed that the immunodominance of this unique epitope(s) in CA215 exists in mice. When mice were immunized with affinity-purified CA215 derived from the shed medium of OC-3-VGH ovarian cancer cells, only five monoclonal antibodies (RCA10, RCA100, RCA104, RCA110 and RCA111) were recovered from about 1000 hybridomas generated by cell fusion between NS-1 myeloma cells and the spleen cells from mice immunized with purified CA215. Unexpectedly, all five were shown to react with carbohydrate-associated epitope(s) which were similar to that of RP215. Judging from comparisons of the primary structures of these five monoclonal antibodies and RP215, three distinct groups of monoclonal antibodies were categorized. Group I including RP215, RCA10 and RCA100 were shown to have identical amino acid sequences and react with the linear epitope of this unique carbohydrate-associated epitope. Group II (RCA104 and RCA111) and Group III (RCA110) monoclonal antibodies were found to recognize only the conformational structure(s) of this carbohydrate-associated epitope and lost their respective CA215 binding upon treatment with methanol or SDS. However, all the monoclonal antibodies were shown to exhibit common characteristics including (1) a decrease in CA215 binding upon the periodate treatment, (2) mutual pairing among monoclonal antibodies for sandwich immunoassays, and (3) loss of CA215 binding by a given monoclonal antibody in the presence of excess of any other monoclonal antibodies (Lee et al., 2011). Furthermore, all of these monoclonal antibodies were shown to induce apoptosis to cancer cells upon incubation with 1 μg/mL of any of these monoclonal antibodies as clearly demonstrated in Figure 3C.

The reason for the existence of immunodominant carbohydrate-associated epitope(s) recognized by RP215 and other CA215-derived monoclonal antibodies in mice is currently unknown (Lee et al., 2011b).

2.12 Chimerization of RP215 and GHR106 monoclonal antibodies

In order to proceed further with preclinical and clinical studies, efforts were made to generate human/mouse chimeric forms of RP215 and GHR106 monoclonal antibodies (Lee et al., 2009; Lee & Ge, 2010a). Details of this genetic engineering process including the elucidation of primary structures of the Fab regions of these two monoclonal antibodies were performed through contract research services (Avantgen, San Diego). Generally speaking, both the murine and chimeric forms of RP215 and GHR106 were found to have almost identical binding affinity to their respective antigens, CA215 and GnRH receptor, on the cancer cells. Successful constructions of chimeric forms of these two monoclonal antibodies are essential to generate humanized forms as effective anti-cancer drugs for treatments of human cancers including that of the ovary.

3. Experimental procedure

3.1 Chemicals

All the chemicals were purchased from Sigma Chemicals Co (St Louis, MD) unless otherwise specified.

3.2 Cell lines

Human ovarian cancer cell lines, including OVCAR-3 and SKOV-3, as well as other cancer cell lines, including Raji and Jurkat were obtained from the American Type Culture Collection (ATCC), Rockville, MD, USA. All cell lines were cultured at 37 °C in a humidified atmosphere consisting of 5% CO_2 and 95% air and maintained by subculturing cells twice a week according to supplier's instructions. OC-3-VGH ovarian cancer cell lines were established in 1986 by Dept. OBS/GYN, Veterans General Hospital, Taipei, Taiwan. This is the cell line of serus origin and has been used to serve as a model for the discovery and studies of RP215 in our laboratory (Lee et al., 1992). This cancer cell line was maintained in RPMI1640 containing 10% fetal calf serum indefinitely.

3.3 Western blot assays

Western blot assay of cell extract from three ovarian cancer cell lines was performed according to the reported procedure (Lee et al., 1992; Liu et al., 1992). RP215 and GHR106 monoclonal antibodies were used as the respective probes to identify the molecular sites of CA215 as well as GnRH receptor in selected cancer cell extract. Briefly, sodium dodecyl sulfate polyacrylamide gel electrophoresis (SDS-PAGE) was performed with cancer cell extract in the presence of reducing agent (β-mercaptoethanol). Indirect Western blot assays were carried out separately by using 10 μg/mL each of RP215 or GHR106 as the respective primary antibody probe for 1 h incubation at room temperature. Subsequently, alkaline phosphatase (ALP)-labeled goat anti-mouse IgG was used as the secondary antibody for an additional 1 h incubation. This was followed by the color development with the substrate, p-nitrophenylphosphate purchased from Bio-Rad Laboratories (Mississauga, ON, Canada). Appropriate positive and negative controls as well as the molecular weight standards (BioRad laboratories, Mississauga, ON, Canada) were included in the routine Western blot assay.

3.4 Immunohistochemical studies

The immunohistochemical staining experiments were performed by using the avidin/biotin complex (ABC) method from Vector Laboratories (Burlingame, CA). Methanol fixed OC-3-

VGH, OVCAR-3 or SKOV-3 ovarian cancer cells were incubated with various primary antibodies (RP215 and GHR106) for 2 h at 37 °C. Normal mouse IgG of the same concentration served as the parallel negative control. The incubation with labeled secondary antibodies as well as the colour staining was performed at room temperature for 1 h by following the protocols and instructions provided in the ABC Kits.

3.5 TUNEL assay for assessment of cellular apoptosis

TUNEL assay was performed to study the apoptotic effects of different monoclonal antibodies including RP215, ChRP215, GHR106 and ChGHR106 on cultured prostate cancer cells. In Situ Cell Death Detection Kit, POD (Roche, Canada) was employed for detection and quantitation of apoptosis at cellular levels. Briefly, OC-3-VGH, OVCAR-3 and SKOV-3 ovarian cancer cells were cultured in RPMI 1640 medium at 37 °C in a CO_2 (5%) incubator for 24 h until all cancer cells became attached to the microwells. Selected antibodies of known concentrations were added separately and co-incubated for 48 h. As the negative control, normal mouse IgG of the same concentration (10 µg/mL) was used for the same incubation period. At the end of the incubation, the attached cells were removed from the tissue culture wells. Apoptosis of treated cancer cells were determined quantitatively by TUNEL assay with the instruction provided by the supplier (Gorczyca et al.,1993).

3.6 Complement-dependent cytotoxicity assay

Complement-dependent cytotoxicity assay was performed according to the standard protocol described previously (Lee et al., 2011a). Briefly, 1 x 10^5 cultured OC-3-VGH cells in 1 mL of appropriate culture medium (RPMI 1640 with 10% FCS) were plated in 24-well plates for 2 h before treatment. RP215, ChRP215, GHR106, and ChGHR106 were added separately to give a final concentration of 10 µg/mL and incubated for 15 min at room temperature, respectively. Three µL of freshly prepared rabbit baby complement (CL3441; Cedarlane labs, Burlington, NC, USA) was added to each well followed by incubation at 37°C for 2 h. After incubation at room temperature, the cells were recovered by centrifugation. Trypan blue (0.4%) (SV30084.01; Thermo Scientific, Waltham, MA, USA) was added and mixed gently. The percentages of cells stained with trypan blue were determined by cell counting under the regular microscope. Normal mouse IgG of the same concentration was used as the negative control. Incubation with the antibody or the complement alone served as the respective negative control for parallel comparisons in this experiment. Statistical analysis was performed to determine the significance of the assay by trypan blue method (Griffioen et al., 2009; Zhao et al., 2010).

3.7 Total RNA extraction and cDNA synthesis

Total RNA was extracted from OC-3-VGH, OVCAR-3, SKOV-3, Raji, and Jurkat cell lines (10^5-10^7 cells) by using QAIGEN RNeasy mini kit (Mississauga, ON, Canada) according to the manufacturer's manual. Total RNA integrity and quality were checked before the reverse transcription. RNase-free DNase set was performed to avoid genomic gene interference. Reverse transcription of total RNA (0.5 µg - 5 µg/20 µL) to cDNA was performed by using oligo $(dT)_{15}$ primer and EasyScript first strand synthesis kit from Applied Biological Materials Inc. (ABM) (Richmond, BC, Canada) following the manufacturer's protocol. Reaction mixtures with RNA template but without reverse-transcriptase were used as the negative controls for cDNA synthesis.

3.8 Semi-quantitative analysis of mRNA expressions of selected genes by RT-PCR

All primers required for PCR amplification were obtained from Integrated DNA Technologies (San Diego, CA) and listed as follows:
IgG: sense: 5′-ACGGCGTGGAGGTGCATAATG -3′; antisense: 5′-CGGGAGGCGTGGTCTTGTAGTT-3′; T cell receptor α chain constant region: sense: 5'-GTGCTAGACATGAGGTCTATGGAC-3' and antisense: 5'-GGATTCGGAAGGGAATCACTGACAGG-3'; T cell receptor β chain constant region: sense: 5′-TCTCGGCCACCTTCTGGC-3′; antisense: 5′-CATCAGCACGAGGGCACTGA-3′; CD3: sense: 5'-CTCTCTGGCCTGGTACTGGC-3' and antisense: 5'-GGCTGATAGACCTGGTCATTCCTCA-3'; CD4: sense: 5' ACTAAAGGTCCATCCAAGCTGA-3' and antisense: 5'-GCAGTCAATCCGAACACTAGCA-3'; CD8: sense: 5'-TTCGAGCCAAGCAGCGTCCT-3' and antisense: 5' CGGCACGAAGTGGCTGAAGTA-3'; CD47: sense: 5'-GAGTGATGCTGTCTCACACAC-3' and antisense: 5'-CTCATCCATACCACCGGATCT-3'; CD54: sense: 5'-CGGCACGAAGTGGCTGAAGTA-3' and antisense: 5'-CGAGGTGTTCTCAAACAGCTCCAG-3'; CD58: sense: 5′-AGAGCATTACAACAGCCATCG-3′ and antisense: 5′-CGCTGCTTGGGATACAGGTT-3′; CD147: sense: 5'-CGAGGTGTTCTCAAACAGCTCCAG-3' and antisense: 5'-CTTCCGGCGCTTCTCGTAGATG-3';
GnRH: sense: 5′-AACCTCTTCACCTTCTGCTGCCT-3′ and antisense: 5′-GATTTCTTCCCAGACCCTCTTACGAG-3′; GnRH receptor: sense: 5′-TGACACGGGTCCTTCATCAG-3′ and antisense: 5′-AAGTGGATCAAAGCATGGGTTT-3′; NFκB: sense: 5′-CACTAAGCAGGAAGATGTGGTGGAG-3′ and antisense: 5′-CATGGCAGGCTATTGCTCATCATGG-3;′ P0: sense: 5′-TTGTGTTCACCAAGGAGG-3′ and antisense: 5′-GTAGCCAATCTGCAGACAG-3′; P1: sense: 5′-CAAGGTGCTCGGTCCTTC-3′ and antisense: 5′-GAACATGTTATAAAAGAGG-3′; P2: sense: 5′-TCCGCCGCAGACGCCGC-3′ and antisense: 5′-TGCAGGGAGCAGGAATT-3′; EGF: sense: 5′-AAGGAAATCCTCGATGAAGCCT-3′ and antisense: 5′-TGTCTTTGTGTTCCCGGACATA -3′; c-fos: sense: 5′-GAGATTGCCAACCTGCTGAA-3′ and antisense: 5′-AGACGAAGGAAGACGTGTAA-3′.
A house-keeping gene, glyceraldehyde-3-phosphate dehydrogenase was amplified and used as an internal control in the experiments. (Sense: 5'-GAAATCCCATCACCATCTTCC-3' and antisense: 5' - CCAGGGGTCTTACTCCTTGG-3').
PCR was performed by using 2×PCR MasterMix kit (ABM, Richmond, BC, Canada) according to the manufacturer's protocols. After denaturing at 94 °C for 4 min, 20-35 cycles were performed under the following conditions: denaturing at 94 °C for 40 s; annealing at 58 °C for 60 s and extension at 72 °C for 60 s. A final complete extension was then executed at 72 °C for 7 min. At the end, the PCR product was checked by 1.5% agarose gel electrophoresis. The negative control from cDNA synthesis was further used in a PCR reaction and served as the negative control.

3.9 Statistical analysis

All experiments were performed in triplicate. All the results were presented as mean ± S.D. Student t-test was performed to estimate the statistical significance.

4. Conclusion

4.1 General conclusion

In this chapter, two monclonal antibodies, RP215 and GHR106, were identified, characterized and assessed to see if they are suitable for development of antibody-based anti-cancer drugs. The target antigens recognized by these two monoclonal antibodies, CA215 and GnRH receptor, were found to be expressed on the surface of cancer cells of many human tissue origins including that of the ovary (Lee et al., 2008). Initially, we have shown by immunohistochemical studies and Western blot assays (Lee et al., 2009) that these two monoclonal antibodies react specifically with antigens of three cancer cell lines, OC-3-VGH, OVCAR-3 and SKOV-3. Immunohistochemical studies with tissue sections of 87 ovarian cancer specimens revealed that the positive staining rates with RP215 can be as high as 64.4% (56/87). These studies have become the basis for further preclinical studies to establish if these monoclonal antibodies are suitable as anti-cancer drugs for the treatment of ovarian cancers.

By *in vitro* apoptosis assay as well as complement-dependent cytotoxicity assay, we have been able to show that these two monoclonal antibodies or their chimeric forms could induce apoptosis to ovarian cancer cells and complement-dependent cytotoxicity reactions upon incubation with cultured cancer cells. Furthermore, *in vivo* nude mouse experiments with implanted OC-3-VGH ovarian cancer cells revealed significant dose-dependent inhibition of the growth of tumor cells by RP215 (Lee et al., 2009). By using MALDI-TOF MS for analysis of tryptic peptides derived from affinity-purified CA215, it can be shown that affinity-purified CA215 consist mainly of glycoproteins including immunoglobulin superfamily proteins and mucins. Therefore, some of the cancer cell-expressed CA215 with unique carbohydrate-associated epitope recognized by RP215 seems to be critical to the growth of cancer cells, *in vitro* or *in vivo* (Lee et al., 2011a).

Efforts have been made to elucidate the primary carbohydrate structures of RP215-specific epitope(s) in CA215 through extensive N-linked and O-linked glycoanalysis and glycosylation site mappings. It was generally concluded that oligosaccharides with terminal NeuGc with structures related to those in mucins might not be crucial in the epitope(s) recognition by RP215 (Lee & Azadi, 2011).

The results of our studies have clearly demonstrated that GHR106, which reacts with the cancer cell-expressed GnRH receptor, can behave like a long acting GnRH analog in its biological actions except with a much longer half life (15-21 days) than the former (Lee & Ge, 2010a). Similar to those of GnRH analogs, apoptosis of many human cancer cells can be induced for effective cancer treatments (Leung et al., 2003). In addition, complement-dependent cytotoxicity and antibody-dependent cell-mediated cytotoxicity reactions could possibly be induced only with antibody-based anti-cancer drugs such as GHR106. We believe that the results presented in this study should provide a strong basis for these two monoclonal antibodies to be developed further in humans as anti-cancer drugs which might potentially target ovarian cancer as well as others in humans.

4.2 Implications to the immunology of cancer cells

It was generally postulated that certain tumor-associated antigens on the surface of cancer cells are overexpressed when compared with those of the normal cells (Rosenberg, 1995; Boon & van der Bruggen, 1996; Topalian, 1994; Lee, 2009). Their specific antibodies can be induced or generated to inhibit the growth of cancer cells through mechanisms of cellular apoptosis, complement-dependent cytotoxicity and/or antibody-dependent cell-mediated cytotoxicity reactions (Oldham & Dillman, 2008; Sanz et al., 2004). These have become the mechanistic basis of almost all the antibody-based anti-cancer drugs currently utilized for clinical treatments of human cancers (Finn, 2010; Wang & Rosenberg, 1999). On the other hand, cancer cells can be neutralized through the mechanisms of T cell activations *in vitro* or *in vivo* (Wang & Rosenberg, 1999) following appropriate processes (Zou, 2006). Based on this principle, the first anti-prostate cancer vaccine, Provenge (Sipuleucel-T) was developed and approved by the US-FDA for use clinically (Kantoff et al., 2010).

Similarly, in this study, we have explored the potential applications of RP215 and GHR106 monoclonal antibodies as antibody-based anti-cancer drugs. In the case of RP215, the molecular nature of CA215 and epitope-specific oligosaccharides were elucidated. Although our knowledge about the immunology of cancer cells has been advanced significantly, more questions arising from this study needs to be addressed here.

During the extensive molecular analysis of cancer cell-expressed CA215 with the unique carbohydrate-associated epitope recognized by RP215 monoclonal antibody, many glycoproteins involved in the normal immune system were identified and found to be highly expressed among many types of cancer cells, but rarely found in non-immune cells in humans. Among these are immunoglobulin superfamily proteins including all immunoglobulins, T cell receptors (α and β) and many cell adhesion CD molecules. The functional significance for the expression of these molecules in cancer cells remains to be explored (Lee et al., 2011a). First of all, the expression of immunoglobulins by cancer cells may be implicated with the existence of innate immunity in these cell types (Lee, 2009; Lee & Ge, 2009). Secondly, the widespread expressions of T cell receptors in cancer cells may also have implications in immune activations of T cells as well as the immune tolerance by T cells on cancer cells (Lee et al., 2011a). Thirdly, the high expression of CD-related cell adhesion molecules may facilitate the metastasis of cancer cells (Lee et al., 2011a). Therefore, more research work needs to be performed to resolve some of these puzzles.

We believe that for cancer cells to survive under the environment of the human immune system, a special protective mechanism should exist among cancer cells. Therefore, much more effort will be required to analyze and study the "immune system" of cancer cells, before any effective immuno-therapy of cancer cells can be achieved (Zou, 2006; Horna & Sotomayor, 2006).

Another question which needs to be addressed is the preferential attachment of RP215-specific carbohydrate-associated epitope(s) in cancer cell-expressed CA215. In the case of immunoglobulin superfamily glycoproteins, the common, but special glycosylations sites might be generated from the conserved and common domain structures of these types of molecules as reported previously (Lee & Azadi, 2011). Mucin proteins, on the other hand, are known to consist of glycosylation sites which are favorable for the unique epitope attachments. However, it is equally difficult to explain the preferential absence of the RP215 recognition sites among the same proteins in normal cells. We believe that the unique RP215-specific epitope(s) is the result of aberrant expressions of certain glycosyltransferases (Yang et al., 1994; Brockhausen, 2000), which are common to all cancer cells. This question can be answered only when the carbohydrate moieties of the epitope(s) structures are completely elucidated in the future (Lee and Azadi, 2011).

In this study, two potential antibody-based anti-cancer drugs were introduced and pre-clinical studies were performed. In view of the high and widespread expressions of the target antigens, namely, CA215 and GnRH receptor among ovarian cancer cells, we are optimistic about their potential in treating ovarian cancers following appropriate research, development and clinical trials in the near future.

5. Acknowledgement

This project was supported in parts by Vancouver Biotech Ltd, the NSERC and IRAP (#743918) kindly.
Suzanne Potzold is a co-op student from Vancouver Biotech Ltd.

6. Conflict of interest statement

GL is co-founder of Vancouver Biotech Ltd.

7. References

Bast, R.C. Jr.; Klug, T.L.; Schaetzl, E.; Lavin, P.; Niloff, J.M.; Greber, T.F.; Zurawski, V.R. Jr. & Knapp, R.C. (1984). Monitoring human ovarian carcinoma with a combination of CA 125, CA 19-9, and carcinoembryonic antigen. *Am J Obstet Gynecol.* 149(5):553-9.

Boon, T. & van der Bruggen, P. (1996). Human tumor antigens recognized by T lymphocytes. *J Exp Med.* 183(3):725-9.

Brockhausen, I.(2000). O-linked chain glycosyltransferases. *Methods Mol Biol.* 125:273-93.

Chien, C.H.; Chen, C.H.; Lee, C.Y.; Chang, T.C.; Chen, R.J. & Chow, S.N. (2004). Detection of gonadotropin-releasing hormone receptor and its mRNA in primary human epithelial ovarian cancers. *Int J Gynecol Cancer.* 14(3):451-8.

Choi, M.; Fuller, C.D.; Thomas, C. R. & Wang, S. (2008). Conditional survival in ovarian cancer: results from the SEER dataset 1988-2001. *Gynecol Oncol.* 109(2): 203-9.

Dragunow, M. & Faull, R. (1989). The use of c-fos as a metabolic marker in neuronal pathway tracing. *J. Neuroscience Methods* 29(3): 261-265.

Finn, O. (2008). Cancer Immunology. *N Engl J Med.* 358:2704-2715

Gorczyca, W.; Bigman, K.; Mittelman, A.; Ahmed, T.; Gong, J.; Melamed, M.R. & Darzynkiewicz, Z. (1993). Induction of DNA strand breaks associated with apoptosis during treatment of leukemias. Leukemia. 7(5): 659-70.

Griffioen, M.; van Egmond, E.H.; Kester, M.G.; Willemze, R.; Falkenburg, J.H. & Heemskerk, M. H. (2009). Retroviral transfer of human CD20 as a suicide gene for adoptive T-cell therapy. *Haematologica.* 94: 1316-1320.

Gründker, C.; Völker, P.; Schulz, K.D. & Emons, G. (2000). Luteinizing hormone-releasing hormone agonist triptorelin and antagonist cetrorelix inhibit EGF-induced c-fos expression in human gynecological cancers. *Gynecol Oncol.* 78(2): 194-202.

Horna, P. & Sotomayor, E.M. (2007). Cellular and molecular mechanisms of tumor-induced T-cell tolerance. *Curr Cancer Drug Targets.* 7(1):41-53.

Huang, J.; Zhang, L.; Ma, T.; Zhang, P. & Qiu, X. (2008). Expression of immunoglobulin gene with classical V-(D)-J rearrangement in mouse testis and epididymis. *J Histochem Cytochem.* 57(4): 339-49.

Jemal, A.; Murray, T.; Samuels, A.; Ghafoor, A.; Ward, E. & Thun, M.J. (2003). Cancer statistics. *Cancer J Clin.* 53, 1, 5-26.

Kang, S.K.; Choi, K.C.; Yang, H.S. & Leung, P.C. (2003) Potential role of gonadotrophin-releasing hormone (GnRH)-I and GnRH-II in the ovary and ovarian cancer. *Endocr Relat Cancer.* 10: 169-77.

Kantoff, P.W.; Higano, C.S.; Shore, N.D.; Berger, E.R.; Small, E.J.; Penson, D.F.; Redfern, C.H.; Ferrari, A.C.; Dreicer, R.; Sims, R.B.; Xu, Y.; Frohlich, M.W. & Schellhammer, P.F. (2010). Sipuleucel-T immunotherapy for castration-resistant prostate cancer. *N. Engl. J. Med.* 363(5): 411-22.

Lee, G.; Chen, K.W.; Sheu, F.S.; Tsang, A.; Chao, K.C. & Ng, H.T. (1992). Studies of a tumor-associated antigen, COX-1, recognized by a monoclonal antibody. *Cancer Immunol Immunother.* 35: 19-26.

Lee, G.; Wu, Q.; Li, C.H.; Ting, H.H. & Chien, C.H. (2006). Recent studies of a new carbohydrate-associated pan cancer marker, CA215. *J Clin Ligand Assay.* 29: 47-51.

Lee, G.; Laflamme, E.; Chien, C.H. & Ting, H.H. (2008). Molecular identity of a pan cancer marker, CA215. *Cancer Biol Ther.*7: 2007-2014.

Lee G. (2009). Cancer cell-expressed immunoglobulins: CA215 as a pan cancer marker and its diagnostic applications. *Cancer Biomark.* 5(3):137-42.

Lee, G. & Ge, B. (2009). Cancer cell expressions of immunoglobulin heavy chains with unique carbohydrateassociated biomarker. *Cancer Biomark..* 5: 177-188.

Lee, G.; Chu, R.A. & Ting, H.H. (2009). Preclinical assessment of anti-cancer drugs by using RP215 monoclonal antibody. *Cancer Biol Ther.* 8: 161-162.

Lee, G. & Ge, B. (2010a). Growth inhibition of tumor cells in vitro by using monoclonal antibodies against gonadotropin- releasing hormone receptor. *Cancer Immunol Immunother.* 59: 1011-9.

Lee, G. & Ge, B. (2010b). Inhibition of in vitro tumor cell growth by RP215 monoclonal antibody and antibodies raised against its anti-idiotype antibodies. *Cancer Immunol Immunother.* 59(9): 1347-56.

Lee, G.; Cheung, A.P.; Ge, B.; Zhu, M.; Li, P.P.; Hsu, E. & Huang, T-K. (2010a). MonoclonalAntiidiotype Antibodies against Carbohydrate-associate Epitope for Anti-Cancer Vaccine Development. *J Vaccin Vaccinat.* 1:106. doi:10.4172/2157-7560.1000106.

Lee, G.; Ge, B.; Huang, T-K.; Zheng, G.; Duan, J. & Wang, I.H. (2010b). Positive identification of CA215 pan cancer biomarker from serum specimens of cancer patients. *Cancer Biomark.* 6(2): 111-7.

Lee G. & Azadi. (2011). Peptide mapping and glycoanalysis of cancer cell-expressed glycoproteins, CA215 recognized by RP215 monoclonal antibody. *The Journal of Carbohydrate Chemistry*, in press.

Lee, G.; Zhu, M.; Ge, B. & Potzold, S. (2011a). Widespread expression of immunoglobulin superfamily proteins in cancer cells. *Cancer Immunol Immunother.* in press.

Lee, G.; Zhu, M.; Ge, B.; Cheung, A. P,; Chien,C.; Chow,S.; Ding. Y. & Yao,H. (2011b). Carbohydrate-associated immunodominant epitope of CA215. *Immunological Investigations*, in press.

Leung, P.C.; Cheng, C.K. & Zhu, X.M. (2003). Multi-factorial role of GnRH-I and GnRH-II in the human ovary. *Mol Cell Endocrinol.* 202(1-2): 145-53.

Li, Q. & Verma, I.M. (2002). NF-kappaB regulation in the immune system. *Nat. Rev. Immunol.* 10: 725-734.

Liu, M.S.; Aebersold, R.; Fann, C.H. & Lee, C.Y. (1992). Molecular and developmental studies of a sperm acrosome antigen recognized by HS-63 monoclonal antibody. *Biol Reprod.* 46: 937-948.

McGuire, W.P.; Hoskins, W.J.; Brady, M.F.; Kucera, P.R.; Partridge, E.E.; Look, K.Y.; Clarke-Pearson, D.L. & Davidson, M. (1996). Cyclophosphamide and cisplatin compared with paclitaxel and cisplatin in patients with stage III and stage IV ovarian cancer. *N Engl J Med.* 334(1): 1-6.

Mørch, L.S.; Løkkegaard, E.; Andreasen, A.H.; Krüger-Kjaer, S. & Lidegaard, O. (2009). Hormone therapy and ovarian cancer. *JAMA* 302(3): 298-305.

Oldham, R.K. & Dillman, R.O. (2008). Monoclonal antibodies in cancer therapy: 25 years of progress. *J Clin Oncol.* 10;26(11):1774-7.

Qiu, X.; Zhu, X.; Zhang, L.; Mao, Y.; Zhang, J.; Hao, P.; Li, G.; Lv, P.; Li, X.; Sun, X.; Wu, L.; Zheng, J.; Deng, Y.; Hou, C.; Tang, P.; Zhang, S. & Zhang, Y. (2003). Human epithelial cancers secrete immunoglobulin G with unidentified specificity to promote growth and survival of tumor cells. *Cancer Res.* 63: 6488-6495.

Rosenberg, S.A.(1995). The development of new cancer therapies based on the molecular identification of cancer regression antigens.*Cancer J Sci Am.* 1(2):90-100.

Sanz L.; Blanco, B. & Alvarez-Vallina, L. (2004).Antibodies and gene therapy: teaching old 'magic bullets' new tricks. *Trends Immunol.* 25(2):85-91.

Tan, A.; De La Peña, H. & Seifalian, A.M. (2010). The application of exosomes as a nanoscale cancer vaccine. *Int J Nanomedicine.* 5:889-900.

Topalian, S.L. (1994). MHC class II restricted tumor antigens and the role of CD4+ T cells in cancer immunotherapy. *Curr Opin Immunol.*6(5):741-5.

Waldmann, T.A. (2003). Immunotherapy: past, present and future. *Nat Med.* 9(3): 269-77.

Wang, R.F. & Rosenberg, S.A. (1999). Human tumor antigens for cancer vaccine development. *Immunol Rev.* 170:85-100.

Zhang, S.; Mao, Y.; Huang, J.; Ma, T.; Zhang, L.; Zhu, X.; Zheng, J.; Wu, L.; Yin, C.C. & Qiu X. (2010). Immunoglobulin gene locus events in epithelial cells of lactating mouse mammary glands. *Cell Mol Life Sci.* 67(6): 985-94.

Yang, J.M.; Byrd, J.C.; Siddiki, B.B.; Chung, Y.S.; Okuno, M.; Sowa, M.; Kim, Y.S.; Matta, K.L. & Brockhausen, I. (1994). Alterations of O-glycan biosynthesis in human colon cancer tissues. *Glycobiology.* 4(6):873-84.

Zhao, X.; Singh, S.; Pardoux, C.; Zhao, J.; Hsi, E.D.; Abo, A. & Korver, W. (2010). Targeting C-type lectin-like molecule-1 for antibody-mediated immunotherapy in acute myeloid leukemia. *Haematologica.* 95: 71-78.

Zheng, J.; Huang, J.; Mao, Y.; Liu, S.; Sun, X.; Zhu, X.; Ma, T.; Zhang, L.; Ji, J.; Zhang, Y.; Yin, C.C. & Qiu, X. (2009). Immunoglobulin gene transcripts have distinct VHDJH recombination characteristics in human epithelial cancer cells. *J Biol Chem.* 284(20): 13610-9.

Zou, W. (2006).Regulatory T cells, tumour immunity and immunotherapy. *Nat Rev Immunol.* 6(4):295-307.

Permissions

The contributors of this book come from diverse backgrounds, making this book a truly international effort. This book will bring forth new frontiers with its revolutionizing research information and detailed analysis of the nascent developments around the world.

We would like to thank Samir A. Farghaly, MD, PhD, for lending his expertise to make the book truly unique. He has played a crucial role in the development of this book. Without his invaluable contribution this book wouldn't have been possible. He has made vital efforts to compile up to date information on the varied aspects of this subject to make this book a valuable addition to the collection of many professionals and students.

This book was conceptualized with the vision of imparting up-to-date information and advanced data in this field. To ensure the same, a matchless editorial board was set up. Every individual on the board went through rigorous rounds of assessment to prove their worth. After which they invested a large part of their time researching and compiling the most relevant data for our readers. Conferences and sessions were held from time to time between the editorial board and the contributing authors to present the data in the most comprehensible form. The editorial team has worked tirelessly to provide valuable and valid information to help people across the globe.

Every chapter published in this book has been scrutinized by our experts. Their significance has been extensively debated. The topics covered herein carry significant findings which will fuel the growth of the discipline. They may even be implemented as practical applications or may be referred to as a beginning point for another development. Chapters in this book were first published by InTech; hereby published with permission under the Creative Commons Attribution License or equivalent.

The editorial board has been involved in producing this book since its inception. They have spent rigorous hours researching and exploring the diverse topics which have resulted in the successful publishing of this book. They have passed on their knowledge of decades through this book. To expedite this challenging task, the publisher supported the team at every step. A small team of assistant editors was also appointed to further simplify the editing procedure and attain best results for the readers.

Our editorial team has been hand-picked from every corner of the world. Their multi-ethnicity adds dynamic inputs to the discussions which result in innovative outcomes. These outcomes are then further discussed with the researchers and contributors who give their valuable feedback and opinion regarding the same. The feedback is then collaborated with the researches and they are edited in a comprehensive manner to aid the understanding of the subject.

Apart from the editorial board, the designing team has also invested a significant amount of their time in understanding the subject and creating the most relevant covers. They scrutinized every image to scout for the most suitable representation of the subject and create an appropriate cover for the book.

The publishing team has been involved in this book since its early stages. They were actively engaged in every process, be it collecting the data, connecting with the contributors or procuring relevant information. The team has been an ardent support to the editorial, designing and production team. Their endless efforts to recruit the best for this project, has resulted in the accomplishment of this book. They are a veteran in the field of academics and their pool of knowledge is as vast as their experience in printing. Their expertise and guidance has proved useful at every step. Their uncompromising quality standards have made this book an exceptional effort. Their encouragement from time to time has been an inspiration for everyone.

The publisher and the editorial board hope that this book will prove to be a valuable piece of knowledge for researchers, students, practitioners and scholars across the globe.

List of Contributors

Antonio Macciò
Department of Obstetrics and Gynecology, Sirai Hospital, Carbonia, Italy

Clelia Madeddu
Department of Medical Oncology, University of Cagliari, Cagliari, Italy

Ana Fernández Montes, Jesús García Gómez, Miguel Nuñez Viejo, Miguel Alonso Bermejo, Susana Alonso Urrutia and Jesús García Mata
Complexo Hospitalario Universitario de Ourense, Spain

Robert Magnusson
Resonant Sensors Incorporated (RSI), Arlington, TX, USA
University of Texas at Arlington, Department of Electrical Engineering, Arlington, TX, USA

Peter Koulen
University of Missouri - Kansas City, School of Medicine, Departments of Ophthalmology and Basic Medical Science, Vision Research Center, Kansas City, MO, USA

Debra Wawro and Shelby Zimmerman
Resonant Sensors Incorporated (RSI), Arlington, TX, USA

Christine Sers and Reinhold Schafer
Institute of Pathology, University Medicine Charité, Berlin, Germany

Irina Nazarenko
Institute of Toxicology and Genetics, Karlsruhe Institute of Technology, Karlsruhe, Germany

Claudine Rancourt, Isabelle Matte, Denis Lane and Alain Piché
Département de Microbiologie et Infectiologie, Faculté de Médecine, Université de Sherbrooke, Canada

Meera Nanjundan
University of South Florida, Department of Cell Biology, Microbiology, and Molecular Biology, USA
Moffitt Cancer Center, Cancer Biology Program, Tampa, Florida, USA

Kyle Bauckman
Moffitt Cancer Center, Cancer Biology Program, Tampa, Florida, USA

Christie Campla
University of South Florida, Department of Cell Biology, Microbiology, and Molecular Biology, USA

Natalia Krawczyk and Tanja Fehm
Department of Obstetrics and Gynecology, University of Tuebingen, Tuebingen, Germany

Malgorzata Banys
Department of Obstetrics and Gynecology, University of Tuebingen, Tuebingen, Germany
Department of Obstetrics and Gynecology, Marienkrankenhaus Hamburg, Hamburg, Germany

Xuan Bich Trinh
Translational Cancer Research Unit, St Augustinus GZA Hospitals, Antwerp, Belgium
Department of Gynaecological Oncology, Antwerp University Hospital, Antwerp, Belgium

Peter A. Van Dam, Luc Y. Dirix and Steven J. van Laere
Translational Cancer Research Unit, St Augustinus GZA Hospitals, Antwerp, Belgium

Wiebren A. A. Tjalma
Department of Gynaecological Oncology, Antwerp University Hospital, Antwerp, Belgium

Yuri Markushin and Noureddine Melikechi
Optical Science Center for Applied Research, Delaware State University, USA

Ryan Serio and Blase Billack
St. John's University, Department of Pharmaceutical Sciences, USA

Fabiola Moretti and Francesca Mancini
Institute of Cell Biology and Neurobiology, National Research Council of Italy (CNR), Italy

Bon Quy Trinh and Honami Naora
University of Texas MD Anderson Cancer Center, USA

Ying Xu
Department of Biochemistry and Molecular Biology, USA
The Institute of Bioinformatics, University of Georgia, Athens, Georgia, USA
College of Computer Science and Technology, Jilin University, Changchun, China

Juan Cui and David Puett
Department of Biochemistry and Molecular Biology, USA

Nicola Lo Buono, Simona Morone, Rossella Parrotta, Alice Giacomino, Erika Ortolan and Ada Funaro
Department of Genetics, Biology and Biochemistry, University of Torino Medical School, Torino, Italy

Seiji Mabuchi, Atsuko Wakabayashi and Tadashi Kimura
Department of Obstetrics and Gynecology, Osaka University, Japan

Stéphanie Gaillard
Sidney Kimmel Comprehensive Cancer Center, Johns Hopkins School of Medicine Baltimore, USA

Janica C. Wong
Center for Diabetes and Obesity Prevention, Treatment, Research and Education, and the College of Pharmacy, Roseman University of Health Sciences (Formerly University of Southern Nevada), Henderson, Nevada, USA
Cancer Molecular Biology Section, Nevada Cancer Institute, Las Vegas, Nevada, USA
Department of Chemistry, University of Nevada Las Vegas, Las Vegas, Nevada, USA

Ronald R. Fiscus and Mary G. Johlfs
Center for Diabetes and Obesity Prevention, Treatment, Research and Education, and the College of Pharmacy, Roseman University of Health Sciences (Formerly University of Southern Nevada), Henderson, Nevada, USA
Cancer Molecular Biology Section, Nevada Cancer Institute, Las Vegas, Nevada, USA

Elaine L. Leung
Center for Diabetes and Obesity Prevention, Treatment, Research and Education, and the College of Pharmacy, Roseman University of Health Sciences (Formerly University of Southern Nevada), Henderson, Nevada, USA
Cancer Molecular Biology Section, Nevada Cancer Institute, Las Vegas, Nevada, USA
State Key Laboratory for Quality Research in Chinese Medicines, Macau University of Science and Technology, Taipa, Macau Special Administrative Region, and Shum Yiu Foon Shum Bik Chuen Memorial Centre for Cancer and Inflammation Research, School of Chinese Medicine, Hong Kong Baptist University, and Department of Pathology, Faculty of Medicine, The University of Hong Kong, Hong Kong Special Administrative Region, China

Steven M. Allin and Alan Richardson
Keele University, UK

John King-Underwood
CompchemRes, UK

Charles W. Redman
University Hospital of North Staffordshire, UK

Gregory Lee, Mingang Zhu and Bixia Ge
UBC Center for Reproductive Health, The University of British Columbia Vancouver, Canada